Occupational Therapy in Acute Care

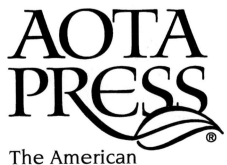

The American
Occupational Therapy
Association, Inc.

AOTA *Centennial Vision*
We envision that occupational therapy is a powerful, widely recognized, science-driven, and evidence-based profession with a globally connected and diverse workforce meeting society's occupational needs.

Vision Statement
AOTA advances occupational therapy as the pre-eminent profession in promoting the health, productivity, and quality of life of individuals and society through the therapeutic application of occupation.

Mission Statement
The American Occupational Therapy Association advances the quality, availability, use, and support of occupational therapy through standard-setting, advocacy, education, and research on behalf of its members and the public.

AOTA Staff
Frederick P. Somers, *Executive Director*
Christopher M. Bluhm, *Chief Operating Officer*

Chris Davis, *Director, AOTA Press*
Ashley Hofmann, *Developmental/Production Editor*
Victoria Davis, *Production Editor/Editorial Assistant*

Beth Ledford, *Director of Marketing*
Emily Zhang, *Technology Marketing Specialist*
Jennifer Folden, *Marketing Specialist*

The American Occupational Therapy Association, Inc.
4720 Montgomery Lane
Bethesda, MD 20814
Phone: 301-652-AOTA (2682)
TDD: 800-377-8555
Fax: 301-652-7711
www.aota.org
To order: http://store

Disclaimers
This publication is designed to provide accurate and authoritative information in regard to the subject matter covered. It is sold or distributed with the understanding that the publisher is not engaged in rendering legal, accounting, or other professional service. If legal advice or other expert assistance is required, the services of a competent professional person should be sought.
—*From the Declaration of Principles jointly adopted by the American Bar Association and a Committee of Publishers and Associations*

It is the objective of the American Occupational Therapy Association to be a forum for free expression and interchange of ideas. The opinions expressed by the contributors to this work are their own and not necessarily those of either the editors or the American Occupational Therapy Association.

ISBN: 978-1-56900-271-1

Library of Congress Control Number: 2011924379

Design by Debra Naylor, Naylor Design, Inc., Washington, DC
Composition by Progressive Information Technologies, York, PA
Printed by Automated Graphics Systems, Inc., White Plains, MD

From little acorns mighty oaks do grow—American proverb

This book is dedicated to FS & LMS A"H

Contents

Contributors

Judy R. Hamby, MHS, OTR/L, BCPR
Clinical Specialist
Acute Care Rehabilitation
Wellstar Kennestone Hospital
Marietta, GA

Suzanne E. Holm, MA, OTR, BCPR
Occupational Therapist
Inpatient Rehabilitation
Medical Center of the Rockies
Loveland, CO

Debra A. Kerrigan, MS, OTR/L
Occupational Therapist
Newton Wellesley Hospital
Newton, MA

Wendy Avery, MS, OTR/L
Occupational Therapist
Bluffton, SC

Kerry Popovich, OT/L
Senior Occupational Therapist
Inpatient Rehabilitation
Portsmouth Regional Hospital
Portsmouth, NH

Rannell Hudson, OTR/L
Occupational Therapist
Emory Health Care
Atlanta
Wellstar Health System
Marietta, GA

Marcy D. Beardon, MS, OTR
Occupational Therapist
Indianapolis, IN

Sharon K. Hennigan, MA, OTR/L, CHT
Consultant
Marietta, GA

Khalilah T. Robinson, MS, OTR/L
Occupational Therapist
Amedisys
Cumming, GA

Mary Shotwell, PhD, OT/L
Associate Professor
Brenau University
Department of Occupational Therapy
Gainesville, GA

Kristen Scola, MS, OTR/L
Occupational Therapist
Newton Wellesley Hospital
Newton, MA

Sonia Smith, BS, OTR/L
Occupational Therapist
Newton Wellesley Hospital
Newton, MA

Natan Berry, MS, OTR/L
Occupational Therapist
Sinai Hospital of Baltimore
Baltimore

Helene Smith-Gabai, OTD, OTR/L, BCPR
Occupational Therapist
Emory Healthcare
Atlanta

Acknowledgments

The authors of *Occupational Therapy in Acute Care* would like to thank their families, friends and colleagues for their patience and support through the writing of this book. We don't think that any of us realized the extent of work and commitment it would take to complete this project. Thanks for believing in us.

Special thanks to our reviewers: Marsha Neville and Susan Halpern, who work well under pressure.

Personal thanks from Debbie, Kristen, and Sonia to the following: Nancy L. Hiltz, who reviewed the orthopedics chapter and provided valuable feedback.

Personal thanks from Judy to the following: Thank you to the following people for reviewing chapters/appendices and providing invaluable feedback: Brenda J. Kramer, Dr. David Villasana, Michelle Rank, Dr. Joseph Hormes, Carolyn Giera, Dr. Dennis Lindenbaum, Orli Weisser-Pike, Meredith Orr, Arlene Kilgore, Carole Prevost, David Williamson, and Allison Haldeman. My patients and their families have provided enormous inspiration to maintain the tenets of occupational therapy as I strive to provide excellent care. I cannot thank them enough for what they have taught me over the years.

Personal thanks from Helene to the following: I would like to thank the following for their unwavering support and encouragement: all the wonderful people I work with in the rehabilitation department at Emory University Hospital, the doctoral program in occupational therapy at Nova Southeastern University, Robin Underwood, and Barbara Schell. Additional acknowledgments to Stephanie Hood, Beth Liakos, Adele Raiz, Sheila Longpre, Pam Latham, and Mallory Sims.

Preface

Four years ago when I took a staff position at a large metropolitan hospital, I was looking for a book that specifically addressed occupational therapy practice in acute care but could not find one. There were many good physical therapy books but no resources explicitly written to help someone like me, a returning therapist, navigate this fast-paced, often chaotic, medical model system. I was fortunate to find like-minded authors who also saw the need for a book on practical information for hospital-based occupational therapists.

Occupational therapy is an allied *health* profession with an underlying belief that engaging in occupations is both health and wellness promoting. Occupational therapists recognize that engagement in meaningful and purposeful occupations is the most effective way to empower patients, facilitate independence, and advance health. Working in a hospital setting can be challenging and frustrating, because the environment remains a predominantly hierarchical and paternalistic *medical* model. Therapists may find it difficult to reconcile values of the medical model system with occupational therapy's core values or the *Occupational Therapy Practice Framework* (American Occupational Therapy Association, 2008). However, they are not incompatible, and working in this setting offers unique opportunities for acute care practice to be both occupation-based and client-centered.

Working within a medical setting also requires an understanding of medical conditions and how illness affects occupational performance areas (the focus of this book). The challenge of acute care practice is looking beyond the specific medical condition and seeing the whole person. Occupational therapists consider their patient's physical, mental, psychosocial, and spiritual needs when planning interventions and making discharge recommendations. What sets occupational therapy apart from other professions is an understanding of the totality of the patient's occupational profile and the importance of helping patients reclaim important roles and routines.

In addition to the diversity of medical conditions seen in acute care, every patient encountered is unique and has his or her own personal story. Unfortunately, for most patients being in a hospital is disrupting to life roles and routines. No one wants to be in the hospital. Patients can experience loss of independence, privacy, comfort, and identity. For example, an *individual* becomes a *patient* once he or she is admitted to the hospital and loses elements of personal control and choice. Medical and nursing procedures override patient choice, because tests have to be done and vital signs must be checked. Working in an acute hospital setting gives one a deeper appreciation and respect for the human condition and spirit.

This book was written specifically for therapists working in a hospital setting. Readers will gain an understanding of the various body systems, common conditions, diseases, procedures, and typical medical management seen in hospitals and how they relate to occupational therapy practice. Chapter 1 discusses the various issues related to the occupational therapy evaluation and provides recommendations for evaluation, interpretation and intervention, commensurate with the *Framework*. Chapters 3–12 review the various body systems (e.g., cardiac, musculoskeletal, nervous), while Chapter 2 deals with the intensive care unit, and Chapters 13–15 discuss working with patients who have dysphagia, organ transplantation, and burns. Appendixes examine important conditions and considerations that are also encountered in acute care practice, such as common diagnostic tests, medications, and laboratory values.

This book is a direct outcome of my search for an increased knowledge base as an acute care occupational therapist. It was written collaboratively by therapists with acute care experience to help demystify medical conditions and issues routinely encountered by occupational therapists working in this practice setting. It is hoped that this information will be useful in laying the foundation for occupation-based practice and in addressing the contextual issues of working within a unique and challenging medical system. Working in acute care is fascinating, fast paced, and certainly never boring.

—*Helene Smith-Gabai, OTD, OTR/L, BCPR*

Reference

American Occupational Therapy Association. (2008). Occupational therapy practice framework: Domain and process (2nd ed.). *American Journal of Occuptional Therapy, 62,* 625–683.

List of Figures, Tables, Boxes, and Appendixes

TABLES

BOXES

APPENDIXES

1

Evaluation of the Acute Care Patient

Khalilah T. Robinson, MS, OTR/L, and
Mary Shotwell, PhD, OT/L

This chapter reviews the evaluation process—including chart review, specific evaluation measures, and making interpretations and recommendations—and the challenges of the evaluation process for occupational therapists in the acute care setting. Contrary to what many acute care therapists may believe, the process of evaluation in acute care is compatible with the tenets of the *Occupational Therapy Practice Framework: Domain and Process* (2nd ed.; American Occupational Therapy Association [AOTA], 2008).

Acute care occupational therapists have little time to administer standardized assessments, but they often rely on occupation-based activities, particularly self-care activities, to perform client evaluations. The acute care occupational therapist typically provides simultaneous evaluation, intervention, and discharge planning. The therapist must consider discharge planning in each treatment session, because hospital stays are typically short, and discharge decisions can be made quickly as the patient's medical status changes. The therapist is cautioned to treat each patient visit as though it might be the last visit before discharge or transfer to another unit or setting. The occupational therapy evaluation in the acute care setting typically follows a sequence that includes

- Chart review
- Interview and occupational profile
- Specific assessment measures (including skilled observations)
- Interpretation and findings
- Recommendations for intervention.

To discuss an evaluation of the acute care patient, we must first define a few terms. Hinojosa, Kramer, and Crist (2009)

differentiated among *screening, evaluation,* and *assessment. Screening* was defined as the process of reviewing data, observing a client, and using screening tools to identify the individual's potential to benefit from further assessment. An *assessment* is a particular tool, systematic observation, or instrument that is used to collect data about the patient during the evaluation process (Hinojosa et al., 2009). An *evaluation* encompasses obtaining, interpreting, and synthesizing data to understand the patient, the situation, or system factors that may or may not influence the therapeutic intervention. Therapists are advised to make themselves aware of specific organizational policies and procedures that influence the process of evaluating patients in this setting. In this chapter, we follow the occupational therapy evaluation sequence described in the preceding paragraph, incorporate recommendations for occupation-based assessment, and highlight specific strategies that may be used in this physical setting.

Challenges in Acute Care Evaluation

Occupational therapists practicing in acute care environments have unique challenges in providing evaluation and intervention. These challenges include the patient's medical instability, limitations in the physical setting, assessing the appropriateness of physician orders, and limited time for evaluation and intervention. The overall focus of interdisciplinary evaluations in medical units is most often based on vital physiological functions to determine whether a less restrictive environment is appropriate for the patient. Similarly, the focus of the occupational therapy evaluation is usually on cognitive and physiological performance factors such as strength, range of motion (ROM), balance, mobility, cardiopulmonary functions, and ability to participate in basic activities of daily living (BADLs).

The purpose of the acute or intensive care unit is to deal with immediate medical (and surgical) care and prepare the patient for discharge to the home or to another setting, whether it is an acute rehabilitation setting, subacute rehabilitation unit, nursing home, or long-term acute care facility. During the evaluation process, the therapist uses observations, screening tools, and assessments, as well as clinical reasoning, to make judgments about a patient's ability to return home or to a setting that provides supervision for safety or necessary medical care.

The acute care setting can be intimidating for an occupational therapist with limited exposure to medically unstable clients. Machines, tubes, and monitors may appear intimidating to the novice occupational therapist. However, a therapist in this setting becomes adept at attending to the alarms of the many different types of medical machinery. The therapist also learns how to use data from these machines or monitors as part of the assessment of the patient's response to intervention or as a baseline measure of physiological responsiveness. Despite the benefit in monitoring the patient, machinery and monitors can also be a limiting factor during the evaluation process. Maneuvering the patient attached to the machines or the need for additional health care providers to move the patient during the evaluation process may affect the therapist's ability to gather data on the patient's current status.

Specific care protocols or patient restrictions may also hinder the therapist's ability to perform an evaluation. For example, post-surgical protocols or precautions may limit the patient's mobility. Questioning the patient about his or her knowledge of these precautions may become part of the assessment process and may provide the occupational therapist with the information necessary to determine the patient's safety awareness. Infection control issues may also interfere with the type of assessment tools used or the time spent in the patient's room. For example, if the therapist must follow isolation procedures before entering and exiting a patient's room, these procedures should be factored into the therapist's schedule and time management. A caseload including many isolation patients may limit the time a therapist has to perform an evaluation or, at the very least, restrict the therapist's ability to fulfill job requirements in a timely manner (i.e., seeing all of the patients on his or her caseload). Specific protocols related to infection control and mobility may also limit the occupation-based assessment choices available to the therapist.

Acute medical settings are characterized by many professionals interacting with patients on an ongoing basis to determine medical status. To the observer, the care provided by the various health care providers may seem chaotic and disjointed, with some assessments repeated multiple times a day or repeated by providers in different disciplines. Therapists may have difficulty finding the patient's medical record or the nurse who is caring for the patient or gaining access to the patient for an occupational therapy assessment because other professionals are working with the patient. Therapists working in acute and intensive care environments must be flexible because their schedules rarely go as planned. Therapists often compete for time to see patients because other services or tests take precedence. Sometimes, having people from more than one discipline (e.g., physical and occupational therapy) evaluating a client at the same time is more time efficient, because it may reduce the need to "compete" for time to see the patient and reduce client fatigue from having to perform the same activities multiple times.

In addition to the chaos of acute care, time becomes one of the most limiting factors in the evaluation process. In the acute care setting, occupational therapists must complete their assessments within the same day or within 24 hours of receiving the referral. A typical evaluation in acute care settings usually takes less than 30 minutes from start to finish. Therapists quickly learn how to gain the most information from a patient interview and task-oriented assessments performed at bedside. An assessment usually begins the minute a therapist walks into the patient's room. Therapists can note how the patient is mobilizing in the hospital bed and whether the patient is able to answer questions. In many cases, occupational therapists extrapolate or use deductive reasoning because the patient may not have the endurance to participate in a detailed evaluation procedure. Occupational therapists are skilled at using activity analysis in combination with their clinical reasoning to ascertain which functional skills the patient can likely perform and which the patient will likely have difficulty or need assistance with, even after discharge.

Chart Review

When evaluating the acute care patient, the primary source of information is the patient's medical record, which includes information from the time of admission to the time of discharge. Medical record information that is useful for occupational therapy includes where and with whom a patient resides, current and new medications, advance directives, orders, precautions, laboratory reports, imaging reports, physician notes, and nursing notes. The chart review not only provides the evaluating therapist with pertinent information about the patient's medical conditions but also shapes the therapist's evaluation and treatment. Reviewing each of these elements, and discussing the patient's disposition with nursing staff or the case manager before evaluation, ensures that the therapist provides the utmost patient care despite differences in opinion regarding medical status or potential disposition.

Physician Orders and Precautions

Orders are written statements, usually written by physicians, physician assistants, or nurse practitioners, that dictate a patient's medical plan of care. The order includes medications, special tests and procedures, surgical precautions, and consultations from other auxiliary services. The occupational therapist must first review and confirm the physician's occupational therapy orders to verify the request for services and determine the type of evaluation (e.g., home safety, splinting, physical agent modalities). The therapist should review and

note any precautions in the physician's order or documentation that need to be observed during the evaluation and treatment session. The therapist should also make recommendations to physicians regarding patients' needs, such as the need for a particular piece of durable medical equipment or splinting or even when occupational therapy services are not indicated.

Patient *precautions* may include those following orthopedic and neurosurgeries such as joint replacement, diskectomies, and fusions. These precautions often restrict patients' ROM and weight-bearing status. Patients with orthopedic or neurologic conditions may also have braces, splints, or fixators that the occupational therapist must attend to during intervention. After cardiac surgery or procedure, patients may have precautions that limit ROM and resistive use of the upper extremities such as avoiding pushing and pulling. Infection control precautions are also common in the acute care setting. Common infection control precautions include contact isolation, airborne precautions, and neutropenic precautions that dictate the use of specific types of personal protective equipment.

Some precautions, such as splinting, wound care, or decisions regarding an ankle–foot orthosis, may be dictated by either the treating therapist or the physician. Roles and responsibilities for writing medical orders may vary in each hospital setting, but in most cases the physician is ultimately responsible for overseeing that the treatment team follows all orders. It is important to consult the facility's policies and procedures regarding the therapist's role in writing patient orders.

Physician orders may also provide available information on special procedures or tests a patient may require that will influence how a therapist administers the evaluation and treatment.

Some common tests include but are not limited to

- *Venous duplex scans,* used to determine locations of deep vein thrombosis or pulmonary embolus;
- *Computed tomography (CT) scan,* which helps determine location of fractures, masses, or fluid retention;

- *Magnetic resonance imaging (MRI),* which provides sophisticated images of tissue and organs; and
- *Ultrasounds,* which provide outlining images of tissue, organs, and blood vessels.

Occupational therapists should check orders before any treatment session because they are frequently revised, and at times new orders may affect intervention. For example, patients must lie flat after returning to their room after undergoing certain diagnostic procedures, such as a cardiac catheterization. If a therapist was unaware of this physician order, he or she might endanger the patient's medical status.

Current and Past Medical History

Each medical chart will contain a complete history and physical examination report, typically written by the admitting physician or house staff. This report generally provides a brief medical overview of the presentation of symptoms, initial labs and vital signs, past medical and surgical history, current medical history, family medical history, review of systems, assessment, and medical plan. This information is especially important for the therapist to be familiar with because it can provide information vital to the occupational therapy evaluation, such as reason for admission (e.g., congestive heart failure, fractures, surgical procedure).

A physician's evaluation of the patient's neurological, vascular, cardiopulmonary, genitourinary, homeostatic, and other physical functions at the time of admission is also critical because it provides information for the therapist to make special considerations during the evaluation. A *special consideration* may include the need to use portable oxygen when mobilizing a patient within or outside of his or her hospital room. Similarly, various monitoring devices such as a Holter monitor (ambulatory electrocardiography monitor) or an oxygen saturation monitor may need to be temporarily disconnected when the patient is performing upper-body dressing.

Depending on the patient's status, the occupational therapist should verify (with the doctor or nurse) that the aforementioned devices can be disabled for the purpose of evaluating activities of daily living (ADLs). Awareness of the physician's physical exam may indicate to the therapist what types of intervention the patient might need. For example, a patient with weakness may need interventions that enhance strength, whereas a patient who has had brain injury may require cognitive remediation and extensive family education.

Vital Signs and Medications

Vital signs and medications vastly affect the course of evaluation and treatment. Medications can influence the body, which is attempting to maintain homeostasis. Medications can also have multiple side effects that may include upset stomach; change in heart rate or rhythm; dizziness; and change in vision, level of alertness, appetite, or metabolism. Two key measures of homeostasis are vital signs and laboratory tests. *Vital signs* include blood pressure, arterial blood pressure, intracranial pressure, respiration rate, heart rate, and oxygen saturation.

Laboratory Values and Imaging Reports

Lab values provide therapists with information regarding a patient's biochemistry. Appendix P describes common lab tests and norms used in acute care and their implications for therapy. These tests and norms include but are not limited to

- Blood cell counts—Red blood cell count, white blood cell count, hemoglobin, and hematocrit
- Arterial blood gases and pH
- Basic metabolic panel—Blood sugar (glucose), potassium (K), calcium (Ca), sodium (Na), creatinine, and blood urea nitrogen
- Coagulation panels—Prothrombin time, international normalized ratio, and partial thromboplastin time
- D-dimer
- Urinalysis.

Each of these values has a range within which functional activity and exercise is appropriate. Functional activity and exercise is contraindicated for values that are critically outside the normal range.

In addition, therapists should refer to the area of the chart containing imaging reports to review any CT, MRI, ultrasound, or X-rays in the event of acute fractures, hemorrhagic events, embolic events, or evidence of metastatic disease. These reports may influence whether the occupational therapist performs specific formalized testing. For example, X-ray results may indicate a fracture or tear of a joint structure; therefore, the occupational therapist will not test ROM or strength in that extremity. Imaging reports may also indicate a need to request clearance for evaluation from a specialist. For example, a patient has been admitted to the hospital after a motor vehicle accident with an X-ray report revealing a tibial plateau fracture, but an orthopedic specialist has not yet seen the patient. The occupational therapist should consult with the occupational specialist, or wait until he or she has seen the patient, to ascertain the appropriateness of an occupational therapy evaluation and clarification of any movement precautions or weight-bearing status.

Physician Progress Notes

Physician progress notes provide the therapist with the day-to-day assessments of and plans for a patient's hospital stay. Reviewing notes daily before intervention is critical. The chart review provides a guideline as to whether participation in occupational therapy services is appropriate for the patient. In the intensive care unit, and when possible on a regular floor, the occupational therapist should first consult with the primary nurse taking care of the patient before initiating the occupational therapy evaluation or intervention regarding changes in medical status, medications, and critical tests. The physician's note will generally include vitals and laboratory values, medical assessment with plan, precautionary notes, and narrative from family or consultations with specialists or other auxiliary services.

When reviewing physician progress notes, the occupational therapist should also refer to progress notes from other disciplines, including physical therapy, speech–language pathology, and nursing, and consultation reports from other clinical specialists. *Physical therapy and speech–language pathology progress notes* are helpful because these notes also afford additional objective findings on functional mobility and receptive and expressive communication. *Nursing notes* are helpful to the evaluating therapist in that they afford information regarding patient's mobility over the course of an entire day, responses to medications and other treatment, and concerns for the patient's family.

Special Considerations

In the acute care setting, patients are more seriously ill and at risk for medical complications; therefore, it is important that the occupational therapist not only be familiar with the specialized equipment used in the various medical units, but also be familiar with specific policies and procedures within medical units. In particular, clinicians should be mindful of infection control concerns as well as cardiopulmonary status of acute care patients.

Isolation and Contact Precaution

An additional issue of great concern to occupational therapists is working with patients who are immunologically compromised, including patients with cancer or HIV/AIDS, as well as transplant organ recipients. Patients with these diagnoses may be categorized as a "contact precaution" patient, meaning that the patient has some form of contagious agent that can be harmful to other patients or that the patient is vulnerable to infection from other patients or hospital staff. The therapist will need to wear protective equipment, including gown, gloves, face mask, or all of these when entering the patient's room. In some cases, therapists and other staff may be asked to cover their hair and shoes. Refer to Chapter 12 for more information on infection control.

Common conditions requiring contact precautions may include methicillin-resistant staphylococcus aureus (MRSA), vancomycin-resistant staphylococcus aureus (VRSA), vancomycin-resistant enterococcus, and *Clostridium difficile* (C. diff.). These bacteria are found in the human system and potentially in any bodily discharge (e.g., urine, blood, saliva, tears). Therapists treating these patients are required to wear personal protective gear, including gowns and gloves. Respiratory infections (e.g., pseudomonas, tuberculosis, some forms of pneumonia) may be categorized as "droplet precaution," thus requiring the therapist to wear not only a gown and gloves but also a proper-fitting mask (e.g., N95) to prevent airborne transmission of disease.

Cardiopulmonary Status

Often when a therapist enters a patient's room, he or she may observe that the patient has a nasal cannula or t-piece or a tracheostomy or is on ventilator support (refer to Chapter 4 for detail). Seeing the intensive care unit or cardiac care unit patient with a tracheostomy or a ventilator is not uncommon. Establishing trust with these patients is important because they are often anxious and may panic because of fear of suffocation, death, or both. Additionally, monitoring oxygen saturation, secretions, respiratory rate, heart rate, and blood pressure remain important in monitoring a patient's response to treatment.

Should the patient have only a nasal cannula and a notation that his or her oxygen saturation is more than 95% at rest, it may be appropriate to remove the cannula and monitor the patient's oxygen saturation on room air while engaging in functional activities. However, facilities may have specific policies such as clearing removal of a respiratory device or monitor with the respiratory therapist, nurse, or doctor beforehand. The patient's desaturation and the recovery time required for the patient to return to more than 90% on room air should be documented and reported to nursing staff. This action will assist the nursing and medical staff in determining the patient's tolerance to activity and his or her oxygen requirements. Oxygen requirements during activities may be helpful in determining whether the patient will require oxygen therapy when being discharged back home. Having an available pulse oximeter or portable oxygen tank accessible during activity may be necessary if the patient has

difficulty recovering from oxygen desaturation (see Figure 1.1).

In some facilities, therapists (occupational, physical, or respiratory) may evaluate a patient using a "6-minute walk test" and a pulse oximeter to assess the patient's oxygen level during this activity. The results of this test may determine whether the patient has the physical endurance to return home with or without supplemental oxygen. Monitoring heart rate, respiratory rate, and oxygen saturation, as well as any physiological changes, will aid in determining the level of activity the patient is able to tolerate, so that families are appropriately educated on how to modify activities for the patient after discharge.

Patients with compromised respiratory function may experience dyspnea and inefficient breathing patterns, often relying on the accessory muscles, such as the scalene muscles, rather than the diaphragm for breathing. Moreover, the therapist may observe forceful expiration, maintaining the chest in an expanded posture, which may also compromise effective inspiration (Migliore, 2004). The therapist should note

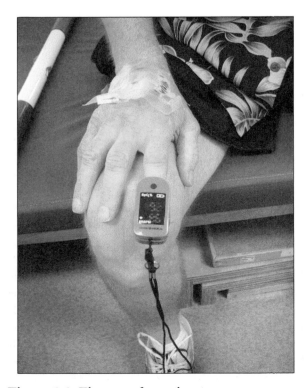

Figure 1.1. Finger pulse oximeter.
Source. K. Robinson.

whether breathing patterns or oxygen saturation changes with activity or changes in body position. For example, patients with emphysema may have difficulty breathing when lying supine.

Evaluation and Assessment in Acute Care Occupational Therapy

Craig, Robertson, and Milligan (2004) studied occupational therapy practice patterns in acute care settings in New Zealand. They found that the top assessment measures included interview, specific assessments of mobility, cognition, and BADLs. Although no such study has been found specific to acute care in the United States, the practice patterns found in the New Zealand study appear to be consistent with those experienced in American occupational therapy practice.

In the acute care environment, evaluation time is quite limited; therefore, the therapist is unlikely to be able to complete many standardized assessments. The therapist will usually use parts of standardized assessments on the basis of patient need. For example, in an interview, the therapist notes that the patient's cognitive status seems to be impaired. The therapist may then choose to follow up with one subtest that is part of a larger cognitive assessment tool.

The therapist should be reminded that although these tools may prove helpful in evaluating a patient, the results (quantitative values) have limited value in terms of interpretation because the test was not administered in its entirety and, therefore, loses validity. Nevertheless, the use of specific test items or subtests can help the occupational therapist quantify clinical observations and provide raw data that may be valuable for monitoring progress. Even if therapists do not use formal standardized assessment tools, they should adopt some "standardization" within their facility or department on how evaluation components are to be assessed (i.e., upper-extremity active range of motion [AROM]) always tested in sitting or upright position or noted as tested in an alternate position). This standardization is particularly important when multiple therapists are evaluating and treating the same patient. Appendix 1.A provides a sample evaluation form and standard protocol for assessing performance areas.

Table 1.1 demonstrates how one might use occupation-based principles in assessment of the acute care patient using the *Framework*. This table shows how the therapist might use interview, observation, and standardized assessments in determining the client's wants and needs and his or her actual performance skills. The *Framework* defines *occupational performance areas* as activities in which people engage, including "activities of daily living (ADL), instrumental activities of daily living (IADL), rest, sleep, work, leisure, play, education, and social participation" (AOTA, 2008, p. 631). If occupational therapists are to help patients be discharged in a timely manner, finding out what activities they need or want to do is critical because patients are more likely to be motivated to perform activities that they perceive as valuable. The therapist interviews the patient, asking him or her to rate his or her perceived ability to complete ADLs, using a rating scale that measures the level of assistance needed and the patient's satisfaction in completing his or her ADLs (e.g., FIM®; Uniform Data System, 2010; Canadian Occupational Performance Measure [COPM]; Law et al., 2005). Table 1.2 also lists evaluation strategies for assessing patient factors, performance skills, performance patterns, context, and environment and activity demands.

Interview and Occupational Profile

A skilled therapist can quickly ascertain multiple patient factors while asking the patient simple interview questions. In acute care, the interview is often conducted informally and is interspersed with physical or task assessments of the patient. The interview is an excellent opportunity to discover what the patient needs or wants to do when he or she leaves the hospital setting. The therapist gathers information about the living environment and the support the patient has at home, critical factors in discharge planning. The interview is an excellent tool for

(Text continues on page 10)

Table 1.1. **Aspects of Occupational Therapy's Domain and Relationship to Occupational Therapy Evaluation Strategies Based on the *Occupational Therapy Practice Framework* (2nd Ed.)**

Domain of Concern	Strategies for Gathering Information
Areas of occupation • Activities of daily living • Instrumental activities of daily living • Rest and sleep • Education • Work, play, leisure, and social participation	• Interview, self-report measures, observational analysis • Model of Human Occupation–based interview tools (Parkinson, Forsyth, & Kielhofner, 2006) • FIM® (Granger et al., 1993; Keith, Granger, Hamilton, & Sherwin, 1987) • Assessment of Motor and Process Skills (Fisher, 1995) • Kohlman Evaluation of Living Skills (subtests)
Client factors • Values, beliefs, spirituality • Body functions • Body structures	• Interview, chart review • Specific assessments and observations (see Table 1.2) • See Table 1.4 for special considerations regarding body structures
Performance skills • Sensory perceptual • Motor and praxis • Emotional regulation • Cognitive • Communication and social skills	Specific assessment measures and observations • Sensory, light touch, sharp–dull • Visual–perceptual: Baylor Adult Visual Perception Test (Baylor University Medical Center, 1980) • Motor and praxis: typically observed during functional activity and specific range of motion tests and manual muscle testing • Cognitive: SLUMS examination (Morley & Turnosa, 2002), Mini-Mental State Examination (Neistadt, 2000), MOAT/GOAT, Rivermeade Behavioural Memory Test (Wilson, et.al., 2008) • Emotional and communication skills typically observed during patient interview
Performance patterns • Habits, routines, roles, rituals	• Interview, self-report measures (occupational questionnaire)
Context and environment • Cultural, personal, physical, social, temporal, and virtual	• Interview, chart review, self-report measures
Activity demands • Objects used, space demands, social demands, sequencing and timing, required actions, required body functions, required body structures	• Task analysis, interview and observation

Note. ROM = range of motion
Source. Table based on AOTA (2008)

Table 1.2. **Body Functions Attended to in the Acute Care Setting**

Body Functions	Assessment Strategies
Mental functions • *Global mental functions*: consciousness, orientation, temperament and personality, energy, and drive and sleep • *Mental functions*: attention, memory, perception, thought, sequencing, emotional, and experience of self and time • *Higher order thinking*: judgment, concept formation, metacognition, mental flexibility, insight, attention, and awareness	Observed during interview and task performance or through cognitive screening tools • Is client alert, arousable, agitated, or lethargic? • Is client oriented to person, time, place, and situation? • Can client recount history of current illness or injury? Past medical history? Family or social history? • Can client attend to task? Can client alternate or divide attention? • Ask client to remember 3 objects, and have him or her recall the objects immediately and then again after 15 minutes. • Is patient able to list and gather items needed for basic activities of daily living (e.g., toothbrush for brushing teeth)? • Does client have awareness of self, situation, and what it might take to go home safely? • Does client have insight regarding limitations and strengths? • Ask client specific safety scenarios and note appropriateness of response. For example, What would you do if your house were on fire? What would you do if you cut yourself and it did not stop bleeding? • Note whether the patient demonstrates ability to comprehend and respond to a joke or abstract phrases such as "don't cry over spilt milk" (information about abstract reasoning has an impact on foresight and planning).

Sensory functions and pain
 	
• Seeing
• Hearing
• Taste
• Smell
• Tactile or touch
• Temperature and pressure
• Proprioceptive
• Vestibular
• Pain
	Observed during interview and task performance
	
	• Seeing
	  • Have client read clock or dry erase board across room.
	  • Have client read the first few lines on the top of your evaluation form.
	• Hearing
	  • Note whether client wears hearing aids or is hard of hearing.
	• Taste and smell
	  • Not typically addressed unless client discusses issues or there is a problem with eating or appetite. Usually assessed by interview.
	• Tactile or touch
	  • Using cotton swab or ball or your fingers, have patient localize touch on their extremities and face; note deficits.

(continued)

Table 1.2. (continued)

Body Functions	Assessment Strategies

	• Temperature and pressure
	  • Not typically addressed except by interview. If client has diabetes or has nerve impairment, should be addressed by interview or by providing a hot and a cold wash cloth and have the patient identify temperature.
	• Proprioceptive
	  • Can be done observationally by observing movement. More specifically done by moving limbs into specific position and having patient identify the direction of movement.
	• Vestibular
	  • Challenge patient balance in sitting and standing, and note deficits.
	  • Interview regarding dizziness and history of falls or loss of balance.
	• Pain
	  • Interview regarding intensity and type of pain.
	  • Visual analog scale or Wong Baker Faces Rating Scale (Loretz, 2005) are often used as self-report measures.

Neuromusculoskeletal
 	
• Tone
• Subluxation
• Motor control
• Synergy
	Observed during task performance and hands on assessment
	• Tone
	  • Assessed during passive ROM, noting amount of resistance to passive movement.
	• Subluxation
	  • Observation and palpation.
	• Motor control.
	• Noted during movement and interaction with objects (refer to Motor Skills in Table 1.4).
	• Synergy
	  • Note muscle imbalances between force couples (e.g., flexors–extensors, adductors–abductors, and internal–external rotators). Note whether flexion or extension synergy is present.

Note. ROM = range of motion.

gaining an overall picture of the patient's cognitive status (and is frequently the best and only method required, thus limiting embedding a cognitive evaluation). Finally and most important, the interview helps establish a rapport with the patient.

Chisholm, Dolhi, and Schreiber (2004) aptly stated, "Putting occupation into your practice is often easier said than done" (p. 5). They asserted that to implement occupation-based practice, the therapist should begin with a client-centered interview. They provided a simple guide for doing a client-centered interview that includes three key areas to ask a client about:

1. Occupations I need to do
2. Occupations I want to do
3. Occupations I am expected to do.

They recommended listing five occupations for each area and then having the client circle the five most important occupations that they want to address. In the acute care setting, this activity may be more practical to perform verbally rather than in writing because both time and the materials one can bring into patient rooms are limited. Once these important occupations are identified, the performance factors contributing to these occupations would be assessed. This step helps the therapist to more accurately assess the appropriate component behaviors the client needs to perform desired occupations.

Similar to the approach advocated by Chisholm et al. (2004), the COPM (Law et al., 2005) uses a semistructured client-centered interview to gain the patient's perspective about his or her current level of function in self-care, productivity, and leisure. The patient is asked to identify activities that are difficult, narrowing this down to the five most important problems in occupational performance. Using a visual analog scale ranging from 1 to 5, the patient is then asked to take each of these problems and rate the activity's level of importance and his or her level of satisfaction with current performance and perceptions about the quality of performance. The value in this assessment in the acute care setting is that patient perception can be used as a measure of progress. For example, a patient may be too debilitated to make significant gains in improvement of functional performance but may be satisfied with his or her enhanced ability to tolerate sitting up to eat or wash his or her face. This enhanced satisfaction could be measured using the COPM and can show that occupational therapy can have an impact on performance when the probability of making significant functional gains in a short period of time is unlikely.

The *Framework* (AOTA, 2008) considers the interview to be an effective tool to ascertain concerns regarding occupational performance and specific body functions influencing occupational performance. Table 1.2 includes these body functions, along with strategies an occupational therapist in acute care might use to gather information. Although the acute care interview is often conducted during physical and functional assessment activities, therapists should ask patients about

- Performance patterns, including habits, roles, and routines;
- Contexts for occupational performance that include cultural, personal, physical, social, temporal, or virtual; and
- Activity demands that take into account objects used, space demands, social demands, sequencing, required actions, and body functions or structures that the patient typically performs in his or her daily life activities.

Occupational therapists from the Cardinal Hill Healthcare System (Skubik-Peplaski, Paris, Boyle, & Culpert, 2008) undertook a project to incorporate occupation into occupational therapy services and occupational therapy documentation throughout their organization. Using the *Framework*, they provided useful forms and structured interview protocols to help ascertain the patient's occupational needs. As part of their initial interview, they had the patient identify five activities that he or she wanted or needed to resume. They also asked the patient about a typical day and when he or she performed routine daily life tasks. Activity demands can be addressed when probing further, for example, when asking about objects, space, and timing of various daily life activities. The Cardinal Hill group also addressed areas of occupation in asking questions beyond basic self-care. For example, their interview guide addressed areas of leisure by asking what people do for fun and how often they engage in these activities. Context can be addressed in a patient interview by asking questions about social support. Appendix 1.A provides a sample evaluation form with ideas similar to those in the Cardinal Hill model.

Areas of Occupation

Evaluation begins with assessment of the patient's wants, needs, and values. This information becomes the structure for all occupational therapy intervention, as opposed to the physical performance factors seen in many settings. By ascertaining what the patient wants or needs to accomplish to go home or to the next level of care, the therapist can then structure the task or performance assessment to the patient's needs. For example, if the patient states "I want to walk again," the therapist might ask the patient to identify some tasks he or she needs to do that incorporate walking. Patients will often state that they need to walk to get in and out of their bathroom or to go into their kitchen to prepare a meal. If appropriate, the therapist can use the task of going to the bathroom as an assessment measure as opposed to performing assessments of patient factors such as ROM or specific sensory tests, which may have little bearing on functional performance.

In a limited-time environment, this approach is preferable to performing a standardized assessment that may not relate to the patient's performance needs on discharge.

> The short stays that characterize acute care settings have led to the focus of occupational therapy in these settings being around self-care. Little time is available for therapists to address patients' leisure and work needs. Occupational therapists in acute care settings rely heavily on referral to other community and rehabilitation setting where these areas can more readily be addressed. (Griffin & McConnell, 2001, p. 194)

In the acute care setting, most patients are concerned with being discharged back home or to a less restrictive setting. Although therapists often have conversations with their patients about engagement in social activities, leisure activities, or IADLs (e.g., money management, shopping, home maintenance), it is rare to have time to address these skills during the patient's acute care stay.

The seasoned therapist can often walk into the patient's room and ascertain his or her functional abilities on the basis of demonstrated bed mobility, ability to transfer from the bed to the chair, or both. Most experienced therapists will use their clinical reasoning skills to ascertain numerous functional abilities. For example, some parts of a standardized assessment protocol may not be performed because the therapist

can use deductive reasoning skills to conclude that a patient who cannot transfer from a bed to a wheelchair without maximal assistance will not be able to get in and out of the shower or on and off of a commode. This use of deductive reasoning is merely one strategy for dealing with acute care time limitations.

Activity Demands and Client Factors

Typically, determining which activities are meaningful for the patient also assesses activity demands. As the occupational therapist is performing the physical and functional portion of the assessment, he or she is asking questions about the patient's living environment and social support, amount of assistance available, and how various daily life tasks are performed. During the evaluation, the therapist should ask the patient about his or her desire to return to various daily life activities and should help the patient identify which activities are most important to him or her. Participating in therapy may also help the patient to recognize that certain activity demands may be beyond his or her current level of performance, thus requiring recommendations for adaptive equipment or alternative support systems to enable occupational performance.

Client factors noted in the *Framework* (AOTA, 2008), such as body systems and body functions, are addressed in Tables 1.2 and 1.3. Often, multiple disciplines are collecting similar patient data. The occupational therapist in acute care becomes skilled at using data from other professionals to support the evaluation process because it saves time and helps to focus the evaluation on occupation-based tasks. The use of existing data sources also helps avoid redundancy of data and fatiguing the patient during the evaluation process.

In acute care, other than occupational performance areas (i.e., ADLs), therapists usually focus on client factors and performance skills. The *Framework* (AOTA, 2008) defined *client factors* as including three main categories: (1) values, beliefs, and spirituality; (2) body functions; and (3) body structures. In the acute care

Table 1.3.   Body Structures and Concerns for the Acute Care Occupational Therapist

Body Structure	Concerns or Considerations
Gastrointestinal	Dysphagia • Aspiration • Diet types • Sitting to eat and staying upright 30 minutes after a meal Nasogastric tubes and drains • Pulling out tubes • Reflux • Oral suctioning Strict intake and output • Closely monitor and record • Fluid restrictions • Collecting urine in the event that nursing is monitoring per physician order
Genitourinary	Continence and scheduling Types of catheters • Indwelling • Condom • Intermittent catheterization Colostomy • Burping the bags • Teaching how to empty • Dressing and clothing management • Rectal bags • Fear of pulling them out
Endocrine and other metabolic functions	Blood glucose • Affects participation and other body structures Osteoporosis • Fracture precautions Obesity • Therapist body mechanics • Equipment needs • Cardiopulmonary function • Skin and hygiene

(continued)

Table 1.3.   (continued)

Body Structure	Concerns or Considerations
	Electrolytes and hydration
	• Cardiac
	• Executive function
Immune system	Isolation
	Presence of infections
	MRSA
	VRE/VRSA
	C. diff.
	CMV
	Immunosuppressed clients (e.g., AIDS, neutropenic)
	Respiratory function
Skin and integumentary system	Skin integrity and wounds
	Decubitis ulcer grades
	Types of ointments and dressings
	Wound VACs
	Burns
	Open wounds vs. graft wounds
	Adhesions
	Sweating and activity grading
	Edema

Note. C. diff. = *Clostridium difficile;* CMV = cytomegalovirus; MRSA = methicillin-resistant staphylococcus aureus; VRE = vancomycin-resistant enterococcus; VRSA = vancomycin-resistant staphylococcus aureus; VAC = vacuum-assisted closure.

situation, the time available to discuss values and beliefs is often little more than a few minutes. Instead, therapists usually focus on the body functions aspect of client factors.

The *Framework* defines *body functions* as including both physiological and psychological functions of body systems. Gutman and Schonfeld (2009) provided excellent examples of observational and screening assessments that might be used with a neurological population. Many of these strategies could also be used with other populations. In their book *Screening Adult Neurological Populations,* Gutman and Schonfeld provided strategies for patients with both high and low cognitive levels. These strategies

are useful to the acute care therapist because many patients have lower cognitive levels secondary to more acute medical conditions. Table 1.2 provides examples of strategies for assessment of body functions, some of which are based on ideas presented by Gutman and Schonfeld.

Body Functions and Structures

The occupational therapist considers body functions and body structures that might influence occupational performance. Specific body functions and assessment strategies to evaluate both specific and global body functions are outlined in Table 1.4. Occupational therapists

Table 1.4. Commands and Movements for Assessing Range of Motion (ROM) and Manual Muscle Testing (MMT)

Movement Being Assessed	Command for ROM	Command for MMT
Scapular elevation	"Shrug your shoulders."	"Shrug your shoulders, and don't let me push down."
Shoulder flexion	"Raise your hands toward the ceiling."	"Move your hands to shoulder level, and don't let me push down."
External rotation and abduction of the shoulder	"Touch the back of your head."	Not typically tested because of frailty
Internal rotation, abduction, and extension of shoulder	"Then touch the small of your back."	Not typically tested because of frailty or if contraindicated
Elbow flexion	"Keep your elbow by your side, and touch your shoulders."	"Keep your elbow by your side, and touch your shoulders; don't let me pull down."
Wrist flexion and extension	"Wave your hand" like a baby.	Wrist in neutral (gravity eliminated): "Don't let me push back/don't let me push in."
Thumb and finger flexion	"Make a fist."	Can use a dynamometer. Place 2 fingers into patient's palm, and say "Squeeze my fingers."
Opposition	"Take each finger and touch your thumb one at a time."	Not typically tested (grip strength generally assesses this)
Hip and knee flexion	*While supine:* "Bend your knee." *While sitting:* "Bend your knee."	"Hold your knee, and don't let me push it down." *Note:* Do this before standing a patient for the first time, so there are no surprises such as one leg buckling.
Hip abduction and adduction	*While supine:* "Bring your leg out to the side and back to the middle."	"Bring your leg out to the side. Hold it, and don't let me push in." "Now, back to the middle; don't let me pull it out."
External rotation of hip	"Roll your knee out to the side" or "turn your toes out."	Not typically tested
Internal rotation of hip	"Roll your knee inward" or "turn your toes in."	Not typically tested
Dorsi or plantar flexion	"Tap your toes."	"Point toes up and hold it." Occupational therapist places hand under forefoot, and instructs patient to push down.

have a working knowledge of body structures as they pertain to occupational performance; however, the goal is not specifically to address the structure but rather the function of these body structures. Body functions and structures may also be improved through engagement in occupation.

The term *body functions* includes the physiologic processes of body systems, and the term *body structures* includes anatomical parts that support function. Body functions include

- Global and specific mental functions
- Sensory functions and pain
- Neuromusculoskeletal and movement-related functions
- Cardiovascular, hematological, immunological, and respiratory system function
- Voice and speech functions
- Digestive, metabolic, and endocrine system function
- Genitourinary and reproductive functions
- Skin and related structure functions.

During evaluation, occupational therapists most specifically address mental, sensory, and neuromusculoskeletal functions.

Mental Processes

The *Framework* (AOTA, 2008) identifies *mental processes* as affective, cognitive, and perceptual functions. It further differentiates mental processes into global and specific mental functions. *Global functions* include orientation, consciousness, temperament, and personality functions. *Specific mental functions* include attention, memory, emotional regulation, and sequencing.

Occupational therapists typically assess mental processes during patient interview and task performance. Therapists are skilled at noting the client's logical flow of conversation and sequencing the client's history, orientation, and emotional state during the interview. Moreover, the client's engagement in simple ADL tasks such as washing one's face, brushing teeth, or toileting can inform the therapist about his or her global and specific mental functions, including attention, memory, and sequencing.

Although some higher order thinking skills can be assessed during ADLs, these skills are typically assessed by means of interview, giving the patient hypothetical or real situations to which to respond. Often, these scenarios are safety related. For example, the therapist might ask "what would you do if" questions to ascertain the client's judgment and insight. Therapists might also ask interview questions such as "Have you noticed a change in your thinking skills recently?" to ascertain the patient's metacognition or his or her ability to have insight into his or her cognition.

Sensory Functions

Sensory functions are often assessed by observation during functional tasks and through hands-on assessment strategies. The five senses—sight, hearing, taste, smell, and touch—are observed during task performance and through questioning. Assessment of these senses is critical in patients with neurological impairment or those patients considered frail elderly because deficits could present difficulties in safety, particularly if the client is returning home to live alone.

Seeing. First and foremost, the therapist should establish whether the client has preexisting visual deficits and whether he or she wears corrective lenses. Age-related changes in vision include having cataracts, glaucoma, diabetic retinopathy, age-related macular degeneration, and yellowing of the lenses (Quintana, 2008). However, in the presence of acute disease or neurological events, the patient may exhibit visual disturbances or oculomotor dysfunction. The therapist may either formally assess or use purposeful activity to determine any of the following dysfunctions: low visual acuity, unilateral neglect, hemianopsia, and visual inattention. Refer to Appendix F for more information on low vision assessment and intervention strategies.

The formal method for assessing peripheral vision and visual tracking involves using two occupational therapists. However, the reality of practice in acute care is that occupational therapists treat their patients alone or with a staff member of another discipline. A quick assessment strategy for an occupational therapist to evaluate peripheral vision includes holding a tongue depressor, toothette, or oral swab along the parietal area of the patient's head, slowly bringing it into the patient's line of vision and asking the patient to indicate when he or she sees it. The therapist can also use a tongue depressor or toothette when assessing oculomotor function with each eye individually. This process involves the occupational therapist positioning himself or herself at the patient's eye level, covering each eye, and mimicking eye movements in all four visual quadrants.

Qualitative indicators of visual deficits can include double vision or obstructed vision, squinting, or closing one eye. The therapist may also observe the patient's eye watering or not attending to either the left or the right side. The therapist may also note that the patient ignores items on the bedside table or dinner tray or tends to under- or overshoot when reaching for an object, which may be indicative of a visual field deficit or double vision.

Hearing. Often, the occupational therapist does not formally assess hearing. In terms of functional independence, the therapist should note whether the patient is hard of hearing and, if so, whether the patient uses hearing aids or hears better with one ear than the other. The occupational therapists should consult with speech pathologists or audiologists if they have a concern regarding a patient's hearing ability.

Smell and Taste. Smell and taste are typically not formally assessed unless the client specifically reports a change in these faculties of recent onset. Nonetheless, therapists may pick up on changes in taste or smell if the client reports having lost his or her appetite or has problems consuming adequate nutrition. Sometimes, the family will also report that the client has difficulties with these body functions in that the client often has spoiled food in the refrigerator or has recently changed food preferences to sweets or spicy foods.

Tactile and Touch. Assessment of tactile abilities is often part of the standard occupational therapy evaluation because it influences motor performance and ultimately patient safety. Inadequate motor control and impaired ability to use objects may be the result of a tactile deficit; therefore, it is imperative that the therapist establish the root cause of a deficit in motor performance. Therapists often use light touch as a quick assessment strategy whereby they use a finger, tissue, or cotton swab to perform light strokes along each sensory dermatome or peripheral nerve distribution, asking the patient to localize where he or she was touched. Similarly, occupational therapists measure recognition of pain sources by using a pin or another sharp object to measure whether the patient can distinguish between sharp or dull sensations. The therapist records the degree of accuracy (e.g., 4 of 5 accurate) and the location of the deficit.

One other form of tactile sensation, *stereognosis,* is much more complex because it involves identifying objects placed in the hand with vision occluded. Should therapists have an opportunity to assess stereognosis, they should choose objects that are familiar but distinctly different (e.g., utensil from tray, toothbrush, comb, pen or pencil, other items typically found in the patient's room).

Proprioception

Proprioception is the ability to know where one's extremities, head, or trunk are in space when the body is static or engaged in movement. A deficit in proprioception impedes quality of movement and the ability to adequately use objects while engaged in tasks. It might also impede safety, particularly during mobility activities in which visual information is limited. For example, getting up in the middle of the night to go to the bathroom requires a keen knowledge of where one's body is in space to navigate in a safe manner. To assess proprioception, therapists use observation, but they may also passively move the client's extremity into a specific position and ask the patient to identify the direction of the limb. For example, the therapist positions the upper extremity toward the ceiling, and the patient must identify whether the limb is pointing up or down.

Pain

The Joint Commission for Accreditation of Healthcare Organizations (JCAHO) requires that all professionals working with patients assess pain with the patient throughout the patient's hospital stay (JCAHO, 2009). Many hospitals have specific measures that are used, but usually practitioners merely ask the patient, "On a scale of 1 to 10, where is your pain right now?"

Another tool is the visual analog scale (see Figure 1.2), which has been shown to be more reliable than verbal-only ratings. Pain is usually assessed via a visual analog scale that might include lines on a continuum from 1 to 10 or a continuum from happy to sad faces (particularly useful for children). Using a visual analog scale helps the therapist take a pre- and postmeasure of pain perception by associating a number with the pain rating, thus allowing therapists to document and compare the response to treatment in terms of pain: remaining the same, increasing, or decreasing after intervention.

Vestibular Function

Many bedridden or deconditioned patients experience vestibular (balance) deficits associated with prolonged bedrest. Many conditions, particularly neurological conditions such as stroke and brain injury, also influence vestibular function. When interviewing a patient, therapists may ask questions regarding whether he or she has had a history of falls in the past year or whether any balance problems or vertigo has been associated with the recent hospitalization.

Always keeping safety in mind (e.g., using a gait belt, assistance of another staff member), occupational therapists typically assess vestibular function while having the patient sit at the edge of the bed supported and unsupported. If the patient can sit unsupported, the therapist may challenge the balance by *perturbing* (gently pushing) the patient side to side or backward and forward, noting how easily the patient corrects his or her balance. Once the therapist has the patient standing unsupported, he or she can also perturb balance to ascertain function. The therapist should also note the client's balance during mobility tasks such as bending, reaching, and twisting side to side and during ambulation.

Neuromusculoskeletal Function

A key focus of occupational therapy intervention in the acute care setting is the neuromusculoskeletal functions associated with occupational performance. Table 1.4 lists specific neuromusculoskeletal functions and strategies for assessing these functions.

To accomplish functional tasks, patients must have adequate muscle tone, ROM, strength, and fine and gross motor coordination, which are associated with effective motor control. Patients with neurological impairment often have muscle tone imbalances that might result in movement synergies that prevent them from demonstrating isolated motor control. For example, the patient with stroke who is influenced by hypertonicity and is bound in a flexion synergy is going to have difficulty feeding himself or herself. A patient may also have a subluxation of a joint that causes pain and inhibits ROM. Subluxation is also common in patients with stroke and may be the result of flaccid musculature or injury to a joint. Because of its anatomical structure (not a true ball-and-socket joint), the shoulder is the most common subluxation seen in patients with neurological impairment.

Motor Functions and Performance

When observing motor behavior, the occupational therapist must consider several components ranging from tone, reflexes, and coordination to postural control, sensation perception, memory, and even judgment. Observation is generally the first line in evaluating motor behavior because keen observation may indicate whether an occupational therapist will use functional versus formal testing for

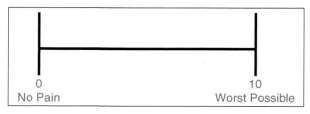

Figure 1.2. Visual analog scale used to assess pain.

ROM. When a patient exhibits normal tone and quality of movement or has a cognitive issue, then functional testing of ROM is used. When patients have a specific injury or a surgical issue that impedes AROM or passive ROM (or PROM), formal assessment measures may be used as a barometer of progress. For example, patients who have had shoulder replacement surgery may be monitored using goniometric measurement.

Rarely does the acute care occupational therapist measure ROM using a goniometer. Instead, functional ROM is measured easily and quickly by instructing the patient to perform the movements described in Table 1.4, which allows for quick assessment of both upper extremities, completing ranges at each major joint (hand, wrist, elbow, and shoulder) and in each plane. An occupational approach would include having the patient "prepare" for additional activity by donning nonskid socks, grooming hair and face, and donning robe or housecoat, in assessing functional mobility and safety. Having the patient complete functional tasks allows the occupational therapist to assess not only ROM but also gross motor and fine motor control, proprioception, stereognosis, sequencing, memory, visual memory, and visual acuity.

An occupational therapist must also consider modifying ROM assessment for patients when a particular range may be contraindicated. Some contraindications include sternotomies, pacer or pacemaker, anterior cervical diskectomies and fusion, shoulder replacement, clavicular fractures, cervical fractures, and humeral and scapular fractures or contractures. If active limitations are found, the therapist could attempt to move the joint through its range passively or as medical orders indicate. If a goniometer is available, the occupational therapist should record the degree to which the patient achieves active range. Commands and movements assessed when evaluating a patient's ROM are reviewed in Table 1.4.

Caution is required in recommending PROM if active limits are found. Some orthopedic conditions may permit only AROM within pain-free ranges, only PROM with no tissue tension, and possibly neither immediately after surgery.

Assessing Strength

Manual muscle testing (MMT) can also be completed formally or informally. Diagnosis and observation, in general, dictates whether the therapist chooses to formally test bilateral upper- and lower-extremity strength. Testing muscle strength against resistance (formally or informally) may be contraindicated for patients who have undergone sternotomies or who have orthopedic precautions. In general, if the therapist observes the patient transfer from supine to sitting and standing at the bedside independently, the therapist may choose to omit a formal MMT because the patient has exhibited the ability to support his or her own weight for functional transfers. Commands for an occupational therapist to use with patients when formally assessing strength are provided in Table 1.4, and MMT grades are provided in Table 1.5.

Tone

Tone is usually assessed during the MMT or when passively moving an extremity through its ROM. The Modified Ashworth Scale (Bohannan & Smith, 1987) is helpful in categorizing tone and is presented in Table 1.6.

Gross and Fine Motor Coordination

Some of the motor dysfunctions that therapists typically treat include weakness, flexor tone patterns, patterns of spasticity, hypotonia or hypertonia, clonus, apraxia, sensory loss, and diminished fractionation (isolation of movement). All of these deficits can ultimately affect fine and gross motor coordination. Knowing whether a patient has a nervous system lesion and where that lesion might be is useful in helping the occupational therapist anticipate what types of motor deficits he or she might have. For example, cortical damage often results in motor planning deficits along with problems executing goal-directed movement (Mathiowetz & Bass-Haugen, 2008).

Cerebellar damage often results in difficulties with timing and force of movement. Patients with cerebellar lesions may present

Table 1.5. Scoring Manual Muscle Testing

Muscle Grade	Definition
0/5	No active movement noted.
1/5	No active movement is achieved, but contraction can be felt.
2−/5	Patient able to initiate movement with gravity eliminated.
2/5	Patient makes incomplete range with gravity eliminated.
2+/5	Patient able to go through entire range with gravity eliminated.
3−/5	Patient able to partially achieve full range against gravity.
3/5	Patient able to complete range against gravity, without any additional external force.
3+/5	Patient able to complete range with light resistance.
4/5	Patient able to complete full range with moderate resistance.
5/5	Patient able to complete full range with maximal resistance.

Table 1.6. Modified Ashworth Scale

Grade	Description
0	No increase in muscle tone
1	Slight increase in muscle tone manifested by a catch and release or by minimal resistance at the end of the ROM when the affected part or parts are moved in flexion or extension
1+	Slight increase in muscle tone manifested by a catch, followed by minimal resistance throughout the remainder (less than half) of the ROM
2	More increase in muscle tone through most of the ROM, but affected parts are easily moved
3	Considerable increase in muscle tone; passive movement difficult
4	Affected part or parts rigid in flexion or extension

Note. ROM = range of motion.
Source. Bohannon & Smith (1987). Adapted with permission.

with dysmetria, ataxia, intention tremor, dysdiadokinesia, and adiadochokinesia. Patients are delayed with initiation or termination of tasks and lack the ability to adjust the timing and accuracy of movement. A patient with damage to the basal ganglia has difficulties with automatic rhythmic and learned movements, often presenting with tremors, bradykinesia, dystonia, festinating gait, or athetosis (Mathiowetz & Bass-Haugen, 2008). Once a therapist establishes the type of motor deficits a client has, he or she can use specific motor assessments or observations in the evaluation process.

Simple coordination tests include

- *Finger-to-nose and gross upper-extremity* dynamic reaching in multiple planes
- *Fine motor:* In-hand manipulation (e.g., buttons, snaps, tying shoes, fastening a hospital gown, twisting a bread tie, opening a tube of toothpaste)
- *Lower extremity:* Heel-to-shin test and checking coordination during transfers and ambulation.

Static and Dynamic Balance

When an occupational therapist assesses static and dynamic balance, whether in sitting or in standing, cognition should also be taken into consideration because processing and attention affect balance. The therapist should be certain to use protective and assistive equipment including gait belts, walkers, or canes as needed. He or she should also ask for assistance from a rehabilitation aide or other staff member (e.g., patient's nursing assistant).

Ask the patient whether he or she can sit at the edge of the bed. Also ask the patient to stand, observing trunk control, weight shifting, and posturing at the shoulders, hips, knees, and ankle. The occupational therapist should be certain to document the level of assistance required for bed mobility and transfers, noting whether the patient has difficulty maintaining an upright position (e.g., leaning heavily right or left as with a cardiovascular accident) in sitting or standing. The therapist should also note other signs of difficulty with balance, including nystagmus with change in position, complaints of dizziness, or change in respiration or heart rate with changes in body position, because these may be indicative of vestibular problems affecting balance.

Functional reach tasks also provide a useful assessment of balance. The occupational therapist should place objects behind, to the right, to the left, and in the midline of the patient and then ask the patient to reach for these objects. The therapist also observes the patient's dynamic sitting or standing balance with weight shifting and should document whether the patient loses balance and in which direction the balance is impaired. The level of assistance needed for client self-correction should also be noted. In addition, the occupational therapist should note whether the patient uses controlled, fluid movements or momentum or propulsion to achieve weight shifting and upright postures. Balance can be further assessed as it pertains to visual–vestibular function by moving objects in various planes and having the patient visually track and reach for the objects while leaning forward, sideways, and backward.

Most hospitals have a system in place to indicate whether a patient is at risk for falls. For example, some hospitals place a marker on the patient's door or chart. Implementing use of nonskid socks or stockings, gait belts, rolling walkers, or canes are several fall prevention measures used in acute care. According to Chronister (2004), different factors may affect balance. "Change the environment or add a complex thinking task and the way we walk changes drastically" (para. 8).

Many programs for fall prevention focus on the physical aspects of maintaining balance. However, a patient's cognitive status may be another important variable to consider. The therapist must also remember that balance can change with normal aging. For example, hair cells located in the labyrinth may decrease, which provides information regarding motion of the head. Diminished visual perception, decreased visual acuity, and diminished visual field may also be present. These visual changes may also explain a patient's inability to change his or her attention from cognitive tasks to balance tasks when unexpected postural changes occur.

Assessment of Other Body Functions

In terms of physiological body functions, occupational therapists attend primarily to cardiovascular and respiratory system functions. Using observation skills, therapists monitor (and record as appropriate) breathing patterns (rate, type, loudness, quality), visible sweating, visible pulse in any blood vessels (particularly in response to straining or strenuous tasks), changes in color (increased pallor or redness), and time engaged in an activity before experiencing fatigue or shortness of breath. If monitors are available, the therapist can use these monitors (e.g., heart rate, blood pressure, respiratory rate) as a measure of response to intervention (i.e., using the quantitative information as pre- and postmeasures).

Occupational therapists do not typically assess voice and speech functions other than by observation. Patients with difficulties producing speech loud enough to be heard may have difficulties with respiration or throat muscles. Therapists also observe the patient's voice quality, such as hoarseness or wet-sounding voice. In particular, a wet-sounding voice after eating may be indicative of dysphagia. Therapists may address oral–motor control as it pertains to eating and speaking. They may note the quality of the muscle tone or the strength of the oral–motor musculature as they watch the patient speak or chew food (refer to Chapter 13 for more information on dysphagia). Recommendations for referral to a speech–language pathologist for further evaluation should be made for patients with significant deficits in speech, language, or both.

Skin and related structure functions are also of concern to occupational therapists. Usually, the nursing staff or a wound care specialist measures aspects of wounds or problems with skin. For example, wound size is measured as the distance across the largest part of a wound, or the depth of a wound is graded. Wound depth is graded on a scale ranging from 1 to 4, with 1 being *the most superficial,* in terms of the layers of skin the wound has penetrated or exposed, and 4 being *destruction of deep tissue that may go as deep as affecting the bone.* Wounds may also be described as partial thickness where the wound affects the epidermis and dermin but not the subcutaneous tissue. Full thickness wounds, which are considered deep, affect the epidermis and the entire dermis.

Function of skin is particularly important in patients with impaired sensation in prevention of development of decubitus ulcers. Surgical wounds also create concern for occupational therapists in terms of mobility and splinting, which might assist or impede wound healing.

All health care professionals attend to skin structure and function for the patients who have been burned. Occupational therapists working with these patients measure the degree of scar formation and work to prevent development of nonmalleable scars, which ultimately inhibit functional mobility (refer to Chapter 15 for more information on burns).

One factor related to both the integumentary system and the vascular system is *edema.* This swelling condition is common in people with circulatory problems, and it can influence mobility and pain while performing functional tasks.

Therapists use observation skills to describe the grading of edema and the type of edema. Table 1.7 presents a scale used to measure

Table 1.7. **Edema Scale**

Grading	Physical Characteristics
0	No edema
+1	Barely discernible pit; normal foot and leg contours
+2	Deeper pit (<5 mm); fairly normal foot and leg contours
+3	Deep pit (5–10 mm); foot and leg swelling
+4	Even deeper pit (>1 cm); severe foot and leg swelling

Source. O'Sullivan and Schmitz (2007). Adapted with permission.

edema. Occupational therapists can also use a tape measure to record the circumference of a joint or extremity in recording the degree of edema. This strategy is useful as a pre–post measure to record the effectiveness of an intervention. Although therapists might not quantify edema, they will typically use descriptive words (e.g., *puffy, pitting, brawny*) to describe edema. These descriptors might change as the client undergoes occupational therapy that influences edema, positively or negatively.

Occupational therapists do not typically evaluate digestive, metabolic, endocrine, genitourinary, and reproductive functions. They should be aware of difficulties or potential difficulties with these body systems and how those difficulties may affect the patient. Examples of how therapists might attend to these body functions and structures in the provision of occupational therapy services are provided in Table 1.3.

Body Structures

The *Framework* states that occupational therapists do not typically address body structures, which are defined as "anatomical parts of the body such as organs, limbs, and their components that support body function" (AOTA, 2008, p. 637). Although occupational therapists do not attempt to "fix" body structures, they may help patients compensate for difficulties with each of these systems. Occupational therapists must also have a keen awareness of these issues because they may affect functional performance and the ability to return to the least restrictive setting in a safe manner. Therapists should also be aware of medical interventions that affect body structures because they must work within these boundaries as functional performance is addressed. Table 1.4 lists examples of problems with specific body structures or systems that might affect or cause concern for occupational therapy.

Additional Systems Influencing Function and Evaluation

When evaluating patients, occupational therapists must also concern themselves with other systems that may influence the method by which they evaluate the patient. These systems may include, but are not limited to, immune system, endocrine, excretory, and integumentary functions. For example, if a patient has an immune system disorder, the therapist would pay close attention to his or her white blood cell levels. If a patient is vulnerable to infection, a good chance exists that he or she will be on contact precautions. Patients with certain disorders may also have associated drains, tubes, or bulbs. For example, a pulmonary patient may have a chest tube to contend with, and a patient with a gastrointestinal disorder may have a nasogastric tube or a suction device.

Performance Skills

The abilities that patients exhibit during engagement in activities are described in the *Framework* (AOTA, 2008) as performance skills. The categories of performance skills include

- Motor and praxis skills
- Sensory–perceptual skills
- Emotional regulation skills
- Cognitive skills
- Communication and social skills.

According to the *Framework*, body functions and structures underline performance skills. *Body functions* are those capacities one possesses when performance skills are "demonstrated." For example, one could have the necessary body functions (upper-body strength or ROM) for a skill such as dressing but may not be able to perform the task because of contextual factors (i.e., performing the activity with a halo vest while supine in the bed).

Occupational therapists in acute care are encouraged to focus on performance skills rather than body functions to help the patient be as independent as possible before discharge. For example, instead of bringing a Thera-Band® to the bedside to ultimately enable the client to be strong enough to engage in a dressing task, he or she would be better served by doing motor and praxis skills related to upper-body dressing (to the extent possible to improve performance in this area). This type of approach is consistent with occupation-based practice and is well suited for the acute care situation because therapists do not have time to help the client achieve the necessary prerequisite skills before discharge. In short, the best way to enhance occupation is to work on occupation. Table 1.8 provides a listing of the specific items in each performance skill category along with strategies for observation and assessment.

Performance Patterns

The *Framework* (AOTA, 2008) defines *performance patterns* as habits, routines, roles, and rituals used during occupational performance. In the acute care environment, occupational therapists interview clients about a typical day to ascertain roles (e.g., expected behaviors such as parent, worker), habits (i.e., automatic behaviors), routines (i.e., established sequences of activities), and rituals (i.e., shared social

Table 1.8. Assessment of Performance Skills

Performance Skills	Assessment Strategies and Key Questions
Motor and praxis	
• Planning, sequencing, and executing new and novel movements • Posture—Stabilizes, aligns, positions • Mobility—Walks, reaches, bends • Coordination—coordinates, manipulates, flows • Strength and effort—Moves, transports, lifts, calibrates, grips • Energy—Endures, paces	Observe during the interview and task performance. • Observe patient during bed-to-wheelchair transfer if this is new learning. • Observe orderly flow of steps to a task or not preparing space or body before execution of a task. Observe at edge of bed and in standing while performing activities of daily living (ADLs) or mobility. Observe during ADLs; set items out of reach and observe patient bending, reaching, or mobilizing self to retrieve objects. Observe as patient interacts with objects and during mobility. • Is patient using too much or too little force? • Is patient working at a too fast or too slow pace? • Is the patient struggling/straining while lifting or carrying objects? • Does patient use one hand or two hands, or is there a delay in stabilizing an object? Does client demonstrate visible signs of fatigue or overexertion (sweating, shortness of breath, stopping in the middle of a task)?
Sensory–perceptual skills	
• Locate, identify, and respond to sensations	Observe during the interview and task performance. • Is patient distracted by external stimuli such that it impedes task performance?

Table 1.8. (continued)

Performance Skills	Assessment Strategies and Key Questions
• Select, interpret, associate, organize, and remember sensory events • Discriminate experiences through a variety of sensations	• Is client aware of time of day (e.g., using external information, clock, window)? • Is client aware of body in space? • Is client able to get back to room after walking in the hallway?
Emotional regulation skills	
• Identify, manage, and express feelings • Responding • Persisting • Controlling • Recovering • Displaying emotions • Using coping strategies	Observe during the interview and task performance • Is client overly emotional or labile? • Does client give up easily or persist? • Is client able to express concern or frustration appropriately? • Is client able to identify emotional coping strategies (e.g., family support, spirituality, goals to get out of hospital)?
Cognitive skills	
• Judging • Selecting • Sequencing • Organizing • Prioritizing • Creating • Multitasking	Observe during task performance • Is client able to select and correctly use appropriate tools or objects? • Can client organize space and materials for task performance? • Can client sequence, prioritize, and multitask? • Can client judge when task is complete? • Can client judge effectiveness of task performance?
Process	
• Energy—Paces, attends • Knowledge—Chooses, uses, handles, heeds, inquires • Temporal organization—Initiates, continues, sequences, terminates • Organizing space and objects—Searches, locates, gathers, organizes, restores, navigates • Adaptation—Notices, responds, accommodates, benefits	Observe during task performance • Can client initiate and continue tasks? Does client appropriately terminate task? • Can the client find needed objects? Does client lose objects or place them in a disorganized array? Does client gather items before commencing a task? Does client clutter his or her space or bump into things? • Does the client notice when tasks are not being completed effectively?

(continued)

Table 1.8. (continued)	
Performance Skills	**Assessment Strategies and Key Questions**
Communication and interaction	
• Physicality—Contacts, gazes, gestures, maneuvers, orients, postures • Information exchange—Articulates, asserts, asks, engages, expresses, modulates, shares, speaks, sustains • Relations—Collaborates, conforms, focuses, relates, respects	Observe during interview and task performance • Is the client able to articulate his or her story, goals? • Does client make eye contact and demonstrate appropriate emotions? • Is client able to maintain a conversation? Is communication and exchange between client and therapist effective?

actions that have meaning) in which the client engages. Of particular importance is establishing which roles, routines, rituals, or habits the client wants or needs to resume when discharged, which should be the priority for intervention. For example, a patient may not care about dressing but be highly motivated to return to receiving Holy Communion in church weekly and therefore want to work on the precursor skills needed to accomplish this ritual.

One caution that the *Framework* (AOTA, 2008) makes is that roles do not define the individual, meaning that stereotyping individuals and guiding interventions and therapeutic activities on the basis of the therapist's perception of that role is a danger. Anyone who has filled the role of parent knows that a parent's activities vary greatly depending on myriad factors that can include the child's age, the parenting setting, and the parent's life situation.

Context and Environment

Using an interview, the acute care therapist attempts to ascertain the cultural, temporal, physical, social, personal, and even virtual contexts in which the patient performs. In the acute care environment, the focus is typically on the physical environment in terms of making sure that the patient will have physical accessibility to home and community

environments. The *Framework* (AOTA, 2008) goes well beyond the physical environment to include exploration of social and cultural factors that might affect performance as well as exploration of the virtual environments in which patients engage. When thinking about teenagers or young adults, for example, the occupational therapist should be mindful that they may place a high priority on resuming activities related to computers and cell phones.

Interpretation of Findings

Interpretation of findings is the evaluation of all of the data gathered and assessment of those factors that might enhance or impede occupational performance (i.e., strengths and weaknesses). The therapist predicts the patient's ability to benefit from occupational therapy rehabilitation and generates goals for the short and long term. In the acute care setting, short-term goals might be accomplished as soon as the next day, and long-term goals might be accomplished in a week, in 2 to 3 days, or by discharge.

The acute care therapist must pay particular attention to the length of stay when interpreting findings. The therapist should assume the patient might be able to go home tomorrow because discharges often happen quickly in the acute care setting. The therapist must also take into account the contextual factors that might influence discharge planning. For example, if the patient requires minimum assistance for functional mobility or ADLs but has no social support in the home, he or she may be deemed unsafe to return home alone. The occupational therapist might then make recommendations for a short-term rehabilitation stay to prepare the patient for a safe return home alone without social or caregiver support. The patient's medical stability might also be a factor in determining the appropriateness of a rehabilitation stay. Therefore, the occupational therapist, when doing his or her assessment and making discharge recommendations, should keep in mind that the patient's medical status can quickly change. Refer to Appendix M for more detail on discharge planning.

Recommendations for Intervention

After the initial evaluation, the occupational therapist's recommendations for intervention should consider both client and contextual factors, including medical instability or deconditioning that may hinder a patient's ability to participate in vigorous or strenuous activities, limiting attainment of occupational therapy goals. Contextual factors such as the patient's needing to walk long distances or up steps once he or she returns home should also be considered. The layout of the patient's home and the degree of social support available might also influence the types of interventions used or recommendations made. For example, if a patient is about to be discharged home but requires moderate assistance in stand–pivot transfers and the spouse or family member is unable to lift the patient, then they may be instructed in a sliding board transfer technique or lift system.

In the acute care setting, occupational therapy interventions typically include helping the client to build strength and endurance to enable participation in BADLs such as dressing, bathing, toileting, grooming, and hygiene that are often necessary for the patient to be able to care for himself or herself once discharged home. Higher level ADLs or IADLs (e.g., cooking) can be managed through community resources such

as Meals on Wheels. IADLs such as home management (e.g., yard work, maintenance, homemaking, cooking, cleaning) or time management can be addressed on an outpatient level once the patient has recovered physical strength and competence in BADLs.

The Joint Commission and Other Mandates

The Joint Commission (formerly JCAHO; 2009) mandates that health care practitioners attend to several issues during the evaluation process. First, occupational therapists must evaluate a patient if an order was received for services. The therapist cannot merely do a chart review and determine that occupational therapy is not indicated. The therapist must visit with the client and perform some level of assessment before determining that therapy may not be indicated. Second (that affects occupational therapy) is that health care providers must attend to the patient's pain. On the initial evaluation, the occupational therapist should record the patient's level of pain. During subsequent treatment sessions, at a minimum, the therapist must assess pre–post levels of pain. If pain is greater than a 5 (on a visual analog scale ranging from 1 to 10; refer to Figure 1.2), the therapist must notify the nursing staff and document that nursing was informed of the patient's pain level. Third, the therapist must document how the patient was left after an evaluation or treatment session with a focus on fall prevention. For example, the therapist could document "Patient placed back in bed to supine position/ bedrails up and all needs within reach."

Another focus of The Joint Commission (2009) has been on patient safety regarding patient and caregiver knowledge of the patient's medications. Although occupational therapists are not specifically responsible for this mandate, they often converse with patients about their medications with regard to medication management. If the therapist becomes aware that the client or caregiver is not fully aware of medication factors, the occupational therapist should at a minimum notify the nursing staff so they can review this information with the client and family as needed.

Many of The Joint Commission's (2009) recent mandates or recommendations are a result of Medicare's mandates for enhancing the quality of patient care. For many years, occupational therapists working with Medicare patients in long-term care facilities needed to have the physician sign off on their plan of care for treatment. More recently, The Joint Commission has been ensuring that this recommendation is also adhered to in the hospital setting. This recommendation ensures that the physician is in agreement with the occupational therapy treatment plan, ultimately ensuring that the patient receives the most optimum care.

One other Joint Commission mandate that has been in existence in long-term care for years is that the patient and caregiver must be in agreement with the plan of care and treatment, ensuring once again that the occupational therapist is collaborating with the patient in addressing his or her concerns and goals and is compatible with occupational therapy's focus on client-centered care. Although these regulations have been put in place to ensure quality care for patients receiving occupational therapy services, they certainly add to documentation time and should be factored into any template evaluations.

Summary

In this chapter, we reviewed the process and the specific assessment strategies used in the acute care setting. Although many of the strategies for the use of standardized assessment tools may not always be appropriate and practical in the acute care setting, occupational therapists are challenged to use objective data sources in collecting data to support the therapist's role in the acute care setting.

Constraints in the evaluation process include the patient's medical instability, competition for the patient's time from other disciplines or procedures, infection control policies and procedures, and lack of time, which inhibits the use of standardized assessment tools. Despite these barriers, many occupational therapists quickly become skilled at using clinical observations and quick assessment tools, combined with their clinical reasoning, to accurately evaluate and predict a client's functional performance abilities. These occupational therapy evaluation results can be invaluable when determining patient discharge disposition.

References

American Occupational Therapy Association. (2008). *Occupational therapy practice framework: Domain* and process (2nd ed.). *American Journal of Occupational Therapy, 62,* 625–683.

Baylor University Medical Center, Department of Occupational Therapy. (1980). *Baylor Adult Visual Perceptual Assessment.* Dallas, TX.

Bohannan, R. W., & Smith, M. B. (1987). Interrater reliability of the Modified Ashworth Scale of Muscle Spasticity. *Physical Therapy, 67,* 206–208.

Chisholm, D., Dolhi, C., & Schreiber, J. (2004). *Occupational therapy intervention resource manual: A guide for occupation-based practice.* Clifton Park, NY: Delmar Learning.

Chronister, K. (2004). Cognition: The missing link in fall-prevention programs. *OT Practice, 9*(12). Available online at www.aota.org/Pubs/OTP/1997-2007/Features/2004/f-112904.aspx

Craig, G., Robertson, L., & Milligan, S. (2004). Occupational therapy practice in acute physical health care settings: A pilot study. *New Zealand Journal of Occupational Therapy, 51,* 5–13.

Fisher, A. G. (1995). *Assessment of motor and process skills.* Fort Collins, CO: Three Star.

Granger, C. V., Hamilton, B. B., Linacre, J. M., Heinremann, A. W. & Wright, B. D. (1993). *Performance profiles of the Functional Independence Measure and Rehabilitation, 72,* 84–89.

Griffin, S., & McConnell, D. (2001). Australian occupational therapy practice in acute care settings. *Occupational Therapy International, 8,* 184–197.

Gutman, S., & Schonfeld, A. (2009). *Screening adult neurological populations: A step-by-step instruction manual* (2nd ed). Bethesda, MD: AOTA Press.

Hinojosa, J., Kramer, P., & Crist, P. (2009). *Evaluation: Obtaining and interpreting data* (3rd ed.). Bethesda, MD: AOTA Press.

The Joint Commission. (2009). *Healthcare issues: Pain management.* Retrieved from http://www.jointcommission.org/NewsRoom/health_care_issues.htm

Keith, R. A., Granger, C. V., Hamilton, B. B., Sherwin, F. S. (1987). *The functional independence measure: A new tool for rehabilitation.* In M. G. Eisenberg & R. C. Grzesiak (Eds.), Advances in clinical rehabilitation (pp. 6–18), New York: Springer Publishing.

Kohlman Thomson, L. (1992). *Kohlman Evaluation of Living Skills (KELS)* (3rd ed.). Bethesda, MD: American Occupational Therapy Association.

Law, M., Baptiste, S., Carswell, A., McColl, M. A., Polatajko, H., & Pollock, N. (2005). *The Canadian Occupational Performance Measure* (4th ed.). Ottawa, Ontario: CAOT Publications.

Lortez, L. (2005). *Primary care tools for clinicians: A compendium of forms, questionnaires, and rating scales for everyday practice.* St. Louis, MO: Elsevier Mosby.

Mathiowetz, V., & Bass-Haugen, J. (2008). Assessing abilities and capacities: Motor behavior. In M. V. Radomski & C. T. Latham (Eds.), *Occupational therapy for physical dysfunction* (pp. 186–211). Philadelphia: Lippincott Williams & Wilkins.

Migliore, A. (2004). Case Report—Improving dyspnea management in three adults with chronic obstructive pulmonary disease. *American Journal of Occupational Therapy, 58,* 639–646.

Morley, J. E., Turnosa, N.: Saint Louis University Mental Status Examination (SLUMS). Aging Successfully, 2002; XII: 4.

Neistadt, M. (2000). *Occupational therapy evaluation for adults: A pocket guide.* Philadelphia, PA: Lippincott Williams & Wilkins.

O'Sullivan, S.B., & Schmitz, T.J. (Eds.) (2007). *Physical rehabilitation: Assessment and treatment* (5th ed.; p. 659). Philadelphia: F.A. Davis Company.

Parkinson, S., Forsyth, K., & Kielhofner, G. (2006). Model of Human Occupation Screening Tool (version 2.0). Authors.

Pierson, F. M., & Fairchild, S. L. (2008). *Basic wound care and specialized interventions in principles and techniques of patient care.* St. Louis, MO: W. B. Saunders.

Quintana, L. (2008). Optimizing vision, visual perception, and praxis abilities. In M. V. Radomski & C. T. Latham (Eds.), *Occupational therapy for physical dysfunction* (pp. 728–747). Philadelphia: Lippincott Williams & Wilkins.

Skubik-Peplaski, C., Paris, C., Boyle, D., & Culpert, A. (Eds.). (2008). *Applying the occupational therapy practice framework: Using the Cardinal Hill Occupational Participation Process in Client Centered Care.* Bethesda, MD: AOTA Press.

Uniform Data System (2010). *About the FIM System.* Available online at http://www.udsmr.org/WebModules/FIM/Fim_About.aspx

Wilson, B., et.al (2008). *Rivermeade Behavioral Memory Test* (3rd ed.). Available online at http://www.pearsonassessments.com/HAIWEB/Cultures/enus/Productdetail.htm?Pid=978-074-9134-761&Mode=summary

Appendix 1.A.

Sample Occupational Therapy Evaluation Form

Patient name: _____ Age: _____ Medical record no. _____

Diagnosis: _____ Precautions: _____

Preadmission Status

Living arrangement: Alone   With family   Other: _____

        _____ Level home _____ Step entry (ramp)   Other: _____

Anticipated living arrangement at discharge: _____

Roles: _____ Worker _____ Student _____ Caregiver/parent

        _____ Homemaker/maintainer _____ Leisure participant   Other: _____

Driving: Yes   No

Prior level of function:

ADLs:	D	Max	Mod	Min	CGA	Sup	Mod I	I
Mobility:	D	Max	Mod	Min	CGA	Sup	Mod I	I

Durable medical equipment before admission: _____

Patient perception of occupational needs/goals: _____

Current level of performance:

Areas of Occupation	Level of Performance/Assistance								Factors Affecting Occupational Performance (check all that apply)							
									Mobility	Sensory-motor	Cognitive-perceptual	Commu-nication	Psycho-social	Environ-ment/Context	Other	Other
BADLs																
Feeding	D	Max	Mod	Min	CGA	Sup	Mod I	I								
Grooming	D	Max	Mod	Min	CGA	Sup	Mod I	I								
Dressing UB	D	Max	Mod	Min	CGA	Sup	Mod I	I								
Dressing LB	D	Max	Mod	Min	CGA	Sup	Mod I	I								
Toileting	D	Max	Mod	Min	CGA	Sup	Mod I	I								
IADL	D	Max	Mod	Min	CGA	Sup	Mod I	I								
Work/school	D	Max	Mod	Min	CGA	Sup	Mod I	I								
Leisure/social	D	Max	Mod	Min	CGA	Sup	Mod I	I								

Neuromusculoskeletal performance:

Left Upper Extremity		Right Upper Extremity	Comments
	ROM		
	Shoulder		
	Elbow		
	Wrist		
	Digits		
	Coordination		
	Gross control—Finger to nose		
	Fine control		
	Sensation		
	Light touch		
	Proprioception		
	Stereognosis		
	Strength		
	Gross grasp		
	MMT—Shoulder		
	MMT—Elbow		
	MMT—Grip		
	Tone		
	Edema		

Left Lower Extremity		Right Lower Extremity	Comments
	ROM		
	Hip		
	Knee		
	Ankle		
	Coordination		
	Heel slide		
	Sensation		
	Light touch		
	Proprioception		
	Strength		
	Hip		
	Knee		
	Ankle		
	Tone		
	Edema		

Comments: _____

Mobility:

Rolling right or left	D	Max	Mod	Min	CGA	Sup	Mod I	I
Supine to sit	D	Max	Mod	Min	CGA	Sup	Mod I	I
Sit to stand	D	Max	Mod	Min	CGA	Sup	Mod I	I
Transfer type	D	Max	Mod	Min	CGA	Sup	Mod I	I
Sitting balance	D	Max	Mod	Min	CGA	Sup	Mod I	I
Standing balance	D	Max	Mod	Min	CGA	Sup	Mod I	I
Ambulation or wheelchair propulsion	D	Max	Mod	Min	CGA	Sup	Mod I	I

Comments: _____

Pain: 1   2   3   4   5   6   7   8   9   10

Location: _____   Type:_____   What relieves pain:_____

Skin integrity: Intact   Decubitus: _____   Surgical incision:_____

Vision: Intact   Glasses/contacts   Complains of visual problems

Hearing: Intact   Hard of hearing   Uses hearing aid(s)

Performance skills:

			Comments:
Cognitive			
Alertness/arousal	Intact/WFL	Impaired	
Orientation/memory	Intact/WFL	Impaired	
Problem solving	Intact/WFL	Impaired	
Judgment/insight	Intact/WFL	Impaired	
Executive function	Intact/WFL	Impaired	
Perceptual			
Visual fields (hemianopsia)	Intact/WFL	Impaired	
Body awareness/neglect	Intact/WFL	Impaired	
Visual figure ground	Intact/WFL	Impaired	
Right/left discrimination	Intact/WFL	Impaired	
Praxis/motor planning	Intact/WFL	Impaired	
Communication			
Receptive language	Intact/WFL	Impaired	
Expressive language	Intact/WFL	Impaired	
Writing/reading	Intact/WFL	Impaired	

Assessment:

Strengths	Factors Potentially Impeding Performance
• Prior level of function • Cognition/perception • Social support	• Prior level of function • Psychological state • Cognition/insight • Physiological function • Physical (strength/ROM) • Social support • ADL function • Safety • Communication • Functional mobility

Rehabilitation Potential

Short-term goals (to be accomplished in _____ visits):

Goal	Measure of Attainment	Comments

Long-term goals (to be accomplished in _____ visits):

Goal	Measure of Attainment	Comments

Plan: Patient to be seen for skilled occupational therapy services for the following modalities:

ADL retraining	Functional mobility/transfer training
Strengthening/endurance/ROM	Cognitive/perceptual remediation
Functional balance training	Splinting/adaptive equipment
Patient/caregiver education for safe discharge	Other: _____

Patient/caregiver informed of treatment plan and in agreement with above-stated goals:

Therapist signature: _____   Date: _____

Note. These pages would take the place of the charts on mobility, sensory–motor performance, and cognitive performance, if one were truly using an occupation-based approach to evaluation.

Areas of Occupation	Intact /WFL	Impaired	Comments
ADLs • Bathing • Bowel and bladder • Toilet hygiene • Dressing • Eating • Feeding • Functional mobility • Personal device care • Personal hygiene and grooming			
IADLs • Care of others • Care of pets • Child rearing • Communication management • Community mobility • Financial management • Health management and maintenance • Home establishment and management • Meal preparation and clean up • Religious observance • Safety and emergency maintenance • Shopping			

Areas of Occupation	Intact/WFL	Impaired	Comments
Rest and sleep • Rest • Sleep • Sleep preparation and participation			
Education • Formal educational participation • Informal personal educational needs or interests exploration • Informal personal education participation			
Work • Employment interests and pursuits • Employment seeking and acquisition • Job performance • Retirement preparation and adjustment • Volunteer exploration and participation			
Play • Play exploration and participation			
Leisure • Leisure exploration and participation			

Body functions:

	Intact/WFL	Impaired	Comments
Mental functions Global mental functions • Consciousness • Orientation • Temperament and personality • Energy and drive • Sleep Specific mental functions • Attention • Memory • Perception • Thought			

	Intact/WFL	Impaired	Comments
• Mental functions of sequencing complex movement • Emotional • Experience of self and time • Higher order thinking: judgment, concept formation, metacognition, mental flexibility, insight, attention, and awareness			
Sensory functions and pain Seeing Hearing Vestibular Taste Smell Proprioceptive Tactile/touch Temperature and pressure Pain			
Neuromusculoskeletal function Tone Subluxation Motor control Synergy			
Cardiovascular, hematological, immunological, and respiratory system function			
Voice and speech functions			
Digestive, metabolic, and endocrine system function			
Genitourinary and reproductive functions			
Skin and related-structure functions			

Performance skills:

	Intact/WFL	Impaired	Comments
Motor and praxis			
Planning, sequencing, and executing new and novel movements			
Posture—Stabilizes, aligns, positions			
Mobility—Walks, reaches, bends			
Coordination—coordinates, manipulates, flows			
Strength and effort—Moves, transports, lifts, calibrates, grips			
Energy—Endures, paces			
Sensory–perceptual skills			
Locate, identify, and respond to sensations			
Select, interpret, associate, organize, and remember sensory events			
Discriminating experiences through a variety of sensations			
Emotional regulation skills			
Identify, manage, and express feelings			
Responding			
Persisting			
Controlling			
Recovering			
Displaying emotions			
Using coping strategies			
Cognitive skills			
Judging			
Selecting			
Sequencing			
Organizing			
Prioritizing			
Creating			
Multitasking			
Process			
Energy—Paces, attends			
Knowledge—Chooses, uses, handles, heeds, inquires			

	Intact/WFL	Impaired	Comments
Temporal organization—Initiates, continues, sequences, terminates			
Organizing space and objects—Searches, locates, gathers, organizes, restores, navigates			
Adaptation—Notices, responds, accommodates, benefits			
Communication/interaction			
Physicality—Contacts, gazes, gestures, maneuvers, orients, postures			
Information exchange—Articulates, asserts, asks, engages, expresses, modulates, shares, speaks, sustains			
Relations—Collaborates, conforms, focuses, relates, respects			

Note. ADLs = activities of daily living; BADLs = basic activities of daily living; CGA = contact guard assist; D = dependent (total assist); IADLs = instrumental activities of daily living; LB = lower body; Max = maximum; Mod = moderate assist; Min = minimum assist; Mod I = modified independence (independent, but uses equipment or task modification); MMT = manual muscle testing; ROM = range of motion; Sup = supervision (usually needed for people w/cognitive limitations); UB = upper body; WFL = Within functional limits (although not "normal")

2

The Intensive Care Unit

Kerry Popovich, OT/L

introduction

As the Baby Boomer generation ages and medical technology improves, the number of intensive care unit (ICU) beds required in the near future is expected to increase significantly. The U.S. Department of Health and Human Services (DHHS), in a report to Congress, has predicted that the number and acuity of hospitalized patients requiring ICU-level care will grow rapidly over the next 8 years (Duke, 2006). In 2006, the Society of Critical Care Medicine estimated the number of ICUs in the United States at approximately 6,000, with more than 55,000 patients receiving care daily. They also noted that, although ICU patients "occupy only 10% of the inpatient beds, they account for almost 30% of acute care hospital costs, amounting to $180 billion annually in the United States alone" (Society of Critical Care Medicine, 2006, p. 1).

The reason for the high cost is the intensity of medical care provided. A high ratio of services to patient is required; for example, nursing requirements may range from 2 patients per nurse to as many as 2 (or more) nurses per patient. In addition, increased primary medicine and consultation hours are needed, as well as heightened monitoring of patients, including internal and external monitoring of the heart and brain. Last, increased intervention delivery is needed in the form of ventilators, potent intravenous solutions, medications, and other therapies (see Figure 2.1). The patients being served are in tenuous situations, with a mortality rate of 12%–17% compared with hospital averages of approximately 1.5% (Duke, 2006, p. 19).

In this environment, occupational therapists have the opportunity to contribute to the healing and quality of life of the patients they encounter. However, providing therapy in the ICU requires not only traditional occupational therapy skills but also a clear understanding of the medical issues surrounding the patient's occupational profile. Because of the fragility of the patient's health, therapists need to be properly oriented to the ICU to maintain the patient's and therapist's safety during interventions. Orientation should include developing familiarity with common equipment, medications, and medical issues, as well as cardiopulmonary rehabilitation principles and the role of occupational therapy in the ICU.

An ICU stay can be the most psychologically and physically challenging part of a patient's recovery. Therapists' unique training in psychology, physiology, neurology, and occupational science positions them to be an essential resource for ICU patients and staff. From range of motion (ROM) exercises to activities of daily living (ADLs), a variety of interventions and meaningful activities can be used therapeutically to assist with patients' physical and psychological recovery from a serious illness.

Among the most appealing reasons for working in acute care, and especially in the ICU, are the endless learning opportunities. This chapter provides the fundamental information needed to function safely and effectively as an ICU therapist.

ICU Staff

More than in most other units, ICU staff must function as a team. Therapists who are assigned to treat in this environment will benefit from being aware of the number and types of staff that are involved in running an ICU. Staff common to the ICU are intensivists and other medical doctors, registered nurses (RNs), licensed practical nurses, licensed nurses' aides, respiratory therapists, pharmacists, registered dietitians, physical therapists, occupational therapists, speech therapists, and administrative support staff such as

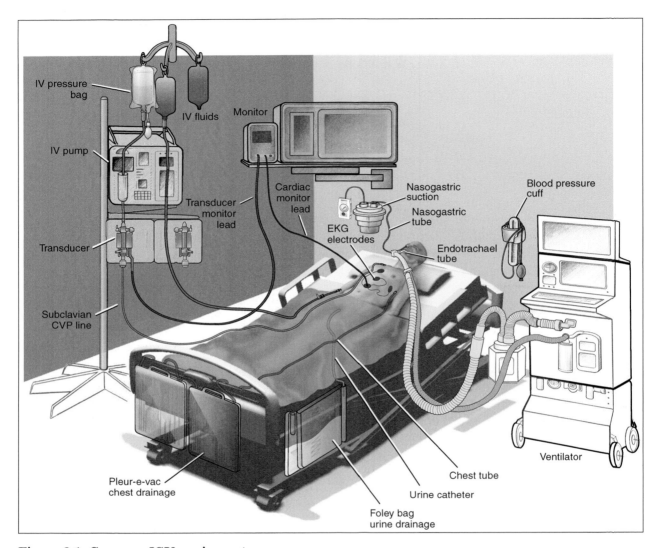

Figure 2.1. Common ICU equipment.
Source. Richard Fritzler, Medical Illustrator Roswell, GA.

unit coordinators. Many ICU clinical staff are required to have extra training and testing to be competent to treat patients in critical care.

Primary Medicine

Critical care became a specialty in the 1980s under the American Board of Medical Specialties, according to the DHHS (Duke, 2006). An *intensivist* is a physician credentialed in critical care medicine and who delivers care primarily in the ICU. He or she may have had primary training in various fields, including internal medicine, anesthesia, surgery, and so forth. Many hospitals nationwide are using intensivists as the primary care doctor in the ICU, meaning they direct all ICU patient care. "Evidence indicates that patient outcomes are improved when intensivists are available around-the-clock for patient consultation" (Duke, 2006, p. 6).

Many hospitals are using *hospitalists*, doctors who specialize in the care of the hospitalized patient. They provide primary care services to some or all of the inpatient population, replacing the need for primary care physicians (PCPs) to round on their patients in the hospital. Depending on the hospital's philosophy on the use of intensivists (as discussed later in this chapter), hospitalists may or may not be directing the care of the ICU patient.

Other hospitals continue to use PCPs to care for patients, following patients from outpatient to inpatient. Similar to hospitalists, they may continue to be the physician directing the patient's care regardless of the ward or unit in which the patient is located. In this case, the PCP is the attending physician in the ICU and will consult specialists, as he or she deems necessary, including a pulmonologist or intensivist (Duke, 2006). In a like manner, patients may be admitted to the hospital with a surgeon or specialist designated as the attending, and these doctors will direct patient care in the ICU. The organization of the ICU's medical staff is further discussed in the ICU Characteristics section.

Nursing

Many *RNs* in the ICU also have critical care specialty certifications. RNs have several options for credentialing in acute or critical care. Among the specialty titles nurses can achieve in the critical care field are *critical care nurse, progressive care nurse, clinical nurse specialist,* and *acute care nurse practitioner in acute and critical care;* subspecialty certifications include cardiac medicine certification and cardiac surgery certification.

Respiratory Therapy

Respiratory therapists have no specific critical care certification. A general advanced credential, registered respiratory therapist, is usually required for supervisory positions and intensive care specialties. However, much of the respiratory therapist's schooling is focused on ventilator management, and many of the respiratory therapists in ICUs today are certified respiratory therapists.

Pharmacy

Pharmacists have multiple options for specialty certification; however, none of the options are specific to intensive care assignments. Clinical pharmacists are often assigned directly to an ICU to improve the speed of providing emergent medications and identifying interactions and contraindications. The clinical pharmacist can also make recommendations for medications expeditiously. The pharmacist can serve as a resource for the therapist if questions arise about a medication's effect on therapeutic intervention.

Nutrition

Dietitians are responsible for managing a patient's nutritional needs. They have several specialty certification options, but none specifically for the ICU. Often, a higher percentage of ICU patients will be placed on supplemental or alternative nutrition such as intravenous total parenteral nutrition or tube feeding.

Physical Therapy

Physical therapists have seven specialty certification options, and of these, the cardiopulmonary clinical specialty is the most helpful in treating ICU patients. However, this certification is not yet common. As of early 2009, 135 physical therapists held cardiopulmonary clinical specialty certification, or 1.6% of all physical therapy clinical specialists practicing in the United States (American Physical Therapy Association, 2009). This certification requires that the therapist have an in-depth knowledge of basic arrhythmias, a certification in advanced cardiac life support, submission of a portfolio including a research project, and a passing grade on the national certification examination.

Occupational Therapy

Specialty clinical certification is a relatively new option for *occupational therapists*. According to the American Occupational Therapy Association (2010), four board certification categories and four specialty certification categories are available. As of September 2010, the total number of certified therapists for all categories was fewer than 150 nationwide.

The most applicable category for occupational therapists treating in the ICU is the board certification in physical rehabilitation, which is a broad category encompassing all levels of care including inpatient and outpatient. It does not ensure that a therapist will be competent for entry-level ICU intervention. The second most applicable category would be the specialty certification in feeding, eating, and swallowing. In the ICU, many patients have *dysphagia*, or difficulty with swallowing. These patients require therapy from either an occupational therapist or a speech–language pathologist to regain this vital function. For more information on dysphagia, see Chapter 13.

Speech Therapy

Speech–language pathologists have one general specialty certification: the Certificate of Clinical Competence that is offered by the American Speech–Language Hearing Association (ASHA). This certification is voluntary and requires that the therapist hold a master's or doctoral degree; have completed a clinical fellowship supervised by a speech–language pathologist certified by ASHA; and have received a passing score on the national exam. Achieving this certification, however, does not indicate that a therapist has had any training in acute care; therapists are able to complete their fellowship in several other settings.

Medical Consultants

Patients in the ICU have varied diagnoses. For each individual's active diagnoses, an equal number of *medical consultants* may be needed. Brief descriptions of the various medical consultants seen in the ICU and their specialty are provided in Table 2.1.

ICU Characteristics

Just as it is valuable to be aware of the staff members who collaborate in the unit, it is also worthwhile to note that not all ICUs are the same. As mentioned earlier, hospitals follow several models regarding the arrangement of medical staff. According to the DHHS report to Congress (Duke, 2006), the three models are open, closed, and comanaged units. In *open units*, patients are admitted to intensive care under an attending physician of record, such as their own PCP or surgeon, who then makes referrals to consultants as needed. In *open units*, the attending physician usually has responsibilities outside of the ICU as well, such as outpatient appointments or other inpatient units. *Closed units* are those in which intensivists are the primary doctors and the patient's own PCP may or may not be invited to be involved in the decision-making process. *Comanaged units* are a blend of care from both the PCP and the intensivist.

The professional literature is beginning to demonstrate that outcomes are improved and costs are kept down when the ICU is managed solely by intensivists. For this reason and because of pressure from payers, many hospitals have begun transitioning to this closed model (Duke, 2006).

A multidisciplinary task force under the direction of the American College of Critical Care Medicine described significant differences in ICUs from hospital to hospital (Haupt et al., 2003). They ascribed these differences to multiple factors such as the population the hospital serves, the internal and external dynamics in the hospital's political and economic environment, and the services and specialties available at the hospital and at its neighboring hospitals. Large centers have multiple ICUs organized according to a specialty or subspecialty practice, acuity, prognosis, or age. Small facilities generally have one ICU in which all populations are cared for, including pediatrics (Haupt et al., 2003).

The wide variety of ICU staffing and organization styles indicates that occupational therapy practice in the ICU can look different from hospital to hospital. For example, a patient who is in a step-down unit for observation in a larger hospital may be admitted to the ICU in a smaller hospital for the same condition to provide that patient with the most appropriate level of care. In the smaller or more rural hospitals, occupational therapists will likely find a larger range of acuity present. Occupational therapy practice could vary significantly, from treating a walking and talking patient with a myocardial infarct to the chronically critically ill patient dependent on a ventilator who is unable to sit up unsupported. The remainder of this chapter focuses on the higher acuity patient. For information regarding the treatment of the lower acuity patient (who, e.g., requires telemetry and observation), please

Table 2.1. **Medical Consultants and Their Specialties**

Consultant	Specialty
Anesthesiologist	Sedation and pain management.
Cardiologist	The heart, with a focus on medical management. Interventional cardiologists perform heart catheterizations.
Cardiovascular surgeon	Surgical management of the heart and large vessels.
Gastroenterologist	Medical management of the gastrointestinal system: stomach, intestines, colon, rectum, pancreas, liver, and gallbladder. Common interventions or procedures performed include endoscopy of the gastrointestinal tract and placement of feeding tubes.
General surgeon or trauma surgeon	Emergency surgery, abdominal surgery, breast surgery, skin or wound surgery, and some vascular surgery. May also place feeding tubes.
Hematologist or oncologist	Blood disorders and cancer.
Infectious disease specialist	Infectious diseases.
Interventional radiologist	Diagnostics, fluoroscopically guided procedures, angiograms, placement of peripherally inserted central catheter or central lines.
Nephrologist	The kidneys and overall renal function.
Neurologist	The central and peripheral nervous systems: brain, spinal cord, and peripheral nerves.
Neurosurgeon	Brain and spinal surgery.
Obstetric–gynecologic surgeon	The surgical management of conditions related to the female sex organs.
Orthopedic surgeon	The musculoskeletal system: bones, joints, ligaments, tendons, muscles, and nerves.
Otolaryngologist (ear, nose, and throat specialist)	Medical and surgical management of head and neck: mouth, ears, nose, throat, and face. Interventions include tracheotomy and repair of trauma to head and neck.
Pathologist	Specialist in diagnostic medicine related to body tissues and fluids.
Pulmonologist	Medical management of the lungs. Interventions include chest tube placement, biopsy, bronchoscopy, and tracheostomy.
Thoracic surgeon	Surgical management of the chest other than the heart.
Urologist	The medical management of the urinary system and male reproductive organs. Interventions include removal of stones in the urinary tract, cystoscopies, and urinary catheter placement.

(continued)

Table 2.1.   (continued)

Consultant	Specialty
Vascular surgeon	Medical and surgical management of peripheral veins and arteries. Interventions include reestablishing blood flow to extremities, for example, femoral–popliteal bypass graft or dialysis catheter placement.

Table 2.2.   Basic Vital Signs

Vital Sign	Normal	Abnormal Ranges
Heart rate	60–100 beats per minute	*Bradycardia:* <60 *Tachycardia:* >100
Blood pressure	*Systolic:* 90–120 mm Hg *Diastolic:* 60–80 mm Hg	*Hypotension:* <90 systolic *Prehypertension:* 120–140/80–89 *Stage 1 hypertension:* 140–159/90–99 *Stage 2 hypertension:* ≥160/≥100
Mean arterial pressure	70–110 mm Hg	
Pulse oximeter oxygen saturation	Percentage of hemoglobin that is bound to another molecule such as oxygen or carbon monoxide	95%–100%
Respiratory rate	12–20 breaths per minute	

Sources. Chobanian (2003); National Heart, Lung, and Blood Institute (2008).

refer to the chapter that best fits the primary admitting diagnosis.

Common Diagnoses

According to the Society of Critical Care Medicine (2006), the top 5 admitting diagnoses are (1) respiratory insufficiency or failure, (2) postoperative management, (3) cardiac ischemia, (4) sepsis, and (5) heart failure. Other common primary diagnoses include gastrointestinal hemorrhage, multiple organ system failure, and shock.

Pulmonary Conditions

As the leading cause for admission into an ICU, respiratory insufficiency fits under the larger umbrella of pulmonary conditions. Therefore, this group of illnesses is arguably the first a therapist should study in preparation for treating patients in intensive care. Familiarity with the mechanisms of disease will assist in the development of appropriate interventions and awareness of precautions related to treatment of these patients. For thorough review of the pulmonary system and common associated illnesses, refer to Chapter 5.

Pulmonary gas exchange is the process of taking in oxygen and releasing carbon dioxide (CO_2). The balance between ventilation and capillary perfusion, commonly referred to as the *V/Q ratio*, is delicate. *Ventilation* can be simply defined as air flow in and out of the lungs. *Capillary perfusion* refers to blood flow in the capillaries surrounding the alveoli in the lungs. In normal respiration, the lungs inflate during inspiration and the alveoli fill with room air, or 20.95% oxygen (Williams, 2009). Blood in the capillaries surrounding the alveoli collect the oxygen and deposit CO_2. On expiration, CO_2-saturated air leaves the alveoli and lungs. In normal pulmonary gas exchange, oxygen and carbon dioxide are balanced in the blood. Refer to the "Clinical Monitoring" section of this chapter for further details on monitoring pulmonary status (see Table 2.3).

Acute respiratory distress syndrome (ARDS) most often occurs 24–72 hours after the onset of a catastrophic illness or injury (Sommers, Johnson, & Beery, 2006). The original illness or injury the patient suffered may or may not have required intubation, but almost 100% of patients who develop ARDS will need life support. According to Sommers et al. (2006), mortality rates are estimated to be between 40% and 50%, although elderly patients and patients with severe infections can have rates higher than this. Sommers et al. also stated that, in general, survivors have near-normal lung function 1 year later.

Herridge et al. (2003) reported that outcomes 1 year later have shown patients continuing to demonstrate muscle weakness. They attributed this muscle weakness to one of several types of myopathy or neuropathy, including critical illness polyneuropathy, which is discussed later in this chapter. For more detailed information on ARDS, refer to Chapter 5.

For the purposes of caring for the ICU patient with ARDS, therapy services are initially limited because of the fragility of the patient's pulmonary status. The medical team can have difficulty with providing effective ventilation because of poor lung compliance. To enhance the patient's ventilatory status, he or she may also require sedation or paralysis for an extended period of time. Initial therapy services would be limited to providing passive range of motion (PROM) in this case.

Once patients are able to participate in interventions, they will follow a course of treatment similar to that outlined at the end of this chapter. Treatment should also include ongoing assessment of cognition, because approximately 45% of ARDS survivors demonstrate neurocognitive deficits 1 year later (Hopkins et al., 2005).

Table 2.3. **Arterial Blood Gases**

Arterial Blood Gases	Measures	Normal Range
PaO_2: Partial pressure of oxygen	Pressure of O_2 dissolved in blood; determines how well O_2 can move from the lungs into the blood	80–95 mm Hg
$PaCO_2$: Partial pressure of carbon dioxide	Amount of CO_2 dissolved in blood and how well CO_2 is able to move out of the body	35–45 mm Hg High $PaCO_2$ (hypercapnia) causes acidosis
pH	Hydrogen ions (H+) in blood	7.35–7.45 <7.35 = acidosis >7.45 = alkalosis
HCO_3: Bicarbonate	HCO_3 keeps blood pH from becoming too acidic	18–23 mEq/L >23 mEq/L is an indicator of CO_2 retention
SaO_2: Oxygen saturation	Percentage of hemoglobin carrying O_2	95%–99%

Source. Leeuwen, Kranpitz, and Smith (2006). Adapted with permission.

Unfortunately, cognitive assessment of survivors has not been consistent. According to Hopkins et al. (2005), after leaving the ICU, 42% received rehabilitation services, but only 12% were identified as having impairment and received cognitive therapy services. Two years later, the group's cognitive performance had not improved, based on longitudinal outcome studies.

Cardiac Conditions

If developing familiarity with the pulmonary system is the place to start in becoming comfortable with treating in the ICU, knowledge of the cardiac system is a close second. Because of ICU patients' tenuous medical status, cardiac performance is closely monitored. All patients are admitted on telemetry, and cardiac enzymes are frequently checked. Chances are that most patients will take one or more cardiac medications during their stay in ICU. For a more in-depth review of the cardiovascular system's anatomy and function, refer to Chapter 3. A better understanding of the physiology of a patient's heart condition leads to more appropriate goal setting and therapeutic interventions in an ICU setting.

Postoperative Management

Patients are sometimes admitted to the ICU after surgery when unexpected complications occur or as a precautionary measure because of a history of significant cardiac or respiratory disorder. As with most ICU admissions, patients often have hemodynamic instability, respiratory distress, or neurological changes. They may require extended time on ventilators, intense monitoring, or treatments that are more demanding. Precautions for therapy are similar to those for all ICU patients, with the addition of the standard precautions for the type of surgical procedure they have undergone. Check the orders carefully for special precautions related to the particular surgery. Precautions may also be related to the reason for ICU admission. Always ask for clarification from the surgeon if any concerns or questions about activity orders arise. The nursing staff may infrequently care for patients with certain postoperative diagnoses such as total hip or knee replacements. They may want review of precautions specific to the surgical repair. Consider posting a sign with the precautions clearly delineated so that all shifts and staff will be kept up to date.

Sepsis

Sepsis is frequently a life-threatening condition compromising cardiopulmonary status, and it can cause multiorgan system failure and death. Mortality rates are from 20%–50% in severe cases, and it is the 10th leading cause of death in the United States (Martin, Mannino, Eaton, & Moss, 2003). Sepsis can cause confusion, significant muscle weakness, and endurance loss in a short period of time. See Chapter 12 for more information.

Neurologic Conditions

Many neurologic conditions may necessitate an ICU stay. These conditions may include traumatic brain injury (TBI), cerebrovascular accidents (CVAs), spinal cord injuries, and other diagnoses requiring neurosurgery. For details on these and other neurological conditions, refer to Chapter 6. Check with the neurologist or neurosurgeon for precautions before working with these patients.

Doctors' orders may include restrictions for head-of-bed angle, intracranial pressure parameters, blood pressure parameters, or activity orders or the need for thromboembolic deterrent (compression) stockings or an abdominal binder when getting out of bed. Primarily in the initial ICU phase, the goal is to stabilize the neurological injury and prevent further secondary injuries. Secondary injuries often come as the result of lack of perfusion, edema, or seizures.

Potential reasons for precautions may include

- *High risk for aspiration:* Keep the head of the bed at 30° or more except for brief changes to assist with scooting up in bed, unless otherwise ordered. Make sure feeding tubes are disconnected or put on hold if bed will be lowered to a flat position.

- *Risk for vasospasm:* A *vasospasm* occurs in the muscles of the cerebral blood vessel walls, causing narrowing of the vessels. It can result in ischemia because of decreased blood flow, or *hypoperfusion*. Vasospasm usually occurs within 3–4 days after a subarachnoid bleed; symptoms can include increasing confusion and decreasing arousal, which may progress to focal neurological deficits, stroke, coma, and death (Murthy, Bhatia, & Prabhakar, 2005). The treatment may include "triple-H therapy," which consists of increasing blood volume (*hypervolemia*), increasing blood pressure (*hypertension*), and dilating the blood vessels (*hemodilation*) to improve perfusion in the areas of vasospasm (Rahimi, Brown, Macomson, Jensen, & Alleyne, 2006). Therefore, if the therapist notes that a doctor has ordered a patient's blood pressure to stay within elevated parameters, a concern for hypoperfusion is likely. Therapists should be aware of the parameters and be cautious in changing the patient's position. An increase in orthostatic stress may result in a drop in blood pressure, compromising blood flow to brain tissue.

- *Risk for seizure:* In TBI, "risk factors include the following: Glasgow Coma Score (GCS) of less than 10 (Teasdale, G., & Jennett, B., 1974), cortical contusion, depressed skull fracture, subdural hematoma (SDH), epidural hematoma, intracerebral hematoma, penetrating head wound or seizure within 24 hrs of injury" (Brain Trauma Foundation, American Association of Neurological Surgeons [AANS], Congress of Neurological Surgeons [CNS], & AANS/CNS Joint Section on Neurotrauma and Critical Care, 2007, p. S83). After stroke, the risk for seizure within 24 hours is 2%–23%, according to the American Heart Association's *Guidelines for the Early Management of Adults With Ischemic Stroke* (American Heart Association [AHA]/American Stroke Association [ASA] Stroke Council, Clinical Cardiology Council, Cardiovascular Radiology and Intervention Council,

& Atherosclerotic Peripheral Vascular Disease and Quality of Care Outcomes in Research Interdisciplinary Working Groups, 2007). Therefore, therapists should be aware that a seizure may occur and be prepared to transfer the patient to a safe location, such as supine in bed. If a patient does appear to be seizing, notify the nurse immediately. See Chapter 6 for more information about seizure.

- *High risk for secondary injury as a result of decreased cerebral perfusion and hypoxemia in TBI:* Hypotension (systolic blood pressure <90 millimeters of mercury [mm Hg]) and hypoxemia (oxygen saturation [SaO$_2$] <90% or partial pressure of oxygen [PaO$_2$] <60 mm Hg) should be avoided because of the high risk for secondary neurological insults after TBI (Brain Trauma Foundation et al., 2007). One incident of hypotension during the acute phase after TBI has been found to result in increased morbidity and a doubled mortality (Brain Trauma Foundation et al., 2007). Therefore, monitor vitals closely, check orthostatic blood pressures during interventions, and verify activity orders before changing a patient's vertical position.

- *Risk for extension of CVA or conversion from ischemic to hemorrhagic CVA:* Five percent to 33% of all ischemic strokes convert to hemorrhagic strokes, but not all hemorrhages are large enough to cause symptoms (AHA/ASA Stroke Council et al., 2007). Therapists need to be alert to potential deterioration of a patient's neurological status and report the changes promptly to the nurse and attending doctor. Hypertension is theoretically a risk factor for conversion and extension of strokes. However, managing hypertension in a person with an acute stroke is done cautiously. Doctors will address high blood pressure gradually and may accept much higher numbers in acute stroke patients than in a general medical patient because of the risk for neurological decline with fluctuations of more than 20 mm Hg (AHA/ASA Stroke Council et al.,

2007). Check orders or ask the doctor or nurse for guidance with blood pressure parameters during treatment.

General neurologic conditions are reviewed in Chapter 6, with the exception of a unique set of neuromuscular disorders that are acquired only in the ICU.

Critical Illness–Acquired Neuromuscular Dysfunction

Neuromuscular dysfunction (NMD) after critical illness has been documented in patients since the late 1970s (Khan, Harrison, & Rich, 2008). Several names have been given to NMD syndromes, such as acquired muscle dysfunction, acute quadriplegic myopathy, thick filament myopathy, acute axonal polyneuropathy, and acute necrotizing myopathy of intensive care (Bercker et al., 2005; Hund, 1999; Khan et al., 2008). Each name is based on a different combination of characteristics involving either muscle or nerve degeneration or both. Khan et al. (2008) divided NMD into two categories: *critical illness myopathy* and *critical illness polyneuropathy.*

Research to improve understanding of the etiology and biochemical mechanisms involved in developing NMD is ongoing, but several risk factors have been identified (Pastores, 2005; Winkelman, 2004). Inactivity and inflammation, use of high-dose corticosteroids, use of neuromuscular blocking agents, renal replacement therapy, hyperglycemia (elevated blood glucose), severe sepsis, multiple organ dysfunction, and elevated acute physiology and chronic health evaluation scores have been linked to the development of NMD (Bercker et al., 2005; Khan et al., 2008; Pastores, 2005; Winkelman, 2004, 2007).

If a patient is still having difficulty weaning from the ventilator after resolution of the condition that initiated its use, it would be reasonable to suspect that they have acquired NMD. Khan et al. (2008) distinguished polyneuropathy from myopathy with a few simple bedside tests (see Table 2.4). Findings in the bedside examination indicating NMD may prompt more formal testing. Electrophysiologic testing and muscle biopsy have, as yet, been the most reliable means of diagnosing and differentiating between the conditions (Bercker et al., 2005; Khan et al., 2008). Fletcher et al. (2003) have found that survivors of extended critical illness commonly experience severe weakness requiring extensive rehabilitation. Up until 5 years after the critical illness episode, patients have a 90% chance of still having neurophysiologic evidence of denervation typical of prior critical illness polyneuropathy (Fletcher et al., 2003).

Table 2.4. **Critical Illness Neuromuscular Disorder Bedside Assessment**

Symptom	Neuropathy	Myopathy
Gross strength	Absent or reduced	Absent or reduced
Spontaneous movement	Reduced	Reduced
Cranial nerves	Intact	Intact
Muscle stretch reflexes	Intact	Absent
Sensation in distal extremities	Absent or reduced	Intact

Source. Khan et al. (2008).

ICU Psychosis and Delirium

ICU patients who are mechanically ventilated have an elevated risk for developing delirium (Ely et al., 2001, 2004; Pustavoitau & Stevens, 2008). "Delirium due to a general medical condition" is a diagnosis defined by the *Diagnostic and Statistical Manual of Mental Disorders* (4th ed., text rev.; American Psychiatric Association [APA], 2000). Diagnostic criteria include a disturbance of consciousness (awareness of environment), change in cognition (memory, disorientation, and language deficit), and acute development with fluctuation during the course of the day (APA, 2000). Many risk factors for developing delirium have been identified, such as preexisting cognitive impairment, advanced age, mechanical ventilation, untreated pain, prolonged immobilization, sleep deprivation, multisystem illness, sepsis, pharmacology, hypoxemia, hypotension, possible metabolic or neurotransmitter dysfunction, and elevated inflammatory response (Ely et al., 2001, 2004; Pustavoitau & Stevens, 2008).

Altered cognition has been observed to result in difficulty with weaning from the ventilator, developing pneumonia, increased length of stay, need for extended rehabilitation, and mortality (Ely et al., 2001). Long-term cognitive impairment has also been associated with delirium experienced during critical illness (Landro, 2007). In fact, Pustavoitau and Stevens (2008) estimated that 30%–80% of survivors of critical illness may be affected by long-term cognitive impairment.

Delirium often goes unidentified in an estimated 50% of patients with the "quiet" subtype of delirium in which patients are alert with a flat affect and calm disposition without any outward behavioral changes (Ely et al., 2004). Research is ongoing regarding how to better identify delirium in mechanically ventilated patients and possible strategies for managing and treating delirium. Occupational therapists can play an integral part in identifying patients with delirium using both standardized and nonstandardized cognitive assessment tools. However, because the topic of ICU-related delirium and its long-term effects is in the early stages of research, attending physicians may express varying levels of interest when an occupational therapist identifies a patient's altered cognitive status. Occupational therapists are recommended to continue with standard reorientation and cognition-based interventions until further evidence is gathered for best practice in treatment of the condition.

Common ICU Equipment

Orientation to ICU-specific equipment is essential. Nurses and other therapists who have been oriented can provide any instruction necessary. Ask the nurse's permission before disconnecting any patient lines or equipment. Before leaving a patient's room after treatment, check that all equipment has been returned to its original setup and everything is reconnected. When reconnecting, be sure lines and tubes have been correctly matched; if unsure, ask the nurse for help.

Ventilators

Of ICU patients, 85%–90% will require mechanical ventilation. Most of these patients will require mechanical ventilation only briefly. *Weaning* is the process of transitioning patients off of the machine. When the reason the patient needed mechanical ventilation has been resolved, most patients wean fairly easily. However, 20%–30% need a more extended time frame to wean (Vassilakopoulos, Roussos, & Zakynthinos, 1999). *Reintubation,* or reinsertion of the endotracheal tube after its removal, is associated with a 30%–40% increase in mortality (Bruton & McPherson, 2004). Table 2.5 contains information about basic ventilator settings and therapeutic implications.

Patients will be connected to the ventilator via tubing that enters the airway in one of three ways, through the mouth, nose, or throat (endotracheal intubation); nasotracheal intubation; or tracheostomy. *Endotracheal intubation* is the most commonly used airway access (see Figure 2.2). *Nasotracheal intubation* is used in cases of jaw, neck, mouth, or facial trauma that preclude use of the mouth for access to the airway. *Tracheostomy* is most often initiated for extended ventilator weaning (see Figure 2.3). Please see the "Tracheostomies" section for more details.

Table 2.5. **Ventilator Settings**

Setting	Type of Support	Description	Therapeutic Implications
Volume control	Total assist.	A preset amount of air is delivered for inflation. Used in modified forms in most other vent settings.	The patient is sedated and most likely paralyzed. Limit activity to gentle passive range of motion.
Pressure control	Total assist.	Air is delivered until a preset amount of air pressure is reached in the lungs.	See above.
Assist-control	Partial assist; often used with patients who are sedated.	Volume cycled (preselected inflation volume) with a preset number of breaths. Patient can initiate each mechanical breath. Does not allow spontaneous unassisted breathing between mechanical breaths.	Minimal work of breathing. Can cause anxiety in patients who are not in synch with the ventilator and fight the control (sometimes called "bucking the vent"). If able to participate, the patient can become short of breath during exercises or activities. Because the rate of breathing is preset, the patient will be unable to increase his or her own respiratory rate to compensate. Watch for signs of increased anxiety and monitor vital signs.
Synchronized intermittent mandatory ventilation	Weaning mode.	Volume cycled with a preset number of breaths. Allows spontaneous unassisted breathing between mechanical breaths. Used as exercise during weaning.	Increased work of breathing. Easy for patients to have respiratory muscle fatigue. Schedule therapy after weaning trials to avoid overtiring the patient because weaning is the priority during this phase.
Pressure support	Weaning mode. Spontaneous breathing required.	The minimum setting only compensates for the resistance of the ventilator tubing. Increased pressure may be provided to decrease the work of breathing.	Increased work of breathing. Schedule therapy carefully during this time because it is more important for the patient to pass the weaning trial. However, the medical team may want to evaluate the patient's ability to perform activity on a lesser vent setting.
Positive end expiratory pressure	Varies. Can be increased or decreased as needed.	Provides a constant amount of baseline positive airway pressure (e.g., 5-cm H_2O) that is maintained even at the end of expiration.	Assists with keeping alveoli open to minimize atelectasis (collapse).

Source. Marino (1998, Chaps. 26 and 27).

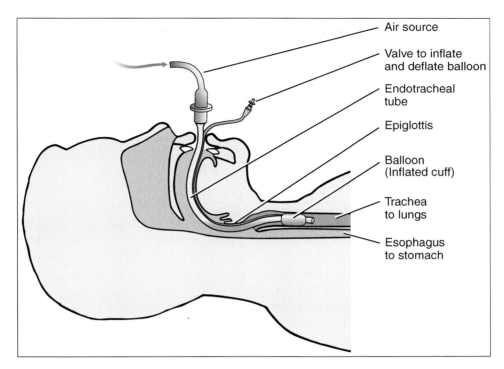

Figure 2.2. Airway with endotracheal tube.
Source. Ritchard Fritzler, Medical Illustrator, Roswell, GA.

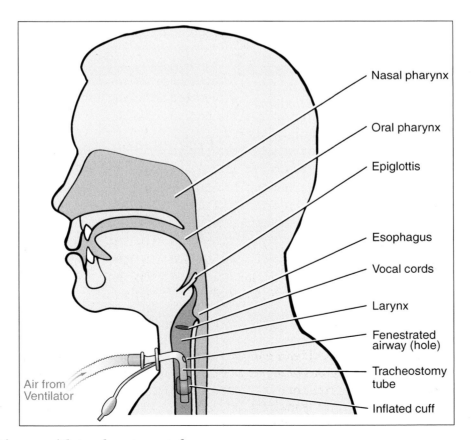

Figure 2.3. Airway with tracheostomy tube.
Source. Ritchard Fritzler, Medical Illustrator, Roswell, GA.

Translaryngeal tubes (endotracheal or nasotracheal) are measured to a specific depth. The tubing has hash marks with numbers indicating the distance in centimeters until the end of the tubing. The tubing should neither go into or out of the body further. Take note of the position of the tubing and the measurement at the lips or nostrils before beginning the treatment. Keep an eye on the tubing during transfers and functional mobility to prevent changes in depth. Often, assigning one person to be responsible for maintaining the position of the tubing during transfers is best.

Beginning to treat patients who require ventilators can be daunting. In truth, an intubated patient who is referred to therapy does require the ventilator to help him or her breathe. Therapists are responsible for preserving the patient's airway during treatment. Bring in the nurse or respiratory therapist for support during initial interventions. Gradually reduce the time the other staff are present as confidence increases. Always ask for help or the stand-by presence of other staff if a question of maintaining the patient's safety arises.

It is worth mentioning that ventilator tubing will inevitably become disconnected. It actually can come disconnected frequently throughout the day depending on how active the patient is. Disconnection is very different from extubation. The patient remains intubated with the translaryngeal tubing in place, but somewhere between the end of that tubing and the ventilator (refer to tubing as illustrated in Figure 2.1), a disconnect occurs, followed by hissing noises, and the ventilator will sound a distinct alarm. Do not panic; the nurse or other staff has enough time to immediately walk to the room and fix the disconnection without detriment to the patient. If the tubing disconnects during a treatment session, reconnect it and continue with the treatment, or call the nurse for help.

If any concern that the tubing became soiled and should be sterilized arises, two options are possible: Either sterilize the tubing quickly (within about 60 seconds) and reconnect it, or wipe it off as best as can be done at the time and reconnect. In both cases, alert the respiratory therapist or nurse so that the tubing can be changed if necessary.

In the event that a patient accidentally becomes extubated during the treatment session, the following procedure is recommended: prepare, prevent, and follow a plan. Prepare for such an occasion by being familiar with the ambu bag's location in the room and have a plan of action in mind. Prevent such occasions by not underestimating the patient's determination to remove the object that is causing them such anxiety and irritation. A patient who has been temporarily released from an arm restraint to participate in a therapeutic activity can be faster than expected at reaching for the endotracheal tube. A recommended plan of action to take if the patient succeeds in self-extubation follows:

- While calling for the nurse, place the patient in a safe position supine in the bed or chair;
- While maintaining the patient's physical safety, retrieve the ambu bag;
- Begin providing respirations to the patient; and
- Attach the ambu bag to oxygen.

Use of an ambu bag is covered in any cardiopulmonary resuscitation course for the health care provider. By the time the therapist retrieves the ambu bag, many staff will most likely have arrived in the room and will take over the process of stabilizing and assessing the patient.

Tracheostomies

A *tracheostomy* is a surgically created artificial airway in the cervical trachea (refer to Figure 2.3). *Tracheotomy* is the name of the surgical procedure used to create the stoma or opening. The two terms are often used interchangeably, however.

Tracheostomies are commonly placed for several reasons. The most common reason is the patient's difficulty weaning from a ventilator (Lindman, Morgan, & Dixon, 2008). Tracheostomies may secondarily be placed for reasons of trauma or catastrophic neurological events. Least common, tracheostomies are sometimes used when treating cancer or infectious disease (Lindman et al., 2008).

During the procedure, the trachea is cut, and the stoma (opening) is secured with stitches.

The outer cannula is then either stitched or taped in place. The outer cannula consists of a tube, which holds the stoma open, the cuff, and the flange (see Figure 2.4). The distal end of the outer cannula tube has the inflatable cuff around it. When inflated, the cuff creates a barrier in the trachea, preventing oral secretions from penetrating the lungs and air from escaping into the larynx. The inflated cuff, sealing the airway, makes the use of pressure ventilation settings possible (refer to Table 2.5). When the cuff is deflated, air can pass up through the larynx and vocal cords, enabling vocalizations and creating increased work of breathing. Secretions can pass around the cuff as well, requiring the patient to manage his or her own saliva and phlegm with swallowing or coughing. A deflated cuff presents a higher risk for aspiration as a result.

The flange, or neck plate, is a small flat piece of plastic that attaches on either side to the proximal outer cannula tube. The outside edges of the flange have holes used to attach cloth or hook-and-loop straps around the neck to help hold the outer cannula in place. The outer cannula with flange provides a secure airway and platform for inserting the inner cannula, which connects to the ventilator tubing.

The inner cannula is a plastic tube a few inches long with a curve at one end. It is inserted through the outer cannula and secured onto it with a built-in clip to prevent it from being coughed out. The inner cannula can easily be removed for cleaning. The inner and outer cannulae can be either solid or fenestrated (having slits in the caudal surface of the tube). When both are fenestrated, some air is able to escape up through the larynx, past the vocal cords, and out the mouth or nose. Similar to deflating the cuff, but on a smaller scale, this fenestration enables more normal secretion management and makes vocalizations possible, but it can increase the work of breathing and risk of aspiration.

Each doctor and each hospital may have different preferences and policies regarding when to use a tracheostomy after a period of prolonged intubation. It eventually becomes necessary and beneficial to change from a translaryngeal tube to a tracheostomy. "The benefits commonly ascribed to tracheotomy, compared to prolonged translaryngeal intubation, include improved patient comfort, more effective airway suctioning, decreased airway resistance, enhanced patient mobility, increased opportunities for articulated speech, ability to eat orally, and a more secure airway" (MacIntyre et al., 2001, p. 11).

When patients have difficulty weaning from the ventilator, a tracheostomy provides increased safety and control. Weaning from the ventilator with a tracheostomy in place makes it possible to have daily trial periods off of ventilator support. These trial periods are often called "trach collar trials" because of the collar-type oxygen

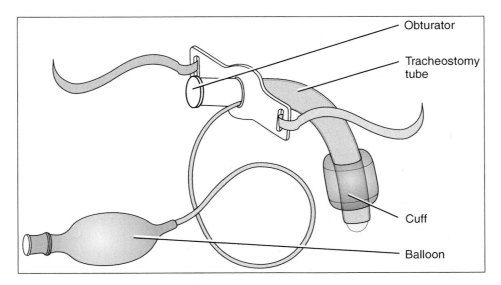

Figure 2.4. Cuffed tracheostomy tube.
Source. Ritchard Fritzler, Medical Illustrator, Roswell, GA.

mask placed in front of the tracheostomy during this phase of weaning. The airway stays protected during the trial because the cannulae in the tracheostomy stay in place; only the ventilator tubing is disconnected. When patients begin trach collar trials, they may initially only tolerate a few minutes. Respiratory therapists will put patients back on the ventilator if they show signs of respiratory fatigue: respiratory rate of more than 30 breaths/minute, use of accessory muscles, or complaints of respiratory distress (Herlihy, Koch, Jackson, & Nora, 2006).

The weaning process takes priority when a patient requires mechanical ventilation. Therapy interventions should be scheduled after trach collar trials, allowing time for the patient to rest after the trial if necessary. Collaborate with the respiratory therapist and nurse to plan a good time for therapy. However, as the patient improves, the medical team may want to try combining trach collar trials with therapy as an increased challenge for the patient.

Oral Suctioning and Yankauer

Most patients will have a *yankauer* at their bedside—a tapered hard plastic tube about 8–10 inches long and with the circumference of pen or marker. A yankauer is used for suctioning excess oral secretions, and it can be a high infection risk if not properly used, cared for, or replaced regularly. Some yankauers come with a sheath that can be slid over the whole tube to keep it clean when not in use. Patients and family members can be taught how to use the yankauer independently if they are comfortable and able to follow infection control precautions.

Precautions are simple: Prevent the yankauer from falling on the floor or into other excretions or waste; follow standard hospital procedures for either cleaning the instrument or acquiring a new one should it become soiled or unusable; and if hospital policy permits use of the yankauer with tracheostomy secretions, do not use the yankauer at the rim of or inside the cannula because of a significantly greater risk of infection at the tracheostomy site and in the lungs. The strength of the suction should already be set by nursing, but if the instrument

is securely attaching itself to the inside of the patient's mouth, check with the nurse for readjustment of the suction settings.

Temperature-Monitoring Devices

Temperature is most commonly monitored via a port on the Foley catheter. Have the nurse provide instruction in how to disconnect and reconnect the temperature line. It is generally not necessary to keep the temperature line connected during a therapy treatment. Reconnect it when the treatment has concluded.

Temporary Pacemaker

Patients commonly have temporary pacemakers after heart surgery. As with any pacemaker, it is used to assist with keeping the heart rate stable. Some patients have a pacemaker attached just in case their heart rate dips below a preset level. Others rely on the pacemaker to initiate every heartbeat.

The pacemaker box itself will be locked; the settings cannot be accidentally changed if a button is pressed by mistake. The electrical leads that attach to the pacemaker are snapped in place; they will only be dislodged by a good pull. However, the point at which the leads enter the body is usually not as secure. The leads will most likely be held in place with tape. The only precaution, therefore, is not to pull on the pacemaker leads. Patients may transfer to a step-down unit with a temporary pacemaker, so it should not be a reason to defer therapy.

ICU Hospital Beds

Beds can be used as a therapeutic tool in the ICU. When encountering an unfamiliar bed, as with anything else in the ICU, ask for help from nursing. Table 2.6 lists types of beds and their therapeutic uses and precautions.

Always remember to return the bed to its intended settings when treatment is finished. For example, if you notice when entering a room that a pulmonary rotation bed is not

Table 2.6. **Hospital Bed Features**

Features	Therapeutic Uses and Settings	Precautions
Air overlay or air mattress	Skin integrity maintenance and healing. Controls are often located at the foot of the bed. Bed can be deflated for cardiopulmonary resuscitation or mobilizing. Using the cardiopulmonary resuscitation setting will deflate the mattress and lower the head of the bed the fastest. For a slower deflation, the pump can usually be turned off, which will allow for a slow leak of air out of the mattress.	*Fall risk*: It is often much easier to transfer a patient from supine to sitting with the bed inflated because the surface provides less friction. However, if the bed is inflated while the patient is sitting at the edge, there is a risk of sliding off the edge or loss of balance. Recommend deflating mattress as soon as possible if patient can tolerate sitting on the hard surface under the air overlay. *Skin breakdown*: The air pressure may be set specifically for the patient; if the therapist changes it, there may be too much or too little support and an increased risk for skin breakdown.
Rotation and percussion	Improve or manage respiratory status. These beds might also have the "turn assist" feature. It uses the bed's rotation ability for the caregiver's benefit when log rolling a patient in bed.	Remember to restart the rotation after treatment.
"Chair position"	Many intensive care unit beds can be moved into chair position, with the head of the bed set almost upright and the legs in a dependent position. This position allows for an intermediate treatment situation when progressing a patient's activity tolerance toward sitting at the edge of the bed. Some beds also allow a patient to stand up from the chair position. These beds are often beneficial for obese patients.	Hemodynamic stability can be compromised with any change in vertical position. Check for orthostasis. Consider using an abdominal binder or compression stockings for patients with poor lower-extremity circulation or low–absent lower-extremity/trunk muscle tone. *Fall risk:* A patient who is short in stature or severely debilitated may be unable to reach to sit back down from this position. The seat is typically high and deep with a >90° angle at the knee position. A patient's feet end up more than a few inches forward of the seat, which can be dangerous when each inch counts. Consider recommending that the nursing staff place the patient's bed in the chair position several times per day as tolerated

(continued)

Table 2.6. (continued)

Features	Therapeutic Uses and Settings	Precautions
Trendelenburg	A position in which the foot of the bed is placed higher than the head of the bed. It is used for shock or in acute cases of hypotension to promote increased blood flow to the organs and brain and in certain surgical procedures as well. When not contraindicated, it can be used to assist with boosting patients up in bed.	Causes difficulty with breathing, increased intracranial pressure, and risk of regurgitation and aspiration. Turn off the tube feed before putting the bed in trendelenburg. This positioning can also be added to the chair position to allow for a more reclined position.
30°	Although not a "feature," keeping the head of the bed at 30° is an important therapeutic tool. It has been shown to decrease regurgitation, aspiration, and ventilator-associated pneumonia. It is not only beneficial for intensive care unit patients but also for patients on a tube feed or with swallow precautions.	Verify that there are no restrictions for head-of-bed angle, for example, in the case of new neurological events.

rotating, check with the nurse first to verify whether this feature should be on. Before leaving a patient's room, remember to put the bed rails in the correct position, reset the bed check alarm, and reapply restraints, if appropriate. Many hospitals need doctor's orders for all four bed rails to be up because they are considered a form of restraint, and all forms of restraint need a doctor's order daily. Verify hospital policy on this issue.

Clinical Monitoring

Clinical monitoring is the essence of intensive care. There are many different ways in which patients are monitored in ICU. There are standard parameters and means of measuring basic vital signs: blood pressure, heart rate, respiratory rate and oxygen saturation, with which all acute care clinicians should be familiar. Vital sign parameters can be found in Table 2.2. In the ICU these are often measured using different equipment than on the regular medical floor. There is also a large amount of monitoring equipment that is specific to the ICU. Clinicians will need to familiarize themselves with the common equipment for clinical monitoring, parameters, and precautions for the devices prior to beginning treatment. Consult with the nurse or other therapists for re-orientation to less familiar devices and parameters as needed.

Pulse Oximetry

It is important to understand the difference between lab values (e.g., SaO_2, PaO_2) and pulse oximeter oxygen saturation (SpO_2) and what the results mean for treatment. Blood gases are drawn frequently in intensive care to monitor a patient's pulmonary status. SaO_2 and PaO_2 are abbreviations used for some of the arterial blood gases. It is not important to memorize the normal blood gas lab values because they are generally available on lab reports. It can be helpful to carry a reference sheet for basic lab values on a clipboard. Refer to Table 2.2 for basic vital signs and Table 2.3 for blood gas values.

Measuring PaO_2 is the most accurate test for blood oxygen level. It requires a blood draw and is a standard part of an arterial blood gases lab order. SpO_2 is the abbreviation for external measurement of oxygen saturation, or pulse oximetry. Normal SpO_2 in a healthy person is 97%–99%. An SpO_2 value of 95% is clinically acceptable in a patient with normal hemoglobin levels (American Association of Critical Care Nurses [AACCN], 2005). A SpO_2 value of 90% is generally equal to a PaO_2 of 60 mm Hg (AACCN, 2005). An external probe with a red infrared light is attached to a finger, nose, ear, or toe. The signal is sent to a computer, which calculates the oxygen saturation percentage.

This method of monitoring blood oxygen is commonly used but inaccurate. First, the monitor does not measure oxygen. Its measurements are based on the percentage of hemoglobin, which has another molecule bound to it. Oxygen is commonly assumed to be the molecule bound to hemoglobin. However, other molecules bind to hemoglobin, creating the non–oxygen-carrying forms of hemoglobin: carboxyhemoglobin or methemoglobin. Carbon monoxide (CO) binds to hemoglobin to create carboxyhemoglobin,

which occurs most commonly after exposure to smoke or exhaust. CO poisoning resolves after 4–5 hours of high-flow oxygen treatment. In rare cases, CO can also be generated in the body as a result of hemolytic anemia or sickle cell disease (Stock, Hampson, & Lavonas, 2007). Methemoglobin can result from exposure to certain drugs and toxins such as benzocaine (local anesthetic), nitrates (such as nitroglycerin), or sulfonamides (a class of antibiotic, e.g., Bactrim).

Other limitations of pulse oximetry may include poor signals because of patients' tremors or poor circulation or because of light interference. In addition, inaccurate readings may be the result of various conditions causing false low readings or false high readings; these conditions are listed in Table 2.7. Because of the inaccuracies inherent to pulse oximetry, it is important to always monitor a patient's symptoms and response to treatment, including respiratory rate, color of lips and nail beds, cognitive status and arousal, anxiety level, and heart rate. Be aware of hemoglobin levels.

Hypoxia will initially cause elevated respiratory rate, heart rate, and anxiety. As patients become more hypoxic, their lips and nail beds will take on a bluish tint called *cyanosis*, they may become pale, and confusion and lethargy are noted. Be aware that patients with poor peripheral circulation may have a small amount of bluish tint in their finger tips at baseline, which may lead to a false low SpO_2 reading. Consult with nursing to verify. If possible, check another location, such as the ear lobe.

Table 2.7. **Pulse Oximetry False Readings Etiology**

False High	False Low
Carboxyhemoglobin	Extremity being tested is cold
Methemoglobin	Peripheral vascular disease—Poor circulation
Low hemoglobin levels	Bruising under the nail or dark nail polish
Fever	Environmental light interference

CO_2 Retention

According to the AACCN (2005), getting a normal value for oxygen saturation (SpO_2) does not necessarily indicate that the patient is able to ventilate adequately. Monitoring SpO_2 in patients with obstructive pulmonary disease does not always provide accurate information about their respiratory status. Normally, the drive to breathe, the biochemical mechanism that controls ventilation, is stimulated by an increase in carbon dioxide (*hypercapnia*) in the bloodstream. When CO_2 levels increase, the body is stimulated to "blow off" the extra CO_2 and return balance to the blood gas levels. As lung disease becomes worse, the drive to breathe switches to being driven by low oxygen levels.

When hypoxia becomes the stimulus for breathing, it can be dangerous to improve the patient's SpO_2. As the SpO_2 increases beyond their baseline range, the drive to breathe decreases because the patient's respiratory system is not stimulated to blow off CO_2 to maintain balance in blood gas levels (AACCN, 2005). This CO_2 retention, if allowed to continue, can result in toxic levels of CO_2. Hypercapnia causes respiratory acidosis, which is characterized by fatigue, lethargy, confusion, and decreased respirations that can lead to coma and death.

Despite the risk for CO_2 retention with supplemental oxygen use, it is far better to avoid hypoxia because the actual risk of developing hypercapnia with carefully controlled supplemental oxygen is low, according to a study by Moloney, Kiely, and McNicholas (2001). They observed that the risk of cardiac arrhythmias and even death is graver if hypoxia is allowed to persist untreated, particularly at night. Patients with chronic obstructive pulmonary disorders have been shown to be able to tolerate 100% oxygen delivery for short periods of time without affecting their ventilation (Moloney et al., 2001). Therefore, Moloney et al. recommended using a brief increase in supplemental oxygen to maintain SpO_2 in a therapeutic range during activity. They argued that because of the increased risk for cardiac events, allowing desaturation during functional activities is more detrimental than allowing brief periods of increase in oxygen delivery (Moloney et al., 2001).

Note that oxygen is a prescribed medication, and increasing or decreasing it will require clearance from the doctor, nurse, or respiratory therapist. If the patient is on a ventilator, the respiratory therapist or nurse can assist with temporarily increasing O_2 delivery if needed. When the session is finished, and the patient has recovered (SpO_2 is within the correct range), the therapist must remember to return the supplemental oxygen to its baseline level.

Telemetry

Telemetry is remote monitoring of vital signs. Unlike in many step-down units or regular hospital rooms, telemetry is visible at all times on a monitor in the intensive care room. On the monitor will be at least one view of the electrocardiogram with the heart rate, SpO_2, blood pressure, and output of any other measuring devices the patient may be attached to, such as arterial line blood pressure, pulmonary artery pressure, intracranial pressure, and electroencephalograph.

The telemetry is usually accurate; however, changes in position and increased patient movement can significantly alter the readings, creating false waves called *artifact*. These false readings will usually cause alarms to go off. Do not become worried by the alarms. Throughout a therapy intervention, cardiac technicians and nurses are watching the telemetry at the nursing station. They will come in and intervene as soon as a reading is concerning. If it is not a concern, they will silence the alarm for a brief time (1–10 minutes). Do not silence the alarm or pause the alarms. Once the therapist develops a rapport with the ICU nurses, some may give him or her permission to silence a specific alarm that has been determined to be false. Be aware that silencing an increased alarm can be dangerous; alarms will remain silenced for a set amount of time, and significant or life-threatening events could be missed while it is silenced. Before leaving the patient's room, make sure to reset all alarms that have been silenced.

Hemodynamic Monitoring

Hemodynamic monitoring refers to monitoring of the cardiovascular system's functioning.

At its most basic, it is the monitoring of blood pressure and heart rate. However, it may also include levels of fluid input and output, mental status, and the heart's internal pressures and efficacy. In general, the more invasive and extensive the measures taken for monitoring a patient are, the more tenuous the patient's cardiovascular status is.

Listed in Table 2.10 are descriptions of some of the lines used for invasive hemodynamic monitoring, such as swan ganz and central venous pressure catheters (see Figures 2.5 and 2.6). Become familiar with the normal ranges of basic hemodynamic values and with the possible symptoms associated with the abnormal ranges. Also be aware that, many times, some values in the abnormal range will be acceptable for individual cases as determined by patient's baseline, medications, past medical history, current medical problems, and the primary diagnosis or surgical procedure. Check with the medical team to determine which values and symptoms are acceptable. In general, only light-headedness is acceptable and only briefly (less than a few minutes) after a change in vertical position. Regardless, if a patient is experiencing any of the symptoms of activity intolerance listed in Table 2.8, a full check of hemodynamic vitals and possibly blood sugar (if the patient has diabetes) should be initiated and the nurse notified.

If the patient is symptomatic but vital signs are good, check with the nurse for permission to continue. If permission is not granted or the vital signs are abnormal, return the patient to supine as soon as safely possible. For more detailed information on managing light-headedness, refer to the "Blood Pressure" section.

Heart Rate

Throughout treatment, pay attention to the heart rate. An abnormal heart rate displayed on the telemetry monitor in the room can be an indicator that other vital signs may be going askew. Be aware, though, that telemetry rhythms can often be inaccurate. Check the patient's radial pulse for confirmation of heart rate if a question about telemetry accuracy arises. Confer with the nurse before entering a patient's room to be aware of any recent problems with the patient's cardiac rhythm such as tachycardia, runs of ventricular tachycardia, rapid atrial fibrillation, or long pauses. Some issues such as tachycardia may simply require giving the patient a brief rest. A new change in rhythm quality will most often require suspending the rest of the treatment. Any change in rhythm will be seen by the nurse on the telemetry, who will advise discontinuing the intervention if necessary. When possible, take advantage of

Table 2.8. **Activity Intolerance**

Warning Signs	Contraindications
Increased anxiety	Acute change in mental status (e.g., somnolence, confusion, agitation)
Increasing discomfort or pain	Acute chest pain
Mild shortness of breath: respiratory rate >20 breaths/min or mild desaturation (pulse oximetry <3%–5%)	Increased work of breathing (use of accessory respiratory muscles, respiration rate >30, increased anxiety)
Light-headedness	Dizziness or feeling faint
Increased fatigue	Changes in vision
Any change in the patients' perception of their body: feeling hot or cold, heavy, "funny," etc.	Acute diaphoresis (sweaty)

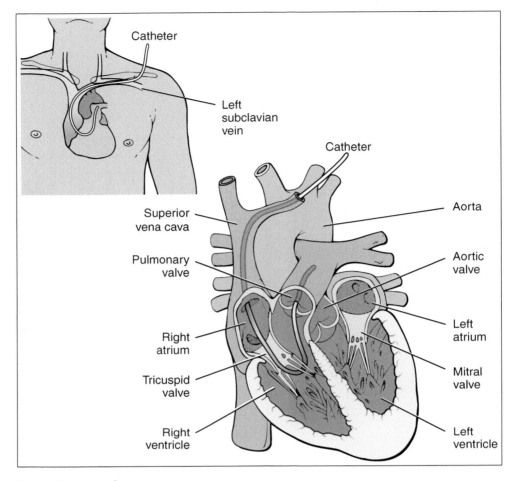

Figure 2.5. Swan Ganz catheter.
Source. Ritchard Fritzler, Medical Illustrator, Roswell, GA.

opportunities to learn basic arrhythmias and symptoms associated with them. It will help with adjusting the demands of the activity during interventions.

Blood Pressure

Make sure to check the patient's blood pressure before and after a treatment. It is always best to know where a patient is starting from and what impact activity had on his or her vital signs. As mentioned earlier, also check the blood pressure if the patient becomes symptomatic (dizzy, change in mental status, cold, clammy, or diaphoretic). It is normal for patients who have been on bed rest to experience a brief period (~30–60 seconds) of light-headedness with any change in position. With this in mind, check orthostatic vitals if the patient experiences more significant or lasting symptoms.

Orthostatic vital signs should include blood pressure and heart rate and be taken first in supine, then in sitting, and finally in standing. According to the Consensus Committee of the American Autonomic Society and the American Academy of Neurology (1996), a patient is considered to be orthostatic when systolic blood pressure drops 20 mm Hg or diastolic blood pressure drops 10 mm Hg within 3 minutes of orthostatic stress. For therapeutic purposes, it is recommended that increased time be spent in each position to determine whether the hemodynamic changes stabilize or not.

When introducing a new change in position, provide the patient with advance warning that he or she may become symptomatic. If a patient is anticipated to be orthostatic, he or she may benefit from more gradual changes in a controlled situation to increase tolerance for orthostatic stress, for example, changing the angle of

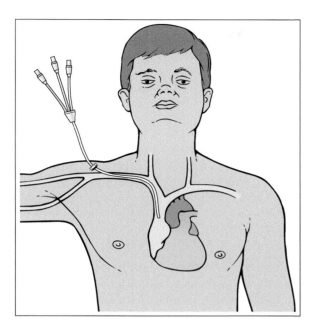

Figure 2.6. Placement of triple lumen nontunneled percutaneous central venous catheter.
Source. Ritchard Fritzler, Medical Illustrator, Roswell, GA.

the head of the bed by 20°–30° as tolerated until upright, putting the bed in the chair position (refer to Table 2.5) so that the feet are in a dependent position, or using a tilt table. It is always best to err on the side of caution when monitoring a patient's hemodynamic status with treatment. Check blood pressure and heart rate with each increase in orthostatic stress, and monitor symptoms closely.

Mean Arterial Pressure

Another important measurement to be aware of is mean arterial pressure. Many times, blood pressure can appear to be too low or too high, but if the mean arterial pressure appears good, the patient is considered stable by the medical team. The mean pressure is an indicator of the heart's ability to perfuse the body's tissues. Most electronic blood pressure monitors in acute care hospitals include mean arterial pressure, or "mean," on their display screen. Mean arterial pressures are considered better for central arterial pressure monitoring than using just systolic pressure as a guide. See Table 2.2 for normal mean arterial pressure parameters.

Cerebral Perfusion Pressure

Cerebral perfusion pressure (CPP) is an indirect measure of cerebral perfusion. It is calculated using mean arterial pressure and intracranial pressure (ICP). A CPP of less than 50 mm Hg is associated with poor outcomes in TBI. A mean arterial pressure of less than 70 mm Hg is also associated with poor outcomes in TBI (Brain Trauma Foundation et al., 2007).

Intracranial Pressure

ICP is measured with an invasive probe inserted into the brain. The purpose of measuring ICP is to calculate and manage cerebral perfusion pressures and to predict outcomes and worsening pathology. During recovery in intensive care, patients with ICP sensors will have the reading displayed on the monitor in their room. Take note of the parameters ordered by the doctor before treating the patient. Pay attention to the readings throughout the session to prevent secondary damage to brain tissue resulting from rising pressure. The *Guidelines for the Management of Severe Traumatic Brain Injury* (Brain Trauma Foundation et al., 2007) recommend that ICP be kept below 20 mm Hg. However, the parameters may be significantly different for acute hemorrhagic or ischemic stroke, so the therapist should check the orders or ask the attending doctor for parameters. During a therapeutic intervention, the following may cause an increase in ICP: an increase in blood pressure, agitation, nausea or vomiting, an increase in physical exertion, supine position with the head of the bed flat, compression of the abdomen, or Valsalva maneuver. If a patient does have an increase in ICP higher than the ordered parameters, discontinuing the treatment is recommended unless the doctor advises otherwise.

Medications Specific to the ICU

Many medications are used in acute care, but some are restricted for use in the ICU because of the powerful nature of the medicine, the critical state of the patient who needs it, and the increased monitoring required. These medications are delivered intravenously, usually through a larger access device than a peripheral IV. A list of medications and precautions for therapy is provided in Table 2.9. Table 2.10 has details on ports and access devices.

Paralytics or neuromuscular blocking agents deserve more attention than I am able to provide in Table 2.10. Patients who are paralyzed by a neuromuscular blockade will be unable to breathe without the ventilator. They will also be unable to communicate because of the paralysis and are likely to be sedated as well. Therapy is contraindicated because the patient is unsafe to mobilize and is usually not medically ready for therapeutic intervention. PROM is the only appropriate choice in this case, but it is also not traditionally performed by therapists. As an intervention, it is considered an unskilled service by insurance providers and is not reimbursable except as a part of the initial evaluation or during training of primary caregivers. Training should be provided to caregivers (including family) before beginning to perform PROM exercises in this setting. Precautions include the following:

- Use caution when working around the ventilator tubing. The patient who is paralyzed and dependent on a ventilator cannot breathe without support, as opposed to the patient who is not paralyzed and dependent on a ventilator who is usually able to breathe briefly, although ineffectively, without support. If the tubing becomes disconnected, the ventilator will sound a distinct alarm. Consider that the patient is now holding his or her breath without having had the luxury of being able to take a deep breath in preparation. Don't panic: The nurse or other staff has enough time to quickly walk to the room and reconnect the tubing without detriment to the patient. Reconnect the tubing and continue with the treatment or call for the nurse to help with it.
- Paralytic medication does not sedate patients or assist with managing anxiety or pain. If the patient is completely paralyzed, he or she will not be able to provide any sign that he or she is alert, anxious, or in pain. Let the nurse know if you have any concerns about the patient.

- Sedated patients cannot express that they are in pain. Be especially careful to protect the joints from painful positions such as hyperextension, subluxation, or impingement and the muscles from overstretching.

Keep in mind, the longer the patient is on paralytics, the longer his or her recovery will be. If the patient had hepatic or renal dysfunction, it may significantly increase the half-life of the paralytic, further prolonging weakness (Khan et al., 2008). Adjust goals appropriately.

Goal Setting

Setting goals for the ICU patient is not very different from setting goals for any other patient. The goals must be measurable and attainable in a reasonable amount of time. Critically ill patients will not all be appropriate for traditional ADL goals; those can be revisited, for example, during reevaluation or transfer to the step-down unit. Setting goals in the ICU may require focus on even the minutest gains to demonstrate progress at this level. Consider setting vital sign goals in combination with task performance. For example, set a goal for improved orthostatic stress tolerance when the patient is asymptomatic and systolic blood pressure remains higher than 95 when the head of the bed is at 60° as the patient performs a grooming task with maximal assist. In cases of severe acquired neuromuscular dysfunction, short-term goals may need to initially focus on the patient's directing some of his or her care.

Treatment Planning

Regardless of a therapist's comfort level with the intensive care environment and an ICU patient, every therapist can follow two basic principles to ensure the treatment plan is safe. First, rely on the nurse to clear the patient to participate in therapy. The nurse has the full picture of the patient's medical status, the patient's activity tolerance, and the medical team's plan for the patient's day. Second, make sure the nurse understands what the treatment's physical demands will be. If the nurse is not made aware of the treatment plan, then you will not have

(Text continues on p. 70)

Table 2.9. Intravenous Medications Particular to the Intensive Care Unit

Medication	Basic Purpose	Conditions Treated	Examples	Precautions
Cardiac medications				
Inotropes	Increase force of heart muscle contraction	Heart failure	Dopamine (Intropin), digoxin, dobutamine, milranone	Used in critical situations to help heart pumping. Monitor vitals closely. Can be changed rapidly by the nurse in response to issues. If the nurse is doing this, the impact of the therapy may be masked.
Angiotensin-converting enzyme inhibitors	Prevent vasoconstriction, lowers blood pressure	Hypertension	Enalapril (Vasotec IV)	Hypotension can occur; monitor vitals.
Beta blockers (beta adrenergic receptor antagonists)	Decrease heart rate	Dysrhythmia, tachycardia, hypertension	Atenolol, metoprolol (Lopressor), labetalol, propanolol	Bradycardia can occur; monitor vitals.
Calcium channel blockers	Decrease muscle contractility	Dysrhythmia, tachycardia	Diltiazem (Cardizem)	Bradycardia can occur; monitor vitals.
Vasodilators	Dilate blood vessels, lowers blood pressure	Perioperative hypertension, unstable angina, acute coronary syndrome	Nitroglycerin	Hypotension can occur; monitor vitals. Often used for unstable angina; monitor for symptoms of myocardial ischemia and terminate session if patient has positive signs or symptoms.

(continued)

Table 2.9. *(continued)*

Medication	Basic Purpose	Conditions Treated	Examples	Precautions
Vasopressors	Cause vasoconstriction, increase blood pressure	Acute hypotension	Dopamine (Intropin), norepinephrine (Levophed), phenylephrine (Neo-Synephrine), antidiuretic hormone (Vasopressin), epinephrine, ephedrine	Used in critical situations to stabilize blood pressure. Patient vitals should be monitored closely, and activity involving orthostatic stress should be limited; consult attending physician for restrictions.
Antiarrhythmics	Convert irregular heart rhythm to normal sinus rhythm; also used to prevent relapse into arrythmia	Arrhythmia	Amioderone (Cordarone), adenosine (Adenocard)	Used to treat life-threatening arrhythmias. Limit strenuous activity, monitor heart rate, and keep rate <100 or the recommended parameter set by the medical team.
Miscellaneous				
Diuretics	Increase urine output	Heart failure, peripheral edema, volume overload	Furosemide (Lasix), mannitol, bumetanide (Bumex), torsemide (Demadex)	Hypotension can occur; monitor vitals. Be prepared for the patient to need to urinate.
Sedatives and hypnotics	Central nervous system depressant, amnesiac	Anxiety, agitation	Lorazepam (Ativan), midazolam (Versed), dexmedetomidine HCL (Precedex), propofol titrated (Diprivan)	Cognition will be impaired. Hypotension can occur; monitor vitals.
Paralytics and neuromuscular blocking agents	Interrupts the transmission of neurotransmitters at the level of the neuromuscular junction	Paralysis of skeletal muscles	Cisatracurium (Nimbex), propofol (Diprivan), vecuronium (Norcuran), atracurium (Tracrium), pancuronium (Pavulon) pipecuronium (Arduan), rocuronium (Zemuron)	The patient cannot communicate and will have little muscle tone. Be careful during passive range of motion exercises: Protect the joints from hyperextension, subluxation, or impingement, and protect the muscles from overstretching.

Table 2.10.　**Ports and Access Devices**

Port or Device	Purpose	Length	Location	Duration	Indications	Precautions
Venous access						
PIV	Infuse a medication or a fluid.	0.25–2 in.	Extremities	≤72 hr	For most noncaustic medications and fluids.	If accidentally disconnected from tubing, occlusion can occur within 4 minutes.
PICC	Long-term medication needs or if unable to establish peripheral intravenous catheter.	20–25 in.	Enters at antecubital fossa and ends in superior vena cava or subclavian or axillary vein. Sutured in place.	≤1 yr	Total parenteral nutrition, prolonged antibiotic needs, continuous pain medication infusion, venous lab draws; can be used to measure central venous pressure if advanced into superior vena cava.	Keep dry. Avoid taking blood pressures over PICC. Caution with using crutches with pressure applied at axilla.
Nontunneled central venous catheter ("triple lumen"; refer to Figure 2.5)	Provides central venous access and multiple access ports.	6–8 in.	Enters at subclavian or IJ and ends in superior vena cava or right atrium.	1 wk (goal) to a few months (possible)	Same as PICC, can also give frequent chemotherapy doses. Can be placed at the bedside quickly.	Highest rate of infection. Keep dry.

(continued)

Table 2.10. (continued)

Port or Device	Purpose	Length	Location	Duration	Indications	Precautions
Tunneled central venous catheter ("Hickman")	Provides central venous access. Used for caustic medications such as chemotherapy.	12 in.	Tunneled subcutaneously from the insertion site (subclavian or IJ) and exits at a site below the nipple line.	≤1 yr	Same capabilities as nontunneled version but with lower infection rate; can safely be used longer term.	Keep dry.
VAD (or Port-A-Cath)	Provides central venous access. Less noticeable; requires less daily care.	~12 in.	Same as tunneled catheter, but port is located under the skin.	Long term, 2,000 punctures	Same as tunneled catheter.	Can get wet without risk of infection.
Arterial access						
CVP (refer to Figure 2.5)	Provides vascular access, measures function and circulatory ability of right side of heart, measures fluid balance.		Enters in subclavian region. Ends just above the right atrium.		Critical illnesses affecting heart function. Also used after heart surgeries.	Needs to be recalibrated by registered nurse after change in position; values will not be accurate until then.

Pulmonary artery catheter (Swan Ganz; refer to Figure 2.4)	Measures intracardiac pressures and oxygen saturation; assists with measuring other hemodynamic parameters such as cardiac output.	Consists of 4–5 lines	Enters in the subclavian or IJ. Winds through the right side of the heart, ending in the proximal left or right branch of pulmonary artery.	Critical illnesses affecting heart function such as shock or acute pulmonary edema. Also used after heart surgeries.	Its use may produce bleeding, vessel rupture, dysrhythmias, and other life-threatening complications (Venes, 2005).
Arterial line (A-line)	For blood pressure monitoring and blood draws: arterial blood gases.		Radial or femoral artery.	Provides more accurate blood pressure than noninvasive techniques; used when patient is getting IV pressors.	Needs to be recalibrated by registered nurse after change in position; values will not be accurate until then. *Femoral artery line:* defer mobility; hip flexion will cause artery occlusion.

Note. CVP = central venous pressure catheter; IJ = intrajugular; PICC = peripherally inserted central catheter; PIV = peripheral intravenous catheter; VAD = venous access device.

obtained informed consent and the activity you were planning may be too difficult for the patient. By collaborating with the nurse, the therapeutic intervention can be adjusted to increase or decrease the challenge, thus providing the patient with the most appropriate intervention.

A patient's condition can change throughout the day. Any plan for treatment must be easily renegotiated minute to minute during the intervention depending on the patient's physiological response to it. At times, the patient may only be able to tolerate a position change and may be unable to participate in a concomitant activity. Simple occupation-based activities can be used with patients whether they are in bed, at the edge of the bed, or out of bed. Basic ADLs can be graded according to the patient's tolerance and interest. Some potential treatment activities are

- *Brushing teeth:* Can be graded to opening the mouth (and keeping it open), holding the toothbrush or toothette, applying toothpaste, hand-over-hand brushing, and so forth.

- *Writing a letter:* Can be graded to pointing to pictures or letters on a communication board; checking off boxes on a daily activities list; writing a note; or making a list of questions to ask the doctor, meals to order, or TV shows or movies to watch.

- *Designing an "about me" or "interests" board:* Can be graded to selecting family pictures to display, selecting pictures of activities the patient likes, or creating a picture collage.

- *Keeping a journal:* Can note visitors, events, meals, progress with therapy, and so forth.

- *Manicure:* Can be graded to a manicure's individual components, including bringing hands to and from the bowl of warm water for soaking or holding the hand out to have nails filed.

- *Applying makeup:* Can be graded to applying any type of makeup or any preparatory tasks.

- *Computing (if available):* Can be graded to watching a family picture slideshow or movies with or without having to hit a button to advance slides or select a movie, reading e-mail, or sending e-mail.

Progression of Therapeutic Activity in Critically Ill Patients

Evidence-based research has provided substantial support for increasing activity in outpatients and general medical ward inpatients, but overall, evidence to guide early activity in the intensive care unit is lacking (Hopkins, Spuhler, & Thomsen, 2007; Morris, 2007; Morris & Herridge, 2007). As the patient stabilizes and is awake, cooperative, and cleared by the medical team for participation in activities, the therapist can begin a more thorough evaluation of the patient's current strength, endurance, and cognitive abilities. For techniques, see Chapter 1. Participation in therapy has a few potential barriers, including hemodynamic stability and the number and type of lines. However, Winkelman, Higgins, and Chen (2005) pointed out that as of yet, little research has assisted in determining whether many of the barriers are definitely contraindications where participation in early activity is concerned.

Daily sessions from 10 to 30 minutes will be more than enough exercise for patients initially. The patient will often require frequent rest periods and vital sign checks during these short treatments. Occasionally, the patient will only tolerate 1 therapy session per day; therefore, a cotreatment with the physical therapist, speech therapist, or both may allow for more aggressive but limited therapy. Consider dovetailing sessions, too. Use the patient's symptoms and vital signs to help determine when rest breaks are needed.

Initially, daily treatments can consist of active assisted and active ROM exercises, orthostatic stress challenges, and assisted participation in basic ADLs such as hand or face washing and mouth care. As the patient's activity tolerance improves, it is appropriate to begin advancing activities from supine to sitting in the chair position (see Table 2.5) to sitting at the edge of the bed and finally to standing. Also consider adding a second treatment so that the patient gets one intervention in the morning and one in the afternoon, as tolerated. If this is not possible, consider scheduling therapy sessions, that is, occupational therapy in the morning and physical therapy in the afternoon. Another possibility might be the addition of a rehabilitation aide program for range of motion, advancing to a full intervention as the patient progresses.

Communication With Nursing

Making contact with the nurses for ICU patients as early in the day as possible is recommended. Many times, this contact can be addressed through ICU rounds with the medical team. During rounds, pay attention to any tests or procedures that may be planned for the day as well as other interventions such as respiratory therapy treatments. If the caseload is large, more coordination and prioritization is needed. The goal is to maximize the patient's participation and responsiveness. If the ICU team is therapy oriented, it may be possible to rearrange the times of many other interventions, such as dialysis.

Providing occupational therapy services in the ICU can be an enriching experience. Among the benefits is the opportunity to collaborate with a wide range of medical staff and to develop highly specialized skills such as familiarity with critical care equipment and being able to monitor and progress activity tolerance in critically ill patients. Other benefits are the interaction with ICU patients. They are experiencing some of the most frightening moments of their lives; they are from varied backgrounds and have a wide range of diagnoses. The patients provide personally meaningful interactions during their recovery while discussing their progress, their fears, and their beliefs about life and death. These moments will be inspiring, troubling, saddening, and amazing. When given the opportunity, despite any reservations, the experience of being a successful therapist in the ICU is one not to be missed.

References

American Association of Critical Care Nurses. (2005). *AACN procedure manual for critical care* (5th ed.). Philadelphia: W. B. Saunders.

American Heart Association/American Stroke Association Stroke Council, Clinical Cardiology Council, Cardiovascular Radiology and Intervention Council, & Atherosclerotic Peripheral Vascular Disease and Quality of Care Outcomes in Research Interdisciplinary Working Groups. (2007). Guidelines for the early management of adults with ischemic stroke. *Circulation, 115,* e478–534. doi: 10.1161/Circulationaha.107.181486

American Occupational Therapy Association. (2010). *Board certified and specialty certified practitioners.* Bethesda, MD: Author. Retrieved September 22, 2010, from www.aota.org/Practitioners/ProfDev/Certification/certified.aspx

American Physical Therapy Association. (2009). *Specialist certification.* Retrieved February 8, 2009, from www.apta.org/AM/Template.cfm?Section=Certification2&Template=/TaggedPage/TaggedPageDisplay.cfm&TPLID=206&ContentID=25738

American Psychiatric Association. (2000). *Diagnostic and statistical manual of mental disorders* (4th ed., text rev.). Washington, DC: Author.

Bercker, S., Weber-Carstens, S., Deja, M., Grimm, C., Wolf, S., Behse, F., et al. (2005). Critical illness polyneuropathy and myopathy in patients with acute respiratory distress syndrome. *Critical Care Medicine, 33,* 711–715.

Brain Trauma Foundation, American Association of Neurological Surgeons, Congress of Neurological Surgeons, & AANS/CNS Joint Section on Neurotrauma and Critical Care. (2007). Guidelines for the management of severe traumatic brain injury. *Journal of Neurotrauma, 24*(Suppl. 1), S1–S106.

Bruton, A., & McPherson, K. (2004). Impact of the introduction of a multidisciplinary weaning team on a general intensive care unit . . . including commentary by Dries DJ, Perry JF. *International Journal of Therapy and Rehabilitation, 11,* 435–440.

Chobanian, A. V. (Ed.). (2003). *JNC 7 Express: The Seventh Report of the Joint National Committee on Prevention, Detection, Evaluation, and Treatment of High Blood Pressure* (NIH Pub. No. 03-5233). Bethesda, MD: National Heart, Lung, and Blood Institute. Retrieved October 5, 2008, from www.nhlbi.nih.gov/guidelines/hypertension/express.pdf

Consensus Committee of the American Autonomic Society and the American Academy of Neurology. (1996). Consensus statement on the definition of orthostatic hypotension, pure autonomic failure, and multiple system atrophy. *Neurology, 46,* 1470.

Duke, E. M. (Ed.). (2006). *Report to Congress: The critical care workforce: A study of the supply and demand for critical care physicians.* Retrieved May 3,

2008, from ftp://ftp.hrsa.gov/bhpr/national center/criticalcare.pdf

Ely, E., Inouye, S., Bernard, G., Gordon, S., Francis, J., May, L., et al. (2001). Caring for the critically ill patient—Delirium in mechanically ventilated patients: Validity and reliability of the Confusion Assessment Method for the Intensive Care Unit (CAM–ICU). *JAMA, 286,* 2703.

Ely, E., Shintani, A., Truman, B., Speroff, T., Gordon, S., Harrell, F., et al. (2004). Caring for the critically ill patient: Delirium as a predictor of mortality in mechanically ventilated patients in the intensive care unit. *JAMA, 291,* 1753–1762.

Fletcher, S. N., Kennedy, D. D., Ghosh, I. R., Misra, V. P., Kiff, K., Coakley, J. H., et al. (2003). Persistent neuromuscular and neurophysiologic abnormalities in long-term survivors of prolonged critical illness. *Critical Care Medicine, 31,* 1012–1016. doi: 10.1097/01.CCM.0000053651.38421.D9

Haupt, M. T., Bekes, C. E., Brilli, R. J., Carl, L. C., Gray, A. W., Jastremski, M. S., et al. (2003). Guidelines on critical care services and personnel: Recommendations based on a system of categorization of three levels of care. *Critical Care Medicine, 31,* 2677–2683.

Herlihy, J. P., Koch, S. M., Jackson, R., & Nora, H. (2006). Course of weaning from prolonged mechanical ventilation after cardiac surgery. *Texas Heart Institute Journal, 33,* 122–129.

Herridge, M. S., Cheung, A. M., Tansey, C. M., Matte-Martyn, A., Diaz-Granados, N., Al-Saidi, F., et al. (2003). One-year outcomes in survivors of the acute respiratory distress syndrome. *New England Journal of Medicine, 348,* 683–693. doi: 10.1056/NEJMoa022450

Hopkins, R. O., Spuhler, V. J., & Thomsen, G. E. (2007). Transforming ICU culture to facilitate early mobility. *Critical Care Clinics, 23,* 81–96.

Hopkins, R. O., Weaver, L. K., Collingridge, D., Parkinson, R. B., Chan, K. J., & Orme, J. F. (2005). Two-year cognitive, emotional, and quality-of-life outcomes in acute respiratory distress syndrome. *American Journal of Respiratory and Critical Care Medicine, 171,* 340–347. doi: 10.1164/rccm.200406-763OC

Hund, E. (1999). Myopathy in critically ill patients. *Critical Care Medicine, 27,* 2544–2547.

Khan, J., Harrison, T. B., & Rich, M. M. (2008). Mechanisms of neuromuscular dysfunction in critical illness. *Critical Care Clinics, 24,* 165–177. doi: 10.1016/j.ccc.2007.10.004

Landro, L. (2007, October 17). The informed patient: Hospitals combat an insidious complication: Delirium in ICU patients, once thought temporary, can inflict lasting damage. *The Wall Street Journal,* p. D1.

Leeuwen, A. M. V., Kranpitz, T. R., & Smith, L. S. (2006). *Davis's comprehensive handbook of laboratory and diagnostic tests: With nursing implications* (2nd ed., pp. 260–271). Philadelphia: F. A. Davis.

Lindman, J. P., Morgan, C. E., & Dixon, S. (2008, September 8). Tracheostomy: Overview. *eMedicine.* Retrieved January 11, 2009, from http://emedicine.medscape.com/article/865068-overview#section~introduction

MacIntyre, N. R., Cook, D. J., Ely, E. W., Epstein, S. K., Fink, J. B., Heffner, J. E., et al. (2001). Evidence-based guidelines for weaning and discontinuing ventilatory support: A collective task force facilitated by the American College of Chest Physicians; the American Association for Respiratory Care; and the American College of Critical Care Medicine. *Chest, 120*(6, Suppl.), 375S–395S.

Marino, P. L. (1998). *The ICU book* (2nd ed.). Philadelphia: Lippincott Williams & Wilkins.

Martin, G. S., Mannino, D. M., Eaton, S., & Moss, M. (2003). The epidemiology of sepsis in the United States from 1979 through 2000. *New England Journal of Medicine, 348,* 1546–1554. doi: 10.1056/NEJMoa022139

Moloney, E. D., Kiely, J. L., & McNicholas, W. T. (2001). Controlled oxygen therapy and carbon dioxide retention during exacerbations of chronic obstructive pulmonary disease. *Lancet, 357,* 526–528. doi: 11229674

Morris, P. E. (2007). Moving our critically ill patients: Mobility barriers and benefits. *Critical Care Clinics, 23,* 1–20.

Morris, P. E., & Herridge, M. S. (2007). Early intensive care unit mobility: Future directions. *Critical Care Clinics, 23,* 97–110.

Murthy, T. V. S. P., Bhatia, M. P., & Prabhakar, B. T. (2005). Cerebral vasospasm: Aetiopathogenesis and intensive care management. *Indian Journal of Critical Care Medicine, 9,* 42–46.

National Heart, Lung, and Blood Institute. (2008). *What is hypotension?* Retrieved October 5, 2008, from www.nhlbi.nih.gov/health/dci/Diseases/hyp/hyp_whatis.html

Pastores, S. M. (2005). Critical illness polyneuropathy and myopathy in acute respiratory distress syndrome: More common than we realize! *Critical Care Medicine, 33,* 895–896.

Pustavoitau, A., & Stevens, R. D. (2008). Mechanisms of neurologic failure in critical illness. *Critical Care Clinics, 24,* 1.

Rahimi, S. Y., Brown, J. H., Macomson, S. D., Jensen, M. A., & Alleyne, C. H., Jr. (2006, October 31). Evaluation treatment of cerebral vasospasm. *Medscape Today.* Retrieved from http://www.medscape.com/viewarticle/545329 February 10, 2009, from Medscape.

Society of Critical Care Medicine. (2006). *Critical care statistics in the United States.* Mt. Prospect, IL: Author. Retrieved April 25, 2008, from http://sccmwww.sccm.org/Documents/WebStatistics PamphletFinalJune06.pdf

Sommers, M. S., Johnson, S. A. P., & Beery, T. A. P. (2006). *Diseases and disorders: A nursing therapeutics manual* (3rd ed.). Philadelphia: F. A. Davis.

Stock, A., Hampson, N., & Lavonas, E. (2007, September 20). *Carbon monoxide poisoning prevention clinical education* [Webcast]. Atlanta, GA: Centers for Disease Control and Prevention. Retrieved July 27, 2008, from www2a.cdc.gov/phtn/COPoisonPrev/default.asp

Teasdale, G., & Jennett, B. (1974). Assessment of coma and impaired consciousness: A practical scale. *Lancet, 2,* 81–84.

Vassilakopoulos, T., Roussos, C., & Zakynthinos, S. (1999). Weaning from mechanical ventilation. *Journal of Critical Care, 14,* 39–62.

Venes, D. (2005). *Taber's cyclopedic medical dictionary* (20th ed.). Philadelphia: F. A. Davis.

Williams, D. R. (2009). *Earth fact sheet.* Retrieved August 15, 2009, from http://nssdc.gsfc.nasa.gov/planetary/factsheet/earthfact.html

Winkelman, C. (2004). Inactivity and inflammation: Selected cytokines as biologic mediators in muscle dysfunction during critical illness. *AACN Clinical Issues, 15,* 74–82.

Winkelman, C. (2007). Inactivity and inflammation in the critically ill patient. *Critical Care Clinics, 23,* 21–34.

Winkelman, C., Higgins, P. A., & Chen, Y. K. (2005). Activity in the chronically critically ill. *Dimensions of Critical Care Nursing, 24,* 281–290. Retrieved April 26, 2008, from www.pubmedcentral.nih.gov/articlerender.fcgi?artid=1469775

3

The Cardiac System

Helene Smith-Gabai, OTD, OTR/L, BCPR

Problems with the heart, which is essential for sustaining life, can have a profound effect on how other organ systems function and on quality of life. Occupational therapists working in hospital settings frequently treat patients who have cardiovascular disease either as their primary diagnosis or as a comorbidity. To be effective as a therapist and provide best practice, occupational therapists need a fundamental knowledge of the cardiovascular system.

According to the American Heart Association (AHA), more than 80 million Americans have one or more forms of cardiovascular disease, including hypertension, coronary heart disease, heart failure, congenital defects, and stroke, with direct and indirect costs of $475.3 billion (AHA, 2009b). Heart disease is the leading cause of death in the United States for both men and women, with a coronary event occurring every 25 seconds and a death approximately every minute (Lloyd-Jones et al., 2009). However, many cardiovascular and heart disease risk factors are modifiable. Occupational therapists take a holistic approach to helping patients with heart disease by facilitating engagement in health and wellness behaviors including activities of daily living (ADLs), improvements in functional capacity, and lifestyle or risk reduction education.

Normal Structure and Function

The heart is the most important muscle in the body and the main organ of the circulatory system. The heart is located in the mediastinum (the central compartment of the thorax) in the middle of the chest and slightly toward the left. It is conical in shape and roughly the size of a clenched fist. The *apex*, the part of the heart that points down, consists primarily of the left ventricle. A fluid-filled sac called the *pericardium* surrounds the heart, protecting it from trauma and infection and helping to lubricate it against friction.

The heart has three layers: the epicardium (outermost layer), the myocardium (middle layer), and the endocardium (innermost layer). The *epicardium* is the inner layer of the pericardium and covers the myocardium. The *myocardium* is the muscle of the heart and contracts to generate pumping action. *Myocardial cells* are also responsible for the heart's automaticity, rhythmicity, and conductivity. The *endocardium* lines the interior of the heart and includes the valves, chordae tendineae, and connected blood vessels. The *chordae tendineae* are thin fiber strands that open and close the valve leaflets and help prevent eversion of the heart valves with ventricular contraction. The chordae tendineae attaches the *atrioventricular (AV)* valves to the *papillary muscles,* which connect to the ventricular walls.

The heart consists of four hollow compartments, two upper chambers called *atria* and two lower chambers called *ventricles*. The atria are smaller and approximately one-third the size of the ventricles. The *left ventricle* is the largest chamber of the heart and the most susceptible to myocardial infarction (MI). The *septum* is the connective tissue that separates the right and left sides of the heart. It also serves a role in cardiac conductivity and ventricular contraction. Another layer of connective tissue also separates the atria from the ventricles. This connective tissue does not conduct electrical impulses but acts as an insulation barrier during the electrical conduction of the cardiac cycle.

The right atrium is where all the action begins. It receives oxygen-depleted blood from the venous system and pumps it through the tricuspid valve into the right ventricle and through to the lungs to be reoxygenated. The left atrium receives the oxygen-rich blood from the pulmonary veins and pumps it through the mitral valve to the left ventricle, which then pumps it through the aorta and on to the rest of the body.

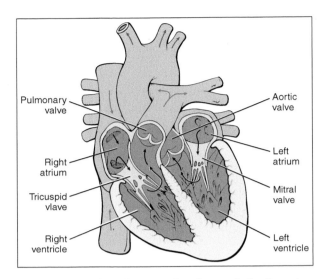

Figure 3.1. Chambers and valves of the heart.
Source. Richard Fritzler, Medical Illustrator, Roswell, GA.

The heart's four valves help transport blood by allowing blood flow in only one direction. Valves work by opening and closing according to pressure on each side. Their names indicate where they are located or how many flaps or cusps they have. Two valves allow blood flow from the atria to the ventricles. These are called *atrioventricular* or *AV valves.* The AV valves consist of the tricuspid and mitral valves. The *tricuspid valve* allows blood flow between the right atrium and right ventricle and has three flaps. The *mitral* or *bicuspid valve* allows blood flow between the left atrium and left ventricle and has two flaps. The aortic and the pulmonary or semilunar valves are moon shaped and separate the right and left ventricles from the pulmonary trunk and the aorta. These valves prevent blood from flowing back into the ventricles. The "lub dub" heartbeat or first (S_1) and second (S_2) heart sounds heard are actually the sound of the AV and semilunar valves closing, respectively (see Figure 3.1).

Circulatory System

Oxygenated blood flows away from the heart through the arterial system and supplies oxygen and nutrients (i.e., glucose and amino acids) to tissue and organs throughout the body. Oxygen-depleted blood returns to the heart via the venous system. The *primary* or *"great"* *blood vessels* are also an important part of the circulation system. They consist of the *superior* and *inferior vena cava, the pulmonary arteries, the pulmonary veins,* and the *aorta.* Both the superior and inferior vena cava blood vessels drain deoxygenated blood from the venous system into the right atrium. The superior vena cava brings blood from the head, neck, and upper body, and the inferior vena cava brings blood from the lower body and viscera. The *coronary venous system* or *coronary sinus* also brings deoxygenated blood back to the right atrium.

Once blood leaves the right side of the heart, it travels to the *pulmonary trunk,* which branches off into the right and left pulmonary arteries, which then branch off into the corresponding lungs. The pulmonary trunk and the aorta are the two main arteries that leave the heart. The pulmonary arteries are the only arteries in the body that carry deoxygenated blood. Once blood is oxygenated in the lungs, it returns to the left atrium of the heart via the four pulmonary veins. Two pulmonary veins carry oxygen from each lung: the *right superior* and *inferior veins* and the *left superior* and *inferior veins.* These are the only veins in the body that carry oxygenated blood. After blood is pumped through the left side of the heart, it exits through the largest artery, the aorta, and then on to the rest of the body. The ascending aorta transports blood to the upper body, and the descending aorta transports blood to the lower body and viscera. Figure 3.2 illustrates how blood circulates throughout the body. Blood travels from the arteries to the smaller arterioles and eventually to the capillaries, where an exchange of gases and nutrients between blood vessels, organs, and tissues occurs. Deoxygenated blood returns to the heart via the capillary and venous system.

Cardiac Cycle and Electrical Conduction System

The heart, unique from other muscles in our bodies, is different in that it possesses these five characteristics:

1. *Automaticity*—The heart initiates its own electrical impulse spontaneously without external stimuli. Cardiac muscle is

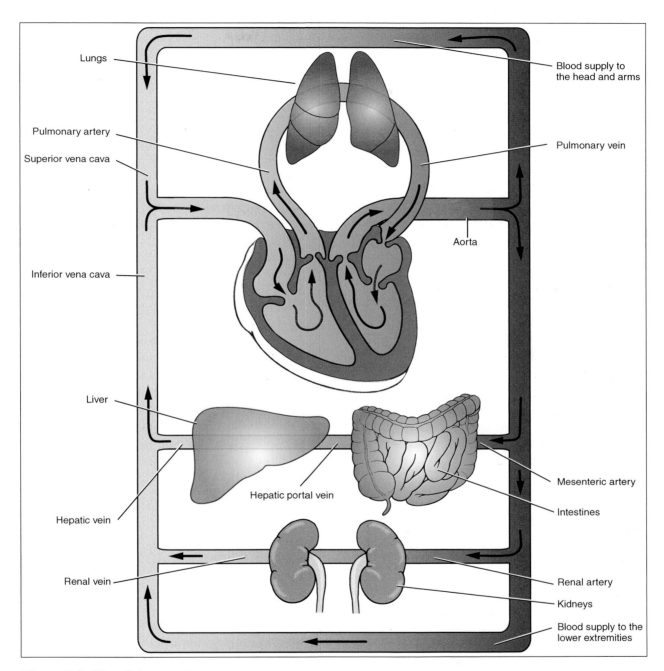

Figure 3.2. Circulatory system.
Source. Richard Fritzler, Medical Illustrator, Roswell, GA.

myogenic, or self-stimulating. It does not require an electrical impulse from the central nervous system to initiate a contraction.

2. *Excitability*—Cardiac cells have the ability to reach a threshold, which causes cardiac muscle to contract.

3. *Conductivity*—The heart has its own pacemaker that generates an electrical impulse that travels from cell to cell through fibers, causing the atria and ventricles to contract.

4. *Contractability*—Electrical impulses stimulate cardiac muscle to contract, causing the heart's chambers to expand and relax, resulting in the heart's pumping action. Contractions occur spontaneously, although the rate can be affected by other

factors (i.e., sympathetic stimulation or hormones).

5. *Rhythmicity*—The cardiac muscle contracts in a set repetitive pattern or rhythm.

Each cardiac cycle begins at the *sinoatrial (SA) node,* a group of specialized cells located on the back wall of the right atrium. The SA node is the heart's natural pacemaker because it generates the first impulse initiating a cardiac cycle. Once the SA node fires, both atria contract, forcing blood into the ventricles. The electrical impulse then passes to the *AV node.* The AV node is located in the bottom of the right atrium near the septum. The AV node passes the impulse along to the septum through the *Bundle of His*. The electrical impulse is delayed at this point, allowing blood from the atria to empty into the ventricles before ventricular contraction. From the Bundle of His, the fibers then branch off into *right* and *left bundle branches*. These bundle branches then split off into the *Purkinje fibers*, located along the bottom of the ventricles. The electrical impulse from the Purkinje fibers then stimulates the ventricles to contract. As both ventricles contract simultaneously, the atria relax (see Figure 3.3).

The entire cardiac cycle takes less than a second based on a HR of 70 beats per minute (BPM). A normal HR is normal sinus rhythm. HRs faster than 100 bpm are called *tachycardia,* and HRs slower than 60 bpm are

called *bradycardia* (refer to the "Arrhythmias" section).

Factors Affecting Cardiac Output

Various factors can affect HR and contractility. One such factor is the autonomic nervous system, which adjusts cardiac output (CO) to meet metabolic demands (Collins & Cocanour, 2004). The parasympathetic system through the vagus nerve slows down cardiac function, thus slowing down HR. The right vagus nerve innervates the SA node, and the left vagus nerve innervates the AV node. Vagolytic drugs that inhibit anticholinergics (e.g., atropine) inhibit the action of the vagus nerve on the heart. Anticholinergic drugs are used to treat bradycardia because they increase HR. The sympathetic nervous system (the system that prepares people for flight or fight), when stimulated, increases HR and therefore CO.

Various hormones also affect HR and vascular resistance. For example, epinephrine vasodilates the coronary arteries, but norepinephrine is a vasoconstrictor. Both hormones can be triggered by stress or exercise. Another factor affecting HR and blood pressure are the cardiac reflexes. Stretch and pressure can trigger the baroreflex, which responds to mechanoreceptors in the heart, main vessels, and cervical and intrathoracic blood vessels, working as a negative feedback loop. When pressure increases, the parasympathetic system is stimulated and the sympathetic system is inhibited, resulting in decreased HR and vasodilation. When pressure is too low, the opposite occurs, and the baroreflex is inhibited, resulting in increased blood pressure.

Another mechanoreceptor called the *Bainbridge reflex* also responds to stretch. When blood volume increases, it also causes an increase in HR. Other factors affecting HR are ions and chemoreceptors. For example, low potassium, low calcium, or high sodium (which blocks calcium intake) can all lower HR. Chemoreceptors in the carotid artery and aorta affect ventilation in response to carbon dioxide levels, which can lead to cardiac arrhythmias.

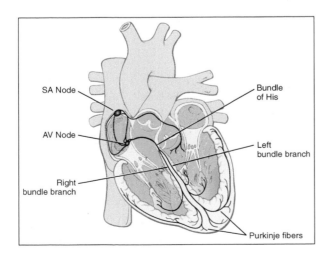

Figure 3.3. Electrical conduction of the heart. *Source.* Richard Fritzler, Medical Illustrator, Roswell, GA.

Heart Rate and Stroke Volume

CO is the volume of blood pumped per minute. CO is typically 5 liters per minute for the average person but can be anywhere between 4 and 8 liters per minute. Two things determine CO: *heart rate (HR)* and *stroke volume (SV)*. HR is the frequency of the cardiac cycle or the number of ventricular contractions per minute. HR is also one of the major vital signs used in monitoring hospital patients. Other vital signs include blood pressure, respiration rate, temperature, pulse oximetry, and pain level.

SV is the actual amount of blood expelled into the aorta with each ventricular contraction, regardless of the initial amount found in the ventricle. CO can be expressed as $CO = HR \times SV$. For example, if SV increases, then CO will increase. If HR increases, then CO will increase until SV goes down.

Other factors affecting CO are Starling's Law, preload, and afterload. *Starling's Law* states that if a muscle wall is stretched more, the contraction will be stronger. Imagine a bow and arrow. If the archer pulls the bow farther back, tension is increased and the arrow shoots forward more forcefully. If the stretch on the ventricle walls is increased, then more blood is ejected. However, when HR is too fast, the ventricles do not have enough time to fill up between contractions, and less volume is ejected.

Preload is the amount of blood in the ventricle before contraction. As preload increases, SV increases. *Peripheral resistance* is the amount of resistance or expansion of the arterial wall in response to circulating blood. *Afterload* is the pressure in the aorta against which the ventricle has to contract to successfully eject blood into the circulatory system. Afterload and SV have an inverse relationship. If the afterload is too high, then SV decreases. However, if the afterload is decreased, then SV increases. Less pressure or resistance to blood entering an artery means the left ventricle can pump out more blood into that artery.

Another factor in heart function is the *ejection fraction (EF*, which is a percentage of the amount of blood ejected relative to the amount received by the ventricle. The EF indicates how well the heart is pumping. In a normal adult, it is approximately 60%; however, an athlete's EF may be even higher. Low EFs (<40%) are usually associated with systolic dysfunction or failure. An EF within the normal range but with signs and symptoms of congestive heart failure (CHF) indicates diastolic failure. Patients with an EF of 5%–10% have severe heart disease and typically present with poor endurance, shortness of breath, and lower-extremity edema.

An additional indicator of heart function and pump performance is the *cardiac index,* which is the measurement of CO in relation to the patient's size and body surface area (Morgan & Dempsey, 2004).

What Is a Heartbeat?

A *heartbeat* is one cardiac cycle consisting of both diastole and systole. *Diastole* is the heart's relaxation phase, during which the four chambers respectively fill up with blood. *Systole* is the phase during which filled chambers pump blood out to the next chamber or blood vessel. For example, during atrial diastole, the atria fill up with blood, but during atrial systole the atria contract and empty blood into the ventricles. When feeling a pulse, what is felt is the wave of the artery wall expanding and then returning to its natural position as blood flows through. The pulse is a reflection of HR because it has the same frequency as a cardiac cycle.

An *electrocardiogram (EKG)* is a graphic recording of the heart's depolarization and repolarization during a cardiac cycle. It traces the route of the heart's electrical conduction. By observing an EKG strip, one can examine each phase of a cardiac cycle, which provides information on cardiac functioning and is useful in detecting abnormalities of rate, rhythm, or regularity. A description of how an EKG is measured is beyond the scope of this chapter; however, Figure 3.4 illustrates an EKG representation of one cardiac cycle.

The different parts of an EKG strip include

- *P wave:* Atrial depolarization, during which the electrical impulse travels through the atria;
- *PR interval:* AV conduction time, during which the impulse travels from the atria,

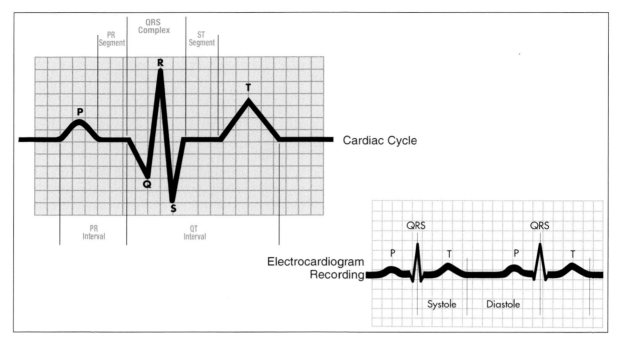

Figure 3.4. Electrocardiogram representation of one cardiac cycle and example of electrocardiogram recording.
Source. Richard Fritzler, Medical Illustrator, Roswell, GA.

to the AV node, and down the bundle branches, to where the ventricles contract;

- *QRS complex:* Ventricular depolarization, during which the impulse travels through the ventricles;

- *T wave:* Ventricular repolarization, during which ventricles return to their resting state; and

- *ST segment:* Early repolarization, during which the ST segment should be at baseline. If it is elevated or depressed it may be an indication of MI or ischemia.

Blood Pressure

Another measure of cardiac function is *blood pressure (BP)*, which provides information on the pressure or force of circulating blood on the walls of arterial blood vessels. A common way of measuring blood pressure noninvasively is with a sphygmomanometer and inflatable cuff, which measures blood pressure in millimeters of mercury (mm HG).

The *sphygmomanometer* is a blood pressure meter that reflects the highest and lowest

values of pressure exerted against the artery wall during a cardiac cycle. When blood pressure is being measured, the cuff feels tight and uncomfortable because it must be sufficiently inflated to occlude the brachial artery. As cuff pressure slowly releases, the pounding sound heard through the stethoscope is the sound of the artery filling up again with blood—the recorded systolic blood pressure. The last sound heard is the recorded diastolic pressure. *Systolic blood pressure* (the higher number) is the amount of pressure exerted at the beginning of a cycle, and *diastolic blood pressure* is the lowest pressure exerted during the relaxation phase of a heart cycle.

Electronic blood pressure machines are more commonly used but are not as accurate as using a manual sphygmomanometer and stethoscope. These machines actually measure mean arterial pressure and then calculate what the systolic and diastolic values should be. *Mean arterial pressure* is the average pressure during a cardiac cycle. Table 3.1 lists general adult blood pressure ranges.

Another method exists for measuring arterial blood pressure, but it is an invasive

Table 3.1. Adult Blood Pressure Ranges

Category	Systolic (top number)		Diastolic (bottom number)
Normal	Less than 120	*And*	Less than 80
Prehypertension	120–139	*Or*	80–89
High blood pressure			
Stage 1	140–159	*Or*	90–99
Stage 2	160 or higher	*Or*	100 or higher

Source. National Heart Lung and Blood Institute Diseases and Conditions.

technique. A needle inserted directly into an artery continuously measures pressure exerted on the arterial wall. Although the needle is usually inserted into the radial artery, it can also be inserted into the axillary, femoral, or pedal arteries. Arterial blood pressure or "art line" measurement is usually restricted to the intensive care unit (refer to Chapter 2) and is often used for patients who are hemodynamically unstable, requiring close monitoring of their blood pressure. An inserted arterial line catheter connects to a transducer, which changes pressure readings into an electrical signal or waveform seen on a bedside monitor. Attached to a bedside pole, the transducer sits level with the fourth intercostal space.

When mobilizing patients with art lines, be aware that changing the patient's position, and therefore the angle of the transducer, may render inaccurate blood pressure readings on the monitor. Most patients who have an art line also have a traditional blood pressure cuff, and the readings should be the same but often are not. Art lines are sewn in, and wrist movements are usually kept to a minimum using an arm board or IV splint; however, the risk of severe bleeding if an art line becomes dislodged is always present.

Risk Factors for Heart Disease

In 1948, the Framingham Heart Study and the National Heart, Lung, and Blood Institute (NHLBI) undertook a long-standing epidemiological project to determine incidence, prevalence, and risk factors contributing to heart disease (Framingham Heart Study, 2009). Many risk factors for heart disease have been identified, and not all are preventable or modifiable. Table 3.2 lists modifiable and nonmodifiable heart disease risk factors. Some common risk factors include being overweight; having a sedentary lifestyle, high cholesterol, and a family history of heart disease; age; and gender. Any one risk factor can contribute to heart disease; however, having more than one risk factor increases the probability of developing a cardiovascular disease.

Making a commitment to a healthy lifestyle and behavioral changes reduce modifiable risk factors and may prevent or reduce the risk of developing heart disease or limit its progression (Lorig et al., 2000). Occupational therapists can be instrumental in reinforcing education addressing modifiable risk factors.

Cardiac Conditions, Diseases, and Disorders

As previously stated, cardiac conditions and diseases, whether a primary diagnosis or a comorbidity, can have a profound effect on other organ systems and quality of life. This section provides

Table 3.2. Heart Disease Risk Factors	
Preventable or Modifiable	**Not Correctable**
<ul><li>High cholesterol</li><li>Cigarette smoking</li><li>Diet high in saturated fat and calories</li><li>Excess alcohol consumption</li><li>High blood pressure or hypertension</li><li>Thrombogenic risk factors (e.g., elevated plasma fibrinogen)</li><li>Diabetes mellitus or hyperglycemia</li><li>Being overweight, obesity</li><li>Left ventricular hypertrophy</li><li>Physical inactivity and sedentary lifestyle</li><li>Psychosocial factors and emotional stress (i.e., anxiety, depression, personality traits and disorders)</li></ul>	<ul><li>Heredity—Family history of heart disease before age 55 in men and age 65 in women</li><li>Age—Older than 60</li><li>Gender—Men have a higher incidence of heart disease</li><li>After menopause in women</li><li>Personal history of coronary artery disease (e.g., stroke or peripheral vascular disease)</li></ul>

Sources. Cassady (2004), Goodman and Smirnova (2009), Roitman and LaFontaine (2006).

an overview of cardiac disorders frequently encountered in the acute care setting.

Coronary Artery Disease

Coronary artery disease (CAD) primarily occurs secondary to atherosclerosis or narrowing of coronary arteries. *Atherosclerosis* is the buildup of fatty deposits and plaque on the lining of blood vessel walls. Narrowed blood vessels restrict blood flow with a consequent reduction of necessary oxygen and nutrients that are unable to reach the heart muscle. The formation of atherosclerosis plaque is a complex and progressive process that may be triggered by injury, rupture, an inflammatory or infectious response, or a structural or genetic predisposition (McConnell & Klinger, 2006). If untreated, *myocardial ischemia* (reduction in blood flow and tissue injury) or *myocardial infarction* (death of heart tissue) occurs.

CAD can also contribute to angina, arrhythmias, heart failure, and sudden death (Gould, 2006; McConnell & Klinger, 2006).

A related disease, *peripheral artery disease (PAD)*, is narrowing of the arteries to the limbs and pelvis but not the heart. A common symptom is intermittent claudication (cramping and pain when walking). Because PAD is a circulatory problem, it can eventually lead to gangrene and amputation if untreated. Refer to Chapter 4 for more information on PAD.

CAD, one of the leading causes of death in the industrialized world (McConnell & Klinger, 2006), is often undiagnosed until a patient has a heart attack. The signs and symptoms of CAD include chest pain (angina), nausea and vomiting, *diaphoresis* (excessive sweating), fatigue, pallor, cool extremities, and shortness of breath ("Cardiovascular Disorders," 2006). Treatment for CAD may consist of medication (e.g., beta blockers, calcium channel blockers, nitrates), surgical intervention, risk factor modification, and exercise (Miller, 2006).

Surgical intervention may include coronary artery bypass graft (CABG), atherectomy, or percutaneous transluminal coronary angioplasty (PTCA) with balloon or stent placement. For more detail, refer to the "Medical and Surgical Management of Heart Disease" section.

Angina

More than 6 million Americans are estimated to have angina, with an incidence of 20%–25% of men and 14%–25% of all women older than age 65 (Miller, 2006). In CAD, narrowed coronary arteries result in reduced blood flow, which causes chest pains known as angina. Pains are described as pressure, tightness, or squeezing in the chest; however, pain can also be felt in the jaw, neck, and left arm. The two common forms of angina are stable and unstable. *Stable angina* is the most common and usually resolves after a few minutes of rest or with medication (e.g., nitroglycerin). Stable angina usually occurs under the same circumstances and with the same level of activity or exercise (Miller, 2006).

Unstable angina has no pattern and is not triggered by any particular activity. It is usually caused by a rupture of plaque with thrombus formation that occludes one of the coronary arteries (Levine, 2006). Unstable angina does not resolve with rest or prescribed medication and requires emergency treatment because it may be indicative of a heart attack.

The third type of angina is the rare *Prinzmetal's* or *variant angina*. Experienced as chest pain at rest and caused by occlusion of the blood vessel by vasospasm and not atherosclerosis, this type of angina occurs in cycles. Prinzmetal's angina is more common among younger women with arrhythmias or conduction defects (Goodman & Smirnova, 2009).

Myocardial Infarction

MI affects more than 1 million people annually and is the leading cause of death in the United States (Goodman & Smirnova, 2009). An MI is also commonly known as a *heart attack* and may result from unstable angina (Miller, 2006). In MI, blood and oxygen to the heart muscle is reduced because of a coronary artery blood vessel plaque rupture or thrombus formation. Reduction in blood supply to the myocardium results in irreversible tissue damage and necrosis.

Acute MI is frequently referred to in medical records as an *ST elevated MI (STEMI)* or a *non-ST elevated MI (NSTEMI)*. ST refers to the segment on an EKG that reflects ventricle repolarization. An STEMI, or transmural MI, usually signifies more profound tissue damage because it implies full thickness necrosis. An NSTEMI, or nontransmural MI, is limited to one or two layers of the heart but not all three layers. The location of the occlusion, the length of time of the occlusion, and the presence of collateral circulation determines the extent of damage from an MI. The endocardium is the layer farthest from the arterial blood supply and the most prone to damage.

The risk factors for MI are the same as for heart disease (e.g., family history of heart disease, smoking, hypertension, obesity). Additional causes include cocaine use, vasculitis, aortic stenosis, and aortic root or coronary artery dissection (Goodman & Smirnova, 2009). An MI may be silent (asymptomatic), or the patient may present with complaints of chest pain, nausea or vomiting, fatigue, shortness of breath, perspiration, cool or clammy skin, anxiety, or restlessness. Pain may be described as a crushing chest pain that radiates to the jaw, neck, or left arm. Women often experience early warning symptoms of unusual fatigue, shortness of breath, anxiety, and sleep disturbances several weeks preceding an MI (McSweeney et al., 2003). Prescribed blood tests look for chemical markers such as creatine kinase or tropinins that are indicative of an MI (refer to Appendix P for more information on cardiac markers). Complications from MI may include arrhythmias, cardiogenic shock, pericarditis, clots, CHF, or sudden death (Goodman & Smirnova, 2009).

The focus of treatment for MI is on limiting damage to the heart muscle, relieving pain, preventing clot formation, and improving blood flow to the area of injury (reestablishing adequate circulation to coronary arteries). Medical

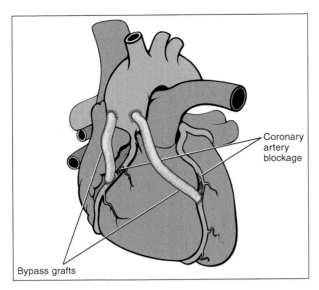

Figure 3.5. View of the heart after bypass surgery.
Source. Richard Fritzler, Medical Illustrator, Roswell, GA.

management includes cardiac monitoring, medication (e.g., nitroglycerin, beta blockers, angiotensis converting enzymes [ACE] inhibitors, aspirin, anticoagulants), supplemental oxygen therapy, or revascularization surgery (i.e., CABG; see Figure 3.5).

It usually takes 4–8 weeks for heart muscle to heal, depending on the extent of damage (Huntley, 2008). Early activity after acute MI should not exceed 1–2 metabolic equivalents (METs), or a 2- to 4-MET range for recommended home exercise programs (Goodman & Smirnova, 2009; Huntley, 2008). Refer to Appendixes 3.A and 3.B for sample MET levels.

Contraindications for therapy may include

- Active signs and symptoms of MI (e.g., nausea, shortness of breath, light-headedness, chest pain),
- Acute MI (<1 day or 2 days after MI),
- Active infection,
- Acute myocarditis or pericarditis,
- Digoxin toxicity,
- Uncontrolled arrhythmias,
- Uncontrolled diabetes,
- Severe CHF,
- Recent pulmonary embolism, and

- Abnormal vital signs and blood counts (O_2 saturation <85%, respiration rate >45 breaths per minute, hemoglobin <8 g/dL or hematocrit <26%; Goodman & Smirnova, 2009).

Cardiomyopathy

Cardiomyopathies, according to the AHA's scientific statement, are a heterogeneous group of diseases of the myocardium associated with mechanical and/or electrical dysfunction that usually (but not invariably) exhibit inappropriate ventricular hypertrophy or dilatation and are due to a variety of causes that frequently are genetic. Cardiomyopathies either are confined to the heart or are part of generalized systemic disorders, often leading to cardiovascular death or progressive heart failure–related disability. (Maron et al., 2006, p. 1809)

Cardiomyopathies may be the result of myocardial contractibility (i.e., systolic or diastolic dysfunction) or diseases that impair the heart's electrical conductivity. According to the AHA, cardiomyopathy is now categorized as either primary (genetic, mixed [genetic and nongenetic], or acquired) or secondary (Maron et al., 2006). Primary cardiomyopathies are largely confined to the heart muscle and affect the heart's ability to pump blood to the rest of the body. The three most common types of primary cardiomyopathy are dilated (mixed), hypertrophic (genetic), and restrictive (mixed; see Figure 3.6).

Dilated cardiomyopathy involves a loss of heart muscle tone, and heart chambers become dilated or enlarged. The left ventricle loses contractability, becomes weaker, and cannot effectively pump blood out to systemic circulation (i.e., systolic dysfunction). As a result, CO decreases, and the risk of blood clot formation is greater. Dilated cardiomyopathy is also the third most common form of heart failure and an indication for heart transplantation (Maron et al., 2006).

Hypertrophic cardiomyopathy involves a thickening of the left ventricle and interventricular septum. Enlargement of the septum can lead

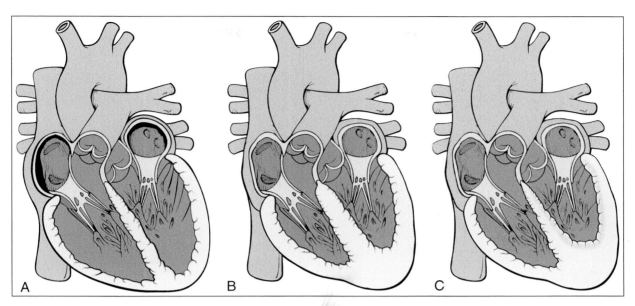

Figure 3.6. A. Dilate cardiomyopathy. B. Hypertrophic cardiomyopathy. C. Restrictive cardiomyopathy.
Source. Richard Fritzler, Medical Illustrator, Roswell, GA.

to obstruction of left ventricle blood flow. The left ventricle becomes stiffer and has less ability to fill up during diastole. Left ventricle volume diminishes, leading to increased pulmonary pressure with resultant dyspnea. Hypertrophic cardiomyopathy is usually hereditary, is the most commonly occurring cardiomyopathy, and is also the most common cause of sudden death in young people, including athletes (Maron et al., 2006).

Restrictive cardiomyopathy, the least common form, involves thickening and rigidity of the ventricles with decreased ventricular filling. As a result, CO falls because of decreased systole and diastole. Severe restrictive cardiomyopathy is irreversible ("Cardiovascular Disorders," 2006).

Acquired cardiomyopathy includes myocarditis, an inflammatory cardiomyopathy. Myocarditis may be caused by virus, bacteria, fungus, parasites, toxins, or drugs. Myocarditis can lead to dilated cardiomyopathy and left ventricular dysfunction (Maron et al., 2006). Two additional forms of acquired cardiomyopathy are those caused by extreme emotional stress or occurring postpartum. Table 3.3 lists the different types of primary cardiomyopathy and their etiology, symptoms, and treatment.

Secondary cardiomyopathies are systemic diseases with myocardial involvement that are not necessarily confined to the heart muscle. These may include

- Infiltrative diseases (e.g., amyloidosis)
- Storage diseases (e.g., hemochromatosis)
- Endomyocardial fibrosis
- Endocrine disorders (e.g., diabetes mellitus, thyroid disease)
- Nutritional deficiencies
- Electrolyte imbalances
- Autoimmune or collagen disorders (e.g., lupus, rheumatoid arthritis, scleroderma)
- Neurological or neuromuscular disorders (e.g., muscular dystrophy)
- Drug or heavy metal toxicity
- Cancer treatment (Maron et al., 2006).

Inflammatory Diseases and Cardiac Tamponade

Bacteria, which enter the heart from the bloodstream, cause an infection in the endocardium and heart valves called *endocarditis*. This bacteria may be introduced through a dental procedure, a urinary tract infection, or IV drug use. However, many other potential causes exist,

Table 3.3.   Types of Primary Cardiomyopathy

Category	Cause	Signs and Symptoms	Treatment
Dilated cardiomyopathy	• Viral or bacterial infection • Hypertension • Ischemic or valvular heart disease • Chemotherapy • Toxic effects of drugs or alcohol on the heart	• SOB • DOE • Orthopnea • Fatigue • Peripheral edema • Peripheral cyanosis • Weight gain • Enlarged liver • JVD • Weight gain • Dry cough at night • Tachycardia	• Treatment of underlying cause • Medication (e.g., anticoagulants, antiarrhythmic drugs, vasodilators, diuretics) • Cardioversion • Pacemaker or ICD placement • Surgery: Revascularization, valve repair or replacement, heart transplantation • Lifestyle modification (e.g., avoidance of alcohol, smoking cessation, dietary changes such as eating a diet low in fat and salt or restricting fluids)
Hypertrophic cardiomyopathy	• Hereditary • Hypertension • Thyroid disease • Obstructive valvular disease	• Angina • Syncope • Dizziness • Dyspnea • Fatigue • Heart murmur • Cardiac arrhythmia	• Medication (e.g., beta blockers, anticoagulant and antiarrhythmic drugs) • Ablation • Cardioversion • Pacemaker or ICD insertion • Mitral valve repair or replacement • Heart transplantation • Septal myectomy or ventricular myotomy
Restrictive cardiomyopathy	• Amyloidosis or sarcoidosis • Hemochromatosis (hereditary iron overload disease) • Infiltrative neoplastic disease (tumors)	• Fatigue • DOE • Orthopnea • Chest pain • Peripheral edema • Ascites • JVD • Liver engorgement • Peripheral cyanosis • Pallor	• Treatment of underlying cause • Medication (e.g., beta blockers, digoxin, vasodilators, diuretics) • Low-sodium diet

Note. DOE = dyspnea on exertion; ICD = implantable cardioverter–defibrillator; JVD = jugular vein distension; SOB = shortness of breath.
Source. "Cardiovascular Disorders" (2006).

including preexisting heart conditions such as rheumatic disease, mitral valve prolapse, existing prosthetic heart valves, Marfan syndrome, hospital-acquired infections, diabetes mellitus, or congenital abnormalities. Poor dental hygiene may also contribute to development of endocarditis.

The same bacteria that cause endocarditis can also cause vegetation (e.g., bacteria, fibrin, platelets) on the heart's valves. These vegetations are at risk of breaking off, forming emboli, which can occlude other blood vessels. Symptoms of endocarditis include fever; fatigue; dyspnea; weight loss; night sweats; joint pain; numbness in the arms or legs; heart murmurs; and splenic, renal, cerebral, or pulmonary infarctions (Malone, 2006). Endocarditis may be treated with antibiotics, bed rest, fluids, or surgery. Those people at risk for endocarditis commonly take antibiotics before dental procedures.

Myocarditis is an inflammation of the myocardium or heart muscle secondary to viral, bacterial, parasitic, or fungal infection. It is associated with immunosuppression (e.g., chemotherapy), allergic reactions, exposure to certain chemicals, and systemic diseases. Signs and symptoms may include dyspnea, orthopnea, fatigue, chest pain, cardiac arrhythmias, fluid retention, or fever. Myocarditis can lead to dilated cardiomyopathy, CHF, or even sudden death. Bacterial infections are treated with antibiotics. Viral infections are treated symptomatically, including steroids for inflammation and diuretics to remove excessive fluid.

Myocarditis is also frequently associated with *pericarditis,* an inflammation of the pericardium. Acute pericarditis may be secondary to a heart attack, open heart surgery, immunologic conditions, uremia, kidney failure, or infection (Malone, 2006). Symptoms include chest pain, fever, dry cough, and fatigue. Pericarditis may lead to cardiac tamponade and heart failure. Treatment consists of nonsteroidal anti-inflammatory drugs, steroids, antibiotics, pericardiocentesis, or surgery.

Cardiac tamponade results from increased pericardial effusion. This fluid buildup exerts a squeezing pressure against the heart muscle, interfering with coronary blood flow. The resultant heart chamber compression prevents normal diastole of the ventricles, leading to decreased CO. Causes of cardiac tamponade include hypothyroidism, trauma, viral pericarditis, chronic renal failure requiring dialysis, cancer, autoimmune conditions, infection, and acute MI, or it may be idiopathic ("Cardiovascular Disorders," 2006). Symptoms include elevated central venous pressure, muffled heart sounds, diaphoresis, cyanosis, anxiety, cough, dyspnea, and tachypnea ("Cardiovascular Disorders," 2006). Treatment may include medication, pericardiocentesis, or pericardectomy.

Valvular Heart Disease

The four valves of the heart open and close in a precise sequence, allowing blood flow in only one direction. For example, when the tricuspid and mitral valves open, the pulmonic and aortic valves close. On an EKG, opening and closing valve movements resemble hands clapping. If the valves do not work properly, then the heart muscle has to work harder to circulate blood. When the malfunction is mild, the heart can compensate; however, when the problem is severe, it can lead to serious consequences such as compromised CO, arrhythmias, and heart failure. *Valvular heart disease* may be caused by endocarditis, rheumatic fever, congenital heart disease, cardiomyopathy, aortic root dilatation, or atherosclerotic heart disease, in which muscles supporting the valves are infarcted (Miller, 2006).

The three categories of valve disorder are stenosis, regurgitation, and prolapse. With *stenosis,* or narrowing of the opening, the valves do not open properly, which restricts blood flow. This stenosis may also cause the chamber behind the valve to hypertrophy, because it has to work harder against the obstructed valve. Blood from the right side of the heart may back up into the veins, and blood from the left side of the heart may back up into the lungs. With *regurgitation* or insufficiency, the valve does not close properly and blood flow, normally in one direction, now leaks back to where it came from. For example, in mitral valve regurgitation, less blood flows from the left atrium into the left ventricle. Moreover, the left ventricle now has to repump the blood that leaked back into the left atrium. *Prolapse* affects only the cusps of the mitral valve and is present in approximately 2% of Americans. In *prolapse*, the valves' leaflets do not close properly; rather, they bulge upward into the left atrium. In most cases, prolapse is not problematic, but it can lead to the more serious condition of mitral regurgitation.

Of the disorders that affect the heart's valves, aortic and mitral valve disorders are more common than pulmonic (rare) or tricuspid disorders. Valvular stenosis and regurgitation cause the sound of the blood flow to be heard as a murmur. Treatment for valvular disorders can include medication to treat symptoms, surgical repair, or replacement if the disorder is severe enough. Repair is preferable to replacement because the heart muscle strength and function are preserved, resulting in a lower risk of endocarditis, negating permanent anticoagulation (NHLBI, 2007). Valve repair may serve to remove or reshape faulty valve tissue, separate fused leaflets, or patch holes or tears in valve tissue (NHLBI, 2007). Valve repair can also be performed through a cardiac catheterization procedure. Valvuloplasty and valvotomy, respectively, dilate or enlarge a narrowed valve (i.e., stenosis) by threading a catheter with a balloon through a heart valve. Annuloplasty, in which placement of a prosthetic ring assists with valve closure, is often performed for regurgitation or prolapse (Malone, 2006).

In replacement surgery, prosthetic valves replace the natural valve and are either tissue or mechanical in nature. Mechanical valves are more durable than tissue valves, but the risk of clot formation increases, and patients must permanently take daily anticoagulation medication. Tissue valves do not have the same risk for clots but do not last as long (approximately 10–15 years; Huntley, 2008; NHLBI, 2007). Tissue valves can come from pigs, cows, or human cadavers.

Valve repair and replacement is usually an open-heart procedure with a traditional sternotomy or thoracotomy; however, more minimally invasive procedures (e.g., transapical approach) are currently being performed. The advantages of minimally invasive procedures include less pain, less bleeding, quicker healing time, shorter hospital stays, and quicker resumption of desired occupations. Table 3.4 includes a list of common valvular disorders, their symptoms, and the traditional treatment approach.

Aortic Aneurysms

An *aortic aneurysm* is a weakening and bulging of a segment of the aorta, which has four parts: the *ascending aorta,* the *aortic arch,* the *descending thoracic aorta,* and the *abdominal aorta.* An aneurysm can occur at any point along the aorta's path. Aneurysms of the ascending aorta, aortic arch, or descending thoracic aorta are all called *thoracic aortic aneurysms.* Abdominal aortic aneurysms are the more common type. Although aortic aneurysms are a vascular issue, they have important repercussions for cardiac functioning.

An aortic aneurysm can lead to aortic dissection or rupture. If an aneurysm ruptures, it can cause internal bleeding, compromise vital functions, and even cause death. Sometimes an infection will cause a pseudo-aneurysm, in which only two of the three layers of the blood vessel are involved; however, a serious risk of rupture still exists. An aortic dissection involves a tear in the inner lining of the blood vessel so that blood leaks between layers. This further weakens the blood vessel, making it susceptible to rupture.

Certain risk factors are associated with aortic aneurysm, including hypertension, atherosclerosis, heredity, and Marfan syndrome, with symptoms including syncope and radiating severe chest or back pain (Goodman & Smirnova, 2009; West, Paz, & Vashi, 2009). Clots from an aneurysm can cause stroke and heart attack. Although thoracic aortic aneurysms account for only 10% of aneurysms, they are more life threatening than other types of aneurysms (Goodman & Smirnova, 2009).

Abdominal aortic aneurysms usually develop slowly, and treatment consists of medication and close monitoring. However, surgical intervention

(Text continues on p. 91)

Table 3.4.   **Valvular Disorders, Symptoms, and Treatment**

Valve Disorder	Causes	Signs and Symptoms	Treatment
Aortic stenosis: Narrowing of the valve between the left ventricle and the aorta; most common valvular lesion in the United States. Occurs more often in men than in women.	• Age-associated degeneration • Atherosclerosis (calcification and hardening of the aortic valve) • Inflammation • Congenital rheumatic fever (rare)	• Palpitations • Angina • Arrhythmia • Syncope • Left-sided heart failure • Decreased cardiac output • Murmur • Dyspnea • Orthopnea • Weakness • Fatigue	• Monitoring if stenosis is mild to moderate • Valve repair or replacement surgery (if stenosis is severe) • Medication to treat symptoms • Oxygen therapy
Aortic insufficiency or regurgitation: Blood leaks back into the left ventricle.	• Idiopathic • HTN • Endocarditis • Congenital deformity (i.e., associated with ventricular septal defect) • Marfan syndrome • Syphilis • Infections (e.g., rheumatic fever)	• Palpitations • Angina • Syncope • Left-sided heart failure • Arrhythmia • Cough • Pulmonary edema • Murmur • Dyspnea • Weakness • Fatigue	• Monitoring if malfunction is mild • Valve repair or replacement surgery if malfunction is severe • Medication to treat symptoms
Mitral stenosis: narrowing of the valve between the left atrium and the left ventricle; results in less blood flow to the left ventricle. More common in women.	• Congenital or rheumatic fever (rare because rates are declining) • Endocarditis	• Orthopnea • Cough • Palpitations • Right-sided heart failure • Atrial fibrillation • Murmur • Lower-extremity swelling • Peripheral edema • JVD • Ascites	• Valve repair (e.g., balloon valvuloplasty) or replacement surgery if malfunction is severe • Medication to treat symptoms • Monitoring if malfunction is mild

(continued)

Table 3.4.   (continued)

Valve Disorder	Causes	Signs and Symptoms	Treatment
		• Hepatomegaly • Dyspnea • Paroxysmal nocturnal dyspnea • Weakness	
Mitral insufficiency and regurgitation	• Rheumatic fever • Hypertrophic obstructive cardiomyopathy • Myocardial infarction • CAD • Marfan syndrome • SLE • Infectious endocarditis • Severe left ventricular failure • Trauma • Myxomatous degeneration • Mitral valve prolapse • Ruptured chordae tendinae • Associated with transposition of great arteries	• Fatigue • Palpitations • Tachycardia • Angina • Right-sided heart failure • Murmur • Peripheral edema • Pulmonary edema • Dyspnea • Orthopnea • Weakness • Fatigue • JVD • Hepatomegaly	• Valve repair or replacement surgery if malfunction is severe • Medication to treat symptoms
Mitral prolapse	• Hereditary • Marfan syndrome • Connective tissue disorders • Ehlers-Danlos syndrome • Polycystic kidney disease	Typically asymptomatic. If symptoms present, usually because of regurgitation and may include • SOB • Dizziness • Fatigue • Palpitations • Arrhythmia	• No treatment if asymptomatic • Medication to treat symptoms • Valve repair or replacement if condition is severe and regurgitation develops

Table 3.4.　(continued)

Valve Disorder	Causes	Signs and Symptoms	Treatment
		• Fatigue • Chest pain • Click-murmur	
Tricuspid regurgitation: Less blood pumped into the right ventricle. Blood leaks back into the right atrium.	• Emphysema • Pulmonary HTN • Right atrium enlargement • Pulmonic valve stenosis	• Arrhythmias • Weakness • Fatigue • Heart failure • Right atrium enlargement • Liver may swell	• Mild regurgitation: little or no treatment • Treatment of underlying cause • Valve repair rarely done unless another valve is also being repaired or replaced (e.g., mitral valve)

Note. CAD = coronary artery disease; HTN = hypertension; JVD = jugular vein distension; SLE = systemic lupus erythematosus; SOB = shortness of breath.
Sources. "Cardiovascular System" (2007), Collins and Dias (2009), Malone (2006).

may be required if the aneurysm enlarges quickly or the risk of rupture outweighs the risks of undergoing surgery. During surgery, an artificial graft replaces the section of damaged blood vessel. This type of open-heart surgery requires a heart bypass machine. In another procedure, a metal or cloth stent may be threaded through a catheter to the damaged area to buttress the weak part of the blood vessel. This less invasive technique is not used with thoracic aortic aneurysm repairs (see Figure 3.7).

Associated risks for surgery include MI, infection at the incision site, renal failure, colon problems, and lower-extremity ischemia. After aneurysm repair surgery, patients are restricted to lifting no more than 10 pounds and are urged to avoid any occupations that require pulling, pushing, or straining (Goodman & Smirnova, 2009).

Arrhythmias

When the heart's conduction system is operating normally, rate and rhythm are regular. However, any conduction disturbances of the heart can lead to changes in rate, rhythm, or regularity, and clinical significance can range from benign to quite serious. As mentioned earlier, the SA node in the right atrium initiates the heart's electrical conduction. It is the heart's natural pacemaker. From there, the impulse travels down to the AV node, on to the Bundle of His, then to the bundle branches, and ultimately to the Purkinje fibers of the ventricles. Conduction problems can occur anywhere along this route. In addition, the autonomic nervous system can affect HR. Increased parasympathetic and decreased sympathetic input can slow HR. Increased sympathetic input and circulating catecholamine hormones result in increased HR.

Arrhythmias are categorized by where the problem originates (e.g., atrium, ventricle, AV junction), the rate (e.g., normal, fast, slow), and regularity. Normal resting HRs are 60 to 100 bpm. A HR below 60 is bradycardia. A HR above 100 is tachycardia. The heart rhythm's pattern can be classified as regular, irregular, regularly irregular, or irregularly irregular. The SA node has the fastest rate of automaticity at 60–100 bpm. The AV node also has automaticity but at a slower rate of 40–60 bpm. The AV node

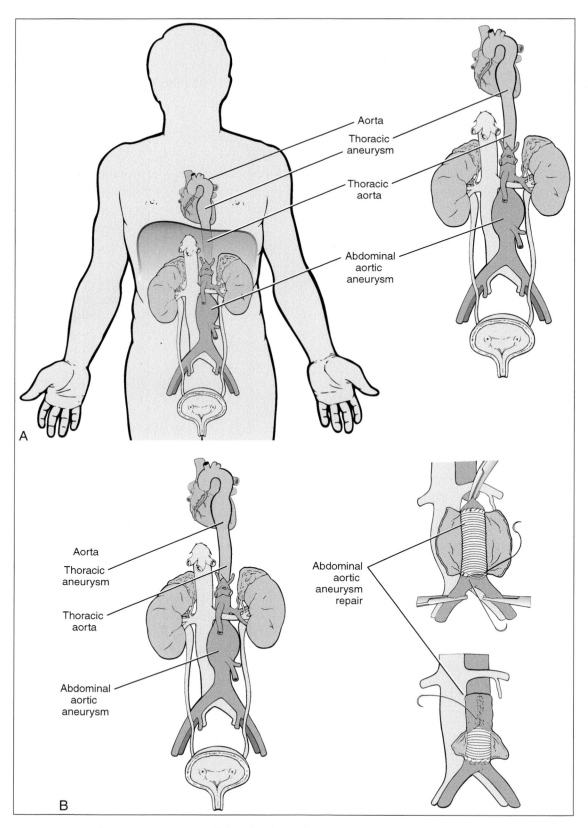

Figure 3.7. A. Aortic aneurysms. B. Abdominal aortic aneurysm repair.
Source. Richard Fritzler, Medical Illustrator, Roswell, GA.

Table 3.5. Heart Rates

Normal Heart Rates	Abnormal Heart Rates
Sinoatrial node: 60–100 bpm Atrioventricular node: 40–60 bpm Ventricular: 20–40 bpm	Bradycardia: <60 bpm Tachycardia: >100 bpm Supraventricular tachycardia: 150–250 bpm Atrial flutter: 250–350 bpm Atrial fibrillation: >350 irregular bpm

Note. bpm = beats per minute.

acts as a backup pacemaker for the heart if the SA node fails to work properly. The ventricles also have their own dangerously slow rate of 20–40 bpm. *Asystole* is the absence of any cardiac electrical activity, resulting in death. Normal and abnormal HRs are listed in Table 3.5.

Uncoordinated, extremely rapid, and irregular contraction of the atria or ventricles is *fibrillation* (see Table 3.6). The heart chamber quivers instead of beating normally. *Atrial fibrillation* is one of the most common arrhythmias, with more than 2 million Americans diagnosed with this condition (AHA, 2009a). Atrial fibrillation rates can be as high as 350–600 bpm (Wung, 2006). Atrial fibrillation may also be a chronic condition that is treated with anti-arrhythmic drugs or shocked back into normal rhythm. When patients with atrial fibrillation are cleared by the physician to work with an occupational therapist, the therapist must first determine whether any activity parameters or precautions exist, then monitor patient tolerance to activity, and modify treatment sessions accordingly.

Atrial flutter is another type of rapid and irregular HR that originates in the atria and has waves on an EKG with a distinctive sawtooth pattern. Atrial rates are usually 250–350 bpm. Treatment consists of atrial pacing at a rapid rate, cardioversion, or medication. Atrial fibrillation and atrial flutter may be sequelae of cardiac surgery or MI.

Ventricular arrhythmias include *premature ventricular contraction (PVC), ventricular tachycardia,* and *ventricular fibrillation.* PVC has an irregular rhythm but a normal rate (e.g., 60–100 bpm). PVC may be triggered by stress, caffeine, smoking, digitalis toxicity, heart disease, or MI (Collins & Dias, 2009). PVC beats may also appear as a couplet (two in a row), bigeminy (every other beat), or trigeminy (every third beat). Ventricular tachycardia has HRs higher than 100 bpm that may be caused by heart disease or acute MI. Therapy should be deferred because the patient is medically unstable. Ventricular fibrillation is very serious because it can lead to cardiac arrest or sudden cardiac death. Table 3.6 lists common cardiac arrhythmias, their etiology, and medical approach.

Causes of arrhythmias may include drug toxicity, electrolyte imbalance, underlying heart disease, hypertension, acid–base imbalances, congenital defects, connective tissue disorders, or emotional stress ("Cardiovascular System," 2007). Even stimulants such as caffeine, nicotine, cocaine, amphetamines, or psychotropic drugs can contribute to arrhythmias. Some arrhythmias are asymptomatic, and others have serious symptoms that may cause death. Symptoms may include palpitation or "fluttering" with premature beats or the sensations of a skipped beat or pause. Symptoms for bradycardia may include fatigue, dizziness, syncope, or presyncope, whereas people with tachycardia may experience palpitations, shortness of breath, chest pain, dizziness, and syncope.

The danger with bradycardia and tachycardia is that the heart beats too slowly or too quickly to meet the body's blood and oxygen demands. When the pumping action is inef-

(Text continues on p. 98)

Table 3.6. Common Cardiac Arrhythmias

Site of Arrhythmia	Origin	Type of Arrhythmia	Cause	Treatment
Sinus node	Sinoatrial node of right atrium	• Sinus bradycardia (regular rhythm; rate <60 bpm) • Sinus tachycardia (regular rhythm; rate >100 bpm)	Bradycardia • Sick sinus syndrome • Hypothyroidism • Inferior wall MI • Increased intracranial pressure • Increased vagal tone • Response to medication Tachycardia • Physiologic response to fever, exercise, pain, anxiety, or dehydration • Left-sided heart failure • Cardiac tamponade • Hyperthyroidism • Anemia • PE • Anterior wall MI • Shock	• Correction of underlying cause • Medication • Pacemaker
Atrial	Right or left atrium	• Premature atrial contractions (irregular rhythm; normal rate 60–100 bpm) • Atrial fibrillation (irregular rhythm; rate >300 bpm) • Atrial flutter (regular or irregular rhythm; rate 250–350 bpm)	Premature atrial contractions • Caffeine • Smoking • Stress Fibrillation • Heart failure or congestive heart failure • Coronary heart disease • Chronic obstructive pulmonary disorder • Cor pulmonale • Ischemic heart disease • PE • RHD • HTN	• Correction of underlying cause • Medication • Ablation • Cardioversion • Possible anticoagulation therapy • Occupational therapy: If cleared for therapy, monitor patient and treat with caution.

Table 3.6.   (continued)

Site of Arrhythmia	Origin	Type of Arrhythmia	Cause	Treatment
		• Supraventricular tachycardia (regular rhythm; rate 160–250 bpm; may be paroxysmal)	• Mitral stenosis • Pericarditis • Medication (e.g., digoxin) Flutter • Heart failure • HTN • CAD • Tricuspid or mitral valve disease • PE • Cor pulmonale • Pericarditis • Inferior wall MI • Digoxin toxicity Supraventricular tachycardia • RHD • Mitral valve prolapse • Cor pulmonale • Digitalis toxicity	
Atrioventricular block	AV node	• First-degree AV block (regular rhythm; normal rate 60–100 bpm) • Second-degree AV block (irregular rhythm; atrial rate > ventricular rate, usually 60–100 bpm)	First degree • Inferior wall MI • Acute myocarditis • Hypothyroidism • Hypokalemia • Digoxin toxicity • Response to medication • Elderly with CHD Second degree • Inferior or anterior wall MI • Acute rheumatic fever	• Correction of underlying cause • Medication • Pacemaker • Discontinuation of digoxin • Occupational therapy: Closely monitor

(*continued*)

Table 3.6. (continued)

Site of Arrhythmia	Origin	Type of Arrhythmia	Cause	Treatment
		• Third-degree AV block (regular rhythm; atrial rate > ventricular rate; total heart block—no transmission of impulse from atria to ventricle)	• Vagal stimulation • Digoxin toxicity • Severe CAD • Acute myocarditis Third degree • Inferior or anterior wall MI • Congenital defect • Rheumatic fever • CAD • Hypoxia • Digoxin toxicity • Lev's disease • Lenegres disease • Complication from mitral valve replacement or ablation • Infection • Electrolyte imbalance	
Junctional	AV junction	• Junctional rhythm	• Inferior wall MI • Hypoxia • Vagal stimulation • Sick sinus syndrome • Valve surgery • Acute rheumatic fever • Digoxin toxicity	• Correction of underlying cause • Pacemaker • Atropine • Occupational therapy: Monitor patient tolerance, consult with medical staff
Ventricular	Right or left ventricle	• Premature ventricular contractions • Ventricular fibrillation	Premature ventricular contractions: • Heart failure • CAD • Previous or acute MI	• Treatment of underlying cause • Electrolytes • Medication

Table 3.6. **(continued)**

Site of Arrhythmia	Origin	Type of Arrhythmia	Cause	Treatment
		• Ventricular tachycardia (V-Tach): Most dangerous arrhythmia because it can cause sudden death	• Hypercapnia • Electrolyte imbalance • Digitalis toxicity • Caffeine, tobacco, alcohol • Stress, anxiety, pain Fibrillation • Severe heart disease • Acute MI • Electrolyte imbalance • Hypoxemia • Alkalosis • Hypothermia • Drug toxicity • Electric shock/ electrocution Tachycardia • MI • Aneurysm • CAD • RHD • Mitral valve prolapse • Heart failure • Cardiomyopathy • HTN • Electrolyte imbalance • Digoxin toxicity • Anxiety	• Discontinuation of drugs causing toxicity • Implantable cardiac defibrillator • Cardiopulmonary resuscitation • Occupational therapy: Defer treatment with V-Tach or ventricular fibrillation. If premature ventricular contractions noted, consult with medical staff, closely monitor

Note. AV = atrioventricular; bpm = beats per minute; CAD = coronary heart disease; CHD = coronary heart disease; CHF = congestive heart failure; CPR = cardiac pulmonary resuscitation; HTN = hypertension; ICD = implantable cardiac defibrillator; MI = myocardial infarction; PE = pulmonary embolism; RHD = rheumatic heart disease.
Sources. "Cardiovascular System" (2007), Collins and Dias (2009).

ficient, it can be a life-threatening condition. With all arrhythmias, the course of treatment focuses on correcting the underlying problem, including use of medication, supplemental oxygen, ablation, pacemaker insertion, implantable cardioverter defibrillator implantation, or cardioversion. Refer to the "Medical and Surgical Management of Heart Disease" section for more information.

Heart Failure and Congestive Heart Failure

Approximately 5 million Americans and 15 million people worldwide currently have CHF (Kavanagh, 2006). *CHF* is a progressive disease that slowly worsens over time. Often, symptoms of heart failure are confused with changes associated with normal aging. However, 1 out of every 10 seniors is diagnosed with heart failure, and heart failure is the most common Medicare diagnosis related group (DRG), with the most medical dollars being spent on diagnosis and treatment (Redman, 2004).

In CHF, the heart is weakened and unable to pump a sufficient amount of blood to meet the body's metabolic needs. Over time, the heart chambers enlarge, making them less and less efficient at pumping blood to the rest of the body, which causes a backup of blood into the venous system, which overloads the tissues (congestion), causing edema. In addition, "vasoconstriction increases total peripheral resistance and thus afterload, adding further to the burden of the failing heart. In short, failure begets failure" (Kavanagh, 2006, p. 141). Heart failure is considered *decompensated* when the heart is unable to maintain adequate circulation but *compensated* when the patient is medically stable (Collins & Dias, 2009).

A variety of conditions contribute to heart failure. These conditions may include hypertension, damage to heart tissue from MI, valvular disease, cardiomyopathy, or congenital heart defects. Hypertension is a predominant risk factor because more than 75% of patients with

CHF have a history of hypertension (Huntley, 2008). Additional risk factors for heart failure include emotional stress, obesity, thyroid disorders, diabetes mellitus, pulmonary disease, renal disease, fever, infection, anemia, drug toxicity, certain medications, or a sedentary lifestyle (Goodman & Smirnova, 2009).

The general symptoms of CHF include dyspnea, orthopnea, fatigue, exercise intolerance, coughing, hepatomegaly, weight gain, and lower-extremity edema from fluid retention. CHF can also lead to pulmonary edema, myopathy, impaired insulin secretion and glucose tolerance, anorexia, malnutrition, and cachexia (Cahalin & Buck, 2004). Heart failure can result in severe debility with a profound effect on quality of life. Most symptoms of heart failure are divided into two general classifications, right-sided or left-sided heart failure. When the right side of the heart fails, blood flows back into the venous system; when the left side of the heart fails, blood flows back to the lungs (Collins & Dias, 2009). The symptoms of both right- and left-sided heart failure are listed in Table 3.7. Cor pulmonale also leads to right-sided heart failure because the right ventricle hypertrophies and dilates in response to a pulmonary circulatory disorder.

Heart failure can also be categorized as systolic or diastolic heart failure. *Systolic heart failure* indicates a problem with systole or ventricular muscle contraction. Systolic dysfunction changes the structure of the ventricles, causing them to enlarge and the muscle to hypertrophy. This remodeling leads to a further deterioration in heart functioning and increased difficulty for the heart to compensate. As a result, the left ventricle cannot pump enough blood out to systemic circulation during systole. Blood backs up into the lungs, and CO falls. EFs usually decrease to less than 40%, and left ventricular end diastolic volume (LVEDV) increases. *Diastolic heart failure* involves an impairment with diastole, or the ventricle relaxation phase when the ventricles fill up with blood before contraction. Afterload increases and SV decreases because the left ventricle cannot fill up sufficiently during dias-

Table 3.7. Types of Heart Failure

Category	Condition	Symptoms
Right-sided heart failure	The right ventricle cannot contract properly. Blood backs up into the peripheral circulation (systemic venous system).	Dyspnea, orthopnea, paroxysmal nocturnal dyspnea, jugular vein distension, cardiac cirrhosis, cyanotic nail beds, hepatomegaly (enlarged liver), ascites, jaundice, right upper-quadrant pain, fatigue, anorexia, nausea, decreased urine output, weight gain, dependent edema in feet and psychological disturbances
Left-sided heart failure	The most common form of heart failure. The left ventricle cannot contract normally. Blood backs up into the lungs, resulting in cardiac output reduction.	Progressive dyspnea, orthopnea, paroxysmal nocturnal dyspnea, cough, pulmonary edema, tachypnea, diaphoresis, enlarged heart, cerebral hypoxia (restlessness, confusion, impaired memory), anxiety, sleep disturbances, fatigue, exercise intolerance, muscular weakness, tachycardia, hemoptysis (coughing up blood), and pallor

Sources. "Cardiovascular Disorders" (2006), Cassady (2004), Goodman and Smirnova (2009).

tole. Left ventricle size and EF may be normal, but the LVEDV decreases.

Over the years, heart failure has been classified in an attempt to make it easier for medical professionals to differentiate between heart failure categories. The New York Heart Association initially classified heart failure into four stages on the basis of functional limitations with physical activity. Although this classification system was originally formulated in 1928, in 1994 the AHA developed a revised and more useful classification system based on functional capacity (see Table 3.8). The American College of Cardiology has also developed a more useful heart failure classification system that also includes management strategies (Collins & Dias, 2009; see Table 3.9).

No matter which classification system is used, the prognosis for CHF is poor, with as much as 50% mortality annually for those with advanced disease (Goodman & Smirnova, 2009). The most common causes of mortality from heart failure are pump failure and development of dangerous arrhythmias. Medical management for heart failure focuses on treating the underlying cause, medication, and lifestyle modification. CHF medications (e.g., ACE inhibitors, beta blockers, digitalis, diuretics, vasodilators) are prescribed to lessen the work of the heart and allow easier blood flow. Surgical intervention for CHF may include revascularization (e.g., CABG), angioplasty, ventricular assist devices (VADs), or heart transplantation. Refer to the "Medical and Surgical Management of Heart Disease" section for more information. Refer to Chapter 14 for more information on heart transplantation.

Table 3.8. **American Heart Association Functional Capacity and Objective Assessment of Patients With Diseases of the Heart**

Class	Functional Capacity	Objective Assessment
Class I	Patients with cardiac disease but without resulting limitation of physical activity. Ordinary physical activity does not cause undue fatigue, palpitation, dyspnea, or anginal pain.	No objective evidence of cardiovascular disease
Class II	Patients with cardiac disease resulting in slight limitation of physical activity. They are comfortable at rest. Ordinary physical activity results in fatigue, palpitation, dyspnea, or anginal pain.	Objective evidence of minimal cardiovascular disease
Class III	Patients with cardiac disease resulting in marked limitation of physical activity. They are comfortable at rest. Less than ordinary activity causes fatigue, palpitation, dyspnea, or anginal pain.	Objective evidence of moderately severe cardiovascular disease
Class IV	Patients with cardiac disease resulting in inability to carry on any physical activity without discomfort. Symptoms of heart failure or the anginal syndrome may be present even at rest. If any physical activity is undertaken, discomfort is increased.	Objective evidence of severe cardiovascular disease

Source. www.americanheart.org. Copyright © 2010 by American Heart Association, Inc. Adapted with permission.

The main goal of treatment is to slow the progression of the disease. In lifestyle management, patients are encouraged to restrict salt intake (≤2 grams per day), weigh themselves daily to see whether they are gaining weight (fluid retention), restrict fluids (<2,000 milliliters per day), exercise regularly to stay active, balance rest and activity, take prescribed medications, and avoid tobacco and limited caffeine and alcohol (Redman, 2004). For therapists working with patients with CHF, allowing them to return to supine after exercise can increase preload, further stressing the heart. Patients should be positioned with the head of the bed elevated or sitting in a chair to minimize pulmonary congestion and improve ventilation. Encourage patients with CHF to engage in their ADLs sitting at the edge of the bed, sitting in a chair, or standing by the sink rather than supine. A cool-down period is also important, and patients should remain upright during exercise recovery.

Congenital Heart Disease

Although most congenital heart defects are addressed in early childhood, these patients may reach adulthood with unresolved or new issues requiring additional medical or surgical treatment. Congenital heart defects are present in 8 of every 1,000 American babies, with more than 1 million adults having a congenital heart disease (Goodman & Smirnova, 2009). Various congenital conditions affect heart function, leading to heart failure or respiratory distress because oxygenated and

Table 3.9. American College of Cardiology Stages of Heart Failure

Stage	Description
A	High risk for heart failure, no structural heart disease or symptoms of heart failure (e.g., patients with hypertension, atherosclerosis, diabetes, metabolic syndrome). Treatment focuses on risk factor modification.
B	Structural heart disease but no symptoms of heart failure (e.g., patients with previous myocardial infarction, asymptomatic valvular disease, left ventricular dysfunction with low ejection fraction). Treatment focuses on risk factor modification and medication. Implantable defibrillator may be indicated.
C	Structural heart disease with prior or current symptoms of heart failure. Symptoms include shortness of breath, fatigue, and exercise intolerance. Treatment focuses on slowing progression of the disease and symptom relief, medication, implantable defibrillator or biventricular pacing (when indicated), and risk factor modification.
D	Refractory heart failure requiring specialized interventions. Patients with marked symptoms at rest despite medical management. Treatment focuses on symptom relief, chronic inotrope medication, permanent mechanical support, heart transplantation, or compassionate end-of-life care or hospice.

Source. Hunt et al. (2001), Collins and Dias (2009).

deoxygenated blood gets mixed. Symptoms can include dyspnea, palpitations, dizziness, fatigue, cyanosis, pulmonary edema, and limited exercise tolerance. Treatment for congenital heart disease may include surgical repair, medication (including oxygen therapy), or heart transplantation.

Common congenital defects include ("Cardiovascular Disorders," 2006)

- *Atrial septal defect:* An opening in the septum allows blood flow from the left to the right atrium instead of between the left atrium and left ventricle. This defect is associated with Down syndrome and may cause right-sided heart enlargement or dilation.

- *Coarctation of the aorta:* Aortic coarctation involves narrowing of the aorta associated with congenital abnormities of the aortic valve and Turner's syndrome. It results in blood vessel pressure changes, which result in left ventricle hypertrophy and dilation of the proximal aorta, and it may limit blood flow to the lower extremities.

- *Patent ductus arteriosus (PDA):* The ductus arteriosus normally closes shortly after birth. In PDA, the duct remains open, allowing a continuous left-to-right flow or shunting. PDA may cause left ventricle hypertrophy, chronic pulmonary artery hypertension, or heart failure.

- *Transposition of the great arteries:* The great blood vessels are in the wrong anatomic position. The aorta exits from the right ventricle, and the pulmonary artery exits from the left ventricle. Pulmonary and systemic circulation do not communicate.

- *Ventricular septal defect:* An opening between both ventricles is present, allowing blood to shunt between the right and left ventricle. Ventricle septal defects normally close on their own and are associated with Down syndrome, premature birth, fetal alcohol syndrome, PDA, and coartication of the aorta.

- *Tetrology of Fallot:* A combination of four cardiac defects associated with fetal alcohol syndrome, Down syndrome, and thalidomide during pregnancy. These defects include pulmonary stenosis, large ventricular septal defect, aortic communication with both ventricles, and right ventricle hypertrophy.

Medical and Surgical Management of Heart Disease

Heart disease is treated in a variety of ways including medication and in some cases invasively through surgical procedures. The following are a list of common encountered procedures, assistive devices, and medications used in the management of heart disease.

Coronary Artery Bypass Graft

CABG surgery involves using a vein or artery from another part of the body to bypass a clogged coronary artery, ensuring adequate blood flow to the heart muscle itself. The two types of CABG surgeries are invasive and minimally invasive. With traditional invasive CABG, an incision is made in the breastbone (a median sternotomy) so the sternum can be pulled apart for easy access to the heart. The heart is attached to a cardiopulmonary bypass machine, and the heart is chemically stopped. The cardiopulmonary bypass allows the body to remain oxygenated even though the heart is no longer beating. The surgeon then takes an artery or vein and attaches it to the aorta and the unclogged portion of the artery. After the graft is completed, the surgeon restarts the heart and closes the incisions.

The advantage of using arteries for grafts is that they remain more patent (open) than veins over time (Levine, 2006). In addition, with a mammary artery graft, only one end is separated and used to bypass the occluded artery; the other end remains in its original position. The left internal mammary artery (LIMA) is usually joined to the left anterior descending artery (LAD). The saphenous vein is often used because it is long and therefore useful for multiple bypasses. In addition, other veins can take over the work of the saphenous vein. However, by 10 years after CABG, most saphenous vein bypass grafts are either occluded or diseased (e.g., saphenous vein graft degeneration; Levine, 2006).

The median incision made through the sternum (sternotomy) is held together with stainless steel wire and usually takes 6 weeks to heal. Until that time, patients are discouraged from engaging in activities that expand the chest or pull the sternum apart. Generally, patients are restricted to lifting no more than 5–10 pounds. Patients are discouraged from using their upper extremities and encouraged to use the stronger muscles of their lower extremities when going from a sitting to a standing position. Patients are also encouraged to splint or brace their chest when coughing (e.g., gently hugging a pillow to their chest). Refer to Appendix 3.C for further therapy guidelines after a sternotomy.

Patients with sternotomy are at risk for infection, mediastinitis, chronic pain, poor wound healing, brachial plexus injury, or posttraumatic stress disorder (Goodman & Smirnova, 2009). Additional postsurgical complications may include diabetes, lung disease (e.g., chronic obstructive pulmonary disease), PAD, or renal disease. In addition, blood clots (deep vein thrombosis), stroke (from a dislodged embolism), sternal wound infections, pneumonia, bleeding, and arrhythmias (atrial fibrillation) are also risks after surgery. Other factors that may influence outcomes are left ventricular EF, urgency (i.e., elective, emergent, or urgent), and prior exercise capacity (Levine, 2006).

"Off-Pump" Coronary Artery Bypass and Endoscopic Atraumatic Coronary Artery Bypass

Two minimally invasive revascularization CABG surgeries include the *"off-pump" coronary artery bypass (OPCAB)* and the *endoscopic atraumatic coronary artery bypass (ENDO–ACAB)*. In both procedures, a heart–lung bypass machine is not used. The advantage is that the heart is not stopped; therefore, the temporary neurocognitive impairments (postperfusion syndrome) that are typically seen with traditional CABG are absent. Neurocognitive changes may be the result of intraoperative hypotension or impaired cerebral profusion (Levine, 2006). An OPCAB procedure is still accessed through a median sternotomy; however, an ENDO–ACAB procedure does not involve sternotomy. Access to the heart is through an incision between the ribs, which allows shorter recovery time and quicker resumption of routine activities. An ENDO–ACAB is performed when only one or two arteries are bypassed.

Atherectomy and Percutaneous Transluminal Coronary Angioplasty

Another procedure to clear clogged arteries is *atherectomy*. A threaded laser catheter or rotating shaver removes plaque from inside arterial walls. Balloon angioplasty is sometimes used after atherectomy. PTCA or balloon angioplasty uses a balloon-tipped catheter threaded through an artery (usually in the groin) until it reaches the location of the blockage. Once inflated, it broadens the narrowed vessel. With vessel blockage reduced, the balloon then deflates.

In addition, placement of a stent (a wire mesh tube) ensures the blood vessel remains open and unobstructed after the angioplasty. Treated stents (e.g., drug-eluting stents or medicated stents) reduce the risk of restenosis. Of MI patients, 20% undergo angioplasty, and 25%–40% with only balloon angioplasty eventually have restenosis (Levine, 2006).

Ablation

Ablation is the process in which the tissue causing an arrhythmia is destroyed. Ablation is a minimally invasive procedure that uses a catheter threaded through a blood vessel (from the groin or neck) to the heart that destroys the site of abnormal electrical impulse (ectopic), thereby restoring normal heart rhythm. The patient is usually on bed rest for 4–6 hours after the procedure. Ablations are used to treat atrial fibrillation, atrial flutter, atrial tachycardia, and AV tachycardia.

Pacemakers and Implantable Defibrillation Devices

A *pacemaker* is a small electronic device that regulates heartbeats when a problem exists in the heart's electrical system. The pacemaker senses when HR slows below a certain set point and sends a signal that induces the heart to beat. A pacemaker can be external (temporary) or internal (permanent) with implantation in the upper chest. The pacemaker is made up of leads attached to the heart and a generator. The generator is a small box with a battery and a programmable chip. It senses the heart's beat and sends out electrical signals that stimulate it to beat in a normal fashion. The different types of pacemakers are single chamber, dual chamber, biventricular, and rate responsive. A single chamber pacemaker carries signals between one chamber of the heart (e.g., right atrium) and the generator. A dual chamber pacemaker carries signals from both right atrium and right ventricle to the generator, coordinating contraction of both chambers. A biventricular pacer has three leads, one to the right atrium, and one to each ventricle. Rate responsive pacemakers are programmed to signal heart rate changes based on physical activity level (NHLBI, 2009).

Pacemaker precautions include no vigorous activity for the first few weeks, no lifting of more than 10 pounds, and no shoulder flexion or abduction greater than 90 degrees of the upper extremity on the side where the pacemaker was implanted. However, patients may engage in their normal ADLs within those parameters. Electrical devices that affect pacemaker function (e.g., iPods, MRIs, magnets, metal detectors) should generally be avoided. Therapy is contraindicated with patients with a temporary pacemaker because mobilization may dislodge pacing wires (Stiller, 2007).

The automatic implantable cardioverter defibrillator is also a device that senses the heart's rhythm. When ventricular fibrillation, ventricular tachycardia, or supraventricular tachycardia occur, the automatic implantable cardioverter defibrillator shocks the heart back into a normal rhythm—an extremely unpleasant sensation for the patient.

Cardioversion

Cardioversion is another technique used to shock the heart back into normal rhythm. It can be chemical or electrical. *Chemical cardioversion* involves taking antiarrhythmia medications. *Electrical cardioversion* is a synchronized electrical shock that disrupts the abnormal rhythm. The patient is sedated, and special pads connected to a defibrillator are placed on the body. The heart is then shocked back into a normal rhythm.

Circulatory Assist Devices: VAD and IABP

A *VAD* is a mechanical device that assists the ventricles' normal pumping action (see Figure 3.8). VADs are used for inpatients with end-stage heart failure as a bridge to transplantation or as destination therapy for those patients who are not candidates for heart transplantation. Various types of VADs are *right ventricle (RVAD), left ventricle (LVAD),* and both *right and left ventricle (BiVAD).* In addition, VADs can be external or implantable and either electric (using a battery source) or pneumatic. Many VADs are portable, and patients return home with them, resuming their everyday activities. However, VAD implantation carries associated risks of renal failure, respiratory failure, infection, or development of clots, leading to stroke. Refer to Appendix 3.D for more information. If a patient has an implantable defibrillator or pacemaker, it is not removed with VAD placement.

Therapy is contraindicated with a VAD rate lower than 50 bpm, volume less than 30 milliliters, systolic blood pressure lower than 80 mm HG, or HR higher than 150 bpm or in the presence of ventricular fibrillation or tachycardia. Resting HR should be less than 100 bpm. Blood pressure is typically measured using a Doppler ultrasound. A traditional blood pressure cuff reading may not be appropriate; there are no systole or diastole sounds (S_1 or S_2) because the VAD pump provides a continuous flow of blood. Tolerance to activity can be monitored by observing CO and HR.

Therapists are cautioned not to pull on drive lines (which connect the VAD to its power source) and to make sure that patients do not step on them during transfers or ambulation, to minimize risk of line dislodgement. Therapists can assist patients with VAD by making sure they have the requisite strength and coordination to carry around battery packs, change the batteries, screw in connections for battery support, and perform any system checks maintenance requirements.

For short-term support, another circulatory assist device called an *intra-aortic balloon pump (IABP)* is used to augment low CO (see Figure 3.8). With this device, a catheter with an attached balloon is threaded through the femoral artery and into the aorta. During diastole, the balloon inflates, and just before systole the balloon deflates, decreasing afterload and thereby increasing the EF and CO. Therapy may be contraindicated with patients with an IABP because they are hemodynamically unstable (Stiller, 2007). Consult with medical staff.

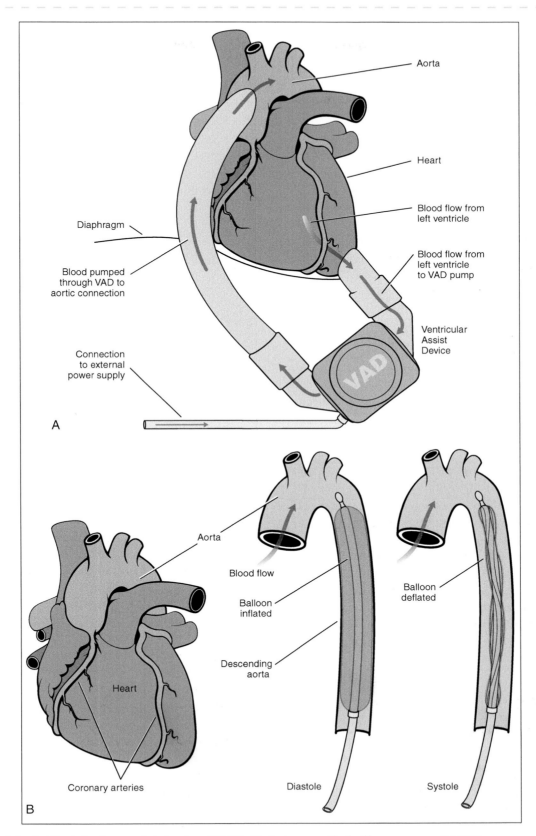

Figure 3.8. A. Ventricular assist device (VAD). B. Intra-aortic balloon pump (IABP).
Source. Richard Fritzler, Medical Illustrator, Roswell, GA.

Medications

Cardiac pharmacology assists by regulating heart function or making the work of the heart easier. Medications are an essential part of medical management for most cardiac diseases. For a list of cardiac medications, refer to Appendix B.

Common medications include

- *Beta-adrenergic blocking agents (beta blockers):* Beta blockers work by lowering blood pressure and slowing down HR by blocking sympathetic conduction of beta receptors on the SA node (Goodman & Smirnova, 2009). They are used to treat angina, high blood pressure, arrhythmias, MI, and CHF.

- *Hypolipidemic agents:* These cholesterol-lowering drugs block bile reabsorption so that the liver can use available cholesterol to make bile acids, thereby lowering blood cholesterol levels.

- *ACE inhibitors:* ACE inhibitors block an enzyme in the body called angiotensin II, which causes vasoconstriction. The result is lowered blood pressure, dilated blood vessels, and increased blood flow.

- *Anticoagulant therapy:* Blood-thinning agents or anticoagulants prevent blood clot formation.

- *Platelet inhibitors:* These inhibitors prevent platelet aggregation and clot formation (Goodman & Smirnova, 2009).

- *Nitrates:* Nitroglycerine taken under the tongue, through a spray, or through a patch dilates coronary blood vessels, thereby increasing blood flow.

- *Calcium channel blockers:* The calcium channel blockers work by relaxing and thereby dilating blood vessels, allowing increased blood flow and lowering blood pressure. They are used in the treatment of hypertension, angina, and arrhythmias. Smoking while taking this medication is contraindicated because it may cause tachycardia.

- *Antiarrythmic medications:* These medications assist in normal conduction of the heart; however, they may exacerbate the very arrhythmia they are intended to correct.

- *Diuretics:* These medications eliminate excess body fluid (fluid retention), thereby decreasing blood pressure.

- *Inotropes:* Inotropes are medications that either strengthen (positive inotrope) or weaken (negative inotrope) cardiac contractibility. Positive agents include catecholamines (e.g., dobutamine, dopamine, epinephrine), are usually prescribed short term, and are administered by IV infusion.

Psychosocial Issues

Patients with heart disease have a strong mind–body connection. With cardiovascular disease, depression has been strongly linked to poorer outcomes, increased morbidity, and increased mortality (Lichtman et al., 2008). The risk of depression is 3 times higher for cardiac patients than for the general population, with 15%–20% of heart patients diagnostically meeting the criteria for major depression (Lichtman et al., 2008). The autonomic nervous system can cause changes in neurotransmitters, elevated lipids, and decreased immune functioning, resulting in a toxic cardiovascular situation (Herridge & Linton, 2006). Chronic stress has also been associated with elevated HR, BP, lipid levels, and blood clotting, which can affect cardiac function and health (Huntley, 2008). Psychological conditions such as depression, anxiety, and stress are strong predictors of health outcomes for patients with heart disease (Herridge & Linton, 2006).

According to Goodman and Smirnova (2009), most patients who experience depression after cardiac surgery generally have a preexisting history of depression. This finding may be a consequence of depression's being associated with cardiovascular risk factors (Lichtman et al., 2008). Depression can lead to engagement in unhealthy behaviors and other psychological factors, including poor diet, sedentary lifestyle, poor coping skills, social isolation, substance abuse, and poor compliance with prescribed medications. All these conditions can contribute to the development of heart disease risk factors.

Patients may feel vulnerable and frightened not only because of their disease but also as a result of being admitted as to the hospital. Therapists should be aware of signs of patient distress, including depression and anxiety. These signs may manifest as flat affect, loss of interest in care or participation in therapy, changes in sleep patterns and eating habits, low energy, poor concentration, restlessness, fear of being alone, or panic attacks. Treatment for depression usually includes antidepressant medication, cognitive–behavioral therapy (or a combination of both), and physical activity. Exercise contributes to increased cardiovascular fitness and diminishes symptoms of depression (Lichtman et al., 2008). Therapists can assist patients by offering support and reassurance or, when warranted, referral to psychosocial services. Patients may also benefit from a referral to support groups such as Mended Hearts, a national organization affiliated with the AHA (Mended Hearts, 2009).

Occupational Therapy Approach

Cardiac functioning has a profound effect on patients' ability to engage in desired and necessary occupations. If the heart does not pump efficiently, circulation of oxygen and nutrients necessary for homeostasis and survival are impaired. Even non–cardiac-related medical treatments can result in arrhythmias, decreased oxygenation, emotional stress, or changes in HR and BP, thereby compromising cardiac function (Goodman & Smirnova, 2009). Appendix 3.E lists tests frequently used in diagnosing cardiac diseases and disorders. Because cardiac functioning is so important for quality of life and the ability to engage in occupations, the therapist needs a basic understanding of it to educate patients on the cardiac system and its effects on all body systems.

Rehabilitation for the cardiac patient occurs in three phases. Phase 1 occurs in the inpatient setting, Phase 2 is a formal outpatient rehabilitation program (usually lasting 6–12 weeks), and Phase 3 is generally an ongoing community exercise program (e.g., joining a gym). This section deals with the inpatient or acute care cardiac patient (Phase 1). Whether a facility has a formal Phase 1 program or not, early intervention focuses on resumption of basic ADLs; early mobilization to reduce the deleterious effects of bed rest; psychological support; simple education about the disease process; and issues regarding recovery, activity tolerance, and cardiopulmonary function. The occupational therapist not only facilitates resumption of normal routines but also acts as a resource person; advocate; and support person.

Occupational therapists focus on increasing functional capacity through education, engagement in ADLs, and exercise. Education can start either before or after scheduled heart procedures or tests. Written handouts along with verbal instruction are preferable. Very often, patients, especially those in the intensive care unit, will not remember or will have only limited recollection of material covered by the therapist.

Patients with heart disease often have limited functional endurance and therefore benefit from instruction in energy conservation principles, including simplifying current lifestyle, organization and modification of the environment, task simplification, and pacing. Refer to Appendix D for more information on energy conservation strategies. Education also focuses on lifestyle and risk factor modification; how the cardiovascular system works; review of the patient's disease process; and, when appropriate, reinforcement of postsurgery precautions in the performance of ADLs.

It is also helpful to encourage patients to learn how to monitor their body's response to activity. For example, instruct patients on how to take their own pulse and use a rate of perceived exertion (RPE) scale (refer to Appendix 3.F). For example, a patient may have a RPE of 6 (*no exertion*) at rest but then have a RPE of 13 (*somewhat hard*) while engaging in a dressing activity. Patients should also be aware of warning signs that may indicate the need for rest or medical attention. These signs may include dizziness, light-headedness, irregular heartbeat, chest pain, nausea or vomiting, diaphoresis, excessive fatigue, shortness of breath (or difficulty breathing), and any unusual weight gain (e.g., gaining up to 5 pounds within 1–3 days; Huntley, 2008). Appendix 3.G lists general precautions and guidelines for working with cardiac patients.

Patients may also benefit from education about stress management and coping strategies, the importance of adequate quality and quantity of sleep, the importance of taking medication as prescribed, and avoidance of certain environmental factors after discharge. Environmental factors may include avoidance of temperature extremes, air pollution, high altitudes, stress, and excess levels of activity. Relaxation breathing, muscle relaxation, guided imagery, visualization, massage, prayer, and meditation are some techniques that may be beneficial. Refer to Appendix J for more information on relaxation techniques.

Engagement in ADLs may begin in the cardiac care unit (or cardiac intensive care unit) with simple hygiene and grooming activities, which can start off bedside and progress to sitting on the edge of the bed, sitting up in a chair, or standing by the sink (refer to Chapter 2 for more information). However, many ADLs may need to be modified to incorporate sternal precautions for patients with a median sternotomy (refer to Appendix 3.C for a comprehensive list of sternal precautions). Therapists can also evaluate equipment needs and make recommendations that will maximize the patient's independent performance of ADLs.

In addition to engagement in self-care and leisure occupations, patients can participate in an exercise program to build up cardiovascular strength and tolerance for activity. Goals for acute care cardiac patients also include improved functional capacity. A cardiovascular or fitness exercise program usually consists of flexibility, endurance, and strengthening. Flexibility and endurance can be addressed through repetitive stretching and range of motion exercises, a home exercise program, or a walking program. Strengthening can be done with light weights or a Thera-Band®; however, strengthening exercises are contraindicated for several weeks for poststernotomy patients. In a cardiac rehabilitation program, exercise intensity should generally fall between 11 and 14 on a RPE scale

(Eckert, 2007). However, the MET system may be more applicable to the acute cardiac patient (refer to Appendix 3.A) than an RPE scale. The patient should work hard enough for effect but not harder than his or her heart can handle.

All exercise sessions should also include a warm-up and a cool-down period, which is especially important with heart transplant patients, whose donor hearts are denervated and rely on circulating catecholamines to increase HR instead of the autonomic nervous system (refer to Chapter 14 for more information). As with all therapeutic interventions, monitor patient's vital signs before, during, and after activity.

Before discharge, the occupational therapist is also instrumental in making recommendations for discharge disposition (i.e., rehabilitation stay vs. home health therapy; refer to Appendix M for more information). Additional benefits of engagement in occupational therapy include improved quality of life, including enhanced self-efficacy (which affects motivation and therefore compliance), psychological well-being, resumption of desired life roles, and wellness promotion. Wellness promotion includes education and activities that prevent and reduce heart disease risk factors and reoccurrence of the cardiac events or symptoms that precipitated the patient's current hospital admission. The occupational therapist working with the cardiac patient performs an important job by enhancing performance skills and performance patterns and assisting the patient with return to a lifestyle that promotes health, wellness, and resumption of important roles and routines.

References

American Association of Cardiovascular and Pulmonary Rehabilitation [AACVPR]. (2004). *Cardiac rehabilitation in the inpatient and transitional settings*. In A.A.O.C.P. Rehabilitation (Ed.), Guidelines for cardiac rehabilitation and secondary prevention programs (4th ed., pp. 31–51). Champaign, IL: Human Kinetics.

American Heart Association. (1994). *Revisions to classification of functional capacity and objective assessment of patients with diseases of the heart.*

Retrieved May 25, 2009, from www.americanheart. org/presenter.jhtml?identifier=1712

American Heart Association. (2007). Physical activity and public health: Updated recommendation for adults from the American College of Sports Medicine and the American Heart Association. *Circulation, 116,* 1081–1093. doi: 10.1161/circulationaha.107.185649

American Heart Association. (2009a). *Arrhythmias.* Retrieved May 21, 2009, from www.americanheart .org/presenter.jhtml?identifier=10845

American Heart Association. (2009b). Heart disease and stroke statistics: 2009 update at a glance. *Learn and Live.* Retrieved August 14, 2010, from http://americanheart.org/downloadable/heart/ 1240250946756LS-1982%20Heart%20and%20 Stroke%20Update.042009.pdf

Borg, G. (1982). Psychophysical bases of perceived exertion. *Medicine and Science in Sports and Exercise, 14,* 377–381.

Cahalin, L. P., & Buck, L. A. (2004). Physical therapy associated with cardiovascular pump dysfunction and failure. In W. E. DeTurk & L. P. Cahalin (Eds.), *Cardiovascular and pulmonary physical therapy: An evidence-based approach* (pp. 493–539). New York: McGraw-Hill.

Cardiovascular disorders. (2006). In J. Munden (Ed.), *Atlas of pathophysiology* (2nd ed., pp. 38–79). Philadelphia: Lippincott Williams & Wilkins.

Cardiovascular system. (2007). In J. Munden (Ed.), *Professional guide to pathophysiology* (2nd ed., pp. 138–226). Philadelphia: Lippincott Williams & Wilkins.

Cassady, S. L. (2004). Cardiovascular pathophysiology. In W. E. DeTurk & L. P. Cahalin (Eds.), *Cardiovascular and pulmonary physical therapy: An evidence-based approach* (pp. 123–150). New York: McGraw-Hill.

Collins, S. M., & Cocanour, B. (2004). Anatomy of the cardiopulmonary system. In W. E. DeTurk & L. P. Cahalin (Eds.), *Cardiovascular and pulmonary physical therapy: An evidence-based approach* (pp. 73–94). New York: McGraw-Hill.

Collins, S. M., & Dias, K. J. (2009). Cardiac system. In J. C. Paz & M. P. West (Eds.), *Acute care handbook for physical therapists* (3rd ed., pp. 1–46). St. Louis, MO: W. B. Saunders.

Eckert, J. (2007). Cardiopulmonary disorders. In B. J. Atchison & D. K. Dirette (Eds.), *Conditions in occupational therapy: Effect on occupational performance* (3rd ed., pp. 195–218). Baltimore: Lippincott Williams & Wilkins.

Framingham Heart Study. (2009). *Framingham Heart Study cohort.* Retrieved May 17, 2009, from www.framinghamheartstudy.org/

Goodman, C. C., & Smirnova, I. V. (2009). The cardiovascular system. In C. C. Goodman & K. S. Fuller (Eds.), *Pathology: Implications for the physical therapist* (3rd ed., pp. 519–641). St. Louis, MO: W. B. Saunders.

Gould, B. E. (2006). Cardiovascular disorders. *In Pathophysiology for the health professions* (3rd ed., pp. 302–361). Philadelphia: W. B. Saunders.

Herridge, M. L., & Linton, J. C. (2006). Psychosocial issues and strategies. In American Association of Cardiovascular and Pulmonary Rehabilitation (Ed.), *AACVPR cardiac rehabilitation resource manual: Promoting health and preventing disease* (pp. 43–50). Champaign, IL: Human Kinetics.

Hunt, S. A., Baker, D. W., Chin, M. H., Cinquegrani, M. P., Feldmanmd, A. M., Francis, G. S., et al. (2001). ACC/AHA Guidelines for the evaluation and management of chronic heart failure in the adult: Executive summary of a report of the American College of Cardiology/American Heart Association Task Force on practice guidelines. *Circulation, 104,* 2996–3007.

Huntley, N. (2008). Cardiac and pulmonary diseases. In M. V. Radomski & C. A. T. Latham (Eds.), *Occupational therapy for physical dysfunction* (6th ed., pp. 1295–1320). Philadelphia: Lippincott Williams & Wilkins.

Kavanagh, T. (2006). Chronic heart failure. In American Association of Cardiovascular and Pulmonary Rehabilitation (Ed.), *AACVPR cardiac rehabilitation resource manual: Promoting health and preventing disease* (pp. 141–147). Champaign, IL: Human Kinetics.

Levine, G. N. (2006). Contemporary revascularization procedures. In American Association of Cardiovascular and Pulmonary Rehabilitation (Ed.), *AACVPR cardiac rehabilitation resource manual: Promoting health and preventing disease* (pp. 11–25). Champaign, IL: Human Kinetics.

Lichtman, J. H., Bigger, J. T., Jr., Blumenthal, J. A., Frasure-Smith, N., Kaufmann, P. G., Lespérance, F., et al. (2008). Depression and coronary heart disease: Recommendations for screening, referral, and treatment. *Circulation, 118,* 1768–1775.

Lloyd-Jones, D., Adams, R., Carnethon, M., De Simone, G., Ferguson, T. B., Flegal, K., et al. (2009). Heart disease and stroke statistics 2009 update. *Circulation, 119,* e21–e181.

Lorig, K., Holman, H., Sobel, D., Laurent, D., Gonzalez, V., & Minor, M. (2000). Understanding heart disease and high blood pressure. In K. Lorig, H. Holman, D. Sobel, D. Laurent, V. Gonzalez, & M. Minor (Ed.), *Living a healthy life with chronic conditions* (2nd ed., pp. 241–259). Palo Alto, CA: Bull.

Malone, D. J. (2006). Cardiovascular diseases and disorders. In D. J. Malone & K. L. B. Lindsay (Eds.), *Physical therapy in acute care: A clinician's guide* (pp. 139–209). Thorofare, NJ: Slack.

Maron, B. J., Towbin, J. A., Thiene, G., Antzelevitch, C., Corrado, D., Arnett, D., et al. (2006). Contemporary definitions and classification of the cardiomyopathies. *Circulation, 113,* 1807–1816.

McConnell, T. R., & Klinger, T. A. (2006). Atherosclerosis. In American Association of Cardiovascular and Pulmonary Rehabilitation (Ed.), *AACVPR cardiac rehabilitation resource manual: Promoting health and preventing disease* (pp. 3–9). Champaign, IL: Human Kinetics.

McSweeney, J. C., Cody, M., O'Sullivan, P., Elberson, K., Moser, D. K., & Garvin, B. J. (2003). Women's early warning symptoms of acute myocardial infarction. *Circulation, 108,* 1–5. doi: 10.1161/01. cir.0000097116.29625.7c

Mended Hearts. (2009). Retrieved May 26, 2009, from www.mendedhearts.org/

Miller, H. S. (2006). Major manifestations of heart disease. In American Association of Cardiovascular and Pulmonary Rehabilitation (Ed.), *AACVPR cardiac rehabilitation resource manual: Promoting health and preventing disease* (pp. xi–xv). Champaign, IL: Human Kinetics.

Morgan, B. J., & Dempsey, J. A. (2004). Physiology of the cardiovascular and pulmonary systems. In W. E. DeTurk & L. P. Cahalin (Eds.), *Cardiovascular and pulmonary physical therapy: An evidence-based approach* (pp. 95–122). New York: McGraw-Hill.

National Heart, Lung, and Blood Institute. (2007, December). *How is heart valve disease treated?* Retrieved May 25, 2009, from www.nhlbi.nih.gov/health/dci/Diseases/hvd/hvd_treatments.html

National Heart, Lung, and Blood Institute. (2009, December). *Pacemaker: How does a pacemaker work? Heart and vascular diseases.* Retrieved August 14, 2010, from http://www.nhlbi.nih.gov/health/dci/Diseases/pace/pace_howdoes.html

Redman, B. K. (2004). Cardiovascular self-management preparation. In *Patient self-management of chronic disease: The health care provider's challenge* (pp. 101–126). Boston: Jones & Bartlett.

Roitman, J. L., & LaFontaine, T. P. (2006). Efficacy of secondary prevention and risk factor reduction. In American Association of Cardiovascular and Pulmonary Rehabilitation (Ed.), *AACVPR cardiac rehabilitation resource manual: Promoting health and preventing disease* (pp. 27–42). Champaign, IL: Human Kinetics.

Stiller, K. (2007). Safety issues that should be considered when mobilizing critically ill patients. *Critical Care Clinics, 23,* 35–53.

West, M. P., Paz, J. C., & Vashi, F. (2009). Vascular system and hematology. In J. C. Paz & M. P. West (Eds.), *Acute care handbook for physical therapists* (3rd ed., pp. 234–235). St. Louis, MO: W. B. Saunders.

Wung, S. F. (2006). Electrocardiography in heart disease. In American Association of Cardiovascular and Pulmonary Rehabilitation (Ed.), *AACVPR cardiac rehabilitation resource manual: Promoting health and preventing disease* (pp. 89–106). Champaign, IL: Human Kinetics.

Appendix 3.A.

Sample Cardiac Rehabilitation Program

A *MET* is a metabolic unit that describes how much oxygen the average person's body needs to perform at rest. The MET system is useful in determining the amount of energy expended to perform different activities. One MET is equal to 3.5 milliliters of oxygen per kilogram of body weight per minute. A 2-MET activity is one that requires twice as much oxygen as the body requires at rest. MET levels increase as the oxygen consumption for the activity increases (i.e., activities that cause an increase in HR or breathing). Patients undergoing cardiac rehabilitation often engage in activities that require a progressive increase in MET levels.

Days	Location	METs	Activities and Average Heart Rate Response
1–2	Cardiac care unit	1.0–2.0	• Bedrest • Generally dependent in self-care • Washing face and performing oral hygiene with arm support • Using a bedpan or urinal in bed • Sitting up in chair as tolerated • Watching television • 5–15 bpm up from RHR
3–4	Floor	2.0–3.0	• Feeding self • Brushing teeth • Combing hair • Bathing upper body • Using bedside commode, urinal in standing • Out of bed as tolerated • Gentle upper-extremity/lower-extremity range-of-motion exercises • Walking around room, or out in hall for 5–10 minutes • 5–15 bpm up from RHR
4–5	Floor	3.0–4.0	• Out of bed as tolerated • Seated shower • Upper-body exercise in standing • Walking in halls (~5–10 minutes) • 10–20 bpm up from RHR
7–10	On discharge	3.0–5.0	• Independent in self-care • Walking 3–5 minutes 4–6 times daily • Walking up and down one flight of stairs • 10–20 bpm up from RHR

Note. bpm = beats per minute; RHR = resting heart rate.
Any approach to cardiac rehabilitation should be individualized according to patient needs and abilities.
Source. American Association of Cardiovascular and Pulmonary Rehabilitation, (2004); Malone (2006).

Appendix 3.B.
Sample Metabolic Unit Levels

Minimal (<1.5)

- Resting, sitting on edge of bed
- Riding in a car
- Listening to the radio
- Watching TV.

Light (1.5–3.0)

- Eating
- Getting in or out of bed
- Dressing and undressing
- Making a bed
- Preparing food
- Washing dishes
- Writing
- Working at the computer
- Knitting, sewing, and crocheting
- Playing cards
- Fishing, seated
- Playing a musical instrument
- Walking at a slow pace.

Moderate (3.0–6.0)

- Having a bowel movement
- General household tasks (e.g., sweeping or mopping floors, carrying light laundry, cleaning the garage)
- Loading or unloading a car
- Raking the lawn
- Gardening
- Moving furniture
- Child care
- Walking 3.0 miles per hour
- Playing table tennis
- Slow dancing
- Bicycling on a flat road (light effort)

- Golfing
- Yoga
- Water aerobics.

Vigorous (>6.0)

- Carrying groceries upstairs
- Climbing stairs rapidly
- High-impact aerobics
- Race walking or running
- Playing basketball or soccer
- Cross-country skiing.

Sources. American Heart Association (2007), Huntley (2008).

Appendix 3.C.

Sternotomy Precautions

Sternotomy (or sternal) precautions may vary at different hospital sites; therefore, good judgment must be used when assisting patients to move, exercise, or engage in activities of daily living (ADLs). Generally, any movements that require asynchronous movement between the two sides of the chest, any excessive shoulder flexion, rotation, abduction, or lifting more than 5–10 pounds are discouraged for the first 4–6 weeks. *Consult the physician or facility policy for specific precautions and restrictions.* The following guidelines are suggested for working with sternotomy patients.

Bed Mobility and Ambulation

- *Scooting up in bed:* Bend knees with feet flat on the bed and push off the bed with legs extended to scoot up. Do not push or pull with arms on bed rails.
- *Rolling side to side:* Bend hips and knees and roll to the side, with the trunk following.
- *Supine to sitting:* Roll onto side, drop legs off the bed, and then push up using elbow. The other hand holds onto the bedrail for support only. Patients may be assisted by supporting their upper back and moving the hips toward the edge of the bed.
- Do not pull on patients' arms when assisting them into an upright position.
- Use the bed controls to raise the head of the bed to assist the patient into an upright position. However, once the patient is sitting on the edge of the bed, flatten the bed back to provide a level seat surface.
- Transferring to a low seat surface should be avoided because of a tendency to push with the arms when coming up to stand.
- Hand-held assistance may be preferable to the patient using an assistive device for ambulation because some patients cannot control the amount of pressure exerted through a walker or other ambulation device.

Activities of Daily Living

- Engage in normal ADLs but minimize excessive shoulder movements (e.g., shoulder retraction, shoulder abduction).
- Avoid holding arms above the head for sustained periods (e.g., washing hair).
- Avoid excessive chest expansion movements with upper-body dressing (e.g., when donning or doffing a shirt or fastening a back-closing bra).
- Avoid upper-body twisting. When reaching for an object (e.g., the telephone), the patient should turn in the direction of the object instead of twisting an arm back behind himself or herself to reach for it.
- Minimize shoulder extension and rotation movements when engaging in toileting hygiene.
- Avoid bending over to don lower-body clothing to minimize inadvertent breath holding when bending forward. Cross one leg over the other to access feet for lower-body ADLs, or consider the use of assistive devices (e.g., reacher, dressing stick).
- Do not lift more than 10 pounds, including grocery bags, children, pets, or trash bags.
- Avoid one-sided pushing, pulling, or lifting (e.g., opening heavy doors, vacuuming).
- Avoid heavy pushing or pulling with both arms (e.g., moving furniture).
- Avoid driving or riding in the front seat of a car. An accident may result in forceful movement or pressure on the sternotomy site.
- Avoid straining, for example, opening tight jars, straining during bowel movements, or activities that may cause breath holding (e.g., Valsalva effect).

Exercise

- Patients may participate in full active range of motion exercise but should not exceed 90 degrees of shoulder flexion with presence of a muscle flap (Goodman & Smirnova, 2009).
- Participants should not participate in resistive exercise, including use of Thera-Band or light weights, until cleared by physician (usually contraindicated the first 4–6 weeks).
- Avoid pushing and pulling activities.
- *Sternal clicking* is a feeling of shifting or snapping of the sternum and indicates instability. Any arm motion that causes clicking, especially shoulder abduction, should be avoided.

Note. Created by Helene Smith-Gabai.

Appendix 3.D.

Ventricular Assist Devices

A VAD may be used as a destination therapy, bridge to candidacy, or bridge to heart transplantation. *Destination therapy* indicates that VAD placement is permanent because the patient is not a good candidate for heart transplantation (e.g., advanced age, diabetes). *Bridge to candidacy* indicates that the patient is not currently on a heart transplant list because of relative contraindications that are currently being addressed (e.g., obesity, other organ system impairment). VAD placement is indicated for patients with refractory arrhythmias, reversible end-organ damage, life expectancy of more than 2 years, EF less than 25%, IV inotrope dependence, increasing oxygen requirements, and reversible acute CHF. The patient must also have the appropriate body size to accommodate the device.

A VAD not only ensures adequate pumping of blood throughout the body but can also assist with heart failure symptom relief. However, patients with VAD placement may be at risk for stroke, infection, blood clots, respiratory failure, kidney failure, or pump failure.

Contraindications for VAD implantation include

- Life expectancy <2 years,
- Mechanical aortic valve,
- Right ventricular failure,
- Irreversible shock,
- Clot in left ventricle,
- Intolerance to anticoagulation therapy (e.g., positive for heparin-induced thrombocytopenia),
- Active infection,
- Ventilator dependence,
- Significant lung disease,
- Active substance abuse,
- Severe mental health issues or psychiatric illness,
- History of poor compliance behavior, and
- Inadequate psychosocial support.

Candidates for VAD implantation undergo an evaluation process including psychological, social support, and medical screening. Patients must also have the financial resources for pump supplies and adequate transportation for follow-up visits.

Diagnostic tests may include

- Echocardiogram,
- Exercise stress test,
- Electrocardiogram,
- Carotid Doppler,
- Right-heart catheterization,
- Pulmonary function test,
- Stool culture,
- Urinalysis, and
- Lab work.

Patient and family education includes

- The underlying disease and the purpose of the device;
- Device function and pump care, including daily system controller check, battery charging, battery maintenance, back-up power source, and recognition of alarms;
- Daily sterile dressing changes (if not performed, patient is at risk for hardware and pump pocket infection);
- Heart failure symptom recognition;
- Lifestyle modifications, including avoidance of alcohol and tobacco, low-sodium diet and fluid restrictions, daily weight monitoring, adherence to medication regimen (e.g., lifelong

anticoagulation therapy), activity restrictions (e.g., avoidance of contact sports), driving restrictions (e.g., airbag or steering wheel compression can compress the graft, leading to decreased blood flow to the body or brain), and restricted water exposure (e.g., avoidance of bathing in a tub or swimming in a pool or lake because water immersion increases the risk of infection; however, patients may shower with a waterproof covering over the driveline);

- Immunization recommendations, including influenza, hepatitis, varicella, and pneumococcal vaccines; and
- Follow-up care (i.e., scheduled medical appointments).

Precautions include

- Contraindication of MRI,
- Adequate electrical system (the patient's life is dependent on an intact power source),
- Availability of reliable telephone (i.e., in case of emergency), and
- Advanced cardiac life support without chest compressions (because they may occlude blood to the brain).

Appendix 3.E.
Diagnostic Tests for Cardiac Diseases and Disorders

- *Auscultation:* A stethoscope is used to listen for heart sounds as blood flows through the heart. Auscultation is useful in detecting murmurs and valve disorders.
- *Electrocardiogram (EKG):* Electrodes placed on the body give a recording of the heart's rate and rhythm.
- *Holter monitor:* This monitor is a small portable or ambulatory EKG machine. It records the heart's rate and rhythm during regular activities over a 24- to 48-hour period.
- *Electrophysiologic test:* This test gives more precise information than an EKG and is used to study the electrical impulses of the heart and location of arrhythmias.
- *Chest X-ray:* An X-ray determines heart enlargement or the presence of fluid in lungs.
- *Echocardiogram:* An echocardiogram is performed with an ultrasound device; sound waves are used to study the size, structure, and movement of the heart. It also provides information on arrhythmias.
- *Transesophageal echocardiogram:* A probe is inserted through the mouth and into the esophagus and sits behind the heart. This type of echocardiogram provides a clearer picture of the heart than a traditional echocardiogram. It is useful in detecting clots, masses in the heart, valvular problems, aortic dissections, and cardiac arrhythmias.
- *Computed tomography and positron emission tomography scans:* Computer imaging (tomography) is used to study coronary artery disease, pericardial disease, aortic diseases, and cardiac masses. Refer to Appendix A for more information on imaging.
- *Stress test:* Heart monitoring is done during exercise on a treadmill to diagnose coronary artery disease and causes of angina and helps to determine a safe level of exercise.
- *Thallium stress test (myocardial perfusion test):* A radioactive substance (thallium) is injected into the bloodstream. Imaging is used to take a picture of the heart while the patient exercises

on a treadmill. This test provides information on damage to the heart muscle, angina, coronary artery occlusion, and safe levels of exercise.

- *Echocardiogram stress test:* This test is used with patients who cannot tolerate a treadmill stress test. Sound waves are used to study the heart at rest and after being given medication (e.g., dobutamine) that simulates the effects of exercise on the heart (increases heart rate and blood pressure).

- *Cardiac catheterization or angiogram:* A catheter inserted into an artery or vein (usually a vein in the leg) is threaded through the blood vessel until it reaches the heart. A dye is injected into the catheter and an X-ray is taken to study narrowing of coronary arteries. This procedure is also used to measure oxygen in the blood and blood pressure of the heart. Patients are usually instructed to remain supine for several hours after cardiac catheterization.

- *Swan–Ganz catheter:* This catheter is used with critically ill patients. A thin tube is threaded through the right side of the heart and used in diagnosing cardiac tamponade, pulmonary hypertension, and restrictive cardiomyopathy. It is also used to monitor consequences of heart attack and effectiveness of medications.

- *Blood tests:* Blood tests are used to measure electrolyte levels, blood counts, lipid profiles, blood clotting time, and cardiac markers (e.g., cardiac enzymes: troponins, creatine kinase, C-reactive protein, brain natruiretic peptide). These tests serve as diagnostic indicators for heart attack and heart disease risk. Refer to Appendix P for more information.

Note. Created by Helene Smith-Gabai.

Appendix 3.F.
Rate of Perceived Exertion (RPE)

Patients can self-monitor how they tolerate certain activities or exercise in several ways. Increased exertion may be experienced as increased respirations, increased heart rate, or fatigue. Rate of perceived exertion (RPE) scales are common tools patients use to judge how hard they are working. Borg's (1982) Rate of Perceived Exertion Scale is probably the most widely known RPE scale. It is an ordinal scale ranging of 6–20 that progressively measures subjective feelings of work intensity and exertion. Exercise experienced in the 12–14 range is considered to be of moderate intensity. On the basis of feelings of exertion, patients can increase or decrease their level of activity accordingly. Borg's (1982) Rate of Perceived Exertion Scale is as follows:

6	No exertion at all
7	Very, very light
8	
9	Very light
10	
11	Fairly light
12	
13	Somewhat hard
14	
15	Hard (heavy)

16	
17	Very hard
18	
19	Very, very hard
20	Maximal exertion

Source. From "Physchophysical bases of perceived exertion," by G. Borg, 1982, *Medicine and Science in Sports and Exercise, 14,* pp. 378–381.

Appendix 3.G.
General Precautions and Guidelines for Working With Cardiac Patients

- Monitor vital signs before, during, and after therapy.
- Be aware of any signs of exercise intolerance or cardiac distress, including complaints of
  — Dizziness
  — Light-headedness
  — Excessive fatigue
  — Shortness of breath
  — Heart palpitations
  — Chest pain described as pressure, burning, or heaviness
  — Indigestion, nausea, or vomiting
  — Sweating
  — Confusion
  — Anxiety or fear
  — Changes in blood pressure (BP; >20 mm HG) or heart rate (HR; >20 bpm over resting heart rate [RHR]).
- Early activity helps prevent cardiopulmonary complications.
- Avoid Valsalva maneuvers or effects. Holding the breath causes an increase in intrathoracic pressure, which decreases venous return, slows heart rate, and increases BP.
- Modify activity requirements per patient tolerance. Gradually grade activities, slowly progressing the patient.
- During the first few weeks after a myocardial infarction, HRs should not exceed 20–30 beats per minute (bpm) over the RHR.
- If the patient's HR is more than 125 bpm with minimal effort, contact the physician.
- Heart transplant patients have a higher-than-normal RHR (e.g., 90–110 bpm) and require a longer warm-up and cool-down period than patients who have had other cardiac surgeries. Refer to Chapter 14 for more detail.
- Patients on beta blockers have lower HR and BP responses; therefore, therapists must be attentive to other symptoms of distress (e.g., shortness of breath, fatigue, complaints of chest pain).

- Upper-extremity exercises tend to increase HR and BP at a faster rate than do lower-extremity exercises.

- Patients with a history of hypertension may have an exaggerated response to exercise, even if medicated.

- At-rest BP should be less than 140 over 90 to be considered normal. If a patient's blood pressure is more than 180 over 90, notify the physician.

- If you are treating a patient with a percutaneous transluminal coronary angioplasty and angina begins, notify medical staff immediately.

- Patients are usually on bedrest precautions for several hours after a cardiac catheterization or angioplasty procedure.

Note. Created by Helene Smith-Gabai.

4

The Vascular System

Rannell Hudson, OTR/L

Vascular diseases encompass a broad spectrum of illnesses and disorders that involve the circulatory, cardiac, peripheral, pulmonary, and cerebral–spinal systems. Vascular diseases commonly seen by occupational therapists practicing in acute care hospitals and reviewed in this chapter include atherosclerosis, peripheral vascular disease (PVD), venous stasis, venous thromboembolism, deep vein thrombosis, superficial thrombophlebitis, pulmonary embolism, compartment syndrome, gangrene, Raynaud's syndrome, heparin-induced thrombocytopenia (HIT), and vasculitis. These diseases and disorders are often managed pharmacologically, surgically, or both. Information on the vascular disorders of coronary artery disease (CAD) and cerebrovascular accident can be found in Chapters 3 and 6, respectively.

Normal Structure and Function

The vascular system consists of blood vessels that circulate blood to the heart and lungs. The heart contracts to drive blood through the arteries, which divide and become arterioles, which further divide to become capillaries. Blood collects in venules and veins that transport the blood back to the heart. Arterioles control blood flow into the capillaries by either *vasoconstriction* (narrowing), which restricts blood flow into the capillaries, or by *vasodilatation* (enlargement), which allows blood to flow into the capillaries. Veins contain valves that allow blood to flow to the heart and restrict blood flow back to the extremities (Venes, Thomas, & Taber, 2001).

Circulatory System

The circulatory system consists of the heart, blood, and blood vessels. However, two types of fluids move through the circulatory system: blood and lymph. Arteries carry blood away from the heart and lungs, and veins carry blood to the heart and lungs. *Blood* consists of *plasma, red blood cells* (erythrocytes), *white blood cells* (leukocytes), and *platelets* (thrombocytes). Plasma is fluid from the intestines and lymphatic system and is the medium that allows cells to move throughout the vascular system (Fischbach & Dunning, 2009). Approximately 5 liters of blood circulate through the body, of which 3 liters are plasma and 2 liters are cells (Fischbach & Dunning, 2009). The types of blood cells and their function are listed in Table 4.1.

Lymph is a watery fluid containing white blood cells and protein. The lymphatic system serves to remove fluid (lymph), protein, and debris that are unable to reenter the blood capillaries. This system returns lymph to venous circulation to prevent edema in the interstitial space. *Lymphedema* is the result of blockage of the lymphatic system (Andrews, Gamble, Gloviczki, Rooke, & Strick, 2005).

Blood vessel walls are made up of three layers of tissues. These layers consist of the tunica interna (innermost layer), tunica media (middle layer), and tunica externa (outermost layer). Arterial wall compositions differ on the basis of the size of the vessels. *Elastic arteries* are large arteries: the aorta, its major branches, the pulmonary trunk, the brachiocephalic trunk, the common carotid artery and its major branches, the proximal parts of the vertebral artery, the internal thoracic artery, the subclavian artery, the thyrocervical trunk, and the common iliac artery.

Arterial walls consist of the three tunics; however, they have three distinguishing features. The innermost layer, or *tunica interna*, is made up of endothelium, a basement membrane, and elastic tissue (internal elastic lamina). The middle layer, or *tunica media*, consists of many elastic and smooth muscle fibers. The outermost

Table 4.1. Type of Blood Cells, Their Count, and Their Function

Type	Normal Count Range	Function
Red blood cells (erythrocytes)	4.5 to 6.0 million cells/µl; usually toward the high end for men and toward the low end for women	Carries oxygen bonded to hemoglobin. Red blood cells travel throughout the body to supply tissues and organs with oxygen.
White blood cells (leukocytes)	5,000 to 10,000 cells/µl	Provides immunity from certain diseases and protects body from infectious diseases. White blood cells are made up of neutrophils, basophils, eosinophils, lymphocytes and monocytes.
Platelets (thrombocytes)	150,000 to 300,000 µl (high-end range may be extended to 500,000)	Platelets are necessary for clot formation and the prevention of blood loss (homeostasis).

Sources. Scalone (2007), West, Paz, and Vashi (2009).

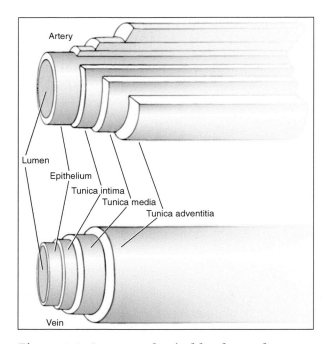

Figure 4.1. Artery and vein blood vessel walls.
Source. Richard Fritzler, Medical Illustrator, Roswell, GA.

layer, or *tunica externa,* consists of collagenous and elastic fibers. The internal elastic lamina lies between the interna and the media layers. The external elastic lamina lies between the media and the externa layers (DeFranco, Hongbao, Kantipudi, & Abela, 2004). Figure 4.1 shows artery and vein blood vessel walls, and Table 4.2. lists the different types of blood vessels and their function.

Veins consist of the same three types of tunica as arteries. The walls of the tunica interna and the tunica media are thinner than those of arteries, and the walls of the tunica externa are thicker. Capillaries unite to form small veins called *venules* (DeFranco et al., 2004). Venules drain blood from capillaries into veins for transport back to the heart. Table 4.2 describes types of blood vessels and their function.

Blood Pressure

Blood pressure (BP) is the pressure that is exerted on the wall of any vessel. BP readings

Table 4.2. Types of Blood Vessels and Their Function

Blood Vessel	Tunica Interna	Tunica Media	Tunica Externa (Adventitia)
Arteries: Carry blood from the heart to arterioles and then to the capillaries	Innermost layer made of endothelium; allows for a smooth blood flow and prevents abnormal blood clotting	Middle layer made of smooth muscle and elastic connective tissue; involved in maintaining normal blood pressure (through constriction and dilation)	Outer layer made of fibrous connective tissue; prevents the rupture of larger arteries that carry blood under high pressure
Arterioles: Smaller arteries; regulate blood flow into the capillaries	Not present	Middle layer; mostly smooth muscle with little elastic tissue	External membrane is lost in the smallest arterioles closest to the capillaries
Capillaries: Communicate between the arterial and venous systems. Allow for blood and gas exchange	Tunica interna surrounds a thin layer of endothelial cells	Not present	Not present
Veins: Carry blood from capillaries to venules and then back to the heart	Innermost layer made of smooth endothelium; includes folds that form valves at intervals, which prevents back flow of blood	Middle layer is a thin layer of smooth muscle; can constrict extensively; important in severe hemorrhage	Outer layer is thin with less fibrous connective tissue because blood pressure in veins is low
Venules: Smaller veins	Innermost layer made of endothelium, surrounded by some fibrous tissue in venules closest to the capillaries	Thin middle layer formed on larger venules that are farther from the capillaries	Not present

Sources. DeFranco, Hongbao, Kantipudi, and Abela (2004), West, Paz, and Vashi, (2009).

consist of two numbers. The higher number, which is recorded as *systole*, refers to pressure exerted by the heart contracting to pump blood to the body. The lower number, which is recorded as *diastole*, refers to pressure of the heart relaxing between beats. During systole, the aorta and elastic arteries, the latter of which serves an important function in blood flow, dilate or stretch as blood flows from the heart. During diastole, elastic arteries return to their original size or recoil to help regulate pressure within the vessel. The pressure is highest in the left ventricle during systole. BP decreases in the arterial system as the distance from the heart increases and is lower in capillaries than in arteries. The *systolic arterial pressure* rises with activity or excitement and falls during sleep. *Diastolic pressure* is the reading obtained during the relaxation phase between heart beats.

BP can be measured in two ways: direct and indirect. *Direct monitoring* uses a sterile needle or small catheter (arterial line), which is placed inside an artery and connected to tubing, a transducer, and an electronic monitor. The changes are recorded graphically and allow frequent monitoring of the patient's cardiovascular status (Venes et al., 2001). *Indirect monitoring* uses an external (noninvasive) method for measuring BP.

Systolic BP can be measured by Doppler, palpatory, or auscultatory methods. The auscultatory method provides both systolic and diastolic readings and is commonly used to measure BP. The auscultatory method is performed with the patient's arm in a relaxed and supported position. Exertion during the examination could result in a higher BP reading. Either the mercury–gravity or aneroid–manometer type of BP apparatus may be used. To prevent inaccurate readings, the BP cuff should be the right size for the extremity. The cuff width should be 40% of the arm circumference, and the cuff length should be 80% of the arm circumference (Prisant, 2008). BP in the upper extremity is taken in the following manner:

- Check for posted signs in the event the patient has precautions regarding which extremity to use for taking BP. For example, BP readings may be contraindicated with the presence of an IV, blood clot, history of lymphedema, or arteriovenous fistulas used for hemodialysis.
- Raise the arm to heart level if the patient is sitting or parallel to the body if the patient is in supine.
- Place the deflated cuff evenly around the upper arm with the lower edge about 1 inch above the brachial artery.
- Inflate the cuff until the pressure is about 30 mm higher than when you can no longer palpate the radial pulse.
- Place the bell of the stethoscope over the brachial artery (just below the BP cuff).

- Deflate the cuff slowly, about 2–3 millimeters of mercury (mm Hg) per heart beat.
- Record the first sound heard as the systolic pressure (the sound is produced when the ventricles contract and causes enough pressure to force blood flow through the artery).
- Continue to listen. As the ventricles relax and the pressure in the artery drops, the cuff again closes the artery and no blood flows in the lower arm.
- Record the diastolic pressure when sounds are no longer heard (the intermittent thumping sounds become dull and muffled with continued reduction of pressure in the cuff).
- Record arterial BP as a fraction, with the numerator being the systolic pressure and the denominator being the diastolic pressure (i.e., 120/80 indicates systolic pressure of 120 and diastolic pressure of 80). Pulse pressure is the difference between systolic and diastolic pressures.

Sounds heard over the brachial artery change in quality at some point before disappearing completely. Some physicians consider this the diastolic pressure. This value should be noted when recording the BP by placing it between the systolic pressure and the pressure noted when the sound disappears (e.g., 120/90/80 would indicate a systolic pressure of 120 with a first diastolic pressure of 90 and a second diastolic pressure of 80). The latter pressure would be the point of disappearance of all sounds from the artery. When the values are so recorded, the physician may use either of the last two figures as the diastolic pressure. When the change in sound and disappearance of all sound coincide, the result should be written as 120/80/80 (Venes et al., 2001).

BP may be referred to as *mean, negative, normal,* or *systolic.*

- *Mean:* BP is half the sum of systolic and diastolic values. For a normal person in good health, this sum is approximately 100 mm Hg.
- *Negative:* BP is less than atmospheric pressure, as in the great veins near the heart.

- *Normal:* BP in healthy young people is 100–140 mm Hg systolic and 60–90 mm Hg diastolic. Loss of resilience in the vascular tree and physiological changes of age must be considered when levels above 140 mm are obtained in apparently healthy older people (Venes et al., 2001). Normal BP may vary between people; therefore, consult patient's health care provider if there are any concerns.
- *Systolic:* Systolic BP is the force caused by the contraction of the left ventricle.

Patients with precautions that limit BPs being taken on either upper extremity may have BPs taken on the lower extremity. The BP cuff should be applied to the thigh area with auscultation at the popliteal artery (Collins & Dias, 2009).

Vascular Disorders and Diseases

Disorders and diseases included in this section are influenced by abnormalities in the vascular system. Occupational therapists working in acute care settings often treat patients diagnosed with these disorders. The focus of this section is to assist therapists with increasing their awareness of signs, symptoms, precautions, and treatment of patients diagnosed with these types of disorders.

Hypertension

The vascular system relies on pressure to produce flow through vessels. High BP contributes to the development of the major vascular diseases through effects on these same vessels. Hypertension is a significant risk factor for CAD, congestive heart failure, cerebrovascular disease, end-stage renal disease, and PVD. *Hypertension* is defined as a systolic BP of 140 mm Hg or greater, a diastolic BP of 90 mm Hg or greater, or both. Hypertension is diagnosed by taking an average of at least two BP measurements on two separate occasions (Gregory & Oparil, 2002). The diagnosis and etiology of hypertension and hypotension are provided in Table 4.3.

Table 4.3. **Diagnosis, Etiology, and Treatment of Hypertension and Hypotension**

Diagnosis	Etiology
Hypertension	
Essential (idiopathic or primary)	Unknown cause (90% of cases)
Secondary	Specific, potentially curable cause; often associated with renal and endocrine diseases, pregnancy, and sleep disorders
Malignant	Progresses rapidly and is associated with papilledema
Hypotension	
Orthostatic	Sudden changes in body position (e.g., from supine to standing)
Neurally mediated	Prolonged standing
Severe	Sudden loss of blood
Postprandial	After eating

Sources. Malone (2006); Venes, Thomas, and Taber (2001).

The three types of hypertension are (1) *essential* (primary or idiopathic), (2) *secondary*, and (3) *malignant*. The etiology of essential hypertension is unknown. However, hypertension may be associated with a genetic predisposition and environmental factors such as increased dietary sodium, obesity, stress, and stimulation of the sympathetic nervous system (Beers & Berkow, 1999). Other risk factors for hypertension include smoking and diabetes (University of Wisconsin Health, 2008).

Hypertension can have devastating effects on other organs of the body (brain, heart, eyes, or kidneys), resulting in cerebrovascular accident, retinopathy, abdominal aortic aneurysm rupture, congestive heart failure, and renal disease (Bockenek, DeJong, Friedland, Lanig, & Mann, 2005). Secondary hypertension is high BP resulting from a habit, medication, or other specific condition. Other causes include alcohol or cocaine abuse, anxiety, stress, atherosclerosis, birth control pills, Cushing syndrome, kidney disease, medications, pain, pregnancy (gestational hypertension), adrenal gland tumor, coarctation of the aorta, retroperitoneal fibrosis, periarteritis nodosa, and primary hyperaldosteronism. Malignant hypertension is a sudden extreme rise in diastolic BP often greater than 130 (a diastolic pressure reading of 80 is usually considered normal). Collagen vascular disorders, toxemia of pregnancy, or kidney failure associated with renal artery stenosis are risk factors for malignant hypertension.

Symptoms of high BP may include

- Fatigue,
- Confusion,
- Chest pain, and
- Visual changes.

Additional symptoms identified for malignant hypertension include

- Anxiety;
- Sleepiness, stupor, lethargy, or decreased ability to concentrate;
- Decreased urinary output;
- Headache;
- Nausea or vomiting;
- Seizure;
- Shortness of breath; and
- Numbness or weakness of extremities or other parts of the body.

Treatment for essential and secondary hypertension may include lifestyle modifications such as losing weight, exercising regularly, reducing sodium intake, and limiting alcohol consumption (Bockenek et al., 2005). Occupational therapists may assist in helping patients in managing hypertension by educating them about lifestyle modifications. Therapists can encourage patients to incorporate measurable goals to assist with making realistic changes (e.g., planning meals, listing possible exercises or activities that may lead to healthy weight loss, keeping a journal to track progress). If lifestyle modifications alone are not successful, then the patient's physician may prescribe medication to lower BP.

Treatment for malignant hypertension includes hospitalization until BP is under control. Intravenous medications are administered to reduce BP. Diuretics are given to remove fluid from the lungs if necessary (University of Wisconsin Health, 2009).

Hypotension

Hypotension or *low BP* is reduced BP resulting from decreased venous return and decreased cardiac output. This sudden fall in BP may be associated with changes in position (e.g., from supine to assuming an upright position) that causes blood to pool in the lower extremities and the trunk.

The four types of hypotension are orthostatic, postprandial (a type of orthostatic hypotension), neurally mediated, and severe. Hypotension may result from medications used for surgery, anxiety, depression, prolonged bed rest, or pain. Hypotension may also be the result of medical conditions including arrhythmias, heart failure, heart attack, dehydration, diarrhea, severe vomiting, shock, and advanced diabetes. Alcohol and diuretics may also cause hypotension.

Orthostatic hypotension or *postural hypotension* is a sudden decrease in BP that occurs when a patient transitions from supine to upright; it is often seen in a patient on prolonged bedrest. Blood pools in the lower extremities and compromises blood returning to the heart (Atkins, 2008). *Postprandial orthostatic hypotension* occurs when BP drops when transitioning from lying down to standing after eating. This type of hypotension usually affects older adults, those with high BP, or those with Parkinson's disease. *Neurally mediated hypotension* is a drop in BP after standing for an extended period of time (it usually affects children and young adults). *Severe hypotension* is caused by a sudden loss of blood (shock; University of Wisconsin Health, 2009). Symptoms frequently seen in patients with hypotension include

- Weakness,
- Sleepiness,
- Blurred vision,
- Confusion,
- Syncope, and
- Light-headedness.

Treatments prescribed by physicians for hypotension may include administering intravenous fluids, blood, antibiotics, or medications that increase BP. The physician may also prescribe *thromboembolic deterrent (TED) stockings* (elastic hose that increase blood flow velocity), sequential compression devices to reduce venous stasis, increased sodium intake, abdominal binders, or elevation of lower extremities (Atkins, 2008; Beers & Berkow, 1999).

Occupational therapists treating patients likely to have orthostatic hypotension should consider the following guidelines (Atkins, 2008; Beers & Berkow, 1999):

- Check the patient's BP in supine.
- Slowly elevate the head of the bed to allow the patient to adjust to gradually sitting upright.
- Evaluate the patient's ability to move to the edge of the bed, assist the patient as needed, or both.
- Recheck the patient's BP, and be aware of signs of orthostatic hypotension, including the patient's report of symptoms.

- If the patient's BP drops more than 20 mm Hg systolic and more than 10 mm Hg diastolic, elevate his or her lower extremities and observe for signs of relief; if the patient reports no relief, return him or her to supine.
- Recheck BP and notify nurse of occurrence and BP recordings.

Occupational therapists can also encourage patients who are cognitively intact to participate in their own health and wellness by gradually and consistently elevating the head of the bed throughout the day. This intervention will allow the patient to adjust to position changes and enhance the possibility of successful outcomes with eventual out-of-bed activities.

Atherosclerosis

The World Health Organization (WHO) defines *atherosclerosis* as a chronic vascular disease of the medium and large arteries that includes thickening and remodeling of the vessel wall leading to reduced or obstructed blood flow through plaque formation and thrombosis (as cited in Coffman & Eberhardt, 2003). Atherosclerosis is characterized by variable changes in the arteries, including the accumulation of lipids, complex carbohydrates, blood and blood products, fibrous tissue, and calcium deposits. It is also associated with changes including occlusions, weakening, and narrowing of the arterial wall (Berry & Vuong, 2002). Atherosclerosis is the most common and serious vascular disease, affecting the heart (CAD), brain (cerebrovascular disease), kidneys (renal artery disease), and other vital organs as well as the extremities (peripheral arterial disease [PAD]).

Peripheral Vascular Disease

The National Institutes of Health has suggested that 60,000 patients are admitted to the hospital each year with PVD, with an average hospital stay longer than 11 days (Jaff, 2004a). PVD is also referred to as *PAD, peripheral arterial occlusive disease, arteriosclerosis obliterans,* and *lower-*

extremity occlusive disease (Bordeaux, Hirsch, & Reich, 2003). PAD is associated with

- Significant morbidity and mortality;
- Increased prevalence with age; and
- Increased risk for cardiovascular disease, CAD, and aneurysms (Jacoby & Mohler, 2004).

An estimated 50% of PAD patients are asymptomatic, and approximately 25% are undergoing treatment.

PAD may result from modifiable and non-modifiable risk factors (Bordeaux et al., 2003; Jaff, 2004a). Modifiable risk factors are

- Diabetes,
- Smoking,
- Hypertension, and
- Hypercholesterolemia.

Nonmodifiable risk factors are

- Age,
- Gender, and
- Family history.

Other risk factors include

- Obesity,
- Personal history of vascular disease,
- Heart attack,
- Stroke,
- Hyperhomocyteinemia,
- Elevated fibrinogen levels,
- Impaired fibrinolysis, and
- C-reactive protein.

PAD is caused by a lack of blood supply, typically to the lower extremities, as a result of stenosis (narrowing) or occlusion (blockage) within the arteries. This decreased blood flow may be mild or severe and can cause various symptoms of the lower extremities, including (West, Paz, & Vashi, 2009) the following:

- Cold extremities;
- Occasional numbness and tingling of the lower extremities;
- Absence of hair;
- Painful ulcers on pressure points; and

- Claudication, which increases with elevation; pain is classified as intermittent claudication, acute limb ischemia, or critical limb ischemia (Comerota & Schmieder, 2003).

Symptoms of PAD should be distinguished from symptoms of venous disorders, which include

- Painless ulcers of the ankle or leg;
- Aching pain that decreases with elevation;
- Brown discoloration of the skin;
- Warm extremity, especially if thrombosis is present (West et al., 2009); and
- Severe itching.

Table 4.4 describes the signs and symptoms of lower-extremity ischemia. The diagnosis of PAD is made by the physician completing an initial history and physical (H&P) evaluation and by performing noninvasive or invasive procedures.

The initial physician's H&P often includes

- A comprehensive history;
- Patient's exercise limitations;
- Presence of ischemic pain;
- A thorough review of other atherosclerotic risk factors and cardiovascular disease;
- Assessment of extremity pulses;
- Presence of audible bruits;
- Evaluation of skin integrity of legs and feet (absent hair and dystrophic or thickened toenails are not reliable physical findings);
- Presence of nonhealing ulcers over bony prominences of the feet and toes (usually painful, dry, nongranular tissue with black or gray base);
- Presence of gangrene;
- Report of presence of pallor with elevation of feet; and
- Notation of rubor, or redness, of the feet when in a dependent position (Jaff, 2004b).

After the initial H&P, the physician may list in the progress note the results of an Ankle Brachial Index (ABI). The ABI is performed to determine the patient's level of ischemia and severity of PAD. The ABI compares the

Table 4.4. Lower-Extremity Ischemia Signs and Symptoms

Type	Signs and Symptoms
Intermittent claudication	• Pain while walking that is relieved with rest • Fatigue • Cramping • Unilateral gluteal, thigh, calf and foot pain • Activity induced • Pain is relieved when exercise is discontinued • Limited activities of daily living • Diminished quality of life
Acute limb ischemia	• Sudden interruption in blood supply • Sensory–motor symptoms • Potential tissue destruction if perfusion is not restored
Critical limb ischemia	• Limited distal lower-extremity perfusion • Rest pain • Ischemic ulcers • Gangrene • Severe decreased quality of life • High rate of amputation • Marked increased short-term mortality • More intense diagnostic efforts, hospital rates, treatment modalities, and general medical care

Sources. Coffman and Eberhardt (2003); West, Paz, and Vashi, (2009).

BP in the pedal artery to that in the brachial artery (Jaff, 2004b). An ABI value less than .90 defines the presence of PAD ($\geq$.90 is considered normal). An abnormal ABI is also a predictor of cardiovascular morbidity and mortality (Bordeaux et al., 2003).

The occupational therapist's evaluation, treatment, or both may reveal additional information not otherwise obtained from the H&P, but that may be useful to the physician's continued plan of care. Information obtained during an occupational therapy session may include decreased sensation leading to impaired safety awareness during performance of activities of daily living (ADLs), transfers, or functional mobility. The patient may experience increased pain, edema, vascular changes, or decreased standing tolerance because of lack of blood flow to the lower extremities with out-of-bed activities. When documented by an occupational therapist, this information may assist the physician with continued assessments, treatment considerations, and discharge disposition.

Arterial duplex ultrasonography is another noninvasive procedure that can detect the location and severity of arterial stenosis and occlusions in lower-extremity occlusive disease (Jaff, 2004b). Other alternative diagnostic procedures to image peripheral arteries are magnetic resonance arteriography, computed tomography angiography, and contrast arteriography (Kaufman, 2003).

Magnetic resonance arteriography

- Examines blood vessels in various parts of the body;
- Involves a powerful magnetic field, radio waves, and a computer to produce detailed images, not ionizing radiation (i.e., X-rays); and
- May be performed with or without contrast.

The patient is usually able to resume normal activities after the test if sedation is not used (unless otherwise indicated by physician). Contrast may cause the patient to experience nausea or vomiting.

Computed tomography angiography is a radiological test that uses helical computed tomography scanners to obtain multiple images enhanced with contrast. The projected image is three-dimensional. *Contrast arteriography* involves X-ray films obtained while contrast is rapidly injected into the artery (Pagana & Pagana, 2007).

The diagnosis of PAD may also occasionally be verified by exercise testing. Testing may be done by having a patient walk on a treadmill in the vascular lab. The initial *claudication distance*, or pain with initial exercise, and the *maximal walking distance*, or distance walked before pain forces the patient to stop, are recorded. The ankle BP is recorded and should not fall to more than 20% of baseline. It should also not require longer than 3 minutes to return to baseline. Significant decreases in ankle BPs suggest severe claudication (Strandness, 2003).

Treatment of PAD and arteriosclerosis includes medication, surgical intervention, and modification of risk factors such as hypertension, diabetes, obesity, physical inactivity, smoking cessation, and eating a low-fat diet (Maciejko, 2004). Occupational therapists may assist in treatment by educating patients regarding

- Exercising to increase circulation;
- Encouraging diabetic patients to inspect their feet daily for calluses, cracks, corns, or ulcers;
- Avoiding use of constricting garters, adhesive tape, harsh chemicals, over-the-counter corn treatments, or electric pads on skin;
- Providing lower-extremity bathing techniques, such as using assistive devices as needed, using lukewarm water and mild soap, and drying feet gently and thoroughly;
- Instructing patients to change socks or stockings daily;
- Wearing well-fitting shoes without open heels or toes at all times when ambulating (diabetic patients may need off-loading shoes to decrease weight bearing on ulcers; special shoes may be required if patient has a history of hammer toes, bunions, or previous toe amputations); and
- Obtaining a podiatrist referral for continued foot care (Beers & Berkow, 1999).

Venous Stasis

The calf muscles contract to direct blood from the lower extremities toward the heart. *Venous stasis* occurs when blood flow is static or altered in the lower extremities. Lack of calf muscle activity and decreased blood flow can lead to thrombosis in the immobile patient. Loss of vein function or loss of blood flow may occur as a result of trauma or injury to the veins.

Blood clots in superficial veins are known as *superficial phlebitis*. Blood clots in deep veins are referred to as *deep venous thrombosis* (DVT). Superficial veins that become enlarged are called *varicose veins* (may appear as cords). The legs may feel full, ache, or become tired. These symptoms are often worse when standing and become relieved with elevation of the legs.

As the blood continues to collect, the skin becomes red or reddish brown as a result of red blood cell stains. This discoloration is referred to as *venous stasis dermatitis*. Venous stasis can be prolonged and cause venous stasis ulcers to develop. These ulcers have a red base and are seen on the medial side of the lower extremity (Schellong & Schwartz, 2002).

Treatment of venous stasis includes rest, elevation of the lower extremities, and wearing compression stockings. The extremity should be elevated higher than the heart to increase blood flow toward the heart. Occupational therapists can provide education regarding these treatments in preventing edema and alleviating pain.

Venous Thromboembolism

Three factors have become known as Virchow's triad and contribute to thrombosis: venous stasis, endothelial injury, and hypercoagulability of blood (Andrews et al., 2005). *Thrombus* is made up of fibrin, red and white blood cells, and platelets (Venes et al., 2001). Risk factors for thrombosis include

- Prolonged immobilization (including long-distance air travel),
- Surgery,
- Trauma,
- Cerebrovascular accident,
- Fractures of the long bones or pelvis,
- Spinal cord injury,
- Smoking,
- Age older than age 40,
- Malignancy,
- Heart failure,
- Previous venous thrombosis,
- Obesity,
- Pregnancy and contraceptives,
- Anesthesia and chemotherapy,
- Varicose veins,
- Inflammatory bowel disease,
- Renal failure,
- Central venous catheterization,
- Chronic obstructive pulmonary disease, and
- Thrombophilia (Test, 2008).

Deep Vein Thrombosis

According to Comerota and Chahwan (2007), an estimated 2 million people annually are diagnosed with DVT. Pulmonary embolism (PE) is also present in 30% to 50% of this population, with an incidence of 10% fatality within the first hour of development (Comerota & Chahwan, 2007). Blood clots

- May occur in the deep veins of the legs and can occur in the arms or pelvis;
- May occur from injured veins (e.g., surgery, trauma);
- Are asymptomatic in at least 50% of people;
- May break off and travel to the lungs to become a PE;
- Present with swelling, pain, tenderness, and warmth of affected area;
- Cause asymmetric calf edema with measurement taken 10 centimeters below tibial tuberosity (3-cm difference in calf girth is considered significant);
- Cause fever; and
- May present with a positive *Homan's sign* (pain with dorsiflexion of the foot).

Management of patients susceptible to DVT depends on the patient's risk factors, comorbidities, level of thrombus, and clinical presentation (Comerota & Chahwan, 2007). Physicians often prescribe heparin (unfractionated or low-molecular-weight heparin), warfarin (Coumadin), or aspirin. Selection of medication and dosage depends on patient's diagnosis, risk factors, or objective for using each medication. Medication dose is monitored by prothrombin time and the standardized international ratio with ranges of 2.0–3.0 (Bell & Halar, 2005).

The physician will inform the patient regarding the length of time the medication is required on discharge. The physician may also prescribe prophylactic devices such as intermittent pneumatic leg or foot compression or graduated compression stockings. Compression stockings worn for 1 year after the initial occurrence of DVT lowers the risk of postthrombotic syndrome. Pneumatic devices increase blood flow velocity and flow in the femoral vein to assist in the prevention of DVT (Knight & Sokolof, 2008).

Treatment for patients who are positive for DVT includes anticoagulation therapy, including unfractionated heparin, low-molecular-weight heparin, or warfarin (Knight & Sokolof, 2008). *Anticoagulants* are medications that help to prevent blood clots, help to prevent existing clots from enlarging, or both. However, anticoagulant medications do not dissolve blood clots. Patients who have a high risk for bleeding or who have a history of PE in spite of anticoagulation therapy may be treated with vena cava filters. If risk is temporary, then anticoagulants may be prescribed by the physician as soon as possible.

Thrombectomy or embolectomy (surgical removal of acute DVT) is generally used in patients with massive thrombosis, decreased arterial circulation, or contraindications to thrombolytic therapy. Thrombolysis (pharmacologic lysis) is used for patients with massive iliofemoral thrombosis or unstable cardiac or pulmonary disease, with no contraindication to thrombolytic therapy.

The risk of recurrent DVT is serious after treatment; therefore, monitoring and treatment (>12 months) may be indicated for patients with continuous risk factors for thromboembolic disease (Knight & Sokolof, 2008). Postthrombotic damage or syndrome may lead to chronic venous insufficiency, which causes limb edema, cellulitis, pain, stasis pigmentation, stasis dermatitis, or ulceration (Andrews et al., 2005; Beers & Berkow, 1999).

Occupational therapists may encourage patients to engage in ADLs and functional mobility activities once the patient's standardized international ratio returns to a therapeutic range, unless contraindicated by the physician. Early mobilization may improve a patient's symptoms of swelling and pain in the calf muscle; however, it will not completely eliminate the potential for PE. After treatment with heparin and warfarin has been initiated, ambulation may be permitted on the second or third day if the partial thromboplastin time is within the therapeutic range. Recent literature has indicated that bedrest for 5–7 days is not necessary if coagulation is within the therapeutic range (Bell & Halar, 2005). Check with facility protocol, the patient's physician, or both before mobilizing patients with suspected or confirmed DVT.

Superficial Thrombophlebitis

Superficial thrombophlebitis is sudden inflammation and blood clots that adhere to superficial vein walls. These blood clots may form in the arms, legs, or groin. If it occurs in the arm, it may be a result of intravenous catheters. These clots usually do not lead to PEs and usually resolve without treatment. Symptoms of superficial thrombophlebitis are

- Pain and swelling of affected area,
- Redness of skin over vein,
- Warmth,
- Tenderness, and
- Feeling of a hard cord under the skin (Bradbury & Ruckley, 2001).

Treatment of thrombophlebitis may include warm, moist compresses; medications for pain or inflammation; antibiotics if infection is a concern; support stockings to prevent reoccurrence of clots, DVT, or both; and surgery to prevent progression to deep veins (Ferri, 2005).

Occupational therapists may train patients in donning support or compression stockings if the stockings have been prescribed by the physician. Donning strategies include

- Using a plastic bag to increase the ease of sliding the stocking over the extremity: (1) Roll the stocking from proximal to distal before applying, (2) place a plastic bag over foot and leg with the end near the toe cut out, (3) put the stocking on over the plastic bag and pull proximally, (4) pull the plastic bag proximally until it is no longer inside the stocking, and (5) slide the plastic bag off of the extremity toward toes;
- Training patients in the use of assistive devices to increase their ease and success in donning the stockings;
- Instructing patients to inspect their extremity for ulcers, blisters, or wounds; patients should refrain from using these techniques if skin integrity is compromised or if wound care is in progress to prevent interference with wound healing.

Pulmonary Embolism

The incidence of PE in the United States is estimated to be 600,000 each year, leading to between 100,000 and 200,000 fatalities.

Many deaths occur when the PE is not suspected or is misdiagnosed (Test, 2008).

PE is caused by a DVT that breaks loose (embolus) and flows through the venous system toward the pulmonary arterial circulation. The embolus lodges in the lungs and blocks blood flow from the right side of the heart to the lungs. PE can be fatal. However, as many as two-thirds of patients may be asymptomatic. Symptoms of PE include

- Sudden dyspnea,
- Tachycardia,
- Tachypnea,
- Chest pain,
- Syncope,
- Cyanosis,
- Sweats, and
- Low-grade fever (Penner, 2004).

The most frequent treatment of thromboembolic events is intravenous heparin (Bell & Halar, 2005). Additional treatment approaches include vena cava filters, thrombolytic agents, and pulmonary artery embolectomy for patients with massive PE and refractory hypotension. Vena cava filters are indicated for patients with high risk for bleeding, recent central nervous system surgery, recent trauma, or recurrent PE in spite of anticoagulation therapy (National Institute of Health, 2010).

Compartment Syndrome

Compartment syndrome occurs when nerves and blood vessels are compressed within a confined space, and it may be acute or chronic. Acute compartment syndromes are the result of hemorrhage, edema, or both within a closed compartment; external compression; or arterial occlusion that occurs before postischemic reperfusion (Venes et al., 2001). The sudden rise in pressure that occurs results in decreased blood flow, which causes necrosis of the muscles and nerves in the involved compartment. Other causes of acute compartment syndrome include tibial fractures, crush injuries, muscle rupture, direct blow to a muscle, burns, or direct pressure from a cast (Barr, 2008).

Chronic compartment syndromes may occur as a result of increased muscle size during exercise or decreased size of the anatomical compartment (Venes et al., 2001). This condition is also called *chronic exertional compartment syndrome* and is an overuse injury commonly seen in sports requiring running.

Symptoms of compartment syndrome may include

- Pain,
- Swelling,
- Loss of voluntary movement of the involved muscles, and
- Sensory changes and paresthesias in the area supplied by the involved nerve (Barr, 2008).

Treatment of compartment syndrome includes fasciotomy, especially for the acute syndrome. The initial treatment of the chronic syndrome includes rest, ice, and nonsteroidal anti-inflammatory drugs. Occupational therapy is indicated for patients having difficulty with ADLs or functional mobility (Barr, 2008).

Gangrene

Gangrene is tissue death or necrosis caused by an interruption or absent blood supply to an organ or tissue. Blood supplies oxygen and nutrients necessary to feed cells and to assist the immune system in preventing infections. Cells cannot survive without a proper blood supply. Gangrene most commonly affects fingers and toes; however, it can also affect muscles and internal organs.

Signs and symptoms of gangrene include

- Blue or black discoloration of skin,
- Severe pain and numbness, and
- Foul-smelling discharge.

Gas or internal gangrene may also cause swelling and fever.

Septic shock may occur if bacterial infection from gangrenous tissue travels throughout the body. Symptoms of septic shock include

- Confusion,
- Light-headedness,

- Shortness of breath,
- Increased heart rate, and
- Low BP.

The five types of gangrene are dry, wet, gas, internal, and Fournier's. Types, etiology, and risk factors for gangrene are listed in Table 4.5. General risk factors for gangrene include

- Age (occurs more often in older .people);
- Blood vessel disease from blood clots or hardened and narrowed arteries that occlude blood flow;

- Severe injury or surgery causing trauma to skin and underlying tissue;
- Immunosuppression or immunocompromise (e.g., patients with HIV or patients undergoing chemotherapy or radiation); and
- Diabetes, because high blood sugar levels can eventually damage blood vessels, interrupting blood flow.

Gangrene is diagnosed by means of

- Blood tests that may detect the presence of infection (increased white blood cell count);

Table 4.5. Types of Gangrene, Appearance, and Causes or Risk Factors

Type	Appearance	Causes or Risk Factors
Dry	Shriveled, dry skin ranging in color from purplish-blue to black	Loss of blood circulation (i.e., blood vessel disease)
Wet	Edematous, blistering, and wet appearance, with bacterial infection in the tissue	Loss of blood circulation (i.e., severe burns, frostbite, diabetic injury to toe or foot); can be fatal
Gas	Pale skin, becomes gray or purplish-red in color, may have a bubbly appearance; gas in the tissue causes a crackling sound when the skin is touched	Loss of blood circulation due to an injury, trauma, or surgical wound that becomes infected with the bacteria *Clostridium perfringens;* toxins are produced that release gas and cause tissue breakdown and death; can be fatal
Internal	May not be visible; affects internal organs such as intestines, gallbladder, or appendix; may be suspected because of fever and severe pain	Occurs as a result of lack of blood flow to internal organs; can be fatal
Fournier's	Redness and edema in the genital area; rare type of gangrene	An infection in the genital area or urinary tract; mostly affects men; however, may occur in women

Sources. Goodman and Smirnova (2009), Mayo Clinic Staff (2009).

- Surgery to determine the extent of gangrene in the body;
- Imaging tests to view interior body structures, including X-ray, arteriogram, computed tomography, or magnetic resonance imaging; or
- Fluid or tissue culture to detect presence of bacteria clostridium perfringens or to determine signs of tissue death.

Treatment for gangrene includes

- IV antibiotics;
- Surgery to remove dead tissue;
- Surgical repair of damaged blood vessels to increase blood flow to the affected area and to help prevent the spread of gangrene;
- Amputation or surgical removal of an affected body part;
- Using hyperbaric oxygen therapy to treat gas gangrene by allowing arteries under pressure to carry greater amounts of oxygen (blood rich in oxygen helps infected wounds heal by inhibiting the growth of bacteria);
- Adequate nutrition and fluids; and
- Pain medication (Mayo Clinic Staff, 2007).

Raynaud's Syndrome

Raynaud's syndrome is classified as a primary disease of unknown etiology or as secondary to other conditions such as scleroderma, systemic lupus erythematosus, Buerger's disease, nerve entrapment or carpal tunnel syndrome, rheumatoid arthritis, or anorexia–bulimia. Raynaud's disease develops when vascular changes occur as a result of interruption of blood flow to the digits resulting from vasospastic attacks. These attacks occur secondary to the patient's exaggerated vasomotor response to cold or emotional stress.

Symptoms of Raynaud's include color changes of the digits from white (interruption of blood flow) to blue (lack of oxygen in the blood) to red (when arteries resume blood flow). Other fingers or toes (less likely, the thumb) may become involved as the disease progresses. Digital ischemia may result in painful, nonhealing ulcers;

pitting scars; gangrene; and digital infarction (Lakos, Manzi, & Varga, 2007). Sensory changes such as numbness, tingling, and burning may also occur. Raynaud's disease generally affects people younger than age 40 and affects women more than men by a ratio of 4:1 (Benatar, 2005).

Treatment for Raynaud's syndrome and phenomenon is the same (Benatar, 2005; Venes et al., 2001). Treatment for Raynaud's may include vasodilators and is commonly started with calcium channel blockers (Lakos et al., 2007). Occupational therapists may educate patients to limit their cold exposure, including wearing gloves, hats, and warm garments before going into cold environments (e.g., during winter, entering air-conditioned environments, while handling cold items). Additional education may include smoking cessation to decrease the potential for vasoconstriction and support to avoid stressful situations (Benatar, 2005).

Heparin-Induced Thrombocytopenia

Heparin is a common intravenous anticoagulant used in the prevention and treatment of blood clots. *HIT* is a complication of heparin use in which blood clots form as a result of the immune system's response to heparin. HIT causes a low platelet count, referred to as *thrombocytopenia*. A specific blood factor (Platelet 4 [PF4]) released by platelets can form an immune complex with heparin. The body interprets this complex (heparin PF4) as a foreign substance and forms an antibody against the heparin PF4 complex. Platelets are destroyed after the antibody binds to this complex.

The two types of HIT are (1) *nonimmune (HIT I)*, caused by a mild decrease in platelet count, and (2) *immune-mediated (HIT II)*, caused by much lower platelet counts. Patients with HIT II are at risk for major clotting problems (which occur 5–10 days after administering heparin). HIT II may cause thrombosis (i.e., DVT, PE) or venous gangrene (Ferguson, 2004). Symptoms may include vascular skin changes such as bruising or blackening of the fingers, toes, nipples, or the skin around the IV site (Warkentin, 2004).

HIT is treated by discontinuing heparin therapy and initiating alternative anticoagulation (Warkentin, 2004). Before initiating treatment, check the patient's platelet levels to determine whether platelets are within normal range. In addition, consult with the patient's physician to determine whether any contraindications to therapy exist because of the risk of bleeding.

Vasculitis

Vascular inflammation or *vasculitis* is also known as *angiitis, vascular necrosis,* or *necrotizing vasculitis.* Inflamed blood vessels such as arteries, veins, or capillaries may cause the body's immune system to protect itself from its own blood vessels. Inflamed blood vessels may become narrow, occluded, or stretched and weakened to the point of bulging, with the risk of aneurysm or hemorrhage. Vasculitis may also lead to cerebrovascular accident (with central nervous system vasculitis) or myocardial infarct (Roenigk & Young, 1996). Tissue death will occur if blood supply is not sufficient or if blood is not supplied by collateral blood vessels (alternate routes of blood supply).

The two types of vasculitides (plural of vasculitis) are (1) *primary vasculitides* (etiology is unknown) and (2) *secondary vasculitides* (response to infection, disease, or allergic reaction to medication). Table 4.6 describes the types of vasculitis and associated symptoms. Diseases of the immune system that may cause vasculitis include rheumatoid arthritis, systemic lupus erythematosus, or Sjogren's syndrome (Calabrese & Duna, 2002; Roenigk & Young, 1996). Medications that may cause an allergic reaction leading to vasculitis include diuretics and antibiotics (Ball & Bridges, 2002).

Symptoms depend on the type of vasculitis and the size of the blood vessel involved, the type of inflammatory cells, and the absence or presence of necrosis of blood vessel walls. Symptoms may include

- Rash;
- Peripheral neuropathy;
- Gastrointestinal symptoms, including abdominal pain;
- Hypertension (with renal cortical ischemia);
- Loss of appetite and weight loss;

Table 4.6. **Types of Vasculitis**

Type	Description
Behcet's disease	Occurs in any size or type of blood vessel and any part of the body; very common in the eyes, mouth, genital area; often affects those ages 15–45 years
Berger's disease (also known as thromboangiitis obliterans)	Causes inflammation and blood clots to the extremities; may cause pain in upper and lower extremities; may cause ulcers on fingers and toes; associated with smoking
Central nervous system vasculitis	Affects the brain and sometimes the spinal cord
Churg–Strauss syndrome	May affect many organs, including the lungs, skin, kidneys, heart, as well as people with asthma
Cryoglobulinemia	Associated with hepatitis C and lymphoma; causes hemorrhagic rash (purpura) on lower extremities, arthritis, weakness, neuropathy

Table 4.6. **(continued)**

Type	Description
Giant cell arteritis	Inflammation of arteries of the neck, upper body, extremities, head; usually affects people older than age 50; can cause headaches, scalp tenderness, jaw pain, blurred vision, double vision, blindness; associated with polymyalgia rheumatica
Henoch–Schonlein purpura	Caused by inflammation of blood vessels of skin, kidneys, joints, bowel; may cause abdominal or joint pain and blood in urine or stool; hemorrhagic rash (purpura) on buttocks, legs, feet; often occurs in children (however, can occur at any age) and may follow an upper respiratory infection
Microscopic polyangiitis	Generally affects blood vessels in the lungs, kidneys, skin, nerves; however, can affect other organs. Signs and symptoms include skin lesions, glomerulone-phritis (inflammation of the small blood vessels in the kidneys)
Polyarteritis nodosa	Most commonly affects blood vessels in the skin, heart, kidneys, peripheral nerves, muscles, intestines; however, may affect any organ. Signs and symptoms include fever, purpura, skin ulcers, muscle and joint pain, weight loss, kidney problems
Polymyalgia rheumatica	Commonly affects large joints in the body such as shoulders, hips, knees; often occurs with giant cell arteritis; signs and symptoms include pain and stiffness in the muscles of the hips, thighs, shoulders, upper arms, neck
Rheumatoid vasculitis	Associated with severe rheumatoid arthritis; may affect many parts of the body, including eyes, skin, hands, feet
Takayasu's arteritis	Affects the aorta and its branches; typically occurs in women of reproductive age; signs and symptoms include back and arm pain with movement, arm weakness, decreased or absent pulse, light-headedness, headaches, visual disturbances
Wegener's granulomatosis	Causes inflammation of the blood vessels in the nose, sinuses, throat (upper respiratory tract); lungs; and kidneys. Signs and symptoms may include shortness of breath, nasal stuffiness, chronic sinusitis, nosebleeds, frequent ear infections

Sources. Calabrese, Clough, & Hoffman (1996), Kent & Mattheson (2004), Shanahan & St. Claire (2002).

- Loss of energy;
- Fever; and
- Swelling.

Treatment of vasculitis depends on the type and severity of the disorder. Some types of vasculitis resolve without treatment. However, others require the use of medication. These medications have been used for treatment of vasculitis: corticosteroids (e.g., Prednisone), which may require short- or long-term use, and cytotoxic drugs, which may be used if corticosteroids are not effective in treating severe cases of vasculitis (e.g., axathiopine [Imuran] or cycloplosphamide [Cytoxan]). These drugs decrease inflammation in blood vessels (Kissin & Merkel, 2003).

Occupational therapists may intervene in treatment by encouraging patients to learn as much as possible about their condition and educating patients on the importance of

- Consulting a nutritionist regarding eating a healthy diet to prevent medication side effects, including osteoporosis, high BP, diabetes, or all of these;
- Participating in aerobic exercise (i.e., walking) to prevent bone loss, manage diabetes and high BP, and improve heart and lung function; and
- Consulting with their physician before starting any exercise program (Mayo Clinic Staff, 2007).

Medical Management of Vascular Disorders

Medical management of vascular disorders may include endovascular therapy, surgical procedures, and wound care.

Endovascular Therapy

Endovascular therapy has existed since the 1920s. Currently, endovascular therapy is used for purposes of diagnosing and treating vascular diseases. This therapy is the manipulation of pathology by an intraluminal approach (manipulation of clots within a vessel; Biswas & Fogarty, 1998).

Endovascular approaches include

- *Balloon angioplasty:* A balloon-tipped catheter inserted into a blood vessel. The artery is forced open when the balloon is inflated (Venes et al., 2001). Figure 4.2 shows a diagram of balloon angioplasty.
- *Stent:* A small metal mesh tube placed in a blood vessel to support or hold the vessel open. Some stents are inserted in the vessel and expanded by balloons. Figure 4.2 also shows a diagram of a stent (Dougherty & Zvonimir, 2004).
- *Vena cava filter:* A metal filter inserted into the vena cava. The filter traps clots from the lower extremities and prevents them from reaching the lungs. This filter may be used for patients who are not candidates for anticoagulant therapy (Society for Vascular Surgery, 2007). Figure 4.3 shows a diagram of an inferior vena cava filter.

Surgical Procedures

Surgical treatment for PVD may include bypass, endarterectomy, or amputation. *Bypass surgery* may be performed because of a narrowed or

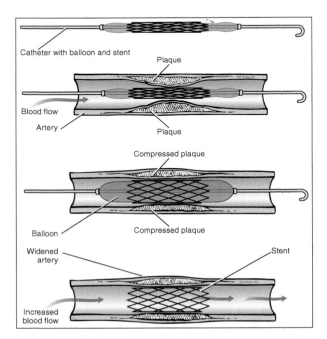

Figure 4.2. Balloon angioplasty and stent.
Source. Richard Fritzler, Medical Illustrator, Roswell, GA.

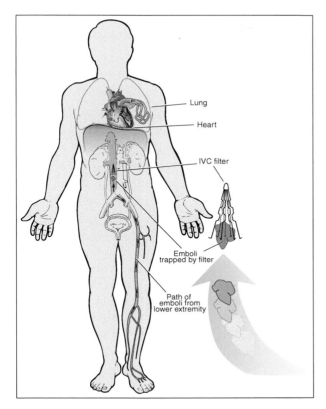

Figure 4.3. Inferior vena cava filter.
Source. Richard Fritzler, Medical Illustrator, Roswell, GA.

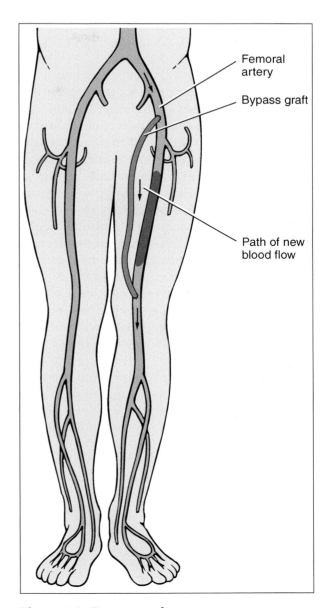

Figure 4.4. Bypass graft.
Source. Richard Fritzler, Medical Illustrator, Roswell, GA.

obstructed artery. Surgeons perform bypasses by attaching a prosthetic tube or a blood vessel above and below the area of obstruction. This bypass provides a detour around the obstructed area, allowing blood to flow through the bypass to the tissues (Beers & Berkow, 1999). Figure 4.4 shows a diagram of a bypass graft. *Endarterectomy* is the surgical removal of obstructions in an artery (Venes et al., 2001). Observe facility or physician precautions before treating patients after these procedures are performed.

Arterial occlusive disease or failed arterial reconstruction leads to lower-extremity *amputations*. Foot complications associated with diabetes also often lead to lower-extremity amputations. Vascular disease accounts for 76%–93% of acquired lower-extremity amputations (i.e., diabetic vascular disease and atherosclerosis). Two-thirds of all lower-extremity amputations are a result of diabetes (Bosker & Gitter, 2005).

Preservation of as much of the limb as possible is considered to promote wound healing and functional prosthetic fitting. Other issues to consider include the severity of the underlying disease process, the patient's medical condition, morbidity associated with wound salvage, and the patient's expected functional level after amputation (Bosker & Gitter, 2005).

Amputees require increased upper-extremity strength and energy expenditure. The patient's premorbid status will greatly influence functional mobility and progression with ADLs after lower-extremity amputation. Weakness, fatigue, phantom and incision pain, and anger and grief may impair the patient's ability to participate in ADLs. Ambulating on one limb with an assistive device requires approximately 60% more energy than normal ambulation. This demand approaches 38%–60% increased energy expenditure for below-knee amputees and 52%–116% increased energy expenditure for above-knee amputees (Gittler, 2008).

Treatment for amputees includes edema control, shaping of the residual limb, splinting to prevent contractures, and pain management. Flexion contractures may occur at the hip, the knee, or both. Surgeons often place a temporary, rigid dressing or use a knee immobilizer for positioning and to prevent contractures for patients with a below-knee amputation. Patients who have (transtibial) below-knee amputations are at risk for knee and hip flexion contractures when lying in bed or sitting. Encourage patients to extend the knee. Patients who have above-knee (transfemoral) amputations are at risk for hip flexion and abduction contractures resulting from sitting. Position the extremity in adduction. Avoid pillows under the residual limb, and promote lying in prone (Gittler, 2008).

The physician may prescribe fabrication of a posterior knee extension splint to prevent knee flexion contractures and to protect the stump from injury. The splint is usually worn at all times except during ADLs, vascular assessments, skin inspections, and dressing changes. Splint wear continues until the residual limb is appropriate for prosthetic training or until use of the splint is discontinued by the physician.

The focus of occupational therapy treatment includes performance of self-care; functional mobility and safety; and assessment of needs including durable medical equipment, assistive devices, or both. Functional mobility training may include safety during ambulation with an assistive device; wheelchair propulsion; and transfers to chair, bedside commode, toilet, tub, or shower stall. Occupational therapists may also educate the patient and family on positioning, splint wear, splint

precautions, skin inspection for vascular changes or wounds, and desensitization techniques such as

- Massaging for desensitization and to loosen adhesions and soften scar tissue;
- Applying sensory stimulation such as tapping, rubbing, or vibration; and
- Wrapping to promote shaping of the limb and desensitization. Wrapping is done in a figure-eight diagonal pattern from distal to proximal. Pressure of the wrap is from distal to proximal to promote shaping for future prosthetic fitting. Avoid wrapping in a circular pattern because of the tourniquet effect and interference with circulation. Figure 4.5 depicts the wrapping sequence for below-knee amputations. The wrap should be removed 2–3 times daily for skin inspection. Bandages can be washed and laid flat to dry (Armstrong & Stubblefield, 2008).

The occupational therapist will also need to monitor the patient's psychosocial presentation

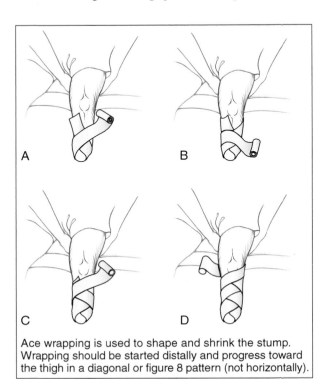

Ace wrapping is used to shape and shrink the stump. Wrapping should be started distally and progress toward the thigh in a diagonal or figure 8 pattern (not horizontally).

Figure 4.5. Below-knee amputation stump wrapping.
Source. Richard Fritzler, Medical Illustrator, Roswell, GA.

to determine whether additional referrals are warranted, including psychology or pastoral services if patient has difficulty accepting the loss of the limb.

Wound Care and Wound Vacuum-Assisted Closure Therapy

Many patients seen for wound care have wounds of a vascular disorder origin (e.g., arterial, venous, diabetic). The evaluation of patients seen by physicians or wound care specialists usually includes a vascular assessment. The success of wound healing is affected by physician assessment and treatment of vascular disease. Wounds may reoccur in the presence of underlying untreated vascular disease.

Vacuum-assisted closure (VAC), referred to as *wound vac*, is also known as *negative pressure wound therapy*. In 1995, the U.S. Food and Drug Administration approved and introduced the V.A.C. Therapy System. The V.A.C. system is used for the management of acute and chronic wounds. An open-cell foam dressing is placed into the wound cavity, and negative pressure is applied. An airtight thin-film secondary dressing distributes the negative pressure over the wound surface and facilitates the drainage of excessive fluid and debris (Gabriel, Gupta, Hiltabidel, & Valenzuela, 2007). This treatment promotes healing because it leads to decreased bacteria, decreased interstitial edema, and increased blood flow. Figure 4.6 shows a picture of a wound vac application.

Pressure ulcers and venous, arterial, and neuropathic ulcers have been proven to be appropriate for treatment with VAC therapy. Contraindications to use of VAC therapy include necrotic tissue, untreated osteomyelitis, malignancy in the wound, and fistulas to organs or body cavities. Precautions to consider include bleeding, anticoagulant use, and exposure of vital organs (Gabriel et al., 2007).

Occupational therapists treating patients who are on VAC therapy should observe the following precautions (KCI, 2007):

- Consult the patient's nurse if the VAC therapy dressing pad tubing is too short to allow patient mobilization. The nurse may

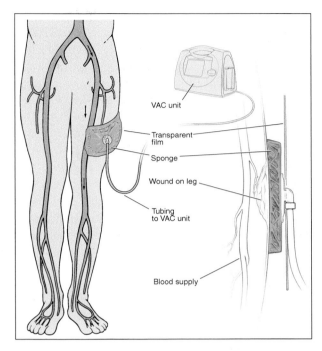

Figure 4.6. Wound vac.
Source. Richard Fritzler, Medical Illustrator, Roswell, GA.

interrupt VAC therapy for occupational therapy treatment (portable battery-operated VAC therapy systems are available).

- Do not turn VAC therapy off without consulting with the patient's nurse because there is a 2-hour (within 24 hours) time limit in which the VAC can be off. The VAC system is recommended to remain on continuously for the first 48 hours and may be intermittent after the initial period. Continuous therapy may be indicated if the patient is at risk of bleeding, the patient experiences discomfort with intermittent therapy, maintaining an airtight seal is difficult, large amounts of drainage are present, grafts or flaps are susceptible to shearing, or a splinting effect is needed (e.g., sternal or abdominal wounds).

- Do not adjust VAC therapy settings.

- Notify the patient's nurse or physician if increased bleeding or leaking occurs at the wound site or if bright red blood is noticed in the tubing or canister.

- Make sure dressing pad tubing is not obstructed or pulled during functional mobility.
- Notify the nurse if the VAC therapy alarm sounds during treatment, indicating a need for adjustment or service.

Occupational Therapy Approach

Occupational therapists serve an important role in treatment of patients with vascular disorders in educating and increasing patients' awareness of their disease, as well as instructing patients on lifestyle modifications, including diet, exercise, and smoking cessation. The following general guidelines are offered to assist occupational therapists working with this population:

- Notice whether extremities show differences in skin color and temperature or edema is present in patients with vascular compromise. Notify the doctor, nurse, or both and document changes.
- Monitor patients' vital signs before, during, and after treatment to determine tolerance to therapy.
- Allow time for position changes in patients with orthostatic hypotension.
- Consider deferring occupational therapy if the physician orders tests such as electrocardiogram, chest X-ray, D-dimer, ventilation perfusion scan, computed tomography angiogram, or computed tomography angiogram with venography to rule out PE or duplex ultrasonography to rule out DVT (Test, 2008).
  - Consult physician or refer to facility policy to determine when to resume occupational therapy if results are pending or positive (and not anticoagulated).
  - Modify or defer treatment pending lab values, physician instructions, or facility policy for patients with abnormal blood counts or coagulation times. Some physicians allow patients who are positive for DVT to engage in activity after low-molecular-weight heparin has been given for at least 24 hours (refer to Appendix P for information on normal lab values and when occupational therapy treatment may be contraindicated).
  - Encourage patients to engage in routine occupation (i.e., ADLs, functional mobility) once their standardized international ratio levels are therapeutic, unless contraindicated by physician.
- Be aware of any contraindications to taking BP on a particular extremity.
- Avoid use of cold water during self-care activities or any treatment that may further constrict blood vessels in the hands or feet (e.g., wrapping Thera-Band® around hands, applying tight socks or tight shoes, maintaining prolonged grip on exercise equipment).

Occupational therapy's role in treating patients with vascular disorders and diseases involves education and training to enhance patients' self-care performance, functional mobility skills, and safety. This role includes educating patients and increasing their knowledge of their specific condition and making appropriate referrals to promote overall health and wellness.

References

Andrews, K., Gamble, G., Gloviczki, P., Rooke, T., & Strick, D. (2005). Vascular diseases. In E. A. J. DeLisa (Ed.), *Physical medicine and rehabilitation* (4th ed., Vol. 1, pp. 797–808). Philadelphia: Lippincott Williams & Wilkins.

Armstrong, A., & Stubblefield, K. (2008). Amputations and prosthesis. In C. T. Latham & M. Radomski (Eds.), *Occupational therapy for physical dysfunction* (6th ed., pp. 1264–1294). Philadelphia: Lippincott Williams & Wilkins.

Atkins, M. S. (2008). Spinal cord injury. In C. T. Latham & M. Radomski (Eds.), *Occupational therapy for physical dysfunction* (6th ed., pp. 1171–1213). Philadelphia: Lippincott Williams & Wilkins.

Ball, G., & Bridges, L. (2002). Pathogenesis of vasculitis. In G. Ball & L. Bridges (Eds.), *Vasculitis* (pp. 39–40). New York: Oxford University Press.

Barr, K. (2008). Compartment syndrome. In T. Frontera, T. Rizzo, & J. Silver (Eds.), *Essentials of physical medicine and rehabilitation* (2nd ed., pp. 325–330). Philadelphia: W. B. Saunders.

Beers, M., & Berkow, R. (Eds.). (1999). *The Merck manual* (17th ed.). Whitehouse Station, NJ: Merck Research Laboratories.

Bell, K., & Halar, E. (2005). Immobility and inactivity: Physiological and functional changes, prevention, and treatment. In E. A. J. DeLisa (Ed.), *Physical medicine and rehabilitation* (4th ed., Vol. 2, pp. 1447–1468). Philadelphia: Lippincott Williams & Wilkins.

Benatar, M. (2005). Raynaud's phenomenon. In F. Ferri (Ed.), *Clinical advisor instant diagnosis and treatment* (pp. 695–696). Philadelphia: Elsevier.

Berry, C., & Vuong, P. (2002). Atherosclerosis. In *The pathology of vessels* (pp. 71–88). Paris: Springer.

Biswas, A., & Fogarty, T. (1998). Evolution of endovascular therapy: Diagnostics and therapeutics. In T. Fogarty & R. White (Eds.), *Peripheral endovascular techniques* (2nd ed., pp. 3–10). Paris: Springer.

Bockenek, W., DeJong, G., Friedland, M., Lanig, I., & Mann, N. (2005). Primary care for persons with disability. In E. A. J. DeLisa (Ed.), *Physical medicine and rehabilitation* (4th ed., Vol. 2, pp. 1469–1492). Philadelphia: Lippincott Williams & Wilkins.

Bordeaux, L. M., Hirsch, A. T., & Reich, L. M. (2003). The epidemiology and natural history of peripheral arterial disease. In J. D. Coffman & R. T. Eberhardt (Eds.), *Peripheral arterial disease diagnosis and treatment* (pp. 21–34). Totowa, NJ: Humana Press.

Bosker, G., & Gitter, A. (2005). Upper and lower extremity prosthetics. In E. A. J. DeLisa (Ed.), *Physical medicine and rehabilitation* (4th ed., Vol. 2, pp. 1325–1354). Philadelphia: Lippincott Williams & Wilkins.

Bradbury, A., & Ruckley, V. (2001). Clinical assessment of patients with venous disease. In P. Glovicki & J. Yao (Eds.), *Handbook of venous disorders* (2nd ed., pp. 71–83). London: Arnold.

Calabrese, L., Clough, J., & Hoffman, G. (1996). Systemic vasculitis. In J. Bartholomew, J. Olin, & J. Young (Ed.), *Peripheral vascular diseases* (2nd ed., pp. 380–406). St. Louis, MO: Mosby.

Calabrese, L. D., & Duna, G. (2002). Vasculitis of the central nervous system. In G. Ball & L. Bridges (Eds.), *Vasculitis* (pp. 445–459). New York: Oxford University Press.

Coffman, J. D., & Eberhardt, R. T. (2003). Clinical evaluation of intermittent claudication. In J. D. Coffman & R. T. Eberhardt (Eds.), *Peripheral arterial disease diagnosis and treatment* (pp. 35–54). Totowa, NJ: Humana Press.

Collins, S. M., & Dias, K. J. (2009). Cardiac system. In J. C. Paz & M. P. West (Eds.), *Acute care handbook for physical therapists* (3rd ed., pp. 10–11). St. Louis, MO: W. B. Saunders.

Comerota, A., & Chahwan, S. (2007). Venous thrombosis. In E. T. Bope & R. E. Rakel (Eds.), *Conn's current therapy* (60th ed., pp. 435–444). Philadelphia: W. B. Saunders.

Comerota, A., & Schmieder, F. (2003). Chronic limb ischemia. In J. D. Coffman & R. T. Eberhardt (Eds.), *Peripheral arterial disease diagnosis and treatment* (pp. 93–119). Totowa, NJ: Humana Press.

DeFranco, A. C., Hongbao, M., Kantipudi, S. C., & Abela, G. S. (2004). Anatomy, physiology, and response to vascular injury. In G. Abelo (Ed.), *Peripheral vascular disease: Basic diagnostic and therapeutic approaches* (pp. 1–22). Philadelphia: Lippincott Williams & Wilkins.

Dougherty, K., & Zvonimir, K. (2004). Endovascular equipment and interventional tools. In R. Heuser & M. Henry (Eds.), *Peripheral vascular interventions* (pp. 35–49). London: Martin Dunitz.

Ferri, F. (2005). Thromboplebitis. In M. Benator, F. Ferri, J. Masci, L. Mercier, P. Petropoulous, I. Tong & T. Wachtel (Eds.), *Ferri's clinical advisor instant diagnosis and treatment*, (7th ed., pp. 685–686, pp. 816–818). Philadelphia: Elsevier Mosby.

Ferguson, L. (2004). Anticoagulant and antiplatelet therapy in peripheral vascular disease. In G. Abela (Ed.), *Peripheral vascular disease* (pp. 200–214). Philadelphia: Lippincott Williams & Wilkins.

Fischbach, F., & Dunning, M., III (2009). Overview of basic bold hematology and coagulation tests. In N. Waltz (Ed.), *A manual of laboratory and diagnostic tests* (8th ed., pp. 56–183). Philadelphia: Wolters Kluwer Health.

Gabriel, A., Gupta, S., Hiltabidel, E., & Valenzuela, A. (2007). Management of the wound environment with negative pressure wound therapy. In C. S. Bates-Jensen (Ed.), *Wound care* (3rd ed., pp. 683–689). Philadelphia: Lippincott Williams & Wilkins.

Gittler, M. (2008). Lower limb amputations. In W. Frontera, T. Rizzo, & J. Silver (Eds.), *Essentials of physical medicine and rehabilitation* (pp. 599–604). Philadelphia: W. B. Saunders.

Goodman, C. C., & Smirnova, I. V. (2009). The Cardiovascular System. In C. C. Goodman & K. S. Fulter (Eds.), *Pathology: Implications for the physical therapist* (3rd ed., pp. 519–641). St. Louis, MO: Saunders/Elsevier.

Gregory, S., & Oparil, S. (2002). Systemic hypertension. In P. Lanzer & E. Topol (Eds.), *Pan vascular medicine* (pp. 1015–1064). Berlin: Springer.

Jacoby, D., & Mohler, E. (2004). Peripheral arterial disease. In G. Abela (Ed.), *Peripheral vascular disease* (pp. 190–199). Philadelphia: Lippincott Williams & Wilkins.

Jaff, M. (2004a). The natural history of peripheral arterial disease: Indication for endovascular therapy. In M. Henry & R. Heuser (Eds.), *Peripheral vascular interventions* (pp.1–4). London: Martin Dunitz.

Jaff, M. (2004b). Peripheral arterial disease. In M. Henry & R. Heuser (Eds.), *Peripheral vasular interventions* (pp. 15–18). London: Martin Dunitz.

Kaufman, J. A. (2003). Vascular imaging with x-ray, magnetic resonance, and computed tomography angiography. In J. D. Coffman & R. T. Eberhardt (Eds.), *Peripheral arterial disease: Diagnosis and treatment* (pp. 75–92). Totowa, NJ: Humana Press.

KCI. (2007). *V.A.C.® therapy safety information.* Retrieved August 15, 2010, from http://www.kci1.com

Kent, P., & Mattheson, E. (2004). Clinical feature and differential diagnosis. In P. Haynes, D. Piesetsky, & E. Williams St. Clair (Eds.), *Rheumatoid arthritis* (pp. 11–25). Philadelphia: Lippincott, Williams, and Wilkins.

Kissin, W. Y., & Merkel, P. A. (2003). Large-vessel vasculitis. In J. D. Coffman & R. T. Eberhardt (Eds.), *Peripheral arterial disease* (pp. 315–346). Totowa, NJ: Humana Press.

Knight, R., & Sokolof, J. (2008). Deep venous thrombosis. In T. Frontera, T. Rizzo, & J. Silver (Eds.), *Essentials of physical medicine and rehabilitation* (pp. 657–664). Philadelphia: W. B. Saunders.

Lakos, G., Manzi, S. M., & Varga, J. (2007). Connective tissue disorders. In E. T. Bope & R. E. Rakel (Eds.), *Conn's therapy* (59th ed., pp. 936–941). Philadelphia: W. B. Saunders.

Maciejko, J. (2004). The management of hyperlipidemia and exercise therapy in the treatment of peripheral arterial disease. In G. Abela (Ed.), *Peripheral vascular disease: Basic diagnostic and therapeutic approaches* (pp. 168–189). Philadelphia: Lippincott Williams & Wilkins.

Malone, D. J. (2006). Cardiovascular diseases and Disorders. In D. J. Malone & K. L. B. Lindsay (Eds.), *Physical therapy in acute care: A clinician's guide* (pp. 139–209). Thorofare, NJ: Slack.

Mayo Clinic Staff. (2007). *Gangrene, vasculitis.* Retrieved April 27, 2009, from www.mayoclinic.com

Mayo Clinic Staff. (2009). *Gangrene.* Retrieved August 16, 2010, from http://www.mayoclinic.com/health/gangrene/DS00993

National Institute of Health. (2010). *Pulmonary embolism.* Retrieved August 18, 2010, from www.nlm.nih.gov/medlineplus/ency/article/000132.htm

Pagana, K., & Pagana, T. (2007). *Diagnostic and laboratory test reference* (8th ed.). St. Louis, MO: Mosby.

Penner, J. P. (2004). Pulmonary embolism. In G. Abela (Ed.), *Peripheral vascular disease* (pp. 461–469). Philadelphia: Lippincott Williams & Wilkins.

Prisant, L. M. (2008). Hypertension. In R. E. Rakel & E. T. Bope (Eds.), *Conn's therapy* (60th ed., pp. 350–360). Philadelphia: W. B. Saunders.

Roenigk, H., & Young, J. (1996). Leg ulcers. In J. Bartholomew, R. Groar, J. W. Olin, & J. R. Young (Eds.), *Peripheral vascular disease* (pp. 605–638). St. Louis, MO: Mosby.

Scalone, V. (2007). Blood. In L. B. Deitch, I. H. Richman, & A. Sorkowitz (Eds.), *Essentials of anatomy and physiology* (5th ed., pp. 250–271). Philadelphia: F. A. Davis.

Schellong, S., & Schwartz, T. (2002). Peripheral vascular disease: Non-surgical approach. In P. Lanzer & E. Topol (Eds.), *Pan vascular medicine* (pp. 1497–1525). New York: Springer.

Shanahan, J., & St. Claire, W. E. (2002). Inflammory diseases of the coronary artery. In P. Lanzer & E. Topol (Eds.), *Panvascular medicine* (pp. 935–970). New York: Springer.

Society for Vascular Surgery. (2007). *Pulmonary embolism.* Retrieved November 16, 2008, from www.vascularweb.org/vascularhealth/Pages/PulmonaryEmbolism.aspx

Strandness, D. E. (2003). Hemodynamics and the vascular laboratory. In J. D. Coffman & R. T. Eberhardt (Eds.), *Peripheral arterial disease: Diagnosis and treatment* (pp. 55–74). Totowa, NJ: Humana Press.

Test, V. (2008). Pulmonary embolism. In E. T. Bope & R. E. Rakel (Eds.), *Conn's current therapy* (60th ed., pp. 267–269). Philadelphia: W. B. Saunders.

University of Wisconsin Health. (2008). *Hypertension*. Retrieved August 23, 2009, from http://apps. uwhealth.org/health/hie/1/000468.htm

University of Wisconsin Health. (2009). *Malignant hypertension*. Retrieved August 23, 2009, from http://apps.uwhealth.org/health/hie/1/000491. htm

Venes, D., Thomas, C. L., & Taber, C. W. (Eds.). (2001). *Taber's cyclopedia medical dictionary* (19th ed.). Philadelphia: F. A. Davis.

Warkentin, T. (2004). Heparin induced thrombocytopenia. *Circulation, 110,* e454–e458.

West, M. P., Paz, J. C., & Vashi, F. (2009). Vascular system and hematology. In J. C. Paz & M. P. West (Eds.), *Acute care handbook for physical therapists* (3rd ed., pp. 219–262). St. Louis, MO: Saunders/ Elsevier.

5

The Pulmonary System

Helene Smith-Gabai, OTD, OTR/L, BCPR

Breathing is a function of the pulmonary system, whose main purpose is inspiration to provide oxygen to tissue and exhalation to remove carbon dioxide from the body. Breathing is both an automatic and a voluntary process, often not thought about until difficulty occurs. Disorders within the pulmonary system may be the result of genetics, infection, or injury from inhaled toxins, such as cigarette smoke, air pollution, or occupational fumes and particles.

Lung function and heart function are essential for life. Any impairment in the pulmonary system can have a profound effect on other body systems. Therefore, it is essential that therapists have a basic understanding of how this system works and of its impact on occupational performance and quality of life.

Normal Structure and Function

Breathing is a dynamic and complex activity requiring coordination between the lungs and the pulmonary tree, the musculoskeletal system (i.e., rib cage and muscles), and the nervous system. *Lung parenchyma* (the functional parts of lung tissue) consists of two lungs. The *right lung* has three lobes, and the *left lung* has two. The pulmonary system is also divided into both an upper and a lower airway. The *upper airway* includes the nose, pharynx, and larynx. The *lower airway* includes the trachea, bronchi, and lungs. The lower airway becomes increasingly narrow and more numerous as it progresses from the two bronchi toward the alveolar sacs (DePalo & McCool, 2003). The lower airway is also referred to as the *bronchial tree*.

The upper airway humidifies and filters air before it descends to the lower airway. Air that is breathed in through the nose or mouth passes into the pharynx. The *epiglottis* (a flap of tissue located in the pharynx) prevents anything swallowed from entering the larynx and trachea, minimizing the risk of aspiration. The *vocal cords* are also located in the larynx, and air passing through the larynx causes the vocal cords to vibrate, creating sound. The *trachea* extends from the base of the larynx and branches off into the two main *bronchi*, which enter each lung. The bronchi further branch off into *bronchioles*, which further branch off into *alveolar sacs*. *Acini* are the gas exchange units of the lungs, which consist of bronchioles, *alveolar ducts,* and the *alveoli* (DePalo & McCool, 2003). The lungs contain approximately 300 million alveoli (Doniger, 2003). Anywhere within the pulmonary system where gas exchange does not occur is considered dead space. Figure 5.1 illustrates the components of the pulmonary system.

The inspiration and exhalation of breathing are generally a function of changes in thoracic pressure attributed to muscular contraction and relaxation. The *diaphragm* is the main inspiratory muscle separating the thoracic and abdominal cavities (DePalo & McCool, 2003). In *inspiration*, the external intercostals, parasternal internal intercostals, scalenes, and sternocleidomastoids contract to move the rib cage up and out while the diaphragm contracts and moves down, resulting in enlargement of the thoracic cavity and a decrease in lung pressure. This decrease in pressure results in air being sucked in.

Expiration is a passive process in which elastic recoil and relaxation of the diaphragm moves the diaphragm back up while the rib cage moves inward and down, forcing air out of the lungs. In addition to this passive process, active contraction of abdominal wall muscles and the internal intercostals can aid in forced exhalation. When inhalation and exhalation are compromised,

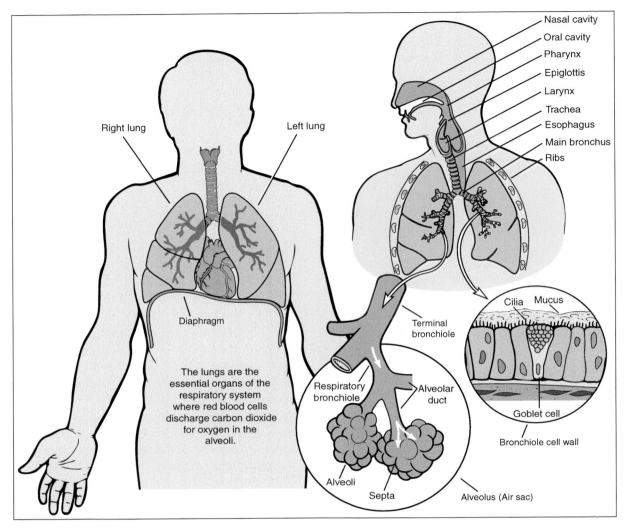

Figure 5.1. The pulmonary system.
Source. Richard Fritzler, Medical Illustrator, Roswell, GA.

accessory muscles can be recruited for respiration. The accessory muscles include the scalenes, sternocleidomastoid, pectoralis, erector spinae, and upper serratus posterior superior muscles (Migliore, 2004b). However, breathing with accessory muscles is generally shallow and inefficient.

The *lung parenchyma* is located within the chest cavity behind the ribs and surrounded by a visceral and parietal pleura membrane. The parietal layer lines the mediastinum and chest wall and folds on itself to form the *visceral membrane,* which surrounds and separates the two lungs. Between these two membranes is the *pleural space* or *pleural cavity,* a thin space containing *serous fluid.* This fluid provides lubrication, allowing for easy movement during respiration, and it also provides surface tension between the lungs and chest wall. In addition, the pleural membranes ensure that the two lungs do not touch, so that if one lung is injured (e.g., through trauma or pneumothorax), the other lung remains airtight.

Ventilation and Perfusion

Two of the most important bodily functions of the cardiopulmonary system are ventilation and perfusion. *Ventilation* is the breathing in and out of air (i.e., inhalation and exhalation).

Ventilation occurs as previously mentioned, through changes in pressure gradients from a high pressure area to a low pressure area (i.e., between inside and outside the body). When the pressure outside the body is higher than the pressure in the lungs, inspiration occurs. When pressure inside the lungs is higher than atmospheric pressure, expiration occurs (Gould, 2006).

Respiration is the gas exchange that takes place between the alveoli and pulmonary capillaries. However, *respiratory rate* refers to the number of times the chest rises and falls with each breath that is inhaled and exhaled (ventilation). Normal respiration is 12–20 breaths per minute. However, ventilation may be affected by the body's requirements for oxygen. For example, during certain activities and exercises, ventilation may be increased to accommodate the body's oxygen needs, which may result in increased rate and depth of breathing. Ventilation can also be affected by emotions (i.e., hypothalamus activity); changes in temperature; or drugs, which depress the central nervous system.

Ventilation is necessary for gas exchange (respiration), which occurs through simple diffusion across the capillary–alveoli boundary. The lungs contain millions of alveoli, which are surrounded by capillaries. Once oxygen crosses from the alveoli to the capillaries, it binds with hemoglobin. Oxygen-rich blood then travels through the pulmonary artery to the left side of the heart, where it is then transported to the rest of the body. The pulmonary vein carries blood containing carbon dioxide from the heart to the lungs, where it is exhaled out of the body.

Perfusion is the blood flow through the pulmonary capillaries. In normal adults, the ventilation to perfusion (V/Q) ratio is closely matched (approximately 0.8; DePalo & McCool, 2003). However, many pulmonary conditions result in a V/Q mismatch (i.e., disorders of ventilation, perfusion, or both) that can interfere with normal respiratory function (e.g., asthma, emphysema, interstitial lung disease). A V/Q mismatch may occur if perfusion is normal but ventilation is not or if ventilation is normal but perfusion is diminished.

The drive to breathe is located within the respiratory center of the autonomic nervous system. Impulses from the medulla oblongata and pons of the brainstem stimulate respiratory muscles to contract. Central chemoreceptors in the medulla oblongata monitor changes in cerebrospinal fluid. When carbon dioxide levels increase (hypercapnia) and pH decreases, the respiratory center is stimulated (Gould, 2006).

The carotid arteries and the aorta also contain peripheral chemoreceptors, which also signal the respiratory center when changes in pH and carbon dioxide level occur. These peripheral chemoreceptors also monitor oxygen levels to stimulate the respiratory center in preventing hypoxia. In addition, stretch receptors in the bronchi and bronchioles signal the respiratory center to halt stimulation of the inspiratory muscles and allow for expiration. This reflex, known as the *Hering–Breuer reflex*, prevents overinflation of the lungs.

Pulmonary Defense System

More than any other organ of the body with the exception of the skin, the lungs are constantly exposed to microorganisms that are breathed in. However, the lower airways are protected through the lung's defense mechanisms. The upper respiratory tract warms, filters, and humidifies inhaled air. Air that is breathed in is predominantly composed of nitrogen (78%), oxygen (~21%), argon (0.9%), and a smaller percentage of other elements and compounds. Additional defense mechanisms are cough, secretions (i.e., mucus and surfactant), and the body's natural antibodies.

- *Cough:* Irritant receptors in the larynx, trachea, and bronchi stimulate the cough reflex, which removes debris and germs from the lungs through a high-velocity response (DePalo & McCool, 2003).
- *Secretions: Mucous* is a sticky substance secreted by the epithelium cells and submucosal glands of the respiratory system. Mucous traps dust, germs, and other unwanted material; the *cilia* (hairlike projections that move

in a wavelike motion) in the epithelium then transport mucous and trapped debris up through the respiratory system to the nose and pharynx, to be removed from the body by sneezing, coughing, or swallowing. *Surfactant* is another substance that lines the alveoli and protects the lungs. Surfactant reduces surface tension and helps maintain the integrity of alveoli, ensuring they remain open for optimal breathing. Without surfactant, atelectasis would occur, and the lungs would collapse.

- *Immune system:* Cellular and humoral immune responses protect the lungs from infection and foreign particles through phagocytosis.

Diagnostic Testing

The pulmonary system can be compromised because of a disease or disorder of the lung structures (i.e., lung parenchyma, respiratory muscles, bones of the rib cage, pleura) or lung function (e.g., impaired ventilation, injury to the respiratory center) or as a consequence of other organ system disorders. Table 5.1 lists common diagnostic tests unique to pulmonary disorders. Two of the most common tests of pulmonary function are measurements of oxygenation (pulse oximetry and arterial blood gas [ABG] panels) and pulmonary function testing.

Oxygenation levels are usually monitored using *pulse oximetry*, a noninvasive, indirect

Table 5.1. Common Diagnostic Tests Unique to Respiratory Disorders

Test	Description
Bronchoscopy	A thin endoscopic tube is inserted through the nose or mouth and down into the airways to visually examine the respiratory tract for abnormalities. Also used to obtain biopsy of tissue samples and remove secretions for analysis. Bronchoscopy may be used therapeutically to remove secretions and foreign objects obstructing the airway or for stent placement to make sure the airway stays patent.
Thoracocentisis	A needle is inserted into the pleural space to aspirate or remove fluid for analysis.
V/Q scan	A ventilation/perfusion scan uses radioisotopes to examine the relationship between ventilation (airflow) and perfusion (blood flow) in the lungs. A mismatch is indicative of disease. A V/Q scan is useful in detecting the presence of pulmonary embolism.
Pulmonary function test	A series of tests that measure lung function. A pulmonary function test assists in determining diffusion abnormalities, obstructions, and restrictive patterns of breathing. Refer to Table 5.3 for more detail.
6-minute walk test	Simple test that measures patient's exercise capacity. A route is predetermined, usually in a hallway or on a track. The patient is asked to walk as far as possible in 6 minutes. The distance is measured and recorded. Frequency and duration of rest stops are also recorded. Speed (miles per hour) and metabolic equivalents (energy required for the body at rest) are also determined from scores. This information can be useful in formulating a plan of care for patients and for monitoring progress.

technique that reflects oxyhemoglobin saturation levels and changes in oxygenation. Oxygenation levels are measured by a probe either wrapped around or clipped on a finger, toe, or ear. Readings are obtained by red and infrared wavelengths of light and a photodetector placed on a pulsating arteriolar bed (Schutz, 2001). Poor readings may be the result of cold fingers or poor circulation, nail polish, bruising under the nail, movement of the probe cord, extreme hypoxia, or increased levels of carboxyhemoglobin. Another disadvantage of pulse oximetry is that it cannot distinguish between oxygen or carbon monoxide bound to hemoglobin and is therefore never used with suspected carbon monoxide poisoning (Schutz, 2001).

A new type of oxygenation monitor for critically ill patients is called an *StO2*. This device is also noninvasive, but differs from pulse oximetry in that it offers continuous monitoring of tissue oxygenation and is an early detector of hypoperfusion.

For a true measure of oxygenation levels, an *ABG panel* is required. In an ABG panel, a sample of blood is taken from an artery, and the concentration of oxygen and carbon dioxide in the blood is checked. An ABG panel is useful in detecting hypoxemia and acid–base imbalances. Table 5.2 lists ABG values (refer to Appendix P for more information).

Pulmonary function testing is used diagnostically for a variety of restrictive and obstructive diseases such as chronic obstructive pulmonary disease (COPD), asthma, sarcoidosis, and fibrosis. A pulmonary function test measures the volume and flow of air during breathing, the strength of respiratory muscles, and how well the lungs function by delivering oxygen to the blood system (lung diffusion capacity). Table 5.3 lists common terms used in pulmonary function testing.

Manifestations of Pulmonary Disorder

Symptoms of pulmonary disorder generally include

- *Dyspnea:* The subjective experience of shortness of breath, often described as air hunger that worsens with activity and may be accompanied by anxiety. It is one of the most important symptoms affecting engagement in daily activities, occupational performance, and quality-of-life issues (Darbee & Ohtake, 2006). Dyspnea management focuses on desensitization, controlled breathing, and educating patients that dyspnea is an ineffective breathing pattern that is not associated with hypoxemia (Migliore, 2004b; refer to Appendix 5.A for detail on dyspnea management). The Medical Research Council has developed a quick dyspnea scale to help quantify the relationship between levels of breathlessness and physical exertion (Darbee & Ohtake, 2006). See Table 5.4 for the Modified Medical Research Council Dyspnea Scale, which may be a useful tool in monitoring patients' progress and patients' perceptions of health-related quality of life.

Table 5.2. **Arterial Blood Gas Values**

Component	Arterial Blood Gas Levels
Partial pressure of oxygen (PaO_2)	80–100 mm Hg
Partial pressure of carbon dioxide ($PaCO_2$)	35–45 mm Hg
Bicarbonate (HCO_3)	20–29 mEq/L
Acid–base balance (pH)	7.35–7.45

Table 5.3.　Pulmonary Function Testing

Title	Description
Vital capacity (VC)	Maximum amount of exhaled air, after a maximal inhalation. Varies with age, gender, and body size. *Decreased VC:* decreased lung tissue elasticity or depression of brain respiratory centers.
Inspiratory capacity (IC)	Largest amount of air inhaled, after a normal exhalation. *Decreased IC:* restrictive disorder, >35%, obstructive disorder.
Inspiratory reserve volume (IRV)	Maximum amount of air that can be inhaled after a normal inhalation. *Decreased IRV:* obstructive lung disease.
Expiratory reserve volume (ERV)	Amount of air that can still be exhaled after a normal exhalation. Decreased ERV: due to ascites, pleural effusion, or pneumothorax.
Functional reserve capacity (FRC)	Amount of air remaining in the lungs after normal exhalation. *Increased FRC:* obstructive respiratory pattern. *Decreased FRC:* restrictive respiratory pattern.
Residual volume (RV)	Amount of air remaining in lungs after a forced exhalation. Used to measure air trapping and hyperinflation. *Increased RV:* obstructive disorder. *Decreased RV:* restrictive disorder.
Tidal volume (TV)	Amount of air inhaled and exhaled during one cycle of normal breathing. *Decreased TV:* atelectasis, restrictive lung disease, or tumor.
Total lung capacity (TLC)	Volume of air in the lungs after a maximal inhalation. *Increased TLC:* obstructive lung disorder. *Decreased TLC:* restrictive lung disorder.
Forced vital capacity (FVC)	Maximum of air that can be forcefully exhaled after a maximal inhalation. May be decreased in obstructive disorders. *Normal values:* ≥80; mild disease, 60−80; moderate disease, 50−60; severe disease, ≥50.
Forced expiratory volume (in 1 second; FEV_1)	Volume of air exhaled over a timed interval from the beginning of a FVC. Looks at the amount of air that can be blown out within 1 second. *Decreased FEV_1:* obstructive or restricted lung disease. *Normal values:* ≥80; mild disease, 60−80; moderate disease, 40−60; severe disease, ≥40.
Maximal voluntary ventilation (MVV)	Largest volume of air breathed per minute by maximal voluntary effort. MVV measures compliance of lung tissue and status of respiratory muscles.

Table 5.3.   (continued)

Title	Description
Diffusing capacity for carbon monoxide (DLCO)	Assists in diagnosis of diffuse infiltrative lung disease and emphysema. Measures gas exchange area of capillaries and alveoli. *Normal values:* 80; mild disease, 60–80; moderate disease, 40–60; severe disease, ≥40.
Dead space volume (VD)	Air that does not participate in gas exchange.

Note. Impaired lung volume and capacity can have a profound effect on occupational performance. Abnormalities can be indicative of obstructive or restrictive lung disease.
Sources. Irion and Goodman (2009); West, Paz, and O'Leary (2009).

Table 5.4.   Modified Medical Research Council Dyspnea Scale

Grade	Degree of Dyspnea	Description
0	None	Not troubled by dyspnea.
1	Slight	Troubled by shortness of breath when hurrying on the level or walking up a slight hill.
2	Moderate	Walks slower than people of the same age on the level because of breathlessness.
3	Moderately severe	Has to stop because of breathlessness when walking at own pace on the level.
4	Severe	Stops for breath after walking about 100 yards or after a few minutes on the level.
5	Very severe	Too breathless to leave the house or breathless when dressing or undressing.

Source. Darbee and Ohtake (2006).

- *Rapid, forceful, or shallow breathing* and use of accessory muscles for breathing.
- *Cough:* A protective mechanism, but it can also be a symptom of disease, especially when chronic. Cough may be productive or nonproductive.
- *Mucous secretions:* Also act as a protective mechanism by trapping germs and debris but become problematic if difficult to clear or if marked by hypersecretions, excessive thickness, or stickiness.
- *Wheezing:* May be a symptom of airway narrowing or obstruction.

Pulmonary Diseases and Disorders

Most lung disorders lead to an increase in the work of breathing. Pulmonary conditions are usually categorized as either *obstructive* or *restrictive* diseases or disorders. Refer to

Appendix 5.B for a list of common symptoms and terms associated with pulmonary disorders.

Obstructive Pulmonary Conditions

These conditions result from a narrowing or blockage of airways, which can result in air trapping and limited surface area for gas exchange, resulting in impaired respiration.

Chronic Obstructive Pulmonary Disease

Chronic obstructive pulmonary disease (COPD) is the fourth leading cause of death in the United States (Doniger, 2003; Hayes & Meyer, 2007; Ikeda & Goodman, 2009; Migliore, 2004a; Petty, 2003; So & Man, 2008; Wisniewski, 2003) and is anticipated to be the third leading cause of death by 2020 (Larsson, 2007; Sin, McAlister, Man, & Anthonisen, 2003). It is a major health care problem in the United States, affecting approximately 16 million adults (Migliore, 2004a; Petty, 2003; Stump, 1999).

COPD is a gradually progressive disorder chiefly defined by chronic airflow limitation that is not fully reversible (Ikeda & Goodman, 2009; West et al., 2009). In COPD, an inflammatory response results in loss of elastic recoil, increased airway resistance, and reduced expiratory airflow, with a deterioration of pulmonary function as the disease progresses (Bauldoff & Diaz, 2006; Hogg, 2004; Petty, 2003). The course of COPD is insidious. A patient may have had the disease for several decades and be asymptomatic until as much as 50%–75% of lung function is lost (Bauldoff & Diaz, 2006; Petty, 2003). As the disease advances, the work of breathing becomes increasingly difficult.

COPD is an umbrella term for a group of diseases that include emphysema, chronic bronchitis, and obstructive bronchiolitis (Hayes & Meyer, 2007; Lindsay & Malone, 2006; Sewell & Singh, 2001). However, some include asthma in this group, even though airway obstruction in asthma is generally reversible. Characteristics of COPD include

- Long history of tobacco use,
- Chronic cough,
- Chronic sputum production,
- History of exposure to dust or chemicals,
- Inhalation of smoke from cooking and heating fuels (Bauldoff & Diaz, 2006),
- Onset in middle age,
- Reduced expiratory airflow and reduced forced expiratory volume in 1 second (FEV_1),
- Rapid and shallow breathing using accessory muscles,
- Lung hyperinflation,
- Dyspnea on exertion,
- Dyspnea-related anxiety, and
- Progressive deconditioning.

The National Heart, Lung, and Blood Institute and the World Health Organization have developed the Global Initiative for COPD, known as *GOLD*, to assist with risk factor reduction and management of symptoms and exacerbations. Information on the GOLD initiative can be found at www.goldcopd.org. Overwhelmingly, the greatest risk factor for developing COPD is a history of tobacco use; however, COPD may also develop from environmental exposure (toxins, dust, fumes), atopy (allergens), or a genetic predisposition (Sewell & Singh, 2001).

Dyspnea and fatigue are two of the most debilitating symptoms affecting patients' general health and ability to engage in desired and meaningful occupations. Dyspnea can often lead to inactivity and deconditioning because patients may not exert themselves for fear of triggering shortness of breath. According to Reishtein (2005) and Kapella, Larson, Patel, Covey, and Berry (2006), as cited in Theander, Jakobsson, Jorgensen, and Unosson (2009), a negative relationship also exists between fatigue and functional performance; as fatigue increases, functional performance decreases. COPD is also associated with age and gender; it is more common in men (Ikeda & Goodman, 2009).

Treatment for COPD focuses on symptom management, prevention of exacerbations, and slowing disease progression. Treatment is usually accomplished through smoking cessation; long-term oxygen use; medication, prophylactic immunizations; airway clearance techniques; and limiting exposure to communicable diseases, environmental pollution, irritants, and allergens (Ikeda & Goodman, 2009; Lindsay & Malone, 2006). Of all these approaches, the most important is encouraging smoking cessation because approximately 4,000 chemicals are inhaled when smoking cigarettes (Bauldoff & Diaz, 2006).

Medications that treat COPD include inhaled bronchodilators, B-agonists, oral corticosteroids, antibiotics, mucolytic agents, and oxygen therapy. Medications are used to open airways, reduce inflammation, and break up secretions. According to the American Lung Association, more than 800,000 COPD patients require chronic oxygen therapy to keep their oxygen saturation levels above 90% (Bauldoff & Diaz, 2006). It is important not to change prescribed levels of supplemental oxygen therapy for COPD patients (who are CO_2 retainers) without first consulting medical staff because too much oxygen can depress the patient's respiratory drive to breathe.

Patients are also encouraged to receive the pneumococcal and influenza vaccines as a preventative measure. Nutritional counseling is also important for COPD patients because they are frequently underweight and malnourished. High-carbohydrate diets are discouraged because they increase carbon dioxide production and the work of breathing (Bauldoff & Diaz, 2006). Fluids can help thin secretions, and patients are encouraged to drink 8 glasses of fluid a day (Doniger, 2003).

Exercise is also an important component of COPD treatment. Maintaining physical activity, increasing exercise tolerance, improving oxygenation, and reducing carbon dioxide retention are important for improving dyspnea and maintaining health, wellness, and quality of life (Ikeda & Goodman, 2009).

Symptoms of COPD progressively influence the patient's ability to engage in self-care and home and community activities; limit performance skills, performance patterns, and important roles and routines; restrict activities; and foster isolation; ultimately, symptoms affect independence and self-esteem (Chi Chung Chan, 2004; So & Man, 2008). According to Eckert (2007), most COPD patients have decreased endurance, limited ability to work, decreased participation in family and social activities, and difficulty sleeping. Occupational therapists

can assist patients by modifying and grading activities, facilitating engagement in basic and instrumental activities of daily living (BADLs and IADLs, respectively), modifying environments, assessing adaptive equipment needs, educating patients on energy conservation strategies and breathing techniques, and offering emotional and psychological support, because many patients with COPD experience anxiety and depression.

COPD may also be treated surgically through lung volume reduction surgery (LVRS), bullectomy, or lung transplantation for end-stage disease. Refer to Table 5.5 for more information on lung procedures. LVRS improves elastic recoil and diaphragmatic function by excising damaged lung tissue, allowing normal tissue to work more effectively. In addition to medical and surgical treatment, pulmonary rehabilitation programs, with their emphasis on patient education, breathing training, and increased exercise tolerance and functional capacity, may also be beneficial in treating patients with COPD (Petty, 2003). Refer to the "Pulmonary Rehabilitation" section.

Emphysema

Emphysema is a common type of COPD in which recurrent inflammation destroys the walls of alveoli causing large *bullae* (air sacs), which leads to air trapping, loss of elastic recoil, hyperinflation, and impaired oxygen exchange. More than 3 million Americans have emphysema (Stoller & Aboussouan, 2005; Twedell, 2007). Smoking and alpha 1 antitrypsin deficiency (α1ATD) are the primary risk factors for developing emphysema ("Respiratory System," 2007). Patients with emphysema are also known as "pink puffers" because they have a redder complexion than patients with chronic bronchitis, another type of COPD.

Symptoms of emphysema include dyspnea on exertion, malnutrition, weight loss, muscle wasting, clubbing of digits, decreased chest expansion, wheezing, and rapid shallow breathing with use of hypertrophied accessory muscles (Wells, 2004). Patients with emphysema may also appear to have a "barrel chest," which occurs because the lungs hyperinflate, partially expanding the rib cage.

Table 5.5. Common Diagnostic Tests Unique to Respiratory Disorders

Procedure	Description
Endotracheal intubation	Insertion of an endotracheal tube through the patient's mouth and into the trachea. Endotracheal tubing may be attached to a ventilator to assist patients who cannot breathe on their own and for removal of secretions patients cannot cough up.
Tracheostomy	An airway is cut in the trachea, and a small tube is inserted. This artificial airway ensures an open airway to lungs, bypassing the nose and mouth.
Bullectomy	Treatment for emphysema and chronic obstructive pulmonary disease. A large oxygen-depleted air space (bullae) is removed, allowing healthy alveoli in the area to expand with resultant improved breathing.
Lung volume reduction surgery (LVRS)	This procedure involves removal of lung tissue consisting of widespread small nonfunctioning air sacs in an attempt to improve elastic recoil and diaphragmatic function. LVRS is also performed on patients with emphysema. LVRS can lead to improvements in forced expiratory volume, forced vital capacity, and total lung capacity.
Wedge resection	The surgical removal of part of a lung. May be performed in early stages of lung cancer.
Lobectomy	Removal of a lobe of a lung
Pneumonectomy	Removal of the whole lung
Lung transplantation	A single lung, both lungs, or a living donor lobe may be transplanted. Refer to Chapter 14 for details.
Decortication	Surgical removal of a restrictive fibrous peel or rind encasing the lung, often found in third-stage empyema. Decortication allows the lungs to reexpand if they have been bound down by scarring and adhesions.
Pleurodesis	Treatment for recurrent pleural effusion or recurrent pneumothorax. After pleural fluid is drained, the two layers of pleura are sealed together through pleurodesis to prevent fluid from building up again.

The most important treatment approach for patients with emphysema is smoking cessation to protect the remaining alveoli. Treatment generally focuses on symptom management and slowing disease progression. This approach includes dietary changes (i.e., small, frequent high-calorie, high-protein meals), adequate hydration to mobilize secretions, oxygen therapy, medication (e.g., bronchodilators, steroids, antibiotics, mucolytics), immunizations for influenza and pneumonia (PNA), and pulmonary rehabilitation ("Respiratory System," 2007). Patients are also instructed to avoid cold, windy weather, which may trigger bronchospasms, and to avoid exposure to inhaled irritants (e.g., exhaust fumes, aerosol sprays, air pollution) and crowds or people with active respiratory infections ("Respiratory System," 2007). Occupational therapists have a role in assisting patients with emphysema through instruction in controlled breathing techniques (e.g., pursed lip and diaphragmatic breathing), energy conservation strategies, and pulmonary rehabilitation. For some patients, LVRS is warranted. Refer to the "Medical and Surgical Treatment of Pulmonary Conditions" section for information on LVRS.

Alpha 1 Antitrypsin Deficiency

α1ATD is a genetic form of emphysema that results from a deficiency of the alpha 1 antitrypsin protein. This protein is produced in the liver, inhibits the release of neutrophil elastase, and has anti-inflammatory properties. A deficiency of alpha 1 antitrypsin protein causes destruction of lung tissue and may also lead to liver disease in middle to late adulthood (Richmond & Zellner, 2005; Stoller & Aboussouan, 2005). α1ATD is often underdiagnosed or underreported; it is believed that as many as 13% of all patients with diagnosed emphysema actually have α1ATD (DeTurk & Cahalin, 2004), and α1ATD is responsible for approximately 3% of all cases of COPD (Richmond & Zellner, 2005).

α1ATD affects patients at a much younger age than does emphysema; onset is generally before age 45. A history of smoking may or may not occur with α1ATD; however, smoking cessation is necessary because smoking accelerates the onset of α1ATD and exacerbates symptoms (American Association of Cardiovascular and Pulmonary Rehabilitation [AACVPR], 1998; DeTurk & Cahalin, 2004; Lindsay & Malone, 2006). Patients with α1ATD are also at risk for liver cirrhosis; vasculitis; bronchiectasis; panniculitis (i.e., inflammatory skin disease); celiac disease; and lung, colorectal, and bladder cancers, as well as intracranial or intra-abdominal aneurysms (Stoller & Aboussouan, 2005).

In addition to smoking cessation, α1ATD is treated with bronchodilators, steroids, and supplemental oxygen when indicated. Additional lifestyle modifications include avoidance of secondhand smoke and air pollution, prompt treatment for respiratory infections, preventative vaccinations (e.g., influenza, pneumococcal, hepatitis A, hepatitis B), nutritional support, and pulmonary rehabilitation (Richmond & Zellner, 2005). Lung transplantation is also indicated for patients with α1ATD, and in some cases LVRS may be performed; however, no definitive evidence supports this approach (Richmond & Zellner, 2005; Stoller & Aboussouan, 2005). Respiratory failure is the most common cause of death for patients with α1ATD.

Chronic Bronchitis

Chronic bronchitis, one of the most common forms of COPD, is characterized by airway resistance (because of inflammation and edema), with impaired mucociliary clearance. Chronic bronchitis, like other COPDs, is largely attributable to cigarette smoking (Bauldoff & Diaz, 2006; DePalo & McCool, 2003; Hogg, 2004). Chronic bronchitis is generally defined as a chronic productive cough that lasts for more than 3 months in a year, during 2 consecutive years, that is not caused by another respiratory disorder, such as bronchiectasis or tuberculosis (TB; Hayes & Meyer, 2007; Wisniewski, 2003). Hallmarks of chronic bronchitis include mucous *hypersecretion* (excess mucous production), prolonged expiration, and periods of exacerbation that result in lung function deterioration. Patients with chronic bronchitis are often described as "blue bloaters" because their lips and skin may have a bluish tinge as a result of poor oxygenation (CO_2 retention) with the presence of edema.

With chronic bronchitis, the lining of the bronchioles becomes inflamed, swollen, and narrowed from long-term lung irritation. An excess of thick mucous is produced that cannot be cleared by normal cough and cilia function. Mucous is trapped, further obstructing the airways and increasing the risk of bacterial infection. As the disease progresses, the smaller airways collapse, with development of hypoxemia, hypoventilation, V/Q mismatch, and eventual right-sided heart failure (Wisniewski, 2003).

Risk factors for chronic bronchitis include exposure to environmental toxins (e.g., tobacco, asbestos, air pollution, occupational fumes, and dust) and recurrent lower respiratory tract infections (Hayes & Meyer, 2007; Wisniewski, 2003). Symptoms of chronic bronchitis include shortness of breath, wheezing, chronic productive cough, and frequent throat clearing. Chronic bronchitis has no cure and a high mortality rate (as much as 30% a year) for patients with acute exacerbations (Little, 2001).

As with other COPD, treatment for chronic bronchitis is aimed at symptom management, prevention of exacerbations, and slowing disease progression. Medications for chronic bronchitis include bronchodilators, steroids, oxygen therapy, and antibiotics for infection. Patients are encouraged to receive the influenza and pneumococcal vaccinations and nutritional support, avoid tobacco and other lung irritants, and practice the use of pursed-lip and diaphragmatic breathing (Wisniewski, 2003). Surgical treatment may include lung transplantation or lung resection. LVRS is performed to excise diseased tissue to reduce lung hyperinflation and improve lung recoil.

Bronchiolitis

Bronchiolitis is an inflammatory disorder that affects the bronchioles and may be present even in young, healthy smokers (Larsson, 2007). In *bronchiolitis obliterans,* the bronchioles are destroyed. This condition is commonly seen as a sequela of chronic rejection in lung transplantation. *Bronchiolitis obliterans organizing pneumonia (BOOP)* is an inflammatory, noninfiltrative disease of the bronchioles, in which connective tissue plugs fill the distal bronchioles, extending to the alveoli, and impairs lung function, decreasing vital capacity (Moore, 2003; White & Ruth-Sahd, 2007).

BOOP may be idiopathic or caused by infection, rheumatologic or connective tissue diseases (e.g., lupus erythematosus, rheumatoid arthritis, scleroderma, ankylosing spondylitis), HIV, environmental toxins (e.g., dust, textile dyes, mold), drugs and medications (e.g., anti-inflammatory drugs, immunosuppressive medications, cocaine), or organ transplantation (i.e., solid organ and stem cell transplantation; Moore, 2003; White & Ruth-Sahd, 2007). Symptoms of BOOP include flulike symptoms, malaise, fever, fatigue, dyspnea, bronchospasm, weight loss, and nonproductive cough (Moore, 2003; White & Ruth-Sahd, 2007).

BOOP is traditionally treated with steroids (e.g., prednisone), nutritional support, exercise, oxygen therapy, instruction in pursed-lip breathing, emotional support, and airway clearance techniques to clear secretions (White & Ruth-Sahd, 2007).

Asthma

Asthma is a reversible or reactive airway disease affecting approximately 14–15 million people in the United States and 7.2% of the world's population (AACVPR, 1998; Doniger, 2003; Lindsay & Malone, 2006; Wells, 2004). In the United States, more than 4,500 deaths each year are attributed to asthma (Ikeda & Goodman, 2009). In asthma, increased airway resistance results from obstruction from mucous, smooth muscle constriction, inflammation, and bronchial edema (DePalo & McCool, 2003). Symptoms can change daily and may include wheezing, dyspnea, early morning or nighttime coughing, and shortness of breath with activity (Bauldoff & Diaz, 2006).

The etiology of asthma is unknown; however, asthma has been associated with several factors, including incidence of childhood asthma, maternal smoking, secondhand smoke, heredity, gender (higher incidence in females), and occupational or environmental exposure (Wells, 2004). It has also been associated with allergies, rhinitis, and eczema. Patients with asthma are at an increased risk of developing COPD (Bauldoff & Diaz, 2006; Ikeda & Goodman, 2009).

Oxygen therapy is a key component of treating acute asthma attacks. Warm-up and cool-down periods are also important with any exercise program because asthma and broncho-spasm can be induced by exercise (AACVPR, 1998; Wells, 2004). Lifestyle modifications for patients with asthma may include

- Recognition and avoidance of triggers (e.g., cigarette smoke, pollen, cold air, people with respiratory infections, flowers and air fresheners with strong scents, stress or anxiety);

- Age-specific patient, family health promotion, and wellness education and training;

- Exercise training emphasizing the importance of exercise warm-up and cool-down;

- Importance of breathing through the nose to humidify and warm air rather than breathing through the mouth;

- Devising a self-management plan, including preparation to prevent and manage symptoms;

- Taking prescribed medications 20–30 minutes before exercise or activity to prevent exercise-induced bronchospasm; and

- Nutritional counseling for patients on long-term steroid medication (AACVPR, 1998; Doniger, 2003; Ikeda & Goodman, 2009; Redman, 2004).

Bronchiectasis

Bronchiectasis is an abnormal dilation of the bronchi resulting in bronchial wall thickening, inflammation, and airway obstruction. Bronchiectasis may be caused by damage to the respiratory system from infection, severe PNA, aspiration of foreign objects or gastric contents, genetics (e.g., cystic fibrosis [CF]), or an immunodeficiency (i.e., autoimmune disease) and eventually leads to chronic infection and bacterial colonization (Bradley, Moran, & Greenstone, 2008; Saavedra & Nick, 2003). Bronchiectasis is marked by purulent sputum, cough, hemoptysis, shortness of breath, and decreased exercise tolerance (Bauldoff & Diaz, 2006; Bradley et al., 2008).

Treatment is aimed at slowing the progression of lung disease, symptom management, and treating the underlying cause. Treatment may include medications and oxygen therapy;

however, at present no evidence exists to support physical exercise as a treatment approach to bronchiectasis (Bradley et al., 2008).

Cystic Fibrosis

CF is a chronic autosomal recessive disease that affects the exocrine glands. A mutation in chromosome 7 of the CF transmembrane conductance regulator gene results in disorder of chloride and sodium transport along cell membranes. Dehydration of the airways occurs with the production of thick, viscous mucous adhering to airway surfaces that is difficult to clear. Mucous accumulation also leads to inflammation, infection, and obstruction of glands, affecting multi-organ systems (e.g., gastrointestinal, respiratory, endocrine, and reproductive systems; Elpern, Patel, & Balk, 2007). Diagnosis is usually early in childhood, although some patients are not diagnosed until adulthood. No matter when diagnosis is established, most patients with CF die from respiratory failure (Yankaskas, Marshall, Sufian, Simon, & Rodman, 2004).

The life expectancy for patients with CF has dramatically increased over the past few decades, with more patients reaching adulthood with an average life expectancy of 32 years (Yankaskas et al., 2004). However, a small percentage survive into their 40s (10%) and 50s (2%), with 78 being the oldest recorded patient in the Cystic Fibrosis Foundation patient registry (Yankaskas et al., 2004). However, by age 21, at least half of patients with CF are hospitalized annually for pulmonary exacerbations (Elpern et al., 2007).

By system, symptoms of CF may include

- *Respiratory system:* Dyspnea, tachypnea, nasal polyps, chronic cough, wheezing, bronchiectasis, emphysema, air trapping, cyanosis, clubbing of fingers and toes, pneumothorax, atelectasis, lung infiltrates, hyperinflation, history of respiratory infections (e.g., *Pseudomonas aeruginosa, Burkholderia cepacia,* influenza, or *Staphylococcus aureus*), and respiratory failure.

- *Endocrine system:* Increased salty sweat resulting in salt depletion and electrolyte imbalances; Vitamin A, D, E, and K deficiencies; and chronic metabolic alkalosis. Older adults may develop CF-related diabetes.

- *Gastrointestinal system:* Failure to thrive, pancreatitis, gastroesophageal reflux, bowel obstruction, gallstones, hepatomegaly, splenomegaly, edema, biliary cirrhosis, ulcers, and rectal prolapse.

- *Reproductive system:* Infertility in 95% of males and decreased fertility in women with delayed *menarche* (initial menstruation).

Traditional treatment for CF includes

- *Exercise:* For airway clearance and to improve cardiovascular fitness, combating the effects of deconditioning;

- *Medication:* Bronchodilators, steroids, expectorants or mucolytic agents (to decrease thickness of sputum), antibiotics or enzyme replacement (to address pancreatic insufficiency and steatorrhea), and supplemental oxygen;

- *Airway clearance techniques:* Percussion and postural drainage, instruction in "huffing" (a weak type of cough that is produced when trying to steam up a mirror);

- *Nutritional support:* High-calorie, high-fat diet; salt tablets; and vitamin supplements; patients should be monitored for dehydration secondary to increased sweating;

- *Annual flu vaccination:* To minimize risk of infection;

- *Education:* Infection prevention;

- *Emotional support:* May include referral to a local Cystic Fibrosis Foundation chapter;

- *Surgical intervention:* Lung, liver, or pancreas transplantation may be required, with lung transplantation the treatment of choice for advanced CF; and

- *Palliative care:* For patients with end-stage disease when a donor organ is not available or transplantation is not appropriate (Philip et al., 2008).

Occupational therapists can assist patients with CF by encouraging engagement in routine occupations and lifestyle modification to increase quality of life and functional capacity.

Therapists must adhere to strict infection control practice to prevent transmission of multidrug resistive organisms such as cepacia (Yankaskas et al., 2004). Refer to Chapter 12 for more information on multidrug resistive organisms.

CF is a chronic progressive disease with no cure. It has ramifications for multiple organ systems and emotional and psychological effects requiring a multidisciplinary approach. CF often entails multiple hospital admissions for exacerbation of symptoms and lung function deterioration.

Restrictive Pulmonary Conditions

Restrictive diseases make it harder for the lungs to move and breathe. These ventilation disorders result in a reduction of lung capacity or total lung volume secondary to decreased lung compliance and elasticity. Restrictive lung disease may be the result of changes in the lung parenchyma from inflammation and scarring or from disorders of the chest wall, pleura, or respiratory muscles. Desaturation and rapid or shallow breathing are common symptoms of restrictive lung disorders.

Atelectasis

Atelectasis is the partial or complete collapse of a lung, usually caused by lung compression or an obstruction of a bronchus (e.g., from a mucus plug, infection, or cancer). Potential causes may include prolonged bed rest, heavy sedation, obesity, smoking, lung compression by fluid (i.e., pleural effusion) or air in the pleural space (i.e., pneumothorax), or foreign objects obstructing the airway (e.g., swallowed small toys or tumors) that obstruct the airway. Symptoms may include tachypnea, shallow respirations, and shortness of breath. Treatment may include removing any obstructions, ensuring airways remain *patent* (open), deep breathing with incentive spirometry, supplemental oxygen, functional mobilization, and bronchopulmonary hygiene (West et al., 2009).

Idiopathic Pulmonary Fibrosis

Idiopathic pulmonary fibrosis (IPF) is a progressive lung disease of unknown etiology; it has a poor prognosis and no cure. Life expectancy is approximately 3–5 years from time of diagnosis. Inflammation may be a contributing factor because lungs become fibrotic, scarred, and stiff, making ventilation difficult, with resulting hypoxemia and severe loss of lung function. IPF is also associated with an extensive smoking history. Signs and symptoms may include chest pain, cyanosis, cough, severe dyspnea, pulmonary hypertension (PH), and clubbed fingers and toes ("Respiratory Disorders," 2006; Schriber, 2008).

Patients with IPF often have difficulty breathing without supplemental oxygen therapy, such as high-flow oxygen or use of nonrebreather masks. When working with patients with IPF, activity tolerance and oxygen saturation levels should be closely monitored. Therapy focuses on increasing activity tolerance and incorporating energy conservation strategies, even though rehabilitation potential is severely limited. Response to conservative treatment is typically poor and generally includes use of supplemental oxygen and medication (e.g., corticosteroids, cholchicine). Lung transplantation is often indicated.

Adult Respiratory Distress Syndrome

Adult respiratory distress syndrome (ARDS) is marked by bilateral pulmonary infiltrates unrelated to left-sided heart failure or left atrial hypertension (Delong, Murray, & Cook, 2006). In ARDS, increased alveolar–capillary permeability and loss of surfactant activity leads to alveolar flooding and collapse. As a result, lung compliance is decreased as the lungs become fibrotic, thereby increasing the work of breathing. Edema further narrows airways, which increases resistance to airflow and results in increased consolidation or atelectasis (Pruitt, 2007). ARDS is not a disease but a syndrome that develops from systemic or pulmonary disorders. Medical treatment focuses on addressing the underlying cause of ARDS because it carries a high risk of respiratory failure. Risk factors may include sepsis, shock, infection, trauma, lung contusion, near drowning, multiple blood product transfusions, or aspiration of gastric contents ("Respiratory Disorders," 2006).

With ARDS, multiple organ failure may occur, and the mortality rate for this syndrome is approximately 30%–40%. For survivors, recovery is slow, but generally without permanent loss of lung function. Symptoms include dyspnea, tachypnea, and hypoxemia that is resistant to oxygen therapy.

Treatment usually consists of low tidal volume mechanical ventilation, which keeps patients alive while their lungs heal. Positive end expiratory pressure (PEEP) for improved oxygenation, conservative fluid management, and kinetic bed therapy may also be beneficial (Bream-Rouwenhorst, Beltz, Ross, & Moores, 2008; Pruitt, 2007). Occasionally, noninvasive ventilation is used because mechanical ventilation can lead to ruptured alveoli and air leaks, causing further lung injury (Delong et al., 2006). Acute lung injury is a less severe form and may be a precursor to ARDS.

Pneumonia

PNA is an inflammation of lung tissue; in 2000, it was the 7th leading cause of death in the United States (Eckert, 2007). Different categories of PNA are classified according to cause (e.g., bacterial, viral, fungal) or location (e.g., lobes, bronchioles). Two general types of PNA are seen in acute care: *community-acquired PNA (CAP)* and *hospital-acquired PNA (HAP),* also known as *nosocomial PNA.* Approximately 20% of patients with CAP require hospitalization. The two most common forms of HAP are ventilator-acquired PNA and aspiration PNA. HAP may account for 10%–15% of nosocomial infections. For the critically ill patient, it may account for a 25%–30% increase in mortality risk (Brozek et al., 2007; Holcomb, 2007). Table 5.6 lists characteristics of the different types of PNA.

Risk factors for developing PNA include

- History of smoking,
- Compromised immune system,
- History of chronic lung disease,
- Antibiotic use within the past 3 months,
- Age (older and young people are at greatest risk for developing PNA),
- Patient hospitalization longer than 5 days,
- Use of mechanical ventilation,
- Loss of consciousness,
- Aspiration of food or liquids,

Table 5.6. Comparison of CAP and HAP

CAP	HAP	Aspiration Pneumonia
• *Cause:* Bacterial or viral. • *Bacterial:* Infection causes alveoli inflammation and swelling, which can lead to atelectasis. • *Influenza:* Streptococcus pneumonia is the most common cause of CAP. • *Viral:* Bronchiolar epithelial cells, bronchial mucous glands, and alveoli may be affected. Viruses account for 10%–31% of CAP in adults.	• Occurs 48 hours after hospital admission. • Mortality rate up to 50%. • Leading cause of death from hospital-acquired infections. • As many as 25% of intensive care patients acquire HAP. • VAP occurs within 48 hours of intubation and mechanical ventilatory support. • 90% of hospital nosocomial infections are attributed to VAP, because placement of an endotrachial tube or tracheotomy bypasses the body's normal defenses against respiratory infection.	• Aspiration is a leading cause of HAP and VAP. • May occur from inhalation of food, liquids, or gastric contents or aspiration of colonized secretions or bacteria. • Aspiration causes lung inflammation and may be difficult to detect. • Poor oral hygiene and dental disease are risk factors for aspiration pneumonia. • Predisposing conditions may include dysphagia secondary to a neurological disorder, glottic closure compromise, ineffective coughing mechanism, or a mechanical obstruction (e.g., nasal-gastric tubes, endotracheal intubation, or tracheostomy).

Note. CAP = community-acquired pneumonia; HAP = hospital-acquired pneumonia; VAP = ventilator-acquired pneumonia.
Sources. Brozek et al. (2007); Holcomb (2007); O'Keefe-McCarthy (2006).

• Therapies that elevate gastric pH,

• Presence of nasogastric tubing,

• Patients undergoing chest surgery, and

• Hospitalization in the fall or winter months (Holcomb, 2007).

Signs and symptoms of PNA may include cough, malaise, dyspnea, tachypnea, fever, and chills. The typical treatment approach to PNA is rest, antibiotics, oxygen therapy, fluids and, in some cases, mechanical ventilation ("Respiratory Disorders," 2006). It may take up to 6 weeks for PNA to clear the lungs (West et al., 2009).

Preventative measures that therapists can use include adhering to good hand hygiene, keeping the head of the patient's bed at a 30°–45° angle to minimize aspiration, and ensuring that patients perform good oral hygiene. Occupational therapy focuses on increasing activity tolerance and functional endurance, strengthening, and education in energy conservation strategies (Eckert, 2007).

Pulmonary Edema

Pulmonary edema is the buildup of fluid in the extravascular spaces of the lungs resulting from changes in hydrostatic pressure forcing fluid into the alveoli ("Respiratory Disorders," 2006). This fluid buildup impairs gas exchange, causing difficulty with breathing. If untreated, pulmonary edema can progress to acute respiratory failure.

The two categories of pulmonary edema are cardiogenic and noncardiogenic. *Cardiogenic pulmonary edema* is an increase in transmural pressure and is often associated with cardiovascular disorders, such as myocardial infarction, left-sided heart failure, cardiomyopathy, mitral or aortic valve disorders, or hypertension. *Noncardiogenic pulmonary edema* results from an increase in alveolar capillary membrane permeability, resulting in alveolar flooding and is associated with ARDS (Beattie, 2007). Noncardiogenic pulmonary edema is also associated with impairment of the lymphatic system, capillary injury, and damage to the lungs through poisoning or infection ("Respiratory Disorders," 2006).

Symptoms may include pink and frothy sputum, dyspnea on exertion, cough, orthopnea, tachypnea, tachycardia, hypotension, or cardiac arrhythmias. Medical treatment includes medications (e.g., diuretics, vasopressors, inotropics, antiarrhythmics, morphine) and supplemental oxygen to address hypoxemia ("Respiratory Disorders," 2006). Modes of oxygen delivery may include mechanical ventilation or noninvasive ventilation, such as continuous positive airway pressure (CPAP), bilevel positive airway pressure (BiPAP), or PEEP ("Respiratory Disorders," 2006).

Diseases of Pulmonary Vasculature

The following section lists two serious lung conditions related to the pulmonary vascular system: pulmonary hypertension and pulmonary embolism. Narrowing or obstruction of pulmonary blood vessels can have a devastating effect on the heart.

Pulmonary Hypertension

Pulmonary hypertension (PH), the "other high blood pressure," is a rare but progressive disease characterized by an elevation in pulmonary artery pressure often associated with heart, vascular, or lung parenchymal disease. PH is also referred to as *pulmonary arterial hypertension (PAH)*, because of its effects on the pulmonary arteries. PH results from increased pulmonary vascular resistance

from hypoxic vasoconstriction and remodeling or destruction of pulmonary blood vessels (i.e., hardening and narrowing of pulmonary arteries and capillaries; Steinbis, 2004). With PH, the right side of the heart has to work harder to pump blood to the lungs, which can cause *cor pulmonale,* a condition in which the right ventricle hypertrophies and weakens, eventually leading to complete heart failure. PH has no cure. Treatment focuses on symptom management and improving quality of life.

In the past, PH was classified into two groups: *primary PH* and *secondary PH* (Steinbis, 2004). It has since been reclassified by the World Symposiums on PAH into 5 groups (Simonneau et al., 2004):

1. *Group I:* PAH
   - Idiopathic PAH
   - Familial PAH
   - PAH associated with
     - Collagen vascular diseases (e.g., scleroderma, lupus erythematosus, rheumatoid arthritis)
     - Congenital heart defects (congenital systemic to pulmonary shunts)
     - Portal hypertension (e.g., liver disease)
     - HIV infection
     - Drugs and toxins (e.g., cocaine, amphetamines, diet pills [fen-phen])
   - PAH associated with venous or capillary involvement (e.g., pulmonary veno-occlusive disease).
2. *Group II:* Pulmonary venous hypertension with left heart disease (e.g., left atrial or left ventricle heart disease, left-sided valvular disease)
3. *Group III:* PAH associated with lung disease, hypoxemia, or both
   - COPD
   - Interstitial lung disease
   - Sleep-disordered breathing (e.g., obstructive sleep apnea [OSA])
   - Alveolar hypoventilation disorder
   - Chronic exposure to high altitude
   - Developmental abnormalities.

4. *Group IV:* PAH resulting from chronic thromboembolic disease, embolic disease, or both
   - Obstruction of proximal and distal pulmonary arteries
   - Pulmonary embolism (PE)
5. *Group V:* Miscellaneous (e.g., sarcoidosis, compression of pulmonary vessels).

Diagnostic testing for PH includes right heart catheterization (to measure right-sided heart pressure), vasodilator testing, echocardiogram, and the 6-minute walk test (6MWT). In vasodilator testing, the patient's response to fast-acting, short-duration vasodilator medications (e.g., nitric oxide or prostacyclin—epoprostenol or adenosine) is monitored. The 6MWT is generally included because it is a simple test but a good indicator of exercise tolerance, disease severity, and response to therapy. In the 6MWT, the patient sees how far he or she can walk within 6 minutes on a hard flat surface. The 6MWT also correlates with cardiac output and oxygen consumption. Walking less than 150 meters is associated with a poor prognosis (McLaughlin & McGoon, 2006).

If untreated, PH eventually leads to decompensated heart failure with an average survival rate of 2.8 years from the time of diagnosis (Berkowitz & Coyne, 2003). Symptoms of PH can include dyspnea, angina, lower-extremity edema, heart palpitations, syncope, cyanosis, and fatigue (McLaughlin & McGoon, 2006). Initially, patients may be asymptomatic or symptoms may be mild. However, usually by the time of diagnosis, the disease is in an advanced stage (Adiutori, 2000; Berkowitz & Coyne, 2003). Table 5.7 is a modified version of the New York Heart Association heart failure classification system and the World Health Organization functional classification system, which is used in staging PH.

Table 5.7. Modified New York Heart Association and World Health Organization Functional Classification System for Pulmonary Hypertension

Class	Description
Class I	Patients with pulmonary hypertension but without resulting limitation of physical activity. Ordinary physical activity does not cause undue dyspnea or fatigue, chest pain, or near syncope.
Class II	Patients with pulmonary hypertension resulting in slight or mild limitation of physical activity. These patients are comfortable at rest, but ordinary physical activity causes increased dyspnea or fatigue, chest pain, or near syncope.
Class III	Patients with pulmonary hypertension resulting in marked limitation of physical activity. These patients are comfortable at rest, but less-than-ordinary physical activity causes undue dyspnea or fatigue, chest pain, or near syncope.
Class IV	Patients with pulmonary hypertension resulting in inability to perform any physical activity without symptoms. These patients manifest signs of right heart failure. Dyspnea, fatigue, or both may be present at rest, and discomfort is increased by any physical activity.

Sources. Berkowitz and Coyne (2003), McLaughlin and McGoon (2006).

Treatment for PH aims at reducing the work of the right ventricle and the lungs (Adiutori, 2000; Widmar, 2005). Treatment includes supplemental oxygen to maintain saturation levels above 90%–92%, anticoagulation (e.g., coumadin) because these patients are susceptible to thromboembolism, diuretics for edema (to reduce volume overload), and vasodilators (e.g., calcium channel blockers, nitrous oxide, prostacyclin analogues; Berkowitz & Coyne, 2003). Epoprostenol (Flolan), a prostacyclin analogue, is a powerful and effective vasodilator administered intravenously through an indwelling catheter or central line. The patient carries an ambulatory infusion pump in a small pouch, which also keeps the medication cold (this medication is unstable at room temperature; Adiutori, 2000; Widmar, 2005).

Although epoprostenol is very effective in slowing the progression of PH, it is expensive and has adverse side effects (e.g., headache, jaw pain, nausea, diarrhea, musculoskeletal pain), and a sharp decrease in dosage or a complete cessation can result in a strong PH rebound effect that can be life threatening (McLaughlin & McGoon, 2006; Widmar, 2005). Therapists working on self-care activities with patients on epoprostenol will often have to work around their pouch.

Treatment for PH also focuses on lifestyle modifications, including low-level aerobic exercise (e.g., walking), a diet low in salt (<2,400 milligrams per day), avoidance of high altitudes (because of the risk of hypoxia), flu and PNA immunization (to minimize risk of respiratory infection), and avoidance of pregnancy, which is associated with a high mortality rate (McLaughlin & McGoon, 2006). For patients who do not respond to conventional therapy, an atrial septostomy or lung transplantation may be indicated. With septostomy, a shunt is created between the two atria that may improve cardiac output and decrease the symptoms of right heart failure (McLaughlin & McGoon, 2006). Atrial septostomy may also be performed as a palliative measure or as a bridge to lung transplantation.

Often, patients are not diagnosed until the disease is well advanced, and therefore many patients do not survive the wait time for a donor lung (Steinbis, 2004). Refer to Chapter 14 for more information on lung transplantation.

Pulmonary Embolism

PE is a serious medical condition in which a clot, air bubble, or fat particle travels through the venous system into the right side of the heart and out to the pulmonary vasculature where it causes an obstruction. Lung tissue deprived of blood infarcts (Peate, 2008). A *saddle PE* obstructs at the level of the bifurcation of the pulmonary trunk extending into both the right and the left pulmonary arteries. Ninety percent of PE is attributed to deep vein thrombosis of the lower extremities. PEs may be undetected because symptoms mimic those of other diseases or they may be very mild or absent.

Heart failure and obesity are risk factors for PE, along with other common risk factors for deep vein thrombosis (DVT). However, the three main categories of risk factors for PE include

1. *Hypercoaguability:* From malignacies, pregnancy, oral contraceptives, hormone replacement therapy, or genetic mutations;
2. *Stasis:* Immobility from prolonged bedrest, long airplane and car trips, or use of casts or external fixators; and
3. *Venous injury:* From surgeries or trauma, especially those of the lower extremities (e.g., long bone fractures, hip or knee replacement surgeries) or damage from a previous DVT.

Symptoms of PE may include sudden tachypnea, dyspnea, pleuritic chest pain, syncope, tachycardia, anxiety, restlessness, or cyanosis ("Respiratory Disorders," 2006). If the PE is treated early, the prognosis is good; however, if it is left untreated, it can be fatal (Peate, 2008). Prognosis depends on the underlying disease or cause of the PE. Preventative measures include early ambulation after surgery, anticoagulation medication, use of antiembolitic stockings (e.g., thromboembolic deterrent hose), or use of lower-extremity sequential compression devices.

Treatment for PE generally includes

- Anticoagulation therapy with unfractionated heparin and warfarin;
- Oxygen therapy;
- Antibiotics or vasopressor medication;

- Placement of an inferior vena cava filter to prevent lower-extremity clots from reaching the lungs;
- Thrombolysis—Introduction of "clot-busting" agents; and
- Embolectomy—Surgical removal of a clot or embolism.

Diseases of the Pleura

Pleura is the membrane that lines the inside of the chest cavity and wraps around the outside of the lungs. The thin space between these two layers is known as the pleural space. Normally a small amount of fluid is contained within the pleural space, to minimize friction between the two layers when the lungs breathe in and out. Pleura disorders can involve the membrane or the pleural space.

Pneumothorax

A *pneumothorax* occurs when air gets between the lungs and chest wall, causing a change in the intrapleural pressure within the chest cavity. Air that leaks into the pleural space can cause the lungs to collapse, usually in proportion to the amount of air that enters the pleural cavity. A pneumothorax may be caused by trauma or injury to the chest wall itself (as in a stab or gunshot wound), a broken rib that punctures the lung, or a surgical procedure that involves the chest wall or lung.

Pneumothorax may also occur spontaneously through the rupture of an air-filled blister, predominantly seen with tall, thin men between the ages of 20 and 40. Symptoms may include chest pain, shortness of breath, tachypnea, fatigue, or tachycardia. Closure of the parenchymal air leak is done by suture, staple, ligature, or chemical pleurodesis. A chest tube may also be inserted to evacuate air.

Hemothorax

Hemothorax occurs when bleeding into the pleural cavity occurs. Treatment of hemothorax focuses on determining the source of the bleeding. If intrathoracic hemorrhage accumulates slowly and does not cause cardiovascular instability, a drain may be placed to assess the rate of blood loss. An explorative thoracotomy is indicated if blood loss persists. If a hemothorax cannot be evacuated by drainage within a few days, then operative evacuation is necessary.

Pleural Effusion

Pleural effusion is the buildup of fluid within the pleural space. Pleural effusion can be the result of a variety of conditions related to the lungs or other organs, including PNA, lung cancer, chest trauma, sarcoidosis, PE, TB, congestive heart failure, liver disease (with ascites), or pancreatitis. Symptoms may include pleuritic chest pain, cough, shortness of breath, tachypnea, fever, or malaise.

Treatment focuses on treating the underlying cause and may include draining fluid through thoracentesis or placement of a chest tube. Additional procedures may include decortication or pleurodesis (refer to Table 5.6). Patients may also receive oxygen therapy and medications, such as diuretics and antibiotics. Infected pleural fluid is known as *empyema*.

Empyema

Empyema is a collection of pus (containing bacteria, fibrin, and debris) caused by an infection found within the pleural cavity. It is often associated with bacterial PNA but may also be caused by bacteria entering the pleural space from trauma, surgery, or aspiration PNA (DeTurk & Cahalin, 2004). Empyema has three stages:

1. *Exudative:* Fluid containing pus fills the pleural cavity.
2. *Fibrinopurulent:* The fluid thickens, and a fibrous coagulation protein (fibrin) begins to accumulate in the cavity.
3. *Organizing:* The lung is encased within a thick covering of fibrous material that can entrap the lung.

Empyema carries the risk that the infection or abscess can rupture into the patient's airway or may spread to the tissue around the heart. Empyema can lead to restricted or even total loss of pulmonary mobility with a corresponding decrease in vital capacity. Empyema is primarily treated with antibiotics to treat the infection, or a chest tube may be inserted to drain pus. In addition, thoracocentesis aspiration may be used either diagnostically or as an intervention. If lung expansion becomes restricted by fibrous adhesions, then decortication, a type of surgical debridement in which the rind of fibrous material is peeled away, may be performed, freeing the lung tissue.

Additional Respiratory Disorders and Conditions

Other conditions can compromise the pulmonary system, resulting in respiratory failure:

- Chest wall restrictions secondary to ankylosing spondylitis, rheumatoid arthritis, kyphoscoliosis, osteoporosis, or pectus excavatum;
- Infectious diseases such as TB;
- Inflammatory disorders such as sarcoidosis;
- Lung cancer; and
- Nervous system disorders such as Guillain–Barré syndrome, myasthenia gravis, high-level spinal cord injuries, or drug overdose.

Pectus Excavatum

Pectus excavatum is a congenital and possibly genetic chest wall deformity in which the anterior chest has a sunken-in or concave appearance. This condition may compromise cardiac function, lung function, or both and is treated surgically for all but mild cases. Symptoms often do not appear until adolescence, when rapid bone and cartilage growth takes place. Mitral valve prolapse is seen in 20%–60% of cases. In the United States, the incidence is 1 in 300 to 400 births with a 3:1 ratio of male to female (Hebra, 2007).

Occupational therapists may be asked to fabricate an orthoplast chest shield, worn during the daytime to protect the chest after surgical repair. Good posture is also advocated while the patient heals. Lifting restrictions and avoidance of contact sports are usually in place for 4 weeks after surgery. Consult with the patient's physician regarding specific precautions and restrictions.

Tuberculosis

Evidence has shown that *TB* has been around since ancient times. The 2007 U.S. incidence of active TB was 4.4 cases per 100,000 people, with 2 billion cases of *active* and *latent* TB worldwide (Centers for Disease Control and Prevention [CDC], 2008). TB manifests as an active disease, or it can be latent, where it lays dormant for many years but is reactivated when the immune system weakens. TB is an infectious disease that usually affects the lungs but can affect other parts of the body, such as the brain, kidneys, or bones (CDC; 2008; DeTurk & Cahalin, 2004).

TB is spread by the inhalation of droplets from a cough or sneeze of someone infected with mycobacterium TB (DeTurk & Cahalin, 2004; Lindsay & Malone, 2006). Once a patient is exposed, the immune system usually surrounds the TB bacteria in the alveoli within a nodule or fibrotic cavity called a *tubercle* (Lindsay & Malone, 2006; "Respiratory Disorders," 2006). However, when the immune system is overwhelmed, the TB bacterium breaks out of the tubercles, becomes active, and spreads to the lungs and other parts of the body through the lymphatic or circulatory system ("Tuberculosis," 2008). Those people with a compromised immune system, as in HIV, are at a greater risk of developing the active form of TB. In addition, people living in crowded conditions with poor health care, including those who are homeless, are also at greater risk.

Symptoms of TB include cough, fatigue, weight loss, malaise, night sweats, and hemopytosis. Untreated TB can lead to pneumothorax, bronchiectasis, and fibrosis or destruction of lung tissue and death. The survival rate is high if treated (90%); however, if untreated, 60% of cases are fatal. Treatment may include antibiotics, chemotherapy, and bedrest. Medications are usually taken over several months.

Hospital precautions generally include use of an air droplet mask and isolation in a negative pressure room (refer to Chapter 12 for more information). Health care workers are generally required to be screened annually with a positive purified protein derivative skin test. Not everyone who has a positive purified protein derivative skin test has an active form of the disease. Some have the latent form of the disease and are asymptomatic and not contagious (CDC, 2008). However, those with a latent form of the disease may be treated to minimize the risk of active infection (DeTurk & Cahalin, 2004). As with other infections, drug-resistant forms of TB exist.

Sarcoidosis

Sarcoidosis is a systemic inflammatory disease of unknown etiology that can affect almost any organ in the body. Sarcoidosis can manifest as skin lesions or musculoskeletal or liver disorders; however, it predominantly affects the lungs (Baughman & Lower, 2005; "Respiratory Disorders," 2006). This disease is marked by a localized accumulation of granulomas or clusters of immune cells. Sarcoidosis can be chronic or acute but is often asymptomatic.

Although the cause of this disease is unknown, it may be linked to heredity, environmental triggers, or a hypersensitive inflammatory response (Baughman & Lower, 2005; "Respiratory Disorders," 2006). This disease carries a low risk of death or organ failure (Baughman & Lower, 2005).

Symptoms can include fever, cough, dyspnea, fatigue, glaucoma, or weight loss. Acute sarcoidosis generally resolves on its own; however, patients with the chronic form of the disease are treated with steroids or possibly immunosuppressant medications. Patients with sarcoidosis may develop obstructive or restrictive lung disorders such as interstitial lung disease, pulmonary fibrosis, or PH (Baughman & Lower, 2005; "Respiratory Disorders," 2006).

Obstructive Sleep Apnea

OSA has been identified in 4% of men and 2% of women but is largely undiagnosed in 80%–90% of cases (Holman, 2005). OSA is marked by recurrent periods of breathing cessation for at least 10 seconds, resulting in sleep fragmentation, hypoxia, and hypercapnia, and may lead to cardiovascular disease (Holman, 2005). Risk factors include gender (male), obesity,

nasal problems, and hypertension. OSA is also associated with PH, cerebrovascular disease (including stroke), cardiac arrhythmias, and myocardial infarction (Berry, 2008; Holman, 2005).

Treatment for OSA usually consists of sleeping with a CPAP machine, which works by maintaining a patent airway. Evidence has strongly suggested that CPAP lowers the danger of cardiovascular risk and improves quality of life (Holman, 2005). However, despite the benefits of CPAP, compliance is an issue because the mask may not be tolerated. Patients complain of claustrophobia, noise from air leakage, nasal dryness, conjunctivitis, or facial abrasions (Berry, 2008; Holman, 2005). Lifestyle modifications recommended for patients with OSA include losing weight, avoidance of alcohol and sedatives, and sleeping in a side-lying position with the head of the bed elevated (30°–45°; Holman, 2005).

Lung Cancer

Lung cancer is responsible for approximately 1.2 million deaths worldwide, making it the most common cause of death from cancer, with a 15% survival rate of 5 years in the United States (Parkin, Bray, Ferlay, & Pisani, 2005). Lung cancer is considered one of the leading causes of preventable death because it is strongly associated with exposure to tobacco (primary and secondhand smoke); in the United States, cigarette smoking is responsible for approximately 90% of all lung cancers (Alberg & Samet, 2003; "Respiratory Disorders," 2006). However, lung cancer has also been linked to environmental and occupational carcinogen exposure such as air pollution, radon, arsenic, asbestos (also associated with mesothelioma and asbestosis), polycyclic aromatic hydrocarbons (which are associated with combustion of fossil fuels), nickel, and exposure to chromates (Alberg & Samet, 2003). Heredity and previous lung injury may also be risk factors for developing lung cancer (Alberg & Samet, 2003).

The two main types of lung cancer are *small cell lung cancer* and *non–small cell lung cancer (NSCLC);* however, the incidence of NSCLC predominates (80%). NSCLC includes squamous cell carcinoma, adenocarcinoma, and large cell undifferentiated carcinoma ("Respiratory Disorders," 2006). Lung tumors are a cause for concern because they can obstruct airways, hemorrhage, or metastasize. The most common sites for metastases are the liver, adrenal glands, brain, and bones (refer to Chapter 11 for more information).

Lung cancer symptoms include cough, chest pain, dyspnea, weakness, and weight loss. Symptoms may also include reduced endurance for activities of daily living (ADLs), anxiety, and depression (AACVPR, 1998). Medical treatment traditionally includes chemotherapy, radiation treatment, surgery (e.g., lobectomy, wedge resection, pneumonectomy), or all of these. Unfortunately, these treatments can themselves cause restrictive pulmonary function (Lindsay & Malone, 2006).

Occupational therapy interventions for patients undergoing radiation and chemotherapy may need to be modified to patient tolerance. Treatments usually focus on breathing retraining and education on pacing and energy conservation strategies (AACVPR, 1998). A holistic treatment approach also includes lifestyle modification, including smoking cessation programs and diets high in antioxidants (i.e., fruits and vegetables), which are believed to neutralize free radicals, protecting cells from damage associated with cancer (National Cancer Institute, 2004).

Medical and Surgical Treatment of Pulmonary Conditions

The medical approach to lung conditions may include a combination of medication, incentive spirometry, supplemental oxygen, surgery, or lifestyle modification education.

Pharmacology usually consists of bronchodilators to dilate airways, anti-inflammatory medications, antibiotics, and mycolytics to thin secretions and assist with expectoration (Lindsay & Malone, 2006).

Incentive Spirometry

Incentive spirometry provides visual feedback and encourages long, slow, deep breaths to improve inspiration, lung expansion, respiratory muscle function, and prevention of atelectasis. Incentive spirometry is usually prescribed after surgery to help clear the lungs.

Patients place their lips around the spirometer's mouthpiece and breathe in slowly and deeply, while raising the piston up a column. Progress is observed by moving a gauge or indicator on the outside of the column to the height the piston reaches. Patients then hold their breath as long as possible before letting the piston return to the bottom of the spirometer. Patients are encouraged to use the spirometer repeatedly throughout the day for bronchial hygiene and to monitor their progress.

Flutter Valve

A *flutter valve* is a small, plastic handheld device that is used for airway clearance of mucous. A small metal ball inside the device causes vibrations with exhalations, which helps loosen mucous from the lungs so it can be coughed out. A flutter valve may be prescribed for patients with COPDs such as bronchitis, asthma, or CF.

Oxygen Therapy

Supplemental oxygen is usually indicated when concentrations of inspired oxygen in room air are insufficient for respiration and patients are at risk for hypoxia and hypoxemia ($O_2 < 88\%$–90%, arterial partial pressure of $O_2 < 55$ millimeters of mercury [mm Hg]). Oxygen therapy focuses on ensuring adequate oxygen levels in blood, reducing shortness of breath, and reducing the work of the heart. Flow rates should not be readjusted before checking with medical staff, especially with patients who retain carbon dioxide because increased oxygen may decrease hypoxic ventilatory drive (Lang & West, 2009).

If patients complain of skin irritation behind the ears from oxygen tubing, apply gauze or foam for cushioning. Always ensure tubing is long enough (or obtain extra tubing) for increased patient mobility. Patients with supplemental oxygen should avoid exposure to combustible material. Check with facility policy; some centers may discourage the use of electrical devices (e.g., electric shaver) that can spark.

Modes of Oxygen Delivery. Various oxygen delivery systems are used in acute care. The source of oxygen is typically plugged into a wall outlet and has a meter attached to regulate flow. A canister of sterile water may also be attached to provide moisture. Patients with high fraction of inspired oxygen (FiO$_2$) requirements have more severe respiratory function compromise, and activities should be modified accordingly. Oxygen tanks are recommended for patients who ambulate outside their hospital room. Before attaching the patient's oxygen tubing to the oxygen canister, ensure the tank has sufficient oxygen and is set on the prescribed liter amount. Modes of delivery are

- *Nasal cannula:* The most common route for supplemental oxygen is through a nasal cannula. Oxygen is delivered via plastic tubing attached to the wall, with prongs inserted into the patient's nostrils and secured under the patient's chin. With a nasal cannula, supplemental oxygen is mixed with room air.

- *Face mask:* The mask is placed over the nose and mouth with ventilation holes on the sides. It provides supplemental oxygen and room air, which is inspired through the nose and mouth. However, the mask may be a barrier to the patient's ability to talk, cough, eat, or engage in light hygiene and grooming activities.

- *Nonrebreather mask:* This apparatus consists of a mask that covers the nose and mouth and provides high concentrations of oxygen (high FiO$_2$). The patient breathes in oxygen from the attached reservoir bag but exhales through valves on the side of the mask, thereby preventing inhalation (e.g., rebreathing) of expired air. This mask also interferes with the ability to talk, cough, eat, or engage in light hygiene and grooming activities.

- *Venturi mask:* This mask fits over the nose and mouth and provides a fixed concentration of oxygen using a high-flow system. Valves may be used to mix a certain percentage of room air with specific oxygen concentrations (Lang & West, 2009). This mask also interferes with the ability to talk, cough, eat, or engage in light hygiene and grooming activities.

- *Tracheostomy collar:* Oxygen is delivered to a tracheal tube (inserted into the trachea), bypassing the mouth and nose. Humidification is usually required for this method of oxygen delivery. For ambulatory patients, adapted tubing may be applied to an oxygen tank instead of the wall unit, allowing patients greater freedom in functional mobility.

- *CPAP:* CPAP is a type of ventilation used to maintain a patent airway, often used for patients with OSA. A mask is placed over the patient's face and is attached to a machine that blows air at a prescribed pressure. Complications of CPAP can include nightmares and excessive dreaming, dry nose, sore throat, nosebleeds, nasal congestion, eye and skin irritation, headaches, abdominal bloating, and air leakage around the mask (Essig, 2007).

- *BiPAP:* BiPAP helps decrease the work of breathing by providing positive inspiratory pressure and PEEP. It may be used to deliver room air or supplemental oxygen. If the BiPAP interferes with engagement in occupational therapy interventions, check with medical staff to see whether patients can be taken off BiPAP or other forms of oxygen delivery methods during the therapy session. The BiPAP mask fits tightly over the face, so patients may complain of claustrophobia (Lang & West, 2009).

- *Hyperbaric chamber:* In hyperbaric oxygen therapy, the patient receives oxygen therapy by entering a specialized closed chamber. This method may be indicated for patients with decompression sickness, embolism, or carbon monoxide poisoning.

Mechanical Ventilation (Invasive and Noninvasive). The purpose of a ventilator is to reduce the work of breathing and ease respiratory distress. Mechanical ventilation sends a controlled flow of oxygen into a patient's lungs (Delong et al., 2006). The ventilator can be adjusted for rate, pattern, and duration of gas delivery. Ventilators are set for either volume control or pressure control. The three general types of mechanical ventilation are assist–control, intermittent mandatory ventilation, or pressure support ventilation. Refer to Chapter 2's Table 2.5, which highlights the different modes of mechanical ventilation.

Noninvasive Positive-Pressure Ventilation. A nasal, or oronasal, facial mask or mouthpiece is used as an interface between the ventilator and the patient's upper airway. This method may be desirable because it is noninvasive and does not require intubation or use of an artificial airway. However, this method is not as effective with late-stage respiratory failure (Penuelas, Frutos-Vivar, & Esteban, 2007). CPAP, although not a true ventilation mode, is still considered the most common form of noninvasive ventilation by delivering constant positive pressure during both inhalation and exhalation (Penuelas et al., 2007).

Lung Volume Reduction Surgery

In LVRS, damaged tissue from the lungs is excised, which allows the remaining healthy tissue to function more effectively with improved expiratory airflow, reducing hyperinflation and facilitating more effective ventilation (Twedell, 2007). LVRS may be performed with a sternotomy, thoracotomy, or a minimally invasive video-assisted thoracic (VATS) procedure (refer to Chapter 3 for details on sternotomy precautions). Risks associated with LVRS include air leaking or other common complications associated with any surgical procedure (Brenner et al., 2004). LVRS has been shown to be beneficial for symptom management, improved lung

function, and improved health-related quality of life (Appleton, Adams, Porter, Peacock, & Ruffin, 2003; Twedell, 2007).

Thoracotomy

Lung surgery is usually performed as an open thoracotomy or as a minimally invasive VATS. A *thoracotomy* is an invasive procedure in which the lungs are accessed through an incision from the back to the side (*posteriolateral*), through the front (*anterolateral*), or between two ribs (*intercostal*). This type of surgery may be performed for a wedge resection, lobectomy, or pneumonectomy. Associated risks include air leaking, bleeding, atelectasis, or infection.

A *VATS procedure* is a type of endoscopic or "keyhole" surgery in which a small incision is made between the ribs for placement of a camera and another incision is made for insertion of surgical tools. As surgeons perform this surgical procedure, they monitor their movements by looking at a closed-circuit monitor, as opposed to observing directly inside the patient. VATS procedures are traditionally performed for recurrent spontaneous pneumothorax, pleural effusions, and pulmonary wedge resections. A VATS procedure is usually desirable because it is less invasive than a traditional thoracotomy, and therefore less pain, fewer complications, and quicker healing times are expected. The VATS procedure also allows therapists to mobilize patients quicker with fewer complaints of pain and discomfort (Smith-Gabai, 2008). VATS can be converted to an open thoracotomy if needed (see Box 5.1).

Box 5.1.	**Comparison of Open Thoracotomy and Video-Assisted Thoracic (VATS) Procedure**	
	Open Thoracotomy	**VATS**
Size of incision	10–14 inches	~1 inch
Average hospital stay	10–12 days	<2 days
Return to work/normal routine	6–8 weeks	7–10 days
Major complications	30%	<5%

Lung Transplantation

Single- and double-lung transplantation is indicated for patients with end-stage pulmonary disease. Lung transplantation is not a panacea for pulmonary disease because many extenuating factors exist. One of the biggest obstacles is the shortage of available donor lungs. Even when patients do undergo lung transplantation, they must forever remain on immunosuppression medication to prevent organ rejection while minimizing risk of infection. Lung transplant recipients are more vulnerable to infection than other organ transplant recipients because every breath they take exposes the lungs to the environment (e.g., air pollution, fumes, irritants, bacteria). Refer to Chapter 14 for detail on lung transplantation.

Pulmonary Rehabilitation

The primary focus of pulmonary rehabilitation is a multidisciplinary approach to treatment of activity limitations. Pulmonary rehabilitation can assist with fatigue, anxiety, breathing, activity tolerance, and renewed confidence in ability to engage in occupations (Norweg, Bose, Snow, & Berkowitz, 2008). Pulmonary rehabilitation traditionally focuses on increasing functional capacity, patient–family education, and psychosocial support in an effort to improve quality of life.

Pulmonary rehabilitation generally includes a cardiovascular exercise program based on the three types of exercise required for a complete program: flexibility, endurance, and strengthening. Exercises are tailored to increase the individual patient's tolerance to activity. Education supports patients' understanding of their disease, its pathophysiology, and medication use and highlights lifestyle modification, energy conservation strategies, breathing retraining, stress management, coping strategies, and nutritional counseling. Occupational therapists are instrumental in pulmonary rehabilitation by designing programs that are appropriately challenging and purposeful to maximize patients' functional capabilities and perceived control over their pulmonary condition (Migliore, 2004b).

However, for all the benefits of pulmonary rehabilitation, it may not be affordable and accessible to all patients, and it may not address the issues of chronicity typical of pulmonary diseases (Bourbeau, 2003). Bourbeau (2003) advocated, in conjunction with pulmonary rehabilitation, developing a disease-specific self-management program for patients in which patients learn to recognize the signs of acute exacerbation and develop an action plan, thereby potentially minimizing hospital readmissions. A self-management program can result in improved coping skills, increased medication compliance, and increased functional capacity to engage in ADLs and facilitate engagement in a healthier lifestyle. However, although evidence has shown that self-management programs are beneficial in addressing chronic health conditions, further research is required to support this approach for patients with COPD (Blackstock & Webster, 2007).

According to the AACVPR, a leading organization in cardiac and pulmonary rehabilitation, professionals (including occupational therapists) should meet certain competency guidelines when working in pulmonary rehabilitation. Rehabilitation therapists should

- Demonstrate an understanding and knowledge of pulmonary anatomy, physiology, and pathophysiology and comorbidities that may influence physical activity. Comorbidities may include metabolic disorders; musculoskeletal, cardiovascular, and neuromuscular conditions; and psychiatric or mood disorders.
- Identify medical barriers and environmental factors that may limit optimal rehabilitation.
- Establish professional communication with all stakeholders.
- Facilitate patient education and training, including addressing specific patient needs, developing an individualized plan of care and a self-management education program, and incorporating adult learning theories and health promotion strategies.
- Assess patient's exercise tolerance, devise an individual exercise prescription, and monitor patient's response and progress to the program.
- Address psychosocial issues by providing support, counseling, and instruction

in self-help techniques. Make appropriate referrals to mental health professionals, support groups, or home care and community services.

- Continue to monitor the patient's progress, collect outcomes data, and revise or modify programs accordingly (Nici et al., 2007).

Occupational therapists play an important role in pulmonary rehabilitation by addressing issues of functional endurance, incorporation of proper breathing techniques during activity, stress management, relaxation techniques, adaptation of leisure activities, and instruction in energy conservation strategies in performance of ADLs (Huntley, 2008).

Occupational Therapy Approach

Dyspnea and other symptoms of pulmonary disease can become an obstacle to patients' participation in therapy and normal occupations, severely limiting their functional abilities and affecting their quality of life. Occupational therapists can address these issues by

- Increasing patients' understanding of their disease and the disease process;
- Increasing activity tolerance through graded activity;
- Prioritizing occupations;
- Instructing patients in controlled breathing (e.g., diaphragmatic and pursed-lip breathing) and dyspnea relief strategies (refer to Appendix 5.B for detail);
- Educating patients on incorporating principles of energy conservation, work simplification strategies, and use of proper body mechanics in daily occupations;
- Instructing patients in problem-solving strategies and coping skills;
- Educating patients on avoiding environmental toxins and minimizing risk of infection (e.g., avoiding crowds or people with active respiratory infection);
- Assessing equipment and recommending home modifications;
- Offering emotional support for breathing disorder–related anxiety;

- Increasing patients' ability to engage in leisure skills; and
- Instructing patients in relaxation and stress management techniques (e.g., guided imagery, relaxation breathing, progressive muscle relaxation).

Occupational therapy is unique as a profession that recognizes the importance of activity and how engagement in occupation can be used to achieve goals and increase self-esteem, which are especially important with breathing disorders, which can make even the simplest task challenging (Stump, 1999).

Therapists should monitor patients' vital signs (e.g., oxygen saturation levels, respiration, heart rate) before, during, and after occupational therapy sessions to determine tolerance for therapeutic activities and interventions. Therapists should also note patient use of accessory muscles and presence of shallow breathing or whether the patient holds his or her breath during activity (Stump, 1999). Ascertain whether any signs of distress are present, including tachypnea, cyanosis, fatigue, or any decrease in oxygen saturation rates, and length of recovery time.

Breathing

Therapy should focus on maintaining optimal oxygen saturation levels and reducing the work of breathing while engaging in occupations. Instructing patients in proper breathing techniques during activity results in deeper breathing with reduced dyspnea. Abdominal or diaphragmatic breathing helps cue patients to increase diaphragmatic motion and decrease use of accessory muscles while breathing. This type of deep breathing minimizes the level of dyspnea on exertion by ensuring more efficient gas exchange at the alveolar level (Migliore, 2004a). Patients are typically instructed to exhale during the hard or strenuous part of an activity or exercise, which allows for a deeper breath, ensures that patients are not holding their breath during an exertional activity, and prevents a Valsalva effect. For some patients, this type of breathing may seem backward and confusing. Patients can be instructed to count out loud, sing, or talk to ensure they are not holding their breath during the activity. If patients become light-headed during this type of breathing, they should be instructed to stop and breathe normally.

Another breathing technique called *pursed-lip breathing* buttresses the small bronchioles, prevents premature airway collapse, and improves breathing control (Lindsay & Malone, 2006). By pursing the lips, the airway is narrowed, which increases resistance to airflow, increasing positive pressure generated by the airways and lengthening expiration time, which helps the lungs to empty (Ford & Weaver, 2000). Pursed-lip breathing is also thought to reduce respiration rate and improve quiet breathing or breathing at rest. Table 5.8 describes several breathing exercises.

Table 5.8. **Breathing Exercises**

Exercise	Description
Abdominal breathing	1. Place one hand on your stomach. 2. Imagine a balloon filling up with air as air is blown into it and collapsing when the air is let out. 3. Focus on your stomach rising when you breathe in, just as the balloon gets bigger as it fills with air. 4. Using the hand on your stomach, tap or gently press in with exhalation to cue the stomach to contract or pull in as air is being pushed out or exhaled (just as the balloon collapses when air is let out).
Pursed-lip breathing	1. Inhale through the nose as if smelling flowers. 2. Exhale gently and slowly through pursed lips as if blowing bubbles through a bubble wand, or blowing kisses. Exhalations should not be forceful. 3. Coordinate abdominal and pursed-lip breathing together.
Lower rib breathing (Ford & Weaver, 2007)	1. Hands are placed on both sides of the body, on the lower section of the rib cage. 2. With each exhalation, tactile resistance is provided to the ribs (to facilitate rib expansion with inhalations).
Relaxation breathing	1. Exhale (breathe out) longer than inhale (breathe in). For example, if breathing in to a count of 2, breathe out to a count of 3, 4, or 5, finding your own rhythm, and repeat. Relaxation breathing is helpful in slowing down respiratory rate.
The accordion (this exercise is similar to the movements of a bellows)	1. Tuck elbows into body. Place hands with palms parallel to each other. 2. As you inhale, move hands out to sides (as if pulling an accordion out). 3. As you exhale, move hands back toward each other (as if pressing in a bellows). 4. Breathing should be slow and relaxed.

Note. Sit comfortably before beginning exercises.

Lifestyle Modifications

Lifestyle modifications focus on making changes in performance patterns, which facilitate patient engagement in meaningful and purposeful activities (e.g., ADLs, leisure, work) while minimizing dyspnea and conserving energy. Some suggestions for performing self-care activities follow.

Grooming

- Prop elbows on countertop (supporting upper extremities) when washing face, brushing teeth, combing hair, or shaving. Organize all utensils ahead of time.
- Dressing
  - Avoid tight clothing, which restricts trunk–chest expansion.
  - Incorporate abdominal and pursed-lip breathing into dressing routine.
  - Sit to dress and avoid unnecessary steps (e.g., don underwear and pants at the same time to avoid standing and sitting multiple times to pull garments up over hips).
  - Use adaptive equipment when warranted (e.g., long-handled reacher, long-handled shoe horn, elastic laces, sock aid, or dressing stick).
- Bathing
  - Sit to bathe.
  - Use adaptive equipment (e.g., long-handled sponge for bathing, bath chair, hand-held shower, wrapping a wash cloth over a long-handled sponge to dry feet).
  - Dry self off by donning a terry cloth robe or draping a large towel around body patting self dry.
  - Avoid hot water for bathing and showering because steam and humidity may make it more difficult to breathe. Steam may also be minimized by leaving the door open or using a ventilation fan.
- Meal preparation
  - Sit whenever possible.

- Use an exhaust fan for fumes, which may interfere with breathing.
- Organize all materials ahead of time. (Huntley, 2008; Stump, 1999)

Patients with lung disease progressively adopt a sedentary lifestyle because engaging in activities often leads to feelings of breathlessness and dyspnea. This lifestyle often spirals to include decreased exercise capacity, psychosocial and behavioral issues, and increased risk of recurrent respiratory infections (Blackstock & Webster, 2007). Interventions may include exercise training and graded activity to increase tolerance and capacity for functional activities.

Energy conservation education is another approach that provides patients with strategies to assist them in engaging in their daily activities but in a more economic, efficient manner. This approach assists by decreasing dyspnea and the amount of energy expended to accomplish the activity (Velloso & Jardim, 2006). Energy conservation strategies include pacing, sitting to do activities rather than standing, and resting before getting too tired or overfatigued. Refer to Appendix D for a list of energy conservation and work simplification strategies. Stump (1999) suggested scheduling occupational therapy sessions after breathing treatments, after patients have taken their medication, and at least 1 hour after meals so the metabolic requirements of digestion will not compete with the energy demands of the therapy session.

Occupational therapists can also be instrumental in instructing patients in relaxation techniques to lessen anxiety and experiences of dyspnea. Guided imagery and relaxation exercises can affect the parasympathetic nervous system, lowering heart rate, blood pressure, and rate of respirations, resulting in increased relaxation and decreased anxiety (Wai-Shan Louie, 2004). Cognitive distraction techniques are also helpful in diverting the mind from the trigger or source of anxiety, affording temporary relief and relaxation. Biofeedback, relaxation breathing (i.e., slow rhythmic breathing), use of nature sound tapes, progressive muscle relaxation exercises, visualization, imagery, and meditation are all strategies that foster relaxation (Ford

& Weaver, 2000). Refer to Appendix J for more information on relaxation techniques.

General Guidelines

The following are general guidelines that may assist therapists working with pulmonary patients:

- Monitor vital signs before, during, and after activity because they reflect the patient's cardiopulmonary function.
- Note any signs of cyanosis, pallor, clubbing of fingers and toes, use of accessory muscles, or signs of abnormal breathing patterns.
- Modify activities if oxygen saturation levels fall below 90% (or other parameters set by medical staff).
- Ensure patients maintain good oral care: The body has several normal defenses against respiratory infection, including cough and saliva, which removes plaque and microorganisms from the mouth (O'Keefe-McCarthy, 2006). Good oral care is essential for reducing bacterial colonization, which can lead to HAP. Oral hygiene includes brushing teeth and tongue and using an antiseptic mouth rinse. Some patients may be prescribed a special mouth rinse (e.g., chlorhexidine).
- Adhere to all aspiration and swallowing precautions posted in patients' chart or in their room.
- Encourage oral suctioning when needed. Notify nursing when patients require tracheotomy suctioning.
- Adhere to infection control protocols, including good hand hygiene and disinfecting equipment. This adherence is especially important for patients with a compromised pulmonary or immune system.
- Work with patients with the head of the bed elevated (30°–45°) or in an upright position.
- Promote engagement in activity. Immobility is detrimental to good respiratory function. Refer to Appendix C for more information on the detrimental effects of bedrest.
- Avoid resistive exercise with thoracotomy or sternotomy patients. Check with the physician because patients may have a lifting restriction for the first 4–6 weeks after surgery.
- Patients who are being discharged with oxygen saturation levels lower than 88% with activity may require home oxygen therapy. Notify medical staff, because home oxygen therapy must be prescribed by a physician.
- Supplemental or increased oxygen may be used to prevent hypoxia; however, do not adjust oxygen levels with patients who are hypercapnic (CO_2 retainers) unless first consulting with medical staff.

The goal of occupational therapy is to facilitate the patient's engagement or reengagement in routine occupations and life roles, within the patient's tolerance. The previously mentioned techniques can foster increased participation in meaningful and purposeful activities; minimize symptoms; increase independence and self-esteem; and improve quality of life, preserving the patient's occupational identity.

References

Adiutori, D. M. (2000). Primary pulmonary hypertension: A review for advanced practice nurses. *Medsurg Nursing, 9*(5), 255–264.

Alberg, A. J., & Samet, J. M. (2003). Epidemiology of lung cancer. *Chest, 123*(1, Suppl.), 21S–49S.

American Association of Cardiovascular and Pulmonary Rehabilitation. (1998). *Guidelines for pulmonary rehabilitation programs* (2nd ed.). Champaign, IL: Human Kinetics.

Appleton, S., Adams, R., Porter, S., Peacock, M., & Ruffin, R. (2003). Sustained improvements in dyspnea and pulmonary function 3 to 5 years after lung volume reduction surgery. *Chest, 123*, 1838–1846.

Baughman, R. P., & Lower, E. E. (2005). *Sarcoidosis*. Retrieved October 5, 2008, from www.accessmedicine.com/content.aspx?aID52863005

Bauldoff, G. S., & Diaz, P. T. (2006). Improving outcomes for COPD patients. *Nurse Practitioner, 31*(8), 27–43.

Beattie, S. (2007). Bedside emergency: Respiratory distress. *RN, 70*(7), 34–38.

Begany, T. (2001). *COPD guidelines go global.* Retrieved April 19, 2007, from www.respiratory reviews.com/jul01/rr_jul01_copd.html

Berkowitz, D. S., & Coyne, N. G. (2003). Understanding primary pulmonary hypertension. *Critical Care Nursing Quarterly, 26*(1), 28–34.

Berry, D. (2008). Case study: Obstructive sleep apnea. *Medsurg Nursing, 17*(1), 11–16.

Blackstock, F., & Webster, K. E. (2007). Disease-specific health education for COPD: A systematic review of changes in health outcomes. *Health Education Research, 22,* 703–717. doi:10.1093/her/cyll50

Bourbeau, J. (2003). Disease-specific self-management programs in patients with advanced chronic obstructive pulmonary disease: A comprehensive and critical evaluation. *Disease Management and Health Outcomes, 11,* 311–319.

Bradley, J., Moran, F., & Greenstone, M. (2008). Physical training for bronchiectasis [Review]. *Cochrane Database of Systematic Reviews,* 2010, CD002166.

Bream-Rouwenhorst, H. R., Beltz, E. A., Ross, M. B., & Moores, K. G. (2008). Recent developments in the management of acute respiratory distress syndrome in adults. *American Journal of Health-System Pharmacy, 65,* 29–36.

Brenner, M., Hanna, N. M., Mina-Araghi, R., Gelb, A. F., McKenna, R. J., Jr., & Colt, H. (2004). Innovative approaches to lung volume reduction for emphysema. *Chest, 126,* 238–248.

Brozek, J., McDonald, E., Clarke, F., Gosse, C., Jaeschke, R., & Cook, D. (2007). Pneumonia observational incidence and treatment: A multidisciplinary process improvement study. *American Journal of Critical Care, 16,* 214–219.

Centers for Disease Control and Prevention. (2008). *The difference between latent TB infection and active TB disease.* [Fact Sheet]. Retrieved August 15, 2010, from http://www.cdc.gov/tb/publications/factsheets/general/LTBIandActiveTB.htm

Chi Chung Chan, S. (2004). Chronic obstructive pulmonary disease and engagement in occupation. *American Journal of Occupational Therapy, 58,* 408–415.

Darbee, J. C., & Ohtake, P. J. (2006). Research corner: Outcome measures in cardiopulmonary physical therapy: Medical Research Council (MRC)

Dyspnea Scale. *Cardiopulmonary Physical Therapy Journal, 17*(1), 29–37.

Delong, P., Murray, J. A., & Cook, C. K. (2006). Mechanical ventilation in the management of acute respiratory distress syndrome. *Seminars in Dialysis, 19,* 517–524.

DePalo, V. A., & McCool, D. (2003). Evaluation of the patient with pulmonary disease: Pulmonary anatomy and physiology. In M. E. Hanley & C. H. Welsh (Eds.), *Current diagnosis and treatment in pulmonary medicine* (pp. 1–15). New York: Lange Medical Books.

DeTurk, W. E., & Cahalin, L. P. (2004). *Cardiovascular and pulmonary physicaltherapy: An evidence-based approach.* New York: McGraw-Hill.

Doniger, S. B. (2003, October). The trouble with breathing. *RDH Magazine,* pp. 42–47. Retrieved April 16, 2009, from http://www.dentistryiq.com/index/display/article-display/190877/articles/rdh/volume-23/issue-10/feature/the-trouble-with-breathing.html

Eckert, J. (2007). Cardiopulmonary disorders. In B. J. Atchison & D. K. Dirette (Eds.), *Conditions in occupational therapy: Effect on occupational performance* (3rd ed., pp. 195–218). Philadelphia: Lippincott Williams & Wilkins.

Elpern, E. H., Patel, G., & Balk, R. A. (2007). Antibiotic therapy for pulmonary exacerbations in adults with cystic fibrosis. *Medsurg Nursing, 16,* 293–297.

Essig, M. G. (2007). *Continuous positive airway pressure (CPAP) therapy for obstructive sleep apnea.* Sleep Apnea Health Center. Retrieved June 21, 2009, from www.webmd.com/sleep-disorders/sleep-apnea/continuous-positive-airway-pressure-cpap-for-obstructive-sleep-apnea

Ford, J., & Weaver, F. H. (2000). Breathing retraining and relaxation techniques for clients with pulmonary disease. *OT Practice, 5*(13), 33–34.

Gould, B. E. (2006). Respiratory disorders. In *Pathophysiology for the health professions* (3rd ed., pp. 362–420). Philadelphia: W. B. Saunders.

Hayes, D., Jr., & Meyer, K. C. (2007). Acute exacerbations of chronic bronchitis in elderly patients: Pathogenesis, diagnosis and management. *Drugs Aging, 24,* 555–572.

Hebra, A. (2007). Pectus excavatum. *eMedicine.* Retrieved October 5, 2008, from www.emedicine.com/PED/topic2558.htm#Multimediamedia1

Hogg, J. C. (2004). Pathophysiology of airflow limitation in chronic obstructive pulmonary disease. *Lancet, 364,* 709–721.

Holcomb, S. S. (2007). Critical care: When your patient has pneumonia. *Nursing, 37*(6), 48cc1–48cc3.

Holman, M. L. (2005). Obstructive sleep apnea: Implications for primary care. *Nurse Practitioner, 30*(9), 38–43.

Huntley, N. (2008). Cardiac and pulmonary diseases. In M. V. Radomski & C. A. T. Latham (Eds.), *Occupational therapy for physical dysfunction* (6th ed., pp. 1296–1320). Philadelphia: Wolters Kluwer.

Ikeda, B., & Goodman, C. C. (2009). The respiratory system. In C. C. Goodman & K. S. Fuller (Eds.), *Pathology* (3rd ed., pp. 742–827). St. Louis, MO: W. B. Saunders.

Irion, G. L., & Goodman, C. C. (2009). Laboratory tests and values. In C. C. Goodman & K. S. Fuller (Eds.), *Pathology: Implications for the physical therapist* (3rd ed., pp. 1637–1667). Philadelphia: W. B. Saunders.

Lang, E. F., & West, M. P. (2009). Medical-surgical equipment in the acute care setting. In J. C. Paz & M. P. West (Eds.), *Acute care handbook for physical therapists* (3rd ed., pp. 441–462). St. Louis, MO: W. B. Saunders.

Larsson, K. (2007). Aspects on pathophysiological mechanisms in COPD. *Journal of Internal Medicine, 262,* 311–340.

Lindsay, K. L. B., & Malone, D. J. (2006). Pulmonary diseases and disorders. In D. J. Malone & K. L. B. Lindsay (Eds.), *Physical therapy in acute care: A clinician's guide* (pp. 211–273). Thorofare, NJ: Slack.

Little, C. (2001). What you need to know about chronic bronchitis. *Nursing, 31*(9), 52–55.

McLaughlin, V. V., & McGoon, M. D. (2006). Contemporary reviews in cardiovascular medicine: Pulmonary arterial hypertension. *Circulation, 114,* 1417–1431. doi: 10.1161/circulationaha.104.503540

Migliore, A. (2004a). Improving dyspnea management in three adults with chronic obstructive pulmonary disease. *American Journal of Occupational Therapy, 58,* 639–646.

Migliore, A. (2004b). Management of dyspnea guidelines for practice for adults with chronic obstructive pulmonary disease. *Occupational Therapy in Health Care, 18*(3), 1–20.

Moore, S. L. (2003). Bronchiolitis obliterans organizing pneumonia: A late complication of stem cell transplantation. *Clinical Journal of Oncology Nursing, 7,* 659–662.

National Cancer Institute. (2004). *Antioxidant and cancer prevention* [Fact Sheet]. Retrieved June 27, 2009, from www.cancer.gov/cancertopics/factsheet/antioxidantsprevention

Nici, L., Limberg, T., Hilling, L., Garvey, C., Normandin, E. A., Reardon, J., et al. (2007). Clinical competency guidelines for pulmonary rehabilitation professionals: American Association of Cardiovascular and Pulmonary Rehabilitation position statement. *Journal of Cardiopulmonary Rehabilitation and Prevention, 27,* 355–358.

Norweg, A., Bose, P., Snow, G., & Berkowitz, M. E. (2008). A pilot study of a pulmonary rehabilitation programme evaluated by four adults with chronic obstructive pulmonary disease. *Occupational Therapy International, 15,* 114–132.

O'Keefe-McCarthy, S. (2006). Evidence-based nursing strategies to prevent ventilator-acquired pneumonia. *Dynamics, 17*(1), 8–11.

Parkin, M., Bray, F., Ferlay, J., & Pisani, P. (2005). Global cancer statistics, 2002. *CA: A Cancer Journal for Clinicians, 55,* 74–108.

Peate, I. (2008). Caring for the person with a pulmonary embolism. *British Journal of Healthcare Assistants, 2,* 318–322.

Penuelas, O., Frutos-Vivar, F., & Esteban, A. (2007). Noninvasive positive-pressure ventilation in acute respiratory failure. *Canadian Medical Association Journal, 177,* 1211–1218.

Petty, T. L. (2003). Chronic obstructive pulmonary disease. In M. E. Hanley & C. H. Welsh (Eds.), *Current diagnosis and treatment in pulmonary medicine* (pp. 82–91). New York: Lange Medical Books.

Philip, J. A. M., Gold, M., Sutherland, S., Finlayson, F., Braithwaite, M., Kotsimbos, T., et al. (2008). End-of-life care in adults with cystic fibrosis. *Journal of Palliative Medicine, 11,* 198–203.

Pruitt, B. (2007). Take an evidence-based approach to treating acute lung injury. *Critical Care Insider, 37,* 14–18.

Redman, B. K. (2004). Asthma and chronic obstructive pulmonary disease self-management preparation. *In Patient self-management of chronic* disease: *The health care provider's challenge* (pp. 147–168). Sudbury, MA: Jones & Bartlett.

Respiratory disorders. (2006). In J. Munden & L. M. Bonsall (Eds.), *Atlas of pathophysiology* (2nd ed., pp. 80–117). Philadelphia: Lippincott Williams & Wilkins.

Respiratory system. (2007). In J. Munden (Ed.), *Professional guide to pathophysiology* (2nd ed., pp. 117–120, 227–277). Philadelphia: Lippincott Williams & Wilkins.

Richmond, R. J., & Zellner, K. M. (2005). a1-antitrypsin deficiency: Incidence and implications. *Dimensions of Critical Care Nursing, 24,* 255–260.

Saavedra, M. T., & Nick, J. A. (2003). Chronic bronchiectasis and cystic fibrosis. In M. E. Hanley & C. H. Welsh (Eds.), *Current diagnosis and treatment in pulmonary medicine* (pp. 92–104). New York: Lange Medical Books.

Schriber, A. (2008). *Idiopathic pulmonary fibrosis.* Retrieved September 12, 2008, from www.nlm.nih.gov/medlineplus/ency/article/000069.htm

Schutz, S. L. (2001). Oxygen saturation monitoring by pulse oximetry. In D. J. Lynn-Mchale & K. K. Carlson (Eds.), *American Association of Critical Care Nurses procedure manual for critical care* (4th ed., pp. 77–82). Philadelphia: W. B. Saunders.

Sewell, L., & Singh, S. J. (2001). The Canadian Occupational Performance Measure: Is it a reliable measure in clients with chronic obstructive pulmonary disease? *British Journal of Occupational Therapy, 64,* 305–310.

Simonneau, G., Galiè, N., Rubin, L. J., Langleben, D., Seeger, W., Domenighetti, G., et al. (2004). Clinical classification of pulmonary hypertension. *Journal of the American College of Cardiology, 43*(12, Suppl.), 5S–12S. doi:10.1016/j.jacc.2004.02.037

Sin, D. D., McAlister, F. A., Man, S. F. P., & Anthonisen, N. R. (2003). Contemporary management of chronic obstructive pulmonary disease: Scientific review. *JAMA, 290,* 2301–2312.

Smith-Gabai, H. (2008). VATs, what's that? *Advance for Occupational Therapy Practitioners, 24*(7), 64.

So, C. T., & Man, D. W. K. (2008). Development and validation of an Activities of Daily Living Inventory for the rehabilitation of patients with chronic obstructive pulmonary disease. *OTJR: Occupation, Participation and Health, 28,* 149–159.

Steinbis, S. (2004). What you should know about pulmonary hypertension. *Nurse Practitioner, 29*(4), 8–19.

Stoller, J. K., & Aboussouan, L. S. (2005). Alpha1-antitrypsin deficiency. *Lancet, 365,* 2225–2236.

Stump, J. R. (1999). Treating chronic pulmonary disease. *OT Practice, 4*(6), 28–32.

Theander, K., Jakobsson, P., Jorgensen, N., & Unosson, M. (2009). Effects of pulmonary rehabilitation on fatigue, functional status, and health perceptions in patients with chronic obstructive pulmonary disease: A randomized controlled trial. *Clinical Rehabilitation, 23,* 125–136.

Tuberculosis. (2008). In *Tutorials.* Retrieved October 24, 2008, from www.nlm.nih.gov/medlineplus/tutorials/tuberculosis/htm/index.htm

Twedell, D. (2007). Emphysema and lung volume reduction surgery. *Journal of Continuing Education in Nursing, 38*(4), 150–151.

Velloso, M., & Jardim, J. R. (2006). Study of energy expenditure during activities of daily living: Using and not using body position recommended by energy conservation techniques in patients with COPD. *Chest, 130,* 126–132.

Wai-Shan Louie, S. (2004). The effects of guided imagery relaxation in people with COPD. *Occupational Therapy International, 11*(3), 145–159.

Wells, C. (2004). Pulmonary pathology. In W. E. DeTurk & L. P. Cahalin (Eds.), *Cardiovascular and pulmonary physical therapy: An evidence-based approach* (pp. 151–188). New York: McGraw-Hill.

West, M. P., Paz, J. C., & O'Leary, K. (2009). Respiratory system. In J. C. Paz & M. P. West (Eds.), *Acute care handbook for physical therapists* (3rd ed., pp. 47–86). St. Louis, MO: W. B. Saunders.

White, K., & Ruth-Sahd, L. A. (2007). Bronchiolitis obliterans organizing pneumonia. *Critical Care Nurse, 27*(3), 53–66.

Widmar, B. (2005). When cure is care: Diagnosis and management of pulmonary arterial hypertension. *Journal of the American Academy of Nurse Practitioners, 17,* 104–112.

Wisniewski, A. (2003). Chronic bronchitis. *Nursing, 33*(5), 46–49.

Yankaskas, J. R., Marshall, B. C., Sufian, B., Simon, R. H., & Rodman, D. (2004). Cystic fibrosis adult care: Consensus conference report. *Chest, 125*(1, Suppl.), 1S–39S.

Appendix 5.A.

Guidelines for Dyspnea Relief

Instruction in diaphragmatic and pursed-lip breathing is one of the most important ways in which therapists can assist patients in relieving symptoms of dyspnea and promoting more efficient breathing. Certain positions can help ameliorate dyspnea and facilitate diaphragmatic breathing by placing the diaphragm in a mechanically advantageous position (i.e., pushed upward and outward) and minimizing movement of accessory muscles, resulting in more effective breathing (Migliore, 2004a).

Positions That Minimize Dyspnea

- At rest or after activity, lean forward in sitting as if slouching forward, but avoid moderate to maximum forward trunk bending.
- In standing, support arms on a table or counter with shoulders internally rotated and adducted.
- In supine, bed should be in Trendelenburg position of 10° to 20°.

Breathing at Rest and With Activity

- When instructing patients in controlled breathing, begin at rest, either in supine or slouching forward in sitting. Then progress to controlled breathing with activity exertion.
- Breathe with pursed-lip technique: Inhale through the nose and exhale slowly through pursed lips.
- Breathing should be slow, deep, and fluid.
- Stomach should rise with inspiration and fall with expiration.
- Breathe with minimal movement of the head, upper rib cage, or shoulder girdle.
- Begin breathing cycle with active exhalation.
- Exhalation should be 2–3 times longer than inspiration.
- Avoid forceful expiration; exhalations should be gentle.
- Avoid holding breath during activity.
- Inspiration occurs with body movements against gravity.
- Expiration occurs with exertion or the strenuous parts of an activity.

Miscellaneous

- When engaging in an activity, move slowly; do not rush and stop to rest.
- Avoid maximal forward bending of the trunk while engaging in occupations.
- Incorporate controlled breathing into all activities. Provide opportunities for patients to coordinate proper breathing into their daily occupations. For example, incorporate proper breathing techniques when rising from a chair, carrying laundry, picking items up off the floor, or reaching overhead to access high shelves or kitchen cabinets.

Source. Migliore (2004b).

Appendix 5.B.

Common Symptoms and Terms Associated With Respiratory Disorders

Symptom or Term	Description
Orthopnea	Shortness of breath while lying down. Usually relieved by being in a more upright position. May be referred to in the chart as 2- to 3-pillow orthopnea, meaning that the patient needs to sleep with 2 or more pillows at night.
Dyspnea	Shortness of breath. *Dyspnea on exertion (DOE)* is shortness of breath with activity. Experiences of dyspnea are subjective but can be debilitating.
Tachypnea	Increased respiratory rate (RR; above normal). Normal adult RR is approximately 12–20 breaths per minute. RR is usually measured by monitoring how often the patient's chest rises in 1 minute. RR is best monitored when the patient is unaware.
Apnea	Brief pauses in breathing. Occupational therapists do not treat obstructive sleep apnea (OSA) as a primary diagnosis, but OSA is a common comorbidity. OSA is usually treated with a continuous positive airway pressure machine used when sleeping.
Hypoxia	Lack of oxygen supply in the body. May lead to unresponsiveness or coma. May be treated with mechanical ventilation.
Hypoxemia	Reduction of oxygen in the blood. May be a symptom of pulmonary fibrosis, pulmonary embolism, pneumonia, pulmonary edema, or other lung disorders. Can be measured through arterial blood gas analysis.
Anoxia	Absence of oxygen, or an extreme form of hypoxia.
FiO_2	*Fraction of inspired air,* which refers to the percentage of oxygen breathed in. Room air is normally 21% oxygen. Supplemental oxygen may be adjusted higher than 21% for patients with increased oxygen requirements.
Stridor and wheezing	*Stridor* is a high-pitched breathing sound caused by an obstruction. Usually requires immediate medical attention. *Wheezing* is a high-pitched whistling usually heard during exhalation and may be caused by narrowed bronchiole tubes. Common in asthma, chronic obstructive pulmonary disorder, and pulmonary edema.
Cheyne–Stokes respiration	Also know as periodic breathing, in which rapid respirations alternate with apnea. This type of breathing pattern may be noted as a patient nears death.
Respiratory insufficiency or failure	A condition in which the lungs cannot take in enough oxygen or remove a sufficient amount of carbon dioxide to meet the metabolic needs of the body. The acid–base balance of the body is disrupted, leading to respiratory acidosis or hypercapnia.
Respiratory arrest	A complete cessation of breathing.

6

The Nervous System

Judy R. Hamby, MHS, OTR/L, BCPR

In the acute care setting, occupational therapists often serve populations who are experiencing the sequelae of neurological diseases and injuries. A clear understanding of the anatomy and physiology that influences and underpins the functioning of the nervous system supports clinicians' application of rehabilitative concepts. Neurological disorders and deficits are vast and cover every part of the body, ranging from traumatic brain injuries to peripheral neuropathies. The sheer variety complicates occupational therapy intervention because no cookbook program can encompass it. Occupational therapists are well suited to bridging neuroscience, medical presentation, and rehabilitative concepts to improve occupational performance. Practical rehabilitation practices discussed in this chapter will maximize functional recovery at the beginning of the continuum of care.

Anatomy and Physiology

What do reading a get-well card, remembering what the doctor said, breathing, and walking to the bathroom all have in common? The nervous system is the one system in the body that meticulously manages the ability to perform all these tasks and is the master controller that monitors and manages all bodily functions. The nervous system is made up of two distinct portions, the central nervous system (CNS) and peripheral nervous system (PNS). Each portion makes specific contributions to functional performance.

Central Nervous System

The *CNS* includes the brain and spinal cord and is encased in the bony structures of the skull and vertebral column. The CNS integrates information from external and internal stimuli, through the PNS, and then controls the response to those stimuli. The brain initiates behavior via body functions such as neuromusculoskeletal and movement-related functions and sensory and mental functions.

Brain

The *brain* is the upper motor neuron control center of the entire body. Clinical features of neurological deficits are entirely contingent on the structures that are affected. Figure 6.1 depicts the anatomical structures of the brain, and Figure 6.2 delineates the functions of the major lobes of the brain.

The brain has two hemispheres, and each is responsible for the opposite side of the body and for the completion of different aspects of the same task. For instance, the *left hemisphere* generally provides recall and detail information that assists in the identification of objects and is responsible for the language components of a task. The *right hemisphere* focuses more on the attention and judgment skills associated with task completion. The brain contains four *ventricles* and is surrounded by three *meninges*. Together the meninges and the ventricular system provide a fluid-filled protection system for the nervous tissue.

Cerebrospinal fluid (CSF) is produced in the brain's ventricles, which are its aqueduct system. The *choroid plexus* makes 500 cubic centimeters of CSF every 24 hours. Each hemisphere contains one ventricle called the *lateral ventricle*. The third ventricle is located between the two *thalami*. The fourth ventricle produces 70% of the CSF and is located between the *cerebellum, pons,* and the front of the *medulla*. The *cerebral aqueduct* connects the third and fourth ventricles. Figure 6.3 illustrates the brain's ventricular system.

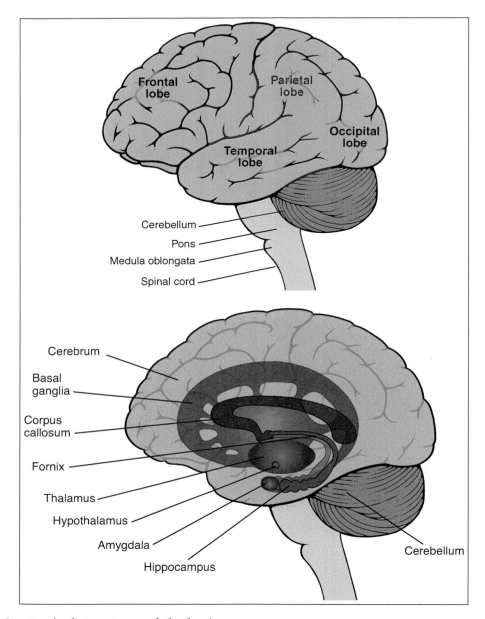

Figure 6.1. Anatomical structures of the brain.
Source. Richard Fritzler, Medical Illustrator, Roswell, GA.

Three meninges provide protective membrane layers around the brain and spinal cord. The *dura mater* is the outermost and most fibrous layer. It surrounds and protects the entire CNS and contains a drainage system and vasculature that ultimately become capillaries in the pia mater. The dura mater also provides separations for specific sections, including the longitudinal fissures between the hemispheres and between the occipital lobes and the cerebellum. The roots of the spinal nerves pierce the dura mater in the spinal canal. The *arachnoid* is the middle layer, which loosely surrounds the brain and provides an additional layer of protection. It looks like a spider web, thus the name's origin. The *pia mater* adheres tightly to the brain and is highly vascularized, supplying blood to the CNS.

Neurological dysfunction is dependent on the location of damage in the CNS. Table 6.1 delineates functional deficits in each hemisphere of the brain. These deficits are not

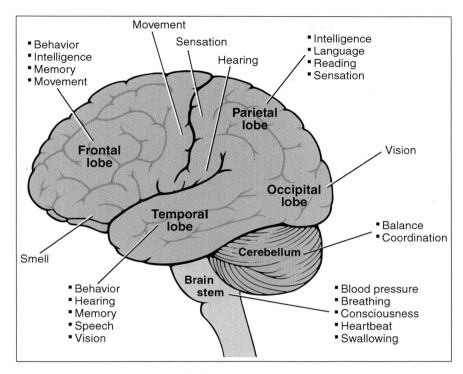

Figure 6.2. Functions of the major lobes of the brain.
Source. Richard Fritzler, Medical Illustrator, Roswell, GA.

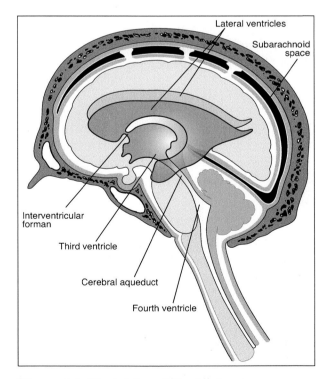

Figure 6.3. Ventricles of the brain.
Source. Richard Fritzler, Medical Illustrator,
Roswell, GA.

diagnosis specific and can manifest in any brain-related diagnosis. Table 6.2 specifies the function associated with each area of the brain and the deficits that can result from injury to each area. Often, the only diagnostic information provided to the acute care therapist is the site of the infarcted vascular distribution of the brain. An understanding of the territory that a particular vessel supplies can assist therapists' focus on identifying deficit areas during evaluation and intervention. Refer to Figure 6.4 and Table 6.3 for a depiction of the vasculature of the brain and associated deficits, respectively.

Spinal Cord

The spinal cord begins and ends the motor and sensory loop associated with volitional and involuntary motor control, and it is considered the core of the lower motor neuron region. The *spinal cord* is a cylindrical tube, approximately 18 inches long, that is encased within the vertebral column and is divided into five distinct sections designated by a letter and a

Function	Left Hemisphere	Right Hemisphere
Extremity	• Right hemiplegia	• Left hemiplegia
Vision–perception	• Right visual field cut (right homonymous hemianopsia) or neglect	• Left visual field cut (left homonymous hemianopsia), neglect, gaze paresis • Spatial awareness
Cognition	• Sequencing deficits • Difficulty with logical progression of thought processes • Decreased ability to distinguish details • Memory deficits of past and recent events	• Significant cognitive deficits, especially safety judgment • Lack of insight and unawareness of deficits • Loss of prosody of speech and impaired pragmatics • Attention deficits
Language	• Receptive aphasia, expressive aphasia, or both	• Dysarthria (resulting from facial and tongue hemiparesis); usually no aphasia
Sensory	• Right-sided sensory deficits	• Left-sided sensory deficits
Praxis	• Ideomotor apraxia (left premotor or parietal)	• Constructional apraxia (usually right parietal)

Table 6.1. **Hemispheric Differentiation by Deficit Areas**

Sources. Littlejohns (2004); Rothstein, Roy, and Wolf (1998); Segal, Levin, Steiger, and Falk (2005).

number. The letter designates the section of the back in which it is located: *cervical* (*C*), *thoracic* (*T*), *lumbar* (*L*), *sacral* (*S*), and the *cauda equina*. The number correlates to the level of the vertebrae at which it is located: C1–C8, T1–T12, L1–L5, and S1–S5. See Figure 6.5 for an illustration of the spinal levels, including the relation of the spinal nerves to the spine. Originating from each level are four spinal roots (ventral and dorsal bilaterally). The ventral and dorsal roots (on each side) eventually merge to form spinal nerves. Once the spinal nerves emerge from the spine, they are considered to be part of the PNS. These nerves contain both efferent and afferent innervation for the entire body, except for the areas the cranial nerves innervate. The spinal cord's ultimate job is to receive and transmit sensory information from the body to the brain. The brain then sends information back through the spinal cord to stimulate a response.

Peripheral Nervous System

The portions of the nervous system outside the skull and vertebral column make up the PNS, which consists of the *PNS* and the autonomic nervous system (ANS). The PNS includes the cranial and spinal nerves that control voluntary skeletal muscle activity and external sensory information. The ANS is further subdivided into the *sympathetic* and *parasympathetic nervous systems* (SNS and PSNS, respectively) and enables the body to control stress reactions

(Text continues on p. 197)

Table 6.2. Anatomical Functional Correlation of Injury in the Brain

Area of the Brain	Functional Areas	Function	Major Deficits Associated With Injury or Disorder
Frontal lobe	• Primary motor (controls voluntary movements) • Premotor (contains programming necessary for movement) • Frontal eye field (conjugate deviation of the eyes to the contralateral side) • Supplementary motor (programming necessary for complex movements involving several parts of the body) • Prefrontal (executive function skills, emotional activities, social behaviors) • Broca's area (motor control of speech)	• Spatial working memory • Oromotor function • Working memory for language assembly • Integrated motor sequences • Planning motor behavior • Bowel and bladder control • Judgment and reasoning • Personality	• Poor executive function skills • Impaired fluency of speech—Telegraphic speech • Impaired pragmatics if right hemisphere is damaged • Personality changes • Initiation deficits, including impulsivity
Temporal lobe	• Primary auditory • Auditory association • Wernicke's area	• Memory • Emotions • Understanding of speech (receptive) • Perception of written language • Auditory discrimination • Visual discrimination • Ability to recognize faces (including one's own)	• Left-sided lesion—Short-term verbal memory loss • Right-sided lesion—Short-term memory loss • Auditory input deficits • Wernicke's aphasia (fluent speech, but not understandable) • Alzheimer's—Intracellular (not externally visible masses) fibrillary tangles flatten inferior temporal lobes, resulting in memory loss

(continued)

Table 6.2.   *(continued)*

Area of the Brain	Functional Areas	Function	Major Deficits Associated With Injury or Disorder
Parietal lobe	• Primary somatosensory (position sense and sensation on contralateral side) • Secondary somatosensory (sensation of pain) • Gustatory (taste) • Association (processes tactile and visual information; concerned with the cognition of peripersonal space, sequencing, and spatial relations)	• Spatial relations • Attention • Behavior • Praxis • Tactile discrimination • Pain } Reflexive • Temperature } response • Modulates and directs motor skills	• Neglect or inattention • Poor personal space boundaries • Emotional or labile behavior • Apraxia • Reading deficits • Spatial relations • Sensory input and integration deficits • Receptive speech deficits
Occipital lobe	• Primary visual cortex (processes visual field received from the retina) • Parastriate cortex and peristriate cortex, which receive visual information and process complex visual perceptions related to color, movement, and direction of objects	• Vision • Perception	• Visual field cuts • Perceptual deficits • Visual input and processing deficits
Cerebellum	Two hemispheres divided by the vermis Cerebral peduncles—Connects the cerebellum to the brainstem • Inferior cerebellar peduncle • Middle cerebellar peduncle • Superior cerebellar peduncle Vestibulocerebellum—Connects to the vestibular system	• All input from spinal cord is from the ipsilateral body • Regulates movement through the timing and force of voluntary muscle • Regulates balance	• Ataxia • Impaired proprioception • Dysdiadochokinesia: Inability to coordinate alternating rapid movements (turning palms up and down, heel up–down shin) • Dysmetria, dyssynergia, hypermetria • Intention tremor

Structure			
	Spinocerebellum connects with the spinal cord and brainstem Cerebrocerebellum connects to the cerebral cortex	• Anterior lobe affected by alcohol abuse—Usually affects legs with an ataxic, wide-stance gait	Nystagmus: Eyes oscillating involuntarily and rhythmically. Can be vertical, horizontal, rotary, or a combination (Honrubia, 2000; Kline & Bajandas, 2004) • Vertigo • Diplopia

Thalamus	Rests on either side of the 3rd ventricle; 4 main nuclear groups containing multiple nuclei:
	• Lateral
	• Dorsomedial
	• Centromedial
	• Ventral
		• Modulates efferent and afferent input and output
		• Receives signals from the following systems:
		  • Somatosensory
		  • Auditory
		  • Visual
		  • Limbic
		  • Gustatory
		  • Vestibular
			• Usually manifests as diffuse pain instead of motor deficits
			• Usually pure sensory deficits
			• Visual field deficits
			• Behavioral changes

Hypothalamus	• Integrally connected to multiple parts of the nervous system • Connects to the pituitary gland; information received from different parts of the brain is transmitted to the pituitary gland via the hypothalamus	• Central regulator of homeostasis • Controls autonomic (sympathetic and parasympathetic) activity • Regulates appetite and thirst • Regulates stress response • Thermoregulatory system • Regulates sleep and wake cycles	• High fever—Neurogenic fevers • Autonomic dysfunction syndrome • Bilateral hypothalamic lesions—Violent and aggressive behavior • Autonomic, emotional, and endocrine dysfunction • Bitemporal visual field cuts with pituitary tumor • Loss of wake–sleep cycle

(continued)

Table 6.2. *(continued)*

Area of the Brain	Functional Areas	Function	Major Deficits Associated With Injury or Disorder
		• Participates in limbic system: Expression of emotions such as fear, anger, and embarrassment • Regulates violent behavior	• Hyperphagia (eats an excessive amount of food) • If in a coma, can lose fluid and develop diabetes
Limbic system	Structures and tracts that encircle the thalamus • Hippocampus • Fornix • Amygdala • Stria terminalis • Habenula • Spetal nuclei	• Central regulator of emotional control and memory encoding • Amygdala—Controls emotional interpretation of environmental and internal stimuli, especially emotional arousal responses to fear and anger (Rubin & Safdieh, 2007)	• Anterograde amnesia • Behavioral changes such as aggression and apathy • Bilateral hippocampal lesions can occur with anoxia—Patients present with amnestic syndromes • Amygdala lesions—Behavioral abnormalities. Bilateral lesions cause emotional blunting, hypersexuality, and hyperphagia
Subcortical	• White matter tracts	• Connects gray matter to white matter	• Multiple sclerosis—Demyelination of white matter tracts
Internal capsule	Large mass of hemispheric white matter; part of the pyramidal system • Anterior limb—Motor • Genu • Posterior limb—Motor and sensory • Retrolintiform part • Sublentiform part	Projection fibers are concentrated in the internal capsule, connecting the cortex and subcortical structures: • Sensory (afferent if carrying information toward the cortex)	• Most commonly called *capsular stroke*, in which the corticospinal and corticobulbar tracts are interrupted • Most common site of cerebral hemorrhage. Symptoms are more widespread

	• Motor (efferent if carrying information away from the cortex)	• Results in contralateral hyperesthesia and spastic hemiplegia, especially in arm flexors and leg extensors • Lower facial paralysis (if corticobulbar tract infarcted) • Volitional movement in contralateral limbs are absent, but return with proximal more than with distal • If retrolenticular part infarcted, then will see contralateral homonymous hemianopsia resulting from interruption of the optic radiations
Corpus callosum	• Rostrum • Genu • Trunk • Splenium	• Connects hemispheres to allow communication • Rostrum and genu connect the anterior frontal lobes • Trunk connects the posterior frontal lobes • Splenium—Interconnects the occipital lobes • Seizure disorder—The corpus callosum is transected surgically to stop seizures moving to the other hemisphere • Exhibits significant language dysfunction if corpus callosum is transected • Bilateral integration may be affected if there is a lesion in the corpus callosum
Optic radiations (geniculocalcarine loop)	• Extends from the lateral geniculate nucleus to the occipital lobe through the parietal and temporal lobe • Meyer's loop goes through the temporal lobe • Parietal loop goes through the parietal lobe	• Lesion of bilateral optic radiations—Cortical blindness • If only the right side is infarcted, then the deficits are as follows (the left side will have the opposite visual field cuts): • Meyer's loop—Carries the upper part of the contralateral visual field

(continued)

Table 6.2. (continued)

Area of the Brain	Functional Areas	Function	Major Deficits Associated With Injury or Disorder
		• Parietal loop—Carries visual information from the inferior visual field. If peripheral fibers are affected, then the lateral visual fields are more affected. If the medial fibers are infarcted, then the central fields are affected	• Combination of Meyer's and Parietal loops • Meyer's loop—Left homonymous superior quadrantanopia • Parietal loop—Left homonymous inferior quadrantanopia
Brainstem	Most internal part of the brain	Living—Homeostasis and automatic functions	Injury to the brainstem is often fatal
Pons	• Near the pontomedullary junction, cranial nerves VI, VII, VIII, V emerge • Largest portion of the brainstem • Reticular formation as central core, continuous with medullary reticular formation and midbrain	• Assists in controlling autonomic functioning • Arousal • Relays sensory information between cerebrum and cerebellum • Sleep • Center for horizontal gaze • Most common site for hypertensive bleed	• Bilateral horizontal gaze paresis • Coma • Locked-in syndrome • Pinpoint pupils • Infarct of the parapontine area of the reticular formation—Patient unable to initiate horizontal gaze and cannot turn his or her eyes past midline

| Medulla oblongata | • Lowest portion of the brainstem
• Pyramids on anterior surface
• Olive (olivary nucleus)
• Post- and preolivary sulcus—Rootlets of cranial nerves XII, IX, X, and XI emerge
• Medullary reticular formation | • Vital respiratory, vasomotor, and cardiovascular centers located in medulla Regulates the heartbeat and adjusts blood flow.
• Controls reflex actions such as vomiting, swallowing, gagging, and coughing
• Medullary reticular formation involved in wakefulness | • Respiratory arrest and death can result from large lesions that compress these structures (Rubin & Safdieh, 2007)
• Medullary reticular formation infarct results in coma
• Wallenberg's syndrome (lesion of posterior inferior cerebellar artery syndrome) is a lesion of the dorsolateral medulla:
  • Nystagmus (Honrrubia, 2000; Keshner, 2007)
  • Diplopia
  • Vertigo
  • Crossed sensory loss (sensory loss on ipsilateral face; poor pain and temperature sensation on contralateral body)
  • Ipsilateral dysmetria

Horner's syndrome:
  • Usually results from carotid dissection
  • Dysphagia
  • Ptosis
  • Meiosis—Constriction of pupil
  • Anhydrosis—Loss of perspiration on the side of the face as a result of losing innervation on that side of the face
  • Hoarseness |

(continued)

Table 6.2.   (continued)

Area of the Brain	Functional Areas	Function	Major Deficits Associated With Injury or Disorder
			• Hiccups • Ipsilateral poor gag • Ataxia
Midbrain	Divided by aqueduct Contains • Nuclei of cranial nerves III and IV. Nerve roots of III emerge from this area • Red nucleus • Superior and inferior colliculi • Substantia nigra • Cerebral peduncles (contain fibers of corticospinal tract)	• Associated with auditory, visual, and papillary reflexes • Center for vertical gaze • Dopamine production center in the substantia nigra • Superior colliculi receive information from the visual cortex and project to the spinal cord to control reflex movement of the head, neck, and eyes • Inferior colliculi mediate auditory input	• Degeneration of substantia nigra results in Parkinson's disease • May have decreased reflexive movement of the head, neck, and eyes in response to visual information • Inability to perform vertical eye movements
Basal ganglia	• Corpus striatum (caudate nucleus, globus pallidum, and putamen) • Subthalamic nucleus • Substantia nigra	• Initiation of voluntary movements • Control of voluntary postural adjustments • Refines coordination of movement; stores frequently used motor programs	• Most common site of hypertensive bleed • Hemiballism—Large flailing movements • Dyskinesias occur at rest • Hypokinetic (Parkinson's disease) or hyperkinetic states (Huntington's chorea)

	• Parkinson's disease (reduced dopamine production): — Akinesia and bradykinesia — Abnormal postural adjustments — Frequent retropulsion (posterior) falls and losses of balance — Pill-rolling — Rigidity–cogwheel tone — Masklike facial expression — Shuffling gait — Micrographia (small writing) — Reduced speech — Multiple visual deficits • Huntington's chorea (degeneration of caudate): • Chorea • Athetosis • Ballismus • Tics • Dementia • Tardive dyskinesias: Involves face, lips, and tongue; manifested by involuntary chewing motion with smacking of lips and tongue	
Meninges	Membranes surrounding the brain and spinal cord: • Dura mater—Outermost layer of the meninges • Arachnoid—Middle layer of the meninges (spider web–like and very thin)	• Along with the ventricular system, the meninges provide a fluid-filled protection system for the nervous tissue • Subdural hematoma occurs between the dura and the arachnoid layer

(continued)

Table 6.2.   *(continued)*

Area of the Brain	Functional Areas	Function	Major Deficits Associated With Injury or Disorder
	• Pia mater—Attached nearest the brain and spinal cord	• Subarachnoid space—Area between the arachnoid and the pia mater and is filled with cerebrospinal fluid • The arachnoid contains no blood vessels	• Subarachnoid hemorrhage—Forms between the arachnoid and pia mater usually as a result of trauma or rupture of an aneurysm of a cerebral artery • Meningitis—Inflammation of the meninges because of an infection (viral, fungal, or bacterial), a reaction to certain medications or medical interventions, or inflammatory diseases such as lupus, cancer, or traumatic brain injury • Meningioma—Arises from the arachnoid

Sources. Littlejohns (2004); Rothstein, Roy, and Wolf (1998).

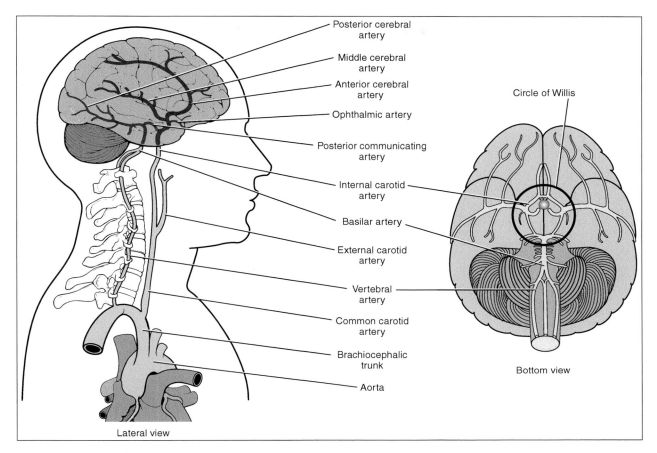

Circle of Willis

Bottom view

Lateral view

Figure 6.4. Vasculature of the brain.
Source. Richard Fritzler, Medical Illustrator, Roswell, GA.

and the homeostatic capabilities of the human body, respectively.

The PNS (sometimes called the *somatic nervous system*) is made up of all the nerves in the body that originate or terminate outside the CNS. The CNS relies on information provided by this system to formulate the appropriate afferent or efferent reaction. There are 31 pairs of *spinal nerves* and 12 pairs of *cranial nerves*. The cranial nerves, their functions, and testing procedures are listed in Table 6.4. They can be remembered with the mnemonic "*On Old Olympus' Towering Top A Famous Vocal German Viewed Some Hops.*" The 31 pairs of spinal nerves continue to divide, ultimately terminating into peripheral nerves throughout the body. The three primary peripheral nerves that affect the occupational therapist in acute care are those of the upper extremity: the median, radial, and ulnar nerves (see Table 6.21

for further information regarding these nerves and the associated deficit areas).

Autonomic Nervous System

The *ANS* ensures homeostasis of body systems. Through the innervation of the internal organs, automatic physiological responses occur, including heart rate, breathing, pupillary reflex, hair growth, body temperature, and metabolism. The ANS is divided into two segments: parasympathetic and sympathetic. See Figure 6.6 for a depiction of the ANS.

The SNS originates at spinal levels T1 to L2 or L3 in the intermediolateral cell column. The primary function of the SNS is the mobilization of energy, stimulating (remember the *s—sympathetic = stimulates*) the internal organs and inhibiting digestion. It prepares the body for fight or flight (Barron & Blair, 1999). The PSNS

Table 6.3. **Deficits Associated With the Brain's Vasculature**

Vessel	Site of Origin	Territory	Deficits Associated With Infarct of Circulation Area
Internal carotid artery	Carotid artery	Supplies the anterior parts of the brain, including parietal, lateral temporal, frontal, internal capsule, thalamus, hippocampus, and basal ganglia	• Contralateral and sensory loss • Transient contralateral monocular blindness • Contralateral hemianopsia • Aphasia • Contralateral hemineglect
Anterior cerebral artery	Internal carotid	• Frontal lobe (interior and inferior) • Medial cortical structures (frontal and parietal cortex) • Caudate (interior)	• Confusion • Personality change • Incontinence • Contralateral motor or sensory loss; leg greater than arm • When left sided, presents with ideomotor apraxia
Middle cerebral artery	Internal carotid	• Lateral portions of the parietal and temporal lobes and some portions of the frontal lobe • Deep branches supply most of basal ganglia and posterior limb of internal capsule	• Contralateral motor or sensory loss; arm greater than leg • Contralateral motor loss in lower face • Contralateral visual field loss • Language loss (if the dominant hemisphere is affected); Wernicke's aphasia • Spatial–perceptual loss (if the nondominant hemisphere is affected)
Vertebro-basilar artery (paired vertebral arteries join to form the basilar artery)	Subclavian artery	Supplies the posterior parts of the brain, including cerebellum, spinal cord, occipital lobe, temporal lobe, brainstem, and thalamus	• Cranial nerve deficits, III–XII • Brainstem and cerebellar impairment • Bilateral blindness, hemianopsia, or diplopia • Vertigo • Confusion • Ataxia • Bilateral limb weakness

Artery	Origin	Supplies	Signs/symptoms
(continued)			• Bilateral paresthesias • Dysarthria • Dysphagia
Posterior cerebral artery	Basilar artery	• Occipital lobe • Inferior temporal lobe • Thalamus	• Contralateral motor or sensory loss • Quadraparesis • Vision deficits; can cause contralateral visual field loss, cortical blindness, or diplopia • Dysarthria • Dysphagia
Posterior inferior cerebellar artery	Branch of vertebral artery	Supplies inferior part of the cerebellum and dorsolateral medulla	• Crossed sensory loss • Vertigo • Dysarthria • Dysphagia • Horner's syndrome
Anterior inferior cerebellar artery	Branch of basilar artery	• Anterior portions of inferior cerebellum • Dorsolateral pons • Portions of midbrain	Incidence is rare but is usually associated with brainstem stroke: • Bleeding can cause pressure on cranial nerves • Hearing loss • Weak or numb face • Ataxia (loss of coordination) • Vertigo • Changes in blood pressure

Note. **Bolded** arteries denote origin of vessels.
Sources. Littlejohns (2004); Rothstein, Roy, and Wolf (1998); Rubin and Safdieh (2007).

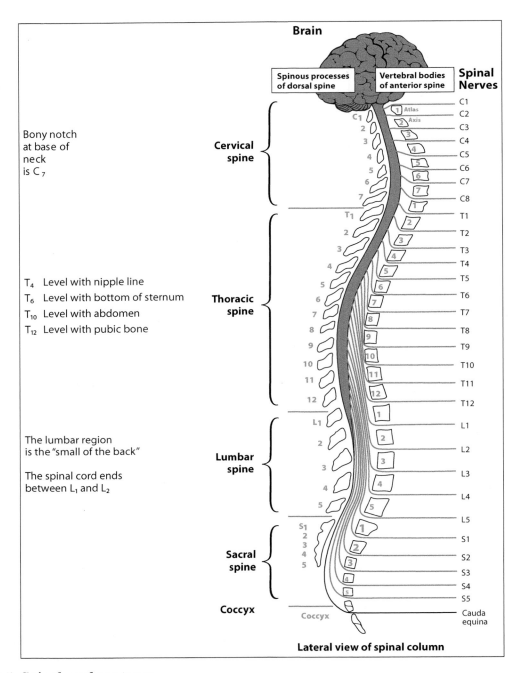

Brain

| Spinous processes of dorsal spine | Vertebral bodies of anterior spine | **Spinal Nerves** |

Bony notch
at base of
neck
is C_7

Cervical spine

T_4 Level with nipple line
T_6 Level with bottom of sternum
T_{10} Level with abdomen
T_{12} Level with pubic bone

Thoracic spine

The lumbar region
is the "small of the back"

The spinal cord ends
between L_1 and L_2

Lumbar spine

Sacral spine

Coccyx

Atlas
Axis

C1
C2
C3
C4
C5
C6
C7
C8
T1
T2
T3
T4
T5
T6
T7
T8
T9
T10
T11
T12
L1
L2
L3
L4
L5
S1
S2
S3
S4
S5
Cauda equina

Lateral view of spinal column

Figure 6.5. Spinal cord anatomy.
Source. Richard Fritzler, Medical Illustrator, Roswell, GA.

is usually inhibitory in nature, conserving and restoring body functions. It arises from the craniosacral region—specifically the oculomotor (III), facial (VII), glossopharyngeal (IX), and vagus (X) nerves and spinal segments S2 to S5 and is most involved in sedentary, digestive conservation and restoration, and voiding activities (Barron & Blair, 1999).

Neurological Diseases and Disorders

The variety of neurological diseases and injuries encountered in the acute care setting often appeals to clinicians but is conversely also the biggest hurdle because every patient presents

(Text continues on p. 205)

Table 6.4. **Cranial Nerve Testing and Function**

No. and Cranial Nerve	Function	Functional Deficits	Appearance	Test
I: Olfactory (only nerve to have a direct connection to the cerebrum)	Sensory; smell	• Unable to accurately identify scents and odors. • More prevalent with frontal lobe impairment or diffuse cerebral edema.	No abnormal appearance.	• Patient identifies various scents (e.g., vanilla, peppermint, coffee, garlic). • Patients on a ventilator or with a tracheostomy are typically unable to smell or taste.
II: Optic nerve	Sensory; vision	Complete visual loss in the affected eye.	No abnormal appearance.	Test visual fields in all quadrants binocularly and monocularly.
III: Oculomotor	Motor; innervates muscles of the eye: • Levator palpebrae superioris—Elevates the eyelid • Superior rectus—Elevation, intorsion, and adduction • Inferior rectus—Depression, extorsion, and adduction • Inferior oblique—Extorsion, elevation, and abduction • Medial rectus—Adduction	• Decreased vertical movement and inward movement. • Decreased ability to converge eyes (adduction). • Diplopia for near visual tasks and in horizontal (images side by side). • If ptosis is present, then binocularity of the eyes is impossible; thus, no diplopia. • Accommodation decreased. • Pupil may be dilated if the parasympathetic nucleus is affected.	• Ptosis. • Eye is generally deviated "down and out" because elevation, depression, and adduction of the eye are impaired.	Test both eyes at the same time: • Tracking and smooth pursuits • Convergence: Instruct patient to watch your finger and move it toward the nose; eyes should adduct smoothly and equally. • Pupillary response: Shine flashlight into one eye at a time to observe pupil constriction.

(continued)

Table 6.4.   *(continued)*

No. and Cranial Nerve	Function	Functional Deficits	Appearance	Test
IV: Trochlear	Motor • Innervates superior oblique—Depression (down) and adduction (in) of the eye • Controls eye movement down, such as in looking down a step	• Vertical diplopia for near vision only. It worsens with downward gaze in the direction opposite to the affected eye. The image may also be tilted because the superior oblique muscle abducts and medially rotates (intorts) the eye (Pelak, 2004). • Primarily associated with trauma and basilar skull fractures.	The affected eye may be looking toward the tip of the nose, and chin will be depressed with head tilted to side opposite of injury.	Test both eyes at the same time. • Tracking and smooth pursuits
V: Trigeminal (3 branches)	Sensory and motor; facial sensation	• Unable to clench jaw. • Deficits with biting, chewing, and rotary jaw movement. The jaw may deviate to the paralyzed side when opened. • Patient may experience sudden and severe neuropathic pain on one side in trigeminal neuralgia.	No abnormal appearance unless the mouth is open; the jaw may then be deviated to the paralyzed side.	• Facial sensation: Sharp or dull, light touch, hot or cold. • Clench mouth—Palpate masseter. • Corneal reflex—Blinks with light touch of cotton to cornea. • Jaw jerk—Strike middle of the jaw with a reflex hammer. Should note slight jaw closing.
VI: Abducens	Motor • Innervates lateral rectus—abduction (out toward the temple) of the eye	• Diplopia with distance vision that is worse when the affected eye is looking to the side (Pelak, 2004). • Horizontal diplopia.	• Posture: Head turned toward the affected side.	Test both eyes at the same time. • Tracking—Move a target in the shape of an *H* so that all cardinal planes of movement are evaluated.

	• Controls eye movement that allows for distance vision		• Affected eye is deviated inward.	
VII: Facial	Sensory and motor; face movement	• Facial droop interferes with articulation and feeding. • Unable to close eye.	Facial droop or asymmetry.	• Wrinkle forehead. • Smile, frown, and puff out cheeks. • Shut eyes tightly and keep them shut while therapist tries to open them manually. • Taste—Use sugar, salt.
VIII: Vestibulocochlear	Sensory; hearing and vestibular function—Position of head in space; provides stable visual image during head movement, postural control	• Cannot hear. • Vestibular system rarely affected, but if it is refer to Appendix H.	No abnormal appearance.	Hearing test: • Rub fingers together loudly or use a ticking watch on one side and ask on which side the patient hears the sound. Repeat on other side. • Tuning fork—Placed on top of head after vibrating. Does patient hear it on one side or the other? (Not usually performed by an occupational therapist). Vestibular test: • Nystagmus: Note response during extraocular musculature testing. • Gait assessment—Looking for ataxia and balance dysfunction.
IX: Glossopharyngeal X: Vagus	Sensory and motor; taste and gag reflex, involuntary muscles (heart, stomach, intestines, throat, chest)	• Voice is hoarse and nasal. • Swallow dysfunction (refer to Chapter 13 on dysphagia).	No abnormal appearance.	• Both nerves are tested together. • Speak without hoarseness. • Stimulate back of throat; should elicit a gag.

(continued)

Table 6.4. (continued)

No. and Cranial Nerve	Function	Functional Deficits	Appearance	Test
		Recurrent laryngeal cough—Bovine cough.		• Say "ah." • Normal response: Palate elevates symmetrically with uvula centered. • Abnormal response: Uvula elevates and deviates unilaterally toward unaffected side. In absence of any other symptoms, may not be pertinent.
XI: Spinal accessory	Motor; voluntary muscles of the shoulders and neck: sternocleidomastoid, trapezius	Unable to turn neck or elevate shoulders.	Atrophy of upper trapezius.	• Resistance to shoulder shrugs (trapezius) and lateral neck flexion with rotation (sternocleidomastoid). Inability to resist may indicate abnormal response. Deficit present in brainstem stroke.
XII: Hypoglossal	Motor; tongue movement	Articulation impaired because of tongue motility deficits.	No abnormal appearance.	Stick out tongue and check for deviation from midline. If abnormal, the tongue deviates to the affected side.

Sources. "Nervous: Cranial Nerve Exam" (n.d.), Flaherty and Rost (2007), Young and Young (1997).

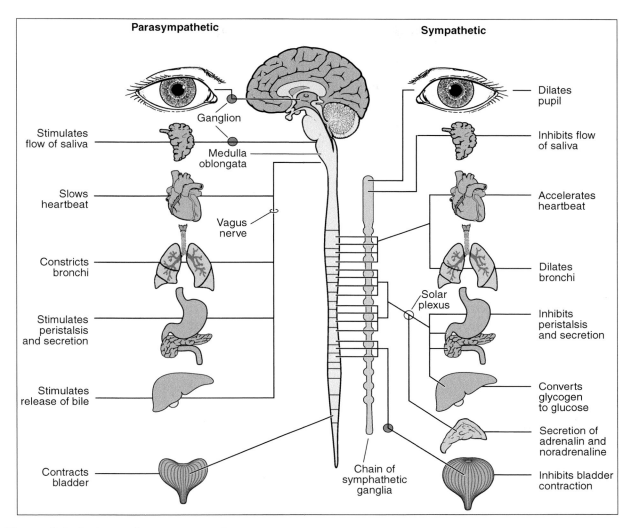

Figure 6.6. Autonomic nervous system.
Source. Richard Fritzler, Medical Illustrator, Roswell, GA.

with a different constellation of symptoms and performance deficits. In addition, patients with a past medical history of neurological disease or injury are admitted for medical reasons that have little to do with neurological issues. These patients may have preexisting residual neurological deficits such as hemiparetic limbs or memory impairments that hinder functional performance. These residual deficits must be considered and treatment plans adjusted accordingly to address new issues.

When working with patients with neurological disorders, therapy focuses on facilitating the patient's transition to the next level in the continuum of rehabilitation. With short hospital stays, understanding the etiology and symptomatology of neurological disorders facilitates efficacious rehabilitative intervention and expedient discharge planning. Because acute care is generally considered the diagnostic phase of a neurological disease or injury, patients receive many tests, which generally include diagnostic tests, reflex testing, and lab work. A clinical understanding of the implications and results of diagnostic tests can improve use of time and resources when preparing to evaluate a new patient. It will also aid in accurate interpretation and analysis of physician and nursing documentation, thus facilitating improved care and outcomes because the patient's medical status is being taken into consideration. Refer to Appendix A for further information on diagnostic tests.

The following sections review the most commonly encountered diagnoses, including their incidence, medical management, symptoms, and precautions. They also discuss acute care therapeutic intervention strategies with regard to the deficits associated with each diagnosis.

Cerebrovascular Accident

The American Heart Association and American Stroke Association have estimated that a *stroke*, or *cerebrovascular accident (CVA)*, occurs once every 40 seconds and ranks third among all causes of death in the United States, behind cardiovascular disease and cancer (Heron, Hoyert, Xu, Scott, & Tejada-Vera, 2008; Lloyd-Jones et al., 2009). Each year, 795,000

new and recurrent strokes occur (Lloyd-Jones et al., 2009).

CVAs occur via two mechanisms, ischemic or hemorrhagic. An *ischemic stroke* is caused by blockage of a blood vessel in one of two ways, embolic or thrombotic. An *embolic stroke* occurs when a clot dislodges and travels to a vessel that is too small to allow it to pass, thus forming a blockage. A *thrombotic stroke,* however, occurs when a clot forms in place, eventually blocking the vessel. A *hemorrhagic stroke* is bleeding in the brain, as in an intracerebral hemorrhage, or around the brain, as in the case of a subarachnoid hemorrhage (SAH). See Figure 6.7 for pictorial interpretations of the three types of strokes, and refer to Table 6.5 for further information on the various types of CVA. Risk factors for stroke are divided into those that cannot be changed and those that are modifiable (American Heart Association,

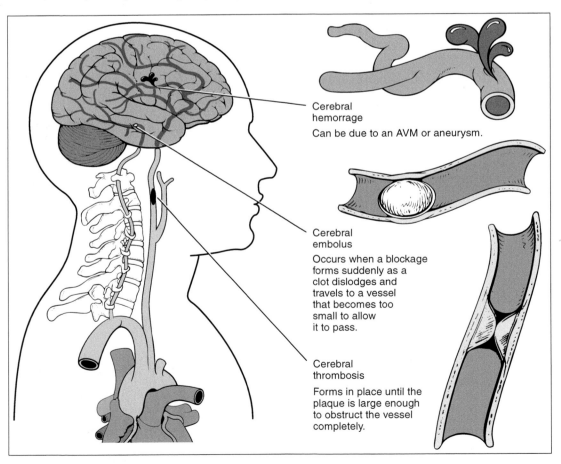

Figure 6.7. Three types of cerebrovascular accident.
AVM = arteriovenous malformation.
Source. Richard Fritzler, Medical Illustrator, Roswell, GA.

Table 6.5.   Types of Cerebrovascular Accident

Type	Traditional Etiology	Symptoms at Onset
Common strokes		
Ischemic—87% of all strokes • Thrombotic • Embolic	Clot • *Thrombotic*: Grows to size sufficient to block artery where it lodges; usually results from atherosclerosis. • *Embolic*: Clot originates in a different site and lodges in a vessel that is too small, blocking arterial blood flow; usually results from atrial fibrillation.	• Focal deficits are usually consistent with specific anatomic distribution. • Sudden mortality: 8%–12%.
Hemorrhagic • SAH; 3% incidence • ICH; 10% incidence	SAH • Trauma • Aneurysm • Hypertension • Carotid or vertebral artery dissection.	• Abnormal vital signs. • Headache. • Nausea and vomiting. • Neurological symptoms that do not correspond to a specific anatomical distribution. • Approximately half of patients with ICH also have intraventricular hemorrhage, which is considered a predictor for poor outcome (Hallevi et al., 2008). SAH • Usually worst headache of a patient's life • Typically results from aneurysm rupture • Initial syncope or seizure but usually resolves quickly • Stiff neck • Cranial nerve III involvement. ICH • Nausea and vomiting • Rapid and prolonged loss of consciousness. Mortality within 30 days • SAH: 33%–50% • ICH: 50%–67% • Overall: 37%.

(continued)

Table 6.5. **(continued)**

Type	Traditional Etiology	Symptoms at Onset
TIA	• Neurological deficits usually last <1 hour. • All deficits resolve completely.	Focal deficits are usually consistent with specific anatomic distribution.
Atypical strokes		
Watershed	Caused by systemic hypoperfusion of the cortical border zone. The *watershed* is the area between different circulatory branches. The central portions of the brain (i.e., the brainstem) are spared (Piper, 2008).	• Deficits are generally more diffuse (not focal) in nature. • Watershed-distribution strokes more common in patients after cardiac surgery. In general, cardiac patients who experience a sudden drop in blood pressure during surgery fare worse than nonsurgical patients who over time develop collaterals, thus preserving cerebral perfusion during chronic hypotensive states (Gottesman et al., 2006). • Nonsurgical patients also generally have a unilateral watershed stroke, which prognostically does better.
Lacunar	Small stroke confined to a single vessel. Usually located in the internal capsule, basal ganglia, thalamus, corona radiata, and paramedian regions (Sacco, 2005).	• Usually presents as pure motor hemiparesis, pure sensory syndrome, clumsy hand, dysarthria, ataxic hemiparesis, and sensory–motor syndrome.
Small vessel infarcts	Generally is considered a lengthy TIA with full-blown stroke symptoms, lasting 24–72 hours with all deficits resolving. These infarcts are not generally seen on computed tomography. Small vessel infarcts are formally called *reversible ischemic neurological deficits*.	• Symptoms will be consistent with the vasculature that was affected. • Because symptoms fully reverse, therapy implications are generally few, if any, but an evaluation would be prudent to ensure no therapeutic discharge needs are present. • Patient is at increased risk of full-blown stroke.

Table 6.5. (continued)

Type	Traditional Etiology	Symptoms at Onset
Aneurysm or AVM	• Aneurysm—Bulging area at a weak portion of the vascular wall. • AVMs are usually congenital, tangled connections between the arteries and veins and can occur in the spinal cord or brain.	The neurological deficits associated with any of the three causative mechanisms depend on the distribution of the vessels. Damage via an aneurysm or AVM occurs in 1 of 3 ways: • Rupture of the AVM (considered a type of ICH if in the interior of the brain and SAH or SDH if in the dural or surface areas)—2%–4% of all AVMs hemorrhage. • Compressing or displacing parts of the brain or spinal cord. • Deficits will occur gradually over time as the amount of blood flow and oxygen to the portions of the brain that the vessels supplied decreases. Treatment • Aneurysm clipping • Endovascular coil embolization • Approximately 300,000 Americans have AVMs; however, only 12% of AVM patients are symptomatic.

Note. AVM = arteriovenous malformation; ICH = intracerebral hemorrhage; SAH = subarachnoid hemorrhage; SDH = subdural hematoma; TIA = transient ischemic attack.

Source. From Casper, M. L., Nwaise, I. A., Croft, J. B., & Nilasena, D. S. (2008). *2008 Atlas of Stroke Hospitalizations Among Medicare Beneficiaries*. Atlanta, GA: Centers for Disease Control and Prevention. Copyright © 2008 by Centers for Disease Control and Prevention. Adapted with permission.

2009). Refer to Table 6.6 for more information regarding risk factors.

According to the American Hospital Association, the average length of stay for patients with stroke is 5.2 days. During that time, a complete medical workup is performed, and the patient is stabilized, ensuring that his or her status does not worsen neurologically (Rosamond et al., 2008). Intervention, both medical and rehabilitation based, depends largely on the type of injury, area of lesion, and presenting symptoms. However, most hospitals have a clinical guideline for stroke pathways. Table 6.7 delineates a typical hospital stroke pathway in order of priority (Gillett, 2007; Rosamond et al., 2008).

Table 6.6. Risk Factors for Cerebrovascular Accident

Nonmodifiable Factors	Modifiable Factors
• Age (older age = higher risk) • Heredity (family history) • Sex (male > female) • Race (African-Americans at highest risk) • History of prior stroke, transient ischemic attack, or heart attack	• Smoking • High blood pressure • Diabetes mellitus • Carotid or other artery disease • Atrial fibrillation • Heart disease • High cholesterol • Obesity and poor diet • Sedentary lifestyle

Table 6.7. Stroke Pathway

Pathway	Components

Medical workup	• Neurological exam and stroke scale (see Appendix A; scored 0–34, the lower the better)
	• Noncontrast brain CT or brain MRI (usually performed in this order)
	• Electrocardiogram
	• Oxygen saturation
	• Lab work (see Chapter 16):
	  — Blood glucose
	  — Serum electrolytes and renal function tests
	  — Markers of cardiac ischemia (CK-MB, troponin)
	  — Complete blood count, including platelet count
	  — Prothrombin time/international normalized ratio
	  — Activated partial thromboplastin time

Medical management of acute complications	• Airway maintenance • Blood pressure and heart rate control • Blood sugar control • Hemorrhagic conversion • Herniation • Increased intracranial pressure • Seizures

Table 6.7.   (continued)

Pathway	Components
Ischemic stroke medication management	• t-PA (if no hemorrhage identified on CT and within 3-hour window from onset) • Heparin—Used to prevent another stroke from a cardioembolic source or coagulopathy. It is preventative, not a therapy for the initial stroke • Long-term anticoagulation if not a hemorrhagic stroke

Swallow evaluation (site dependent on sequence)	• Screen by nursing. If no deficits are noted, then usually no further evaluation is ordered
	• Full swallow evaluation by either occupational therapist or speech–language pathologist, either bedside or via modified barium swallow (refer to Chapter 13)
	• Initiation of nutrition and hydration and medication via one of the following methods:
	  — Mouth with or without modifications to food and liquid consistency
	  — Nasogastric tube through nose
	  — Percutaneous endoscopic gastrostomy tube through stomach
	  — Total parenteral nutrition (IV fluid)

Deep vein thrombosis, pulmonary embolism, infection prophylaxis	• Foot or leg pumps • Compression hose • Universal precautions
Continued treatment of comorbidities	Usually other specialties are consulted, such as cardiology, endocrinology, and pulmonology, to manage comorbid diseases
Evaluation by physical therapist, occupational therapist, and speech–language pathologist	• Early mobilization • ADL evaluation • Cognitive evaluation • Swallow evaluation
Discharge planning initiated	Determine appropriate discharge disposition

Note. ADL = activities of daily living; CK-MB = creatine kinase isoenzyme; CT = computed tomography.
Source. Adams et al. (2007).

Precautions

Patients with acute CVAs often have limitations due to their medical condition. This is especially pertinent in the very early stages of hospitalization, as every patient presents with a different constellation of medical issues. Physicians are the best guide regarding precautions and should be consulted for particular limitations.

Blood Pressure Parameter. Check with the physician first to determine blood pressure parameters, because different specialists may use different parameters. Cardiologists and internal medicine physicians generally want blood pressure to be within the normal range, whereas neurologists and neurosurgeons determine parameters on the basis of the type of stroke the patient sustained. The goal is cerebral autoregulation or maintaining a relatively stable blood flow; however, the American Heart Association and American Stroke Association have recommended further study regarding blood pressure management for the acute stroke patient (Adams et al., 2007). The current recommendations for an ischemic stroke include keeping the blood pressure higher to protect the penumbra, or the area around the ischemic region.

A higher blood pressure allows vasculature to perfuse the ischemic area (Adams et al., 2007; Pugh, Mathiesen, Meighan, Summers, & Zrelak, 2008). The patient with a hemorrhagic stroke, however, needs the blood pressure to be lower to reduce the risk of rebleeding (Broderick et al., 2007). Recommended blood pressure ranges are listed in Table 6.8.

Carotid Artery Stenosis. Be extremely cautious if carotid artery stenosis is 90%–100% bilaterally because blood flow is compromised. Inappropriately aggressive therapy could result in another stroke. However, physicians frequently

Table 6.8. **Blood Pressure Ranges**

Type of Stroke	Systolic Blood Pressure (SBP) Goal	Diastolic Blood Pressure (DBP) Goal	Purpose and Complications
Ischemic CVA	140–180 (possibly as high as 200–220)	<130	Compensatory vasodilation maintains adequate blood flow to protect the penumbra (the ischemic, but still viable, brain tissue around the area of the stroke) and maintain perfusion.
Hemorrhagic CVA	Below 140–160	Below 90	Untreated hypertension allows expansion of hemorrhage. Increased SBP causes enlargement of the CVA in 14% of cases. With a controlled blood pressure of SBP <160 and DBP <90, the rate of neurological degeneration is lower, as is the risk of rebleed.
Ischemic stroke after t-PA administered	<140	<105	Blood pressure needs to be lower to reduce the risk of hemorrhagic conversion.

Note. CVA = cerebrovascular accident.
Sources. Broderick et al. (2007); Brown (2008); Gillett (2007); Pugh, Mathiesen, Meighan, Summers, and Zelak (2008).

explicitly approve therapy despite the presence of the stenosis, especially if the patient is awaiting a carotid endarterectomy. Activity that does not increase blood pressure but also does not allow hypotension is optimal. Basic activities of daily living (BADLs) should be completed, with careful monitoring of vital signs and observation of the patient's symptoms. The patient may have had the stenosis for a long time but may not yet be medically stable enough for a carotid endarterectomy. Therapy may be the medium for improving the patient's overall conditioning so that survival of the surgical procedure is optimized.

t-PA Administration. *t-PA* (sometimes called *recombinant t-PA* or *rt-PA*) is a "super anticoagulant" that breaks up blood clots in the brain. Bedrest is required for 24 hours after administration of the bolus because of potential injury while extremely anticoagulated, but check the hospital's policies and procedures for therapy time restrictions after t-PA administration. With t-PA, frequent nursing assessments are performed, and vital signs are observed during this acute period because of the potential for hemorrhagic conversion. Patients who receive t-PA are generally admitted to the intensive care unit for continuous monitoring of vital signs, symptoms of neurological change, and hemorrhagic transformation (Adams et al., 2007; Pugh et al., 2008).

Symptoms can change rapidly with t-PA; therefore, performing an evaluation may be only an academic endeavor and may not contribute to the patient's final disposition. Anaphylactic reactions occur approximately 2% of the time (Adams et al., 2007; Pugh et al., 2008).

Vasospasm. Approximately one-third of patients who have had a SAH or ruptured aneurysm are at high risk for vasospasm, especially 4–14 days after the initial episode (Mahanes, 2006). *Vasospasm* is narrowing of the cerebral arteries that cause ischemia to the portions of the brain supplied by that vessel. It is usually monitored and evaluated via a transcranial Doppler. Symptoms of vasospasm include

- Neurological decline in status;
- Increased headache;
- New or increased focal neurological signs;

- weakness in the lower extremity more than in the upper extremity;
- Decreased cognition, especially indecision, and decreased attention and initiation;
- Aphasia;
- Decrease in the level of consciousness; and
- Seizure (Adams, del Zoppo, & Kummer, 2006; Flaherty & Rost, 2007; Mahanes, 2006).

Therapy should be suspended when vasospasm is suspected. Evaluation of vasospasm is made via computed tomography scan, transcranial Doppler, and the presence of clinical symptoms. "Triple H therapy"—which includes *h*ypervolemia, *h*ypertension, and *h*emodilution—is used to medically manage vasospasm (Sen et al., 2003).

Traumatic Brain Injury

Approximately 1.4 million people per year experience a *traumatic brain injury (TBI),* of whom approximately 230,000 are hospitalized (National Institute of Neurological Disorders and Stroke [NINDS], 2008b). Length of stay is highly variable depending on injury's severity and cause. Fifteen- to 24-year-olds and adults older than 75 have the highest risk of sustaining a brain injury (NINDS, 2008b). The most common causes of TBI in older people are falls, whereas vehicular accidents are the most common mechanism in teenagers and young adults. Risk factors include age, sex (males more than females), and drug or alcohol abuse.

The four major types of TBI are subdural *hematoma, concussion, contusion,* and *anoxia* (refer to Table 6.9 for further information on these conditions). TBI can range from mild to severe. Patients with a mild TBI have a Glasgow Coma Scale score of 14–15; with moderate TBI, 9–13; and severe TBI, 3–8. See Appendix 6.B for the Glasgow Coma Scale (Teasdale & Jennett, 1974).

Coma

Coma is frequently a sequela of TBI and is defined as "unarousable unresponsiveness" (Flaherty & Rost, 2007, p. 30), but it can also occur after CVA, which is less common. Coma

Table 6.9. Types of Traumatic Brain Injury

Type	Traditional Etiology	Symptoms at Onset
Subdural hematoma	Usually follows trauma such as a fall, but can be caused by cerebral atrophy, alcoholism, or poor or absent blood flow. Symptoms can slowly emerge as long as 2 weeks after injury.	Weakness • Fluctuating levels or loss of consciousness, lethargy • Vision changes • Nausea, vomiting, loss of appetite • Memory deficits • Dizziness • Seizures • Mood changes, irritability
Concussion	Minor head trauma.	• Results in a short loss of consciousness • May cause mild brain injury
Contusion	Bruising of the brain resulting from the brain moving back and forth within the skull. Can result in one or both of the following: • *Coup–contrecoup:* The brain hits opposite sides of the skull (*coup*—initial contusion; *contrecoup*—location where the brain bounced off the other side). The base of the skull is rough, so regardless of the point of impact, a contusion can occur. • Diffuse axonal injury (shearing) caused with contrecoup is damage to the neurons and their connections.	• Symptoms vary according to the severity of the injury • Often associated with a skull fracture
Anoxia	• Absence of oxygen to the brain for more than several minutes. Usually seen in patients with cardiac or respiratory arrest or near drowning.	• Unconsciousness • Memory loss • Vision field losses • Diffuse cognitive and physical symptoms • Deficits are not overtly focal, although one side may be slightly weaker than the other

has several levels, which are generally measured by using the Glasgow Coma Scale (Teasdale & Jennett, 1974) and the Rancho Los Amigos Cognitive Scale (Revised; Hagen, 1998; see Appendixes 6.B and 6.C). Other assessment tools that can be used as part of the initial evaluation include the JFK Coma Recovery Scale–Revised (Kalmar & Giacino, 2005), available at www.tbims.org/combi/crs/CRS%20form.pdf, and the Rappaport Coma/Near Coma Scale in combination with the Disability Rating Scale (Rappaport, 2005), available at www.coma.ulg.ac.be/images/cncs_e.pdf. However, discussion of these assessments is beyond the scope of this chapter.

Coma duration is considered an important predictor of functional recovery in terms of *post-traumatic amnesia (PTA)*, or a permanent gap of memory, from the time of the injury until when the patient starts remembering events (Dixon, Layton, & Shaw, 2005). The severity of a brain injury is classified in the following manner:

- PTA <1 hour = mild brain injury
- PTA 1–24 hours = moderate brain injury
- PTA 1–7 days = severe brain injury
- PTA >7 days = very severe brain injury.

Posturing is frequently observed in the comatose patient and indicates abnormal reflexive activity at the brainstem level. Decerebrate and decorticate posturing are illustrated in Figure 6.8.

Therapeutic Implications

"Rehabilitative management of patients with DOC [disorders of consciousness] continues to be plagued by many unanswerable questions. In the absence of clear-cut guidelines, it is critical that clinicians adopt a systematic approach

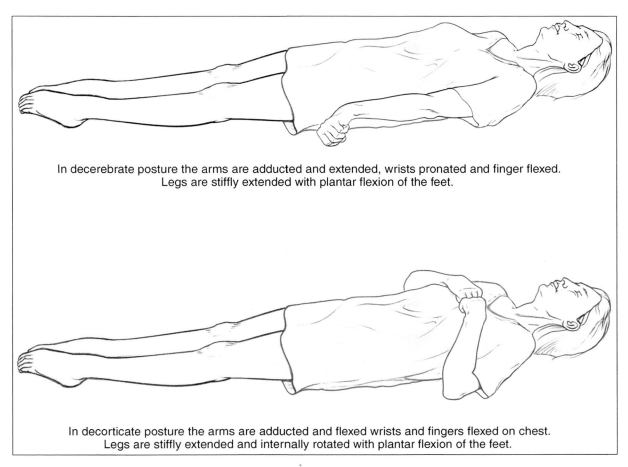

In decerebrate posture the arms are adducted and extended, wrists pronated and finger flexed. Legs are stiffly extended with plantar flexion of the feet.

In decorticate posture the arms are adducted and flexed wrists and fingers flexed on chest. Legs are stiffly extended and internally rotated with plantar flexion of the feet.

Figure 6.8. Comparison of decerebrate and decorticate posturing.
Source. Richard Fritzler, Medical Illustrator, Roswell, GA.

to assessment and rehabilitative treatment" (Giancino & Trott, 2004, pp. 263–264). Although the comatose patient may not engage overtly, he or she may be engaged covertly even initially on an ANS level. Treatment at this stage of consciousness can be likened to the treatment model of "occupational readiness." To prepare the patient for the next level of care, the SNS and ANS must first be normalized.

Evaluation of the coma patient generally focuses on identifying subtle signs in response to sensory stimulation. A typical evaluation of body functions (e.g., passive range of motion [PROM], tone, positioning) should be performed along with careful observation of changes in vital signs in response to task performance. If possible, attempt to increase the patient's upright position, either through a bed–chair position or sitting the patient up on the side of the bed with a two-person assist to assess activation of the reticular activating system.

The following interventions should be addressed:

- Perform PROM, splinting, or both to reduce contractures.
- Educate the family on all interventions and rationale at their level of understanding. The family should also be trained on what reactions should be noted. See Table 6.10 for examples of positive and negative responses to sensory stimulation.
- Inform the patient before performing any intervention.
- Speak positively in the presence of the comatose patient.
- Perform sensory stimulation—Sensory input using all five senses that should be performed daily (Oh & Seo, 2003). Families must be trained to perform a structured sensory stimulation program to augment

Table 6.10. **Examples of Positive and Negative Responses to Coma Sensory Stimulation**

Positive Responses	Negative Responses
• Blinking	• Absence of any response
• Calming effect	• Agitation
• Crying	• Bite reflex or tightly pursed lips
• Direct response to stimulus (pushing stimulus away or attending to it)	• Flushing
• Eye opening	• Increased salivation
• Following commands	• Perspiration
• Grimacing	• Seizure activity
• Increased arousal	• Startle response followed by posturing
• Increased movement	• Sudden decrease in arousal
• Increased muscle tone	• Sustained increase in heart rate, respiration rate, intracranial pressure
• Respiration rate increases, then decreases	
• Swallowing	
• Vocal utterances (e.g., moaning)	

Sources. Gerber (2005), Grüner and Terhaag (2000).

the daily routines of the medical and therapy staff. These techniques are used sparingly in the acute care setting primarily because they have not been shown to be an efficacious and cost-effective treatment strategy and take an inordinate amount of time to administer and achieve results (Oh & Seo, 2003).

Sensory input can include acoustic (music, voices of loved ones, loud clapping, tuning fork, bell, or singing), tactile or kinesthetic (massage, touch, temperature, noxious stimuli such as nail bed pressure, range of motion [ROM] exercises), olfactory (perfume, vinegar, lemon, vanilla, coffee), gustatory (sour, salty, sweet, mouthwash on mouth swab during oral care), and visual (colored paper, light pens, pictures of family faces, manually opening eyes momentarily).

The therapist must meet the patient where he or she is in the continuum of recovery. Other disciplines must also be consulted to avoid duplication of services. At this level, the occupational, speech, and physical therapists are performing many overlapping interventions; however, the outcome goals are different. Consistent reevaluation should be performed with the focus on close observation to determine the patient's response to the various sensory modalities and whether any patterns of behavior are exhibited. Table 6.11 presents examples of occupational therapy goals for the coma patient at Rancho Levels I to III.

Precautions

Patients with a TBI often present with neurological issues that, if overlooked, are medically dangerous and could cause further complications. Careful observation of a patient's medical status before therapy is initiated could avert worsening of these complications.

Neurogenic Fever. An uncontrolled fever is associated with patients with TBI but can also occur in patients with a stroke. A diagnosis of a *neurogenic fever* is usually a diagnosis of exclusion after all sepsis etiologies have been ruled out (Agrawal, Timothy, & Thapa, 2007). Defer therapy if the patient's temperature is higher than 100.9° F (38.27° C),

especially in light of other autonomic abnormalities such as bradycardia, lower respiration rate, increased perspiration, and decreased level of consciousness. Higher mortality rates and increased functional and cognitive disabilities are associated in patients with SAH and fevers higher than 100.9° F that persist for more than 7 days (Fernandez et al., 2007; Redekop, 2007).

Cerebral Perfusion Pressure. *Cerebral perfusion pressure (CPP)* is an indirect measure of perfusion in the brain or the blood pressure of the brain. The brain is susceptible to changes in blood pressure. CPP is usually more associated with TBI but is sometimes measured after a CVA, especially a hemorrhagic CVA. A low CPP can result in further ischemic damage (see Table 6.12 for CPP-level therapeutic implications). The CPP should be kept at more than 60 millimeters of mercury (mm Hg) for best patient outcomes. On an intensive care unit monitor, this number can usually be found near the intracranial pressure (ICP) measurement. CPP is calculated with the formula MAP – ICP = CPP, in which *MAP* is the acronym for *mean arterial pressure* and refers to the heart's ability to perfuse the body's tissues. On an intensive care unit monitor, MAP can usually be found as a separate number on the screen, listed as MAP or mean, and is usually directly next to or under the blood pressure in parentheses. Refer to Chapter 2 for further information.

Intracranial Pressure. *ICP* is defined as the pressure exerted on the brain by extra tissue or fluid (CSF or blood) inside the cranium. Increased ICP can cause brain herniation; therefore, activities that increase the pressure beyond acceptable levels should be ceased immediately. ICP monitors measure ICP. They do not serve as drains but may share the same monitoring system and setup, especially with an intraventricular catheter or lumbar drain. Symptoms of increasing ICP include changes in consciousness, confusion, elevated blood pressure and slowing heart rate, and cranial nerve III involvement, especially ptosis or unilateral pupil dilation, which is usually noted before changes in consciousness (Adams et al., 2006; Fields, Blackshear, Mortimer, & Wallace,

Table 6.11. Goals for the Low-Level Coma Patient at Rancho Levels I–III

Client Factors	Examples of Goals
Mental functions	
Attention and arousal	• Opens eyes for 15 seconds in response to verbal stimulation. • Grasps cold washcloth for 10 seconds when placed in hand. • Arousal noted for >1 minute for motor task.
Direction following	• Responds to 3 of 5 directions for simple motor skill. • Washes face to command with no tactile cues. • Turn head 5 times to verbal stimulation.
Global mental functions	• Family verbalizes 3 methods to appropriately provide stimulation.
Body functions	
Hemodynamics	• Heart rate <130 during verbal stimulation.
Respiratory function	• Respiration rate <25 during face washing performed by therapist.
Sensory functions	
Visual skills	• Maintain visual attention to picture of family member for <10 seconds. • Maintains fixation on grooming or hygiene objects for 10 seconds.
Auditory skills	• Patient will turn head toward name spoken aloud 5 times.
Neuromuscular and movement-related functions	
Balance	• Maximum 2-person assistance to sit on the edge of bed for 5 minutes for grooming and hygiene tasks. • Maintain upright position in bed or chair position during light hygiene or grooming tasks for 5 minutes with no assistance.
Muscle power or reflexes	• Grasp grooming object for 10 seconds. • Family independent with passive range of motion exercise program and positioning of upper extremities.

Table 6.12. Clinical Implications of Cerebral Perfusion Pressure (CPP)

CPP Level	Therapeutic Implication
70–100	Therapy proceeds as normal.
60–70	Therapy can be performed, but should be limited to light activity. Recommend keeping head of bed at 30° to maintain CPP and discuss with nurse, physician, or both (Rangel-Castillo, Gopinath, & Robertson, 2008).
>50	Defer therapy.
>30	Indicates a poor prognosis, resulting in irreversible neuronal hypoxia.

Sources. Hemphill and Smith (2008), Mahanes (2006).
Note. Created by Judy R. Hamby.

2005; Flaherty & Rost, 2007). Normal ICP is 5–13 mm Hg, and life-threatening ICP is more than 30 mm Hg. Pressures higher than 18 mm Hg require medical intervention with either an *external ventricular drain (EVD)* or *ventriculo-peritoneal (VP) shunt,* and the patient will be drowsy or confused (Adams et al., 2006; Fields et al., 2005; Flaherty & Rost, 2007).

Drains. Drains may be inserted to remove excess fluid, either CSF or blood, to prevent a pressure buildup in the CNS (Fields et al., 2005). There are three types of drains, and the rate of flow is determined by the position of the drip chamber. An *intraventricular catheter* is inserted into the ventricles (usually the lateral ventricle) of the brain and drains excess CSF via an EVD. The drip chamber is external and level with the ear at the external auditory meatus or tragus. *Lumbar drains* drain directly from the lumbar region of the spine instead of the ventricles and are level with the bed and the umbilicus. *VP shunts* drain CSF directly from the ventricles, but the drip chamber is located inside the abdominal cavity. These drains do not require leveling. General guidelines for drains follow.

- Do not get the patient up without specific orders if the drip chamber is external and actively draining. Speak directly with the neurosurgeon or neurologist if necessary.
- VP shunts do not require clamping.
- Orders must be written before the drain can be clamped, and the nurse must clamp the drain.
- The nurse will clamp the intraventricular catheter and lumbar drain before all transitional movements—including moving the bed, the patient, or both—because the drainage flow may be disturbed. Raising the bed just a few degrees could cause unrestricted CSF drainage because the drain will then be set to gravity.
- The head of the bed is usually elevated to assist in controlling ICP, but check with the nurse, physician, or both. The patient may need to remain flat to ensure medical stability.

Autonomic Dysfunction Syndrome.

Autonomic dysfunction syndrome—also called *storming, sympathetic storms,* or *neurostorming*—and paroxysmal autonomic instability with dystonia are usually noted in very low-level comatose patients whose ANS is overstimulated (Blackman, Patrick, Buck, & Rust, 2004). If this onset is new, therapy is deferred until etiology (e.g., sepsis, myocardial infarction) has been determined. If symptoms are persistent for several days, monitor vitals and continue with therapy as permitted by the physician. The usual presentation of autonomic dysfunction syndrome includes

- Tachycardia (heart rate >130 beats per minute)
- Increased blood pressure (extremely high)
- Tachypnea (>40 respirations per minute)
- Profuse sweating
- Extensor posturing
- Dilated pupils
- Fever (>101.3 °F; Blackman et al., 2004; Lemke, 2007).

Craniectomy. With *craniectomy*, a portion of the skull is removed and may be placed in a subcutaneous pocket in the abdomen, a flap in the subgaleal space (in the scalp on the other side), or a deep freeze or is discarded. Placement of the bone flap in the abdomen, subgaleal space, or a deep freeze protects the bone flap, preserving the patient's own bone in a less contaminated manner. Discarding the bone flap occurs when infection is noted. Generally, the bone flap is not replaced for 6–12 weeks and as long as 6–12 months depending on functional recovery and medical and infection status. See Table 6.13 for further information regarding precautions specific to a craniectomy and other neurosurgical interventions.

Parkinson's Disease, Normal Pressure Hydrocephalus, and Essential Tremor

Parkinson's disease, normal pressure hydrocephalus, and *essential tremor* appear similar in presentation and symptomatology: These three diagnoses, especially Parkinson's disease, are usually comorbid with the admitting diagnosis but can become the primary factor hindering functional recovery. Worsening of symptoms and interference with activities of daily living (ADLs) associated with these diagnoses may be the

reason for an acute admission or a contributing factor to the admitting diagnosis. In addition, the patient may be admitted to confirm or rule out a particular disease. Parkinson's disease is often exacerbated by illness and worsens significantly. Careful evaluation and appropriate medical and therapeutic intervention can help ameliorate functional implications of the impairments.

Presentation of symptoms for these three diagnoses is not usually the primary admitting factor; therefore, reporting them to the physician may assist in medical management. For these populations, the primary responsibilities of the acute care therapist are to evaluate safety and ADL performance, educate regarding the diagnosis, and recommend disposition plan and adaptive devices. Table 6.14 delineates the functional symptomatology for Parkinson's disease, normal pressure hydrocephalus, and essential tremor and the medical and therapeutic interventions associated with each disease.

Seizure Disorders and Epilepsy

Seizure disorders are common in the neurological population either as the primary diagnosis or as a sequela of a neurological injury (Alberti et al., 2008; Frey, 2003). After TBI and CVA, seizures occur in approximately 50% and 10% of patients, respectively (Bladin et al., 2000; Lowenstein, 2009).

Seizures are abnormal electrical impulses in the brain and manifest in many ways that can involve alterations in sensation, movement, behaviors, levels of consciousness, or all of these. The two general types of seizures are partial seizure and generalized seizure. A *partial seizure* occurs in only one part of the brain, whereas a *generalized seizure* occurs in both sides of the brain, usually producing an absence, tonic–clonic, or atonic seizure.

Therapeutic Implications

Therapists should be aware whether a patient has a history of seizures and what to do if one occurs in their presence. When a patient has two or more seizures, he or she may be diagnosed with *epilepsy* (Epilepsy Foundation, n.d.). Table 6.15 outlines common types of seizures, including

(Text continues on p. 230)

Table 6.13. **Common Neurosurgical Procedures**

Procedure	Definition	Purpose	Therapeutic Precautions
Neurosurgical procedures	Surgeries performed on the central nervous system.	Prevent neurological deficits.	• Check neurosurgical order set. • Avoid bending over for prolonged periods (e.g., when tying shoes or donning pants). • Confirm lifting restriction limits with neurosurgeon. • Avoid Valsalva maneuvers such as straining to have a bowel movement, breath holding, and lifting. • Monitor vital signs including blood pressure, heart rate, and oxygen saturation, especially the first time the patient gets up. • Check for elevated intracranial pressures.
Burr hole	Tiny hole(s) drilled into the skull.	Remove localized fluid collection.	See general neurosurgical precautions.
Clipping	Small metal clip placed around the base of the aneurysm.	Isolate aneurysm from normal blood flow to prevent rupture.	See general neurosurgical precautions.
Craniectomy	A portion of the skull is removed. It is then placed into a subcutaneous pocket in the abdomen or a flap in the subgaleal space (in the scalp on the other side) or a deep freeze or is discarded.	• Relieve pressure. • Reduce intracranial pressure. • Reduce intracranial hypertension. • Allow for unrestricted brain swelling.	• Helmets are generally recommended when getting patients with a craniectomy up. However, some neurosurgeons oppose the use of helmets because the helmets themselves may compress the brain and can cause incisional wounds (Benedict, personal communication, August 2008). • If no helmet is used, be cautious not to press on areas in which there is no bone. • When ordering helmets for patients, measure the circumference of the head approximately 1 inch above the ears.

(continued)

Table 6.13. *(continued)*

Procedure	Definition	Purpose	Therapeutic Precautions
			• Ensure the helmet is not compressing any of the craniectomy areas. • Do not roll the patient onto the side with the craniectomy because it will put pressure on the portion of the brain that is unprotected by the skull. • Restrict the patient from bending forward with activities of daily living (ADLs) or mobility.
Cranioplasty	Replacement of the bone flap in the skull.	• Prevent damage to the brain. • Cosmetic.	See general neurosurgical precautions.
Craniotomy	Removal of a portion of the skull (bone flap) and subsequent opening of the dura.	• Remove a tumor. • Relieve pressure. • Drain blood from a hemorrhagic area. • Repair damaged area.	See general neurosurgical precautions.
Deep brain stimulator	Electrodes are implanted into target areas of the brain that will deliver electrical impulses. A wire then extends down toward the chest, where a pacemaker-like device, called an *impulse generator*, is implanted. This device	Blocks abnormal electrical activity that causes symptoms. Uses • Parkinson's disease	• See general neurosurgical precautions. • If the deep brain stimulator is for Parkinson's disease or dystonia, symptoms may return once the swelling in the brain from the surgery reduces and before the impulse generator is turned back on. • The patient usually does not need any acute care therapy.

	then controls the impulses and is activated automatically or can be activated volitionally if symptoms worsen or the patient feels them coming. The impulse generator is turned on 2–3 weeks after implantation.	• Dystonia • Essential tremor • Multiple sclerosis • Seizure disorders • Depression • Bipolar disorders	• Patients are discharged from the hospital at the same level as at admission because the impulse generator has not yet been turned on. • An ADL, home safety, and durable medical equipment evaluation may be warranted.
Debulking	Surgical excision of a central nervous system mass.	• Prevent further growth. • Reduce neurological deficits. • Improve quality of life.	See general neurosurgical precautions.
Endovascular coil embolization	Coils are placed in an aneurysm or vascular area via a catheter. The body responds by forming a blood clot around the coil, blocking off the aneurysm.	• Block an aneurysm. • Block vascularity that may rupture during a surgery (e.g., preparation for tumor debulking).	See general neurosurgical precautions.
Evacuation	Usually done in conjunction with a burr hole, craniectomy, or craniotomy to remove excess intracerebral blood or a clot.	Reduce intracranial pressure from bleeding in the brain.	See general neurosurgical precautions.

(continued)

Table 6.13. *(continued)*

Procedure	Definition	Purpose	Therapeutic Precautions
Transsphenoidal adenomectomy	Surgical procedure done transnasally.	Removal of pituitary tumor.	• Do not remove nasal packing. • Keep the head of the bed at 30°. • Avoid Valsalva maneuvers. • If clear, thin fluid draining from the nose is noted, alert medical staff immediately because this could be cerebrospinal fluid. Precautions in place for approximately 4–6 weeks (check with the neurosurgeon): • Do not bend or lean forward at the waist. • Do not drink with straws (can increase negative pressure). • Do not sneeze through the nose. • Do not sniffle. • Do not pick nose. • Do not blow nose. Appendix 6.G is a patient handout that delineates these precautions.
Ventriculoperito-neal shunt	Alternate path to redirect excess cerebrospinal fluid from one area to another (from the ventricles to the peritoneal cavity) using an implanted tube.	Relieve intracerebral pressure from excess cerebrospinal fluid.	• Patients may complain of headache or stomachache. • Do not push on shunt that is visible on the head.

Table 6.14. **Symptoms of Parkinson's Disease, Normal Pressure Hydrocephalus, and Essential Tremor**

Symptom	Parkinson's Disease	Normal Pressure Hydrocephalus	Essential Tremor
Prevalence	1% of patients ≥ age 65	Thought to actually be 5% of dementias	• Affects 5% of people ≥ age 65 or 5 million Americans • Can affect children • May erroneously be referred to as *familial tremors*
Etiology	Reduction of substantia nigra cells, thus reduction of dopaminergic cells	Communicating hydrocephalus	Unknown, but usually genetic
Progressive	Yes, with reduction of dopaminergic cells	Yes	Yes, with aging
Tremor	• Resting (pill-rolling) • Intention tremor	Not present	• Bilateral; usually action and postural tremors; disappears at rest • Tremors in arms, legs, head, voice, neck, or all of these • Usually dystonia in neck
Speed of movement	Bradykinetic	Bradykinetic	No slowing
Tone	Cogwheel rigidity	Not abnormal	No rigidity
Voice	Hypophonia—Soft volume and difficulty with vocal production	Not abnormal	• Spasmodic dysphonia occurs because muscles of vocal cords, mouth wall, and tongue are involved • Symptoms worsen on the phone • Can often laugh, sing, and whisper normally. • Symptoms best in the morning on waking

(*continued*)

Table 6.14. **(continued)**

Symptom	Parkinson's Disease	Normal Pressure Hydrocephalus	Essential Tremor
Gait	Shuffling or festinating	• Decreased initiation—Gait apraxia • Short, slow, shuffling gait with wide base of support	Deterioration of tandem gait
Balance	Posterior losses of balance	May experience sudden falls or drop attacks because of lower-extremity weakness	Mild cerebellar changes
Facial features	Masked	Flat affect	Flat affect
Visual deficits	• Marked deficits in oculomotor control, especially restricted upward and vertical gaze • Diplopia or blurry vision possible (convergence insufficiency) • Upper visual field deficits • Reduced blinking causing dry eyes and eye inflammation • Reduced color perception (see Hamby, 2006, for further information)	Blurred or double vision	None
Smell	Diminished in early stages	Not addressed in literature	Mildly diminished

Cognitive deficits	Dementia	• Short-term memory deficits • Progressive dementia	Possibly mild memory, attention, cognitive flexibility, and verbal fluency deficits
Bowel and bladder function	Constipation because of decreased anal and sphincter motility, decreased mobility, abdominal weakness, and diets low in fiber because of dysphagia	Urinary frequency, incontinence, or both	No change
Headache	No	Yes	No
Nausea	No	Yes	No
Psychiatric	No	• Apathetic • Withdrawn	Anxiety prevalent and increases symptoms, further exacerbating them
Weight loss	No	No	Underweight
Diagnostic tests	No definitive tests are available, although CT or MRI may be used to rule out other diagnosis Parkinson's disease is a diagnosis of exclusion and obtained by a careful history	• CT indicates increased volume in the ventricles • Lumbar puncture: If function improves after draining some cerebrospinal fluid, then usually proceed with VP shunt insertion	No definitive tests are available, although several are used (CT, MRI) to rule out other diagnoses. Essential tremor is a diagnosis of exclusion and is obtained by a careful history and writing test (spirography)
Medical treatment	Medicines • Levodopa or dopamine-like drugs (e.g., Sinemet)	Medicines • None	Medicines • Botox for vocal tremor • Beta blockers

(continued)

Table 6.14. **(continued)**

Symptom	Parkinson's Disease	Normal Pressure Hydrocephalus	Essential Tremor
	Surgical intervention	Surgical intervention—VP shunt	• Anticonvulsant drugs
	• *DBS*—Implanted electrical leads that interrupt the signals that cause the abnormal movement		• Anti-anxiety medicines
	• *Thalamotomy*—Destruction of a portion of the thalamus		Surgical intervention
	• *Pallidotomy*—Surgical lesion of the globus pallidus		• DBS
			• Thalamotomy
Therapeutic intervention	• Weighted utensils will quickly be habituated to and should be used judiciously	• Therapist may be asked to complete evaluation before and after lumbar puncture to evaluate effectiveness or pressure relief	• Recommend adaptive devices, especially feeding equipment (weighted utensils)
	• Use conscious cognitive overrides for motor tasks; massed practice		• Brace on supports (such as a table) to increase stabilization
	• Use visual or auditory cues to assist initiation		• Preplan movements
	• Coordinate treatment sessions to occur 45–90 minutes after Parkinson's medications are taken, which will optimize the therapeutic window when the medication is working best	• Reduce cognitive memory and attentional demands	• Massed practice, focusing on the most important tasks, that includes a strengthening component (Plumb & Bain, 2007)
	• Reduce cognitive memory and attentional demands		• Incorporate relaxation techniques because stress increases tremors
	• Use low vision strategies (refer to Appendix F)		

Note. CT = computed tomography; DBS = deep brain stimulator; MRI = magnetic resonance imaging; VP = ventriculoperitoneal.

Table 6.15. Types of Seizures

Type	Presenting Symptoms	Postictal State
Absence seizure (petit mal)	• Patient noted to have a blank stare and eyelids fluttering • Unaware of environment • No changes in vital signs	• Promptly resumes activity • No confusion • Amnesia for seizure events • No need to cancel therapy session, but may need to repeat concepts
Generalized tonic–clonic (grand mal)	Phases • Tonic—Stiffening of extremities; all limbs and spine extend, jaw clamps shut, pupils dilate and are nonreactive, and loss of consciousness. Respiratory muscles spasm, causing apnea • Clonic—Bilateral jerking of limbs, trunk, and neck; labored breathing; profuse sweating; frothing at the mouth; incontinence; and clenched jaw • Postictal state • Probable changes in vital signs	• Deep sleep • Amnesia for seizure events • Confusion • Cancel therapy • Very rarely, patient may have Todd's paralysis—Usually hemiplegia lasting 0.5–36 hours, resolving completely If it lasts longer, then the patient may need therapeutic intervention
Atonic	Sudden abrupt loss of muscle tone resulting in drop attacks that can cause severe injury from the fall	• Uncommon; patient promptly resumes activity • No need to cancel therapy
Simple partial	• No loss of consciousness • Sudden jerking • Sensory phenomena • No change in vital signs	• Possible transient weakness or loss of sensation • Cancel therapy session
Complex partial	• May have an aura • Automatisms (lip smacking, picking at clothes, fumbling) • Unaware of environment	• Amnesia for seizure events • Mild to moderate confusion • Sleepy
	• May wander • Not likely to have a change in vitals, but possible	• Cancel therapy session

Source. Epilepsy Foundation (n.d.).

> ### Box 6.1.   Occupational Therapy Guidelines During and After a Seizure
>
> **During a Seizure**
>
> - Protect the patient's head with something soft.
> - Do not put anything in the mouth.
> - Do not leave the patient alone; press the call light or call for help.
> - Turn the patient on his or her side.
> - Do not try to forcefully position the patient's arms, legs, or neck once the seizure has started.
> - Loosen tight clothing.
> - Be aware that incontinence can occur.
>
> **Therapy Guidelines After a Seizure**
>
> - Speak quietly and calmly to the patient.
> - Cover the patient to keep him or her warm and to protect him or her from the embarrassment of incontinence.
> - Do not give the patient anything to eat or drink until fully awake.
> - Obtain medical assistance; notify the nurse immediately if a seizure occurs.
>
> *Note.* Created by Judy R. Hamby.

the presenting symptoms and postictal sequelae. Refer to Box 6.1 for further information.

If the therapist is the only one who witnesses the seizure, then a detailed description may be necessary, especially if it is the first one on record. If seizures are new for the patient, orders should be obtained to continue therapy. New-onset seizures may indicate a decline in medical status. The form in Appendix 6.D delineates the commonly required information that should be contained in a report of a witnessed seizure.

Precautions

The precautions for patients with seizures include the following:

- The patient can be taken out of the room, but be very aware of sudden changes in demeanor or physical ability and be ready for protective action.
- If the patient is having frequent seizures, have an assistant following you with a chair.
- Pad bedrails with seizure pads or blankets.

- Do not leave the patient unattended out of the bed if seizures are frequent. Return the patient back to bed with bedrails up.
- Avoid flashing lights; even fluorescent lights that are flickering can induce a seizure.
- Illness such as fever, low blood sugar, stress, lack of sleep, and fatigue can increase susceptibility to seizures.
- Pain can cause a seizure; however, it is unusual. After a generalized tonic–clonic seizure, pain can be present because of the massive amount of muscle activity.
- Seizures can occur even while the patient is on antiseizure medication.
- Determine whether the patient has an *aura*— a sensory signal that a seizure is imminent— because the aura may be a warning. An aura may be visual (seeing lines, colors), auditory (ringing), or olfactory (smell of roses, vanilla). If the patient has an aura, return the patient to bed if possible; otherwise, lay the patient down on the nearest surface possible, protecting the head.

Tumors

Acute care occupational therapists are members of the team that provides therapeutic intervention before and after surgery or other medical treatment for patients with CNS tumors. According to the American Cancer Society ("Cancer Facts and Figures," 2008), an estimated 21,810 new cases of brain and nervous system cancer occurred in the United States in 2008. The most common types of *tumors* treated by acute care therapists are *astrocytoma, glioblastoma multiforme,* and *metastatic tumors.* Symptoms depend on where in the CNS the tumor is located. For more information on tumors, refer to Chapter 11. Treatment is determined by the tumor's location. Refer to Tables 6.1–6.3, 6.16, and 6.17 to determine functional deficits and the appropriate therapeutic intervention.

Medical Intervention

The medical treatment for CNS tumors typically depends on the location and the patient's medical status and prognosis for survival. Refer to Table 6.13 and Appendix 6.G for further information regarding neurosurgical interventions. Treatments include debulking via craniotomy, radiation, and chemotherapy.

Spinal Cord Injuries

Most acute care therapists rarely treat patients with acute *spinal cord injuries (SCIs)* for a prolonged period of time because these patients are usually transferred to a model SCI treatment center. However, in some instances, additional medical complications (e.g., fractures, pneumonia) result in an extended acute care stay. The average length of stay in a model SCI treatment center acute care division is 12 days (National Spinal Cord Injury Statistical Center, 2009), and then the patient is transferred to the inpatient rehabilitation division, usually within the same center. The therapist's primary role in a general acute care hospital is focusing on immediate needs such as preservation of ROM and vital sign stability during functional mobility in preparation for discharge to an inpatient rehabilitation facility. The acute care course centers on addressing life-threatening issues by stabilizing the patient's medical status.

Clinical Syndromes

Clinical SCI syndromes include many different types:

- *Anterior spinal cord syndrome:* Loss of all sensation (except proprioception) and motor function below the injury to the anterior spinal artery.
- *Brown–Sequard:* Lateral damage as a result of damage to only one side of the spinal cord, usually because of a stabbing or gunshot wound. The patient experiences motor paralysis and loss of proprioception on the ipsilateral side of the injury and loss of pain, temperature, and touch discrimination on the contralateral side of the injury.
- *Cauda equina syndrome:* Occurs with fractures below L2 with flaccid paralysis as the primary feature.
- *Central cord syndrome:* Destruction of the central cord versus the periphery of the cord. Paralysis and sensory loss are greater in the upper extremities than in the lower extremities. Central cord syndrome is more common in older people because of narrowing of the spinal cord.
- *Complete SCI:* No muscle preservation at and below the level of the injury.
- *Conus medullaris syndrome:* Injury to the sacral cord and lumbar nerve roots, resulting in the loss of bowel and bladder function and lower-extremity function.
- *Incomplete SCI:* Preservation of some sensation or motor capabilities at or below the level of the injury.
- *Paraplegia:* Impaired movement in both lower extremities, but movement in the upper extremities is preserved. The trunk may also be impaired.
- *Quadriplegia (tetraplegia):* Impaired movement in all four limbs.
- *Spinal cord infarct:* Stroke within the spinal cord vascular distribution. The pattern

(Text continues on p. 238)

Table 6.16. **Most Common Types of Central Nervous System Tumors**

Type	Other Names	Description	Medical Intervention
Astrocytoma	• Anaplastic astrocytoma • Malignant astrocytoma • High-grade astrocytoma	• Grade III malignant glioma tumor (Janus & Yung, 2007) • May progress to glioblastoma • Usually in the cerebral hemispheres and frontal lobe • Star-shaped cells throughout the brain • Survival rate: 2–3 years after initial diagnosis (Sathornsumetee, Rich, & Reardon, 2007), but may be longer	• Surgical debulking and resection followed by radiation. • Surgical resection followed by radiation, then chemotherapy. • If significant vascularity is present in the vicinity of the tumor, endovascular coil embolization techniques may be used to reduce risk of intracerebral bleeding. • Treatment dependent on medical status.
Glioblastoma	Glioblastoma multiforme	• Grade IV malignant glioma tumor (Janus & Yung, 2007) • Astrocytoma with associated necrosis • Most frequent, accounting for approximately 12%–15% of all brain tumors (National Cancer Institute, 2008) • Usually located in the cerebral hemispheres • Survival rate: 9–12 months after initial diagnosis (Sathornsumetee et al., 2007), but may be longer	• Surgical debulking and resection followed by radiation. • Surgical resection followed by radiation, then chemotherapy. • If significant vascularity is present in the vicinity of the tumor, endovascular coil embolization techniques may be used to reduce risk of intracerebral bleeding. • Treatment dependent on medical status.
Metastatic tumors	"Mets"	• Can be anywhere in the central nervous system and arise from a different primary site • The most common primary cancer is lung cancer, which accounts for 50% of all brain metastases • Brain metastases occur in 20%–40% of cancer patients (National Cancer Institute, 2008)	• Surgical resection followed by radiation. • Surgical resection followed by radiation, then chemotherapy. • If significant vascularity is present in the vicinity of the tumor, endovascular coil embolization techniques may be used to reduce risk of intracerebral bleeding. • Treatment dependent on medical status.

Table 6.17. **Functional Expectations After Spinal Cord Injury**

Level of Injury	Preserved Muscles and Movements	Patterns of Weakness	Expected Functional Outcomes	Therapeutic Intervention	Adaptive Devices
C1–C3	Face and neck muscles allowing for neck movement and facial expressions, use of mouth	Total paralysis (high-level quadriplegia)	• Dependent with all ADLs • Can use electronic activation devices	• Improve ability to use sip and puff with tasks such as blowing with a straw to push paper across the bedside table. • Neck ROM if allowed by the physician; incorporate isometric exercises when feasible. • Teach caregiver instruction methods. • Move out of bed to a chair using a sling lift (i.e., Hoyer, Invacare) • Monitor vital signs. • Address DME needs.	• Hospital bed • ECU • Electric, tilt-in-space wheelchair with sip-and-puff control and portable respirator
C4	Neck movement, upper traps for scapular elevation, and diaphragm for respiration	Paralysis of trunk and UEs and LEs and inability to cough	• Dependent with all ADLs • May be able to breathe without a respirator	• Focus on scapular elevation to strengthen accessory muscles for respiration and vent weaning and isometrics. • Quad coughing—After maximal inspiration, an assistant exerts pressure at the abdomen to increase the strength of a cough. • Teach caregiver instruction methods.	• ECU • Electric wheelchair • Mouth stick • Hospital bed

(continued)

Table 6.17. (continued)

Level of Injury	Preserved Muscles and Movements	Patterns of Weakness	Expected Functional Outcomes	Therapeutic Intervention	Adaptive Devices
				• Out of bed to a chair using a Hoyer lift. • Monitor vital signs. • Address DME needs.	
C5	Muscles spared • Biceps • Brachialis • Brachioradialis • Deltoid • Infraspinatus • Rhomboid • Supinator Preserved movement • Elbow flexion • Supination • External rotation • Shoulder abduction to 90° but limited shoulder flexion	• No elbow extension • No hand function • Total paralysis of trunk and LEs • Patient at high risk for scapular hiking or winging	• Moderate to maximal assistance with functional mobility • Minimal to moderate assistance for setup, then able to perform BADLs with adaptive devices	• Out of bed to a chair. Monitor vital signs. • Teach caregiver instruction methods. • BADLs. • Prevent elbow tightening resulting from lack of inhibitory action from elbow extensors. Daily PROM is imperative. • Address DME needs.	• Mobile arm supports • Adapted feeding devices (universal cuff) • Hand splints • Manual wheelchair with hand-rim projections • Sliding board • Transfer tub bench or shower seat
C6	Muscles spared • Extensor carpi radialis • Infraspinatus • Latissimus dorsi	• Wrist flexion • Elbow extension	Independent with BADLs with the following exceptions:	• Emphasize scaption depression with lower traps. • Out of bed to chair. • Monitor vital signs.	• Hospital bed • Manual wheelchair with rim projections

Level	Preserved Muscles	Functional Outcomes		Treatment	Equipment
	• Pectoralis major (clavicular portion) • Pronator teres • Serratus anterior • Teres minor Preserved movement • Shoulder movement • Scapular protraction • Horizontal adduction • Supination • Radial wrist extension • Tenodesis grasp	• Hand function with tenodesis spared • Total paralysis from trunk to LEs	• Cutting • Shoe tying • Lower body dressing and bathing • Uneven surface transfers	• Teach the patient to provide effective caregiver instructions. • BADLs. • Especially focus on the wrist to maximize the tenodesis grasp. • Address DME needs.	• Adaptive equipment for all BADLs
C7–C8	• Preserved muscles • All above muscles • Triceps • Pronator quadratus • Extensor carpi ulnaris • Flexor carpi radialis • Flexor digitorum profundus and superficialis • Extensor communis • Thumb muscles • Lumbricals (partially)	• Paralysis of trunk and LEs (low-level quadriplegia) • Limited grasp and dexterity because of partial intrinsic muscle innervation	Independent with all BADLs with adaptive equipment and DME	• Out of bed to a chair. Monitor vital signs. • Teach caregiver instruction methods. • BADLs. • Intrinsic and muscle and shoulder strengthening. • Balance tasks to prepare for safe sliding board transfers or depression transfers. • Address DME needs.	• Manual wheelchair with hand rims • Gloves • Adapted devices • Tub seat • Adapted seat for bowel program • Hospital bed or standard bed • Sliding board

(continued)

Table 6.17.   **(continued)**

Level of Injury	Preserved Muscles and Movements	Patterns of Weakness	Expected Functional Outcomes	Therapeutic Intervention	Adaptive Devices
	Preserved movement • Elbow extension • Strong wrist extension and flexion • Finger flexion and extension • Thumb flexion, extension, and abduction • Good shoulder movement				
T1–T9	Preserved muscles • Intrinsics • Intercostals • Erector spinae Preserved movements • UEs intact • Some patients may be able to ambulate with devices	• Limited trunk stability • Paraplegia	Independent with all ADLs	• Out of bed to a chair. Monitor vital signs. • Teach caregiver instruction methods. • BADLs. • Improve unsupported trunk stability and balance during task performance. • Address DME needs.	• Wheelchair with hand rims • Standard bed
T10–L1	Preserved muscles • Intercostals • External obliques • Rectus abdominus	Weak LEs; may be able to ambulate	Independent with all ADLs	• Out of bed to a chair. Watch vital signs. • BADLs. • Address DME needs.	• May use wheelchair for distances. • Bilateral ankle foot orthoses

Level	Preserved movements/muscles	Status	Function	Interventions	Equipment
	Preserved movements • Good trunk stability				• Standard bed
L2–S5	Preserved muscles • All trunk muscles • Depending on level, some hip, knee, and ankle muscles Preserved movements • Good trunk stability • Partial control of LEs	Weak LEs; may be able to ambulate	• Independent with all ADLs • May have bowel dysfunction but is independent with bowel program.	• Out of bed to a chair. Monitor vital signs. • Teach caregiver instruction methods. • BADLs. • Address DME needs.	• Wheelchair • Standard bed

Note. ADLs = activities of daily living; BADLs = basic activities of daily living; DME = durable medical equipment; ECU = environmental control unit; LEs = lower extremities; PROM = passive range of motion; ROM = range of motion; UEs = upper extremities.

Sources. Adler (2006); Flaherty and Rost (2007); Rothstein, Roy, and Wolf (1998); Rubin and Safdieh (2007); Young and Young (1997).

of deficits is dependent on the level of the infarct.

- *Transverse myelitis:* Inflammation across one level of the spinal cord. The myelin sheath is attacked and causes paralysis below the level of the inflammation, which can progress over the course of several weeks. One-third of patients recover fully, one-third recover partially but are left with significant deficits such as spasticity and bowel and bladder deficits, and one-third demonstrate no recovery at all (NINDS, 2009). Patients are generally treated with corticosteroids and rehabilitation.

Therapeutic Implications

Table 6.17 delineates functional expectations for each injury level to help in determining the most appropriate intervention. However, the therapist's role is primarily preparation for rehabilitation, including

- Preventing the loss of valuable passive and active ROM and strength;
- Preventing the loss of respiratory capacity with trunk and intercostal muscle flexibility for improved vent-weaning potential; and
- Preservation of functional hand position for potential neurological return in the hands (Atkins, Clark & Waters, 2003).

The standard evaluation tool for classification of a SCI is the American Spinal Injury Association (ASIA) Standard Neurological Classification of Spinal Cord Injury (see Appendix 6.E). This evaluation will assist in determining the degree and pattern of paralysis and sensory loss. ASIA testing is crucial for determining the level of injury, which is not always at the same level as the vertebral fracture. The ASIA test is also important for insurance classification for monetary allotments for durable medical equipment and is especially crucial for patients with high quadriplegia. Even if a patient is wearing a halo vest and ASIA testing at the T3–T6 level is obstructed, it is still important to perform the test. In general, unless the therapist is working in a specialized spinal cord unit and is specifically trained, a physician performs the test.

Occupational therapy evaluation and intervention should focus on client factors with respect to level of injury and medical stability. See Table 6.18 for clinical interventions for SCI.

Complications in the Acute Phase

Several complications should be considered when addressing SCIs:

- Spinal shock can last from 24 hours after the injury to as long as 6 weeks (Adler, 2006). Symptoms of spinal shock include *areflexia* (no reflex activity below the level of the injury), flaccid bladder and bowel, decreased deep tendon reflexes, and impaired sympathetic functioning. Diminished sympathetic responses include decreased heart rate and blood pressure, no perspiration below the injury level, and decreased constriction of the blood vessels.

- Spasticity results from the muscles' inability to inhibit messages to contract and tighten, thus forming an overactive muscle response. The brain's more efficient reflex centers are not able to control muscle function below the level of the SCI, so the spinal cord sends messages that do not allow the nerves to control voluntary movement. Spasticity can be very painful. If pain is interfering with therapy, notify the doctor and request antispasticity medicine be considered along with pain medications. Many patients see a spasm for the first time and think the muscle function is returning; handle the situation gently because they are hopeful or desperate for movement. Educate the patient on the nature of spasticity.

- *Autonomic dysreflexia* is the response of the ANS to noxious stimuli. Examples may include distended bladder, fecal mass, an ingrown toenail, a toe pushed against the footboard of the bed, kinked catheter, or overheating. It is frequently characterized by autonomic symptoms such as

Table 6.18. Clinical Interventions for Spinal Cord Injury (SCI)

Client Factors	Occupational Performance	Clinical Intervention
Vital sign stability: Blood pressure, respiration rate, heart rate and rhythm, and oxygen saturation	Implement position changes (especially sitting) and task performance.	• Abdominal binder and thigh-high thromboembolic deterrent hose to maintain blood pressure. If these are not effective, then wrap the legs with elastic bandages. • Expect a drop in blood pressure the first several times the patient is in an upright position. Do not sit patient completely upright the first several times. The patient will likely better tolerate gradual changes in the incline level. • Implement a bed–chair position schedule with the nurses for at least 3 times/day for 15–30 minutes to augment and facilitate therapy efforts. Be sure weight shifts occur at least every 20 minutes. Do not use bed–chair position if spine is unstable; request clarification from physician, especially if spine stabilization surgery is being considered. • Initially use a high-back reclining wheelchair unless a tilt-in-space wheelchair is available. • Watch for autonomic dysreflexia symptoms.
Psychosocial adjustment to injury	Assess.	• Encourage active participation. • Begin education process because knowledge decreases fear of the unknown; take care to not give false hope for recovery. • The patient may be grieving because of a significant loss of his or her body. Acutely, this may present as false hope or disinterest. • Include the family.
Discharge planning	Assess current and previous level of function and psychosocial issues to determine appropriate recommendations.	Anticipate durable medical equipment and home environmental adaptations to allow the family time to begin preparing for discharge. These adaptations may include home modifications such as building a ramp, rearranging rooms for a bedroom on the main level, or moving if the home is inaccessible (i.e., lives in second-story walk-up apartment). Continued therapy recommendation options: • Model SCI unit • Inpatient rehabilitation facility • Home health • Subacute rehabilitation • Nursing home • Long-term acute care (especially if vent weaning is possible).

(continued)

Table 6.18. **(continued)**

Client Factors	Occupational Performance	Clinical Intervention
Basic activities of daily living	Assess whether adaptive devices and positioning can be used to maximize function.	• Using room controls (e.g., call bell, TV remote, bed controls), obtain adaptive devices such as feather-light touch pad or fabricate them. Place it near the most effective movement such as the jaw or hand. See adapted quad bell in Figure 6.9. • Feeding and drinking—Long straw, universal cuff, built-up handle. • Grooming and hygiene—Universal cuff. • Functional mobility—Including log rolling for pressure relief, transfers, maintenance of upright balance.
Bowel and bladder	Assess.	• Generally, nursing staff address bowel and bladder maintenance in acute care. • Educate patient on adaptive devices and options for self-catheterization and bowel management.
Passive and active range of motion	Assess and maintain. Must assess this area first before completing manual muscle testing.	Joint mobility must be maintained to maximize recovery in the future. • *Exercises and stretching:* Include family education, perform within parameters of ability and tolerance levels, and begin muscle reeducation efforts as appropriate. • *Scapulas:* Prone position best if possible. Preserve scaption, prevent adhesions, and prevent overstretching and tearing of posterior shoulder ligaments or impingements. Necessary for preservation of the accessory muscles for breathing, shoulders, elbows, and wrists. • *Neck:* Check with the physician before attempting. Especially important for patients with high quadriplegia. • *Shoulders:* Horizontal abduction is important for pectoralis major stretch. Important to preserve maximum ribcage expansion for vent weaning. Perform internal and external rotation. • *Elbows, wrists, and hands:* Flexion, extension, pronation and supination, and ulnar and radial deviation.
Splinting	Assess on the basis of spasticity and level of injury.	Spasticity usually occurs in the muscles below the level of injury. Muscles are not actually damaged but have no inhibitory influences from neurons above the injury. Careful observation must continue throughout acute hospitalization to prevent the emergence of a nonfunctional spasticity. Initially, splint patients at night who have sustained a C1–C5 and possibly a C6–C7 injury with a static resting splint with fingers flexed halfway to prevent flattening of the palmar

Table 6.18. (continued)

Client Factors	Occupational Performance	Clinical Intervention
		arch and maintain functional hand range of motion and positioning. Judiciously apply the splints because they could inhibit the emergence of tenodesis. If tone increases in the elbows, apply pillow extension splints (Atkins, Clark, & Waters, 2003).
Positioning	Assess skin integrity and hemodynamics.	• Maintain skin integrity: Keep heels off the bed at all times; avoid multipodus boots because they can cause pressure ulcers on the balls of the feet. • Sitting positioning: Pelvis should be all the way back in the seat. Check to ensure proper positioning. • Improve hemodynamics (blood pressure) in the upright position. • Maximize respiratory function.
Pain	Patients with C4–C7 injury frequently experience shoulder pain because of scapular immobilization (Southam & Schmidt, 2006).	• Request premedication before therapy. • Increase joint mobility using traditional strategies. • Undiagnosed fractures, shoulder dislocations, and rotator cuff tears are common in the acute stages. If the patient complains of severe pain, consult with the physician.

Source. Adler (2006), M. Rank, (personal communication, August 2008).

perspiration, flushing, chills, nasal congestion, hypertension, and lowered heart rate. The patient may also be very anxious (Adler, 2006). The cause must be quickly ascertained because autonomic dysreflexia can be a life-threatening situation with rapid onset. Place the patient in a reclined position or return the patient to bed, if possible, and remove any constricting clothing (thromboembolic deterrent hose, abdominal binder) or objects to reduce blood pressure. Check for a kinked catheter, and empty the catheter bag. Notify the nurse immediately.

• Patients with an unstable cervical fracture may have a halo vest applied for stability. This vest will increase safety and neck stability for functional mobility. The halo weighs only 7 pounds even though it feels very heavy to the patient. Encourage the use of button-up shirts. Do not pull or push on the halo, especially when performing bed mobility. The halo is stabilized by being directly screwed into the skull. In the event that the halo becomes dislodged, the therapist should keep the head and neck stable and in midline. This situation is emergent; obtain medical assistance immediately.

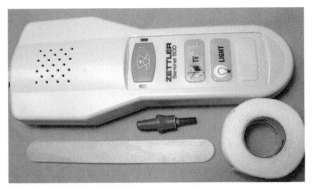

1. Supplies:
   • Tongue depressor
   • Small cylindrical object like a male IV connector or pen lid
   • Silk tape

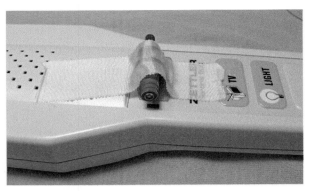

2. Tape the cylindrical object over the call button.

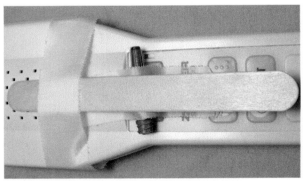

3. Place the tongue depressor over the taped object. Tape one end down, leaving the other end free.

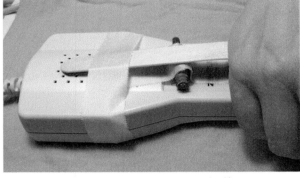

4. Adjust tension for patient's strength. If necessary, place additional tape over the cylindrical object, use 2 tongue depressors, and/or adjust how tightly the tongue depressor is fastened.

Figure 6.9. Adapted quad bell.
Source. Judy R. Hamby

Amyotrophic Lateral Sclerosis

Amyotrophic lateral sclerosis (ALS), or Lou Gehrig's disease, is the most common motor neuron disease that affects adults. Onset generally occurs between ages 40 and 60, and men are affected more than women. According to NINDS (2003), 20,000 Americans have ALS, and 5,000 are diagnosed each year. This disease involves a progressive degeneration of the motor neurons in the brainstem, anterior horn cells of the spinal cord, and motor cortex and eventually affects all voluntary muscles. The disease's name describes the physical symptoms.

> The term *amyotrophic* refers to the muscle atrophy that is seen as a result of degeneration of the anterior horn cells and corticospinal tracts of the spinal cord. . . . *Lateral sclerosis* refers to the demyelination and gliosis occurring in the corticospinal tracts, located in the lateral spinal cord, and corticobulbar tracts. . . . The areas that harden and degenerate cause a *scar* or *sclerosis.* (Barker & Hobdell, 1994, p. 591, *added*)

The disease is eventually fatal with a life expectancy of 2–5 years after diagnosis. ALS has no cure, and treatment is largely supportive care.

To be accurately diagnosed, the patient must have upper motor neuron and lower motor neuron symptoms. The disease is usually diagnosed with an electromyograph and muscle biopsy, but still remains a diagnosis of exclusion. ALS has no standard pattern of progression, but the most common early symptoms are focal weaknesses in the arms, legs, or the facial muscles. Disease progression depends on where the first symptoms occur. Functionally, the most common initial deficits reported by the patient include dyspnea, difficulty with fine motor control, stumbling while walking, swallowing and chewing difficulties, and slurred speech. ALS does not affect autonomic functions, bowel and bladder function, cerebellar extraocular movements, or sensation. As the disease progresses, ALS includes lower motor neuron, upper motor neuron, and bulbar symptoms. Refer to Table 6.19 for more information on these symptoms.

The acute care therapist can establish an occupational profile for patient and family with goals identified to improve quality of life. Consider the patient's and family's readiness for adaptations, and bear in mind that needs continue to evolve because of the disease's continuous progression (Southam & Schmidt, 2006). As needs change, however, therapists in later levels of the continuum of care can assist in determining necessary adaptations. At a time when durable medical equipment or adaptive devices may not be well received, judicious recommendations should not overload the patient (McGovern-Denk, Levine, & Casey, 2005). Tailor recommendations toward equipment that facilitates safety and the most important needs identified by patients and families. Refer to Table 6.20 for more information on acute care intervention for the patient with ALS.

Peripheral Nerve Injuries

Peripheral nerve injuries are frequently treated in the acute care setting; however, they are typically not the primary diagnosis. These injuries are generally the result of complications from surgical procedures or trauma. For instance, during a long surgery, the blood pressure cuff may have been too tight, thus constricting the radial nerve as it passed through the radial groove, which then causes a radial nerve palsy. Follow-up intervention for radial, ulnar, or median nerve injuries can best be served in an outpatient setting, but if intervention is required in acute care, refer to Table 6.21.

Guillain-Barré Syndrome

Guillain–Barré syndrome (GBS) is an acute, rapidly progressing inflammatory demyelination of the peripheral nerves and spinal nerve roots that results in an ascending paralysis (Li, 2008). GBS is considered an autoimmune disease that follows an upper respiratory illness in two-thirds of the affected population. This syndrome has no known cause or cure, and it

Table 6.19. Lower and Upper Motor Neuron and Bulbar Symptoms

Lower Motor Neuron Symptoms	Bulbar Symptoms	Upper Motor Neuron Symptoms
• Progression from weakness to total paralysis of all striated muscles, including the diaphragm • Respiratory failure and dysphagia eventually necessitate ventilator and augmentative feeding support • Atrophy • Flaccidity • Hyporeflexia • Fatigue and stiffness • Muscle cramps and fasciculations	• Absent jaw and gag reflex • Dysarthria • Dysphagia	• Weakness • Hyperreflexia and clonus • Spasticity—"[M]ost prominent in upper extremity flexors and lower extremity extensors" (Bronfin, 2005, p. 386) • Emotional lability and depression (because of the effects on the limbic motor neuron system) • Frontotemporal dementia with resultant changes in behavior, judgment, executive function, and personality has been noted in later stages (Lomen-Hoerth, 2004; Ringholz & Greene, 2006)

affects 5,000 people annually in the United States (Southam & Schmidt, 2006).

The two primary variant types of GBS are Miller–Fisher syndrome and chronic inflammatory demyelinating polyneuropathy. *Miller–Fisher* syndrome is characterized by paralysis of the eye muscles, absence of tendon reflexes, and muscle coordination abnormalities (NINDS, 2008a; Southam & Schmidt, 2006). *Chronic inflammatory demyelinating polyneuropathy* closely resembles GBS and is considered a chronic form of the disease.

Tests generally performed include MRI and computed tomography to rule out a stroke; however, the diagnosis is confirmed by a lumbar puncture in which the opening pressure may initially be elevated, later showing increased fluid proteins. Electromyography may also be performed. The most common medical intervention includes plasmapheresis or high-dose intravenous immunoglobulin. *Plasmapheresis* removes plasma antibodies and is a blood-cleansing procedure, whereas *intravenous immunoglobulin* is a high-dose plasma protein

replacement therapy that works as an immunosuppressant (Shields & Wilbourn, 2007).

The disease's progression is divided into three phases (Li, 2008): initial, plateau, and recovery. In the *initial, acute phase,* patients are generally hospitalized because of the high risk of life-threatening autonomic dysfunction such as respiratory failure, bowel and bladder dysfunction, and fluctuating cardiac rhythms. The initial phase has the highest mortality level because of the autonomic dysfunction, and many patients are intubated during this phase. This phase is marked by the initial onset of the first conclusive symptoms and ends when the progression of weakness ceases. Motor and sensory impairments occur distal to proximal. The first symptoms are generally numbness and tingling in the palms and soles of the feet with eventual progression to the proximal musculature.

The *plateau phase* begins when strength ceases to deteriorate but no recovery has occurred. It generally lasts several weeks (Southam & Schmidt, 2006). The evaluation

(Text continues on p. 248)

Table 6.20. Clinical Interventions for Amyotrophic Lateral Sclerosis

Client Factors	Occupational Performance	Clinical Intervention
Psychosocial adjustment to injury	Assess.	• Encourage active participation. • Begin education process, because knowledge decreases fear of the unknown, taking care to not give false hope for recovery. Do not overwhelm the patient or the family with information. • Include the family. • Request psychiatry, psychology, or social work consults to manage adjustment issues appropriately. • Request palliative care consult if counseling is required to make difficult medical decisions and advanced care planning.

Discharge planning	Assess current and previous level of function and psychosocial issues to determine appropriate recommendations.	• Follow up on continuum of care therapy recommendations.
		• Evaluate safety. Provide strategies to increase safety, especially if frontotemporal dementia is present or the patient is not yet receptive to safer adaptive methods as function changes.
		• Assess durable medical equipment needs.
		  — Anticipate durable medical equipment and home environmental adaptations to allow the family time to begin preparing for discharge. These adaptations may include home modifications such as building a ramp, rearranging rooms for a bedroom on the main level, or moving if the home is inaccessible.
		  — Recommend durable medical equipment that addresses the disease's progression and patient's level of acceptance. Examples might include
		    ▪ Transfer tub bench versus shower stool to allow for safe access when stepping into a tub eventually becomes unsafe.
		    ▪ Hoyer lift to assist with safe transfers and ease the burden of the caregivers
		    ▪ Hospital bed
		    ▪ Wheelchair and cushion; refer patient to a seating clinic if mobility is not sufficient for ambulation.
		• Request palliative care consult if help is required to navigate health care system.
		• Make disposition recommendations:
		  — Home care assistant and therapy if going home
		  — Assisted living facility

(*continued*)

Table 6.20. (continued)

Client Factors	Occupational Performance	Clinical Intervention
		— Nursing home — Hospice.
Basic activities of daily living	Assess whether adaptive devices and positioning can be used to maximize function.	• Recommend adaptive devices such as a buttonhook, long-handled sponge, or adapted call bell (see Figure 6.9). • Provide a catalog or recommend Web sites for family to begin identifying items they may find helpful. • Evaluate feeding and swallowing. Recommend adaptive equipment as needed (see Chapter 13 for further information).
Range of motion and strengthening	Assess and maintain.	• Implement a stretching program to prevent contractures and, if needed, request consideration of antispasticity medicine. • Perform AROM, PROM, and AAROM, but do not fatigue. • Cautious strengthening in the early stages (AROM with light resistance or isometrics) as needed for muscle preservation. The expectation is for joint integrity because muscle mass will likely not increase.
Splinting	Assess.	Hand splinting (to prevent clawing and skin breakdown).
Positioning	Assess skin integrity and edema.	• Maintain skin integrity: — Positioning in the bed or a chair — Cervical neck collar to maintain head positioning (because of neck weakness). • Control edema: — Use techniques such as elevation, slings to prevent arms from hanging down, and seated positioning.
Pain	Reduce pain resulting from contractures and edema.	• Request medical management of pain, including premedication before therapy. • Increase joint mobility using traditional strategies. • Request palliative care consult if symptom management outweighs benefits or pain control is inadequate.
Activity tolerance	Easily fatigued.	• Do not overfatigue the patient. • Teach energy conservation strategies to minimize fatigue. See Appendix D for a handout on energy conservation.

Note. AAROM = active assistive range of motion; AROM = active range of motion; PROM = passive range of motion.

Table 6.21. **Peripheral Nerve Injuries**

Nerve	Primary Mechanism of Injury	Most Common Deficits	Evaluation	Treatment
Median nerve	• Compression. • Overuse. • Laceration. • IV insertion.	Motor • Decreased 3-jaw chuck, opposition, and tip pinch. Sensory • Numbness in thumb, index, and middle fingers.	• Tinel's—Positive if tapping at center of volar wrist crease causes paresthesias • Opposition • Carpal and metacarpal arches are flattened • Pain	• *Splint:* In the acute care setting, situation is not emergent. Instruct patient to obtain a wrist cock-up splint at discharge. • *Referral:* Outpatient hand therapy.
Radial nerve	Compression from the blood pressure cuff or improper positioning during surgery. Most frequently seen after upper-body surgery. Usually the nerve is just "bruised" and needs time to heal. Frequently in this case, movement begins returning in a few days. Also seen after humeral fractures.	Motor • If injury occurs at the forearm or proximally, there is no extension of the wrist, thumb, or finger metacarpals. Proximal interphalangeal extension is preserved. Sensory • Generally preserved but occasionally numb on dorsum of radial side of hand.	• Wrist and finger extension against gravity and gravity eliminated. • Sensation—Ask if any part of the hand, wrist, or arm is numb.	• *Splint:* Fit with a resting mitt splint to preserve extensors. If radial nerve damage is untreated, it can cause lasting damage to the wrist and finger extensors. • *Referral:* Outpatient hand therapy. The hand therapist can continue with dynamic splinting as appropriate • Instruct in PROM exercises.
Ulnar nerve	• Elbow fractures. • Improper positioning during surgery.	Motor • Decreased intrinsics and thumb function. • Will note a claw hand or Benedictine position. • Loss of power grip. Sensory • Numbness in ring and little finger.	• Froment's sign (positive ulnar nerve damage if distal interphalangeal joint of thumb flexes when pulling a piece of paper using lateral pinch).	• Ulnar nerve splint—Figure-8 splint that encircles the hand and little and ring fingers. The little and ring fingers are flexed at 20°–30° (intrinsic + position). • Refer to an outpatient hand therapist.

and treatment during this phase are similar to that for other neurological diseases, with special emphasis on preventing fatigue while increasing activity tolerance and strength.

During the third, *recovery phase,* the patient begins to recover strength, and rehabilitation begins in earnest. This phase can last several years, and sometimes full recovery eludes the patient. Each phase requires a differing level of evaluation and treatment. Refer to Table 6.22 for occupational therapy evaluation and therapeutic implications for patients with GBS.

Multiple Sclerosis

Multiple sclerosis (MS) is a progressive, unpredictable, and chronic demyelinating disorder caused by plaques that form in the white matter of the brain. Plaques can also form on the spinal cord and optic nerve and in the gray matter. Deficits are dependent on the location of the plaques. MS most frequently occurs between ages 20 and 40 and is more prevalent in women than in men (Pirko & Noseworthy, 2007). The disease's effects range from a mild weakness or visual disturbance to complete debility. The primary feature of MS is its unpredictability because exacerbations and remission can occur without warning. Where the next plaque will form is not predictable.

MS has three types. *Relapsing remitting* is the most common type, affecting 85% of those with MS. The deficits are cumulative because the disease enters periods of exacerbation followed by remission. The second most common type is *primary progressive,* affecting 10% of those with MS. The symptoms are continuous with no remission and continue to worsen. Affecting 5% of those with MS, *secondary progressive* is the least common type. It begins as the relapsing remitting type, but then progresses into the primary progressive type.

Table 6.23 delineates the most frequent clinical symptoms and therapeutic interventions for patients with MS. Once the patient is medically stable, discharge to the next level of care should be the primary goal.

Myasthenia Gravis

Myasthenia gravis is an autoimmune disease that affects the acetylcholine receptors of the skeletal voluntary muscles. It affects women more than men, and the usual age of onset is approximately 20. A second peak may occur around age 50, but generally men are more affected at that age (Bartt & Topel, 2007). Clinically, primary symptoms include ocular dysfunction, ptosis, fluctuating muscle weakness, and fatiguability. The disease can be limited to the ocular musculature or can be generalized.

Symptoms and therapeutic intervention are listed in Table 6.24. Medical intervention is generally limited to anticholinesterase medications, plasmaphoresis for those in myasthenic crisis (respiratory distress), or thymectomy (surgical removal of the thymus gland) (Bartt & Topel, 2007). This disease is not curable, but many of the symptoms can be managed with appropriate medical intervention.

Conversion Disorder

Conversion disorder, sometimes called *functional disorder,* is a psychiatric disorder listed in the *Diagnostic and Statistical Manual of Mental Disorders* (4th ed.; American Psychiatric Association, 1994) as a subset of somatoform disorders. Conversion disorder requires an interdisciplinary, focused intervention plan to facilitate recovery. This diagnosis is amenable to therapy if it is performed in the appropriate manner. Conversion disorder is more common in women than in men and generally occurs between the ages of 10 and 35 (Smith et al., 2007). Six factors must be present to accurately diagnose conversion disorder:

1. No pathophysiological rationale for a clinical diagnosis can be detected through a thorough medical testing, symptoms are not a culturally acceptable behavior (e.g., fainting during a religious service), or both. With detailed modern medical testing, only 4% of those initially diagnosed with conversion disorder are misdiag-

(Text continues on p. 253)

Table 6.22. **Phases of Guillain–Barré Syndrome**

Process	Initial Acute Phase	Plateau Phase	Recovery Phase
Evaluation—Standard evaluation with additions as noted	• Swallow-dysphagia. • Hemodynamics (especially lowered blood pressure) associated with performance of self-care.	• Swallow-dysphagia. • Pain. • Careful documentation of results of manual muscle training in the beginning of the plateau phase. • Discharge disposition.	• Swallow-dysphagia. • Pain. • Careful documentation of results of manual muscle training.
Treatment	• Daily passive range of motion to minimize contractures. • Positioning and splinting to minimize contractures, deformity, and wounds. • Pain management. • Adaptations of call bell (see Figure 6.9) and environmental controls. • Self-care as able. • Family education.	• Continue with treatment as in the initial acute phase, but monitor closely for increasing strength. If noted, then move on to the recovery phase.	• Increasing independence with self-care. • Strengthening with increased resistance. • Energy conservation and work simplification. • Adaptive devices and durable medical equipment.
Precautions	• Careful observation of hemodynamics during treatment. • Notify medical staff immediately if difficulty with breathing increases; it may indicate imminent respiratory failure. • Pain control. • Do not fatigue.	• Monitor for muscle belly tenderness. • Do not fatigue. • Do not irritate inflamed nerves.	• Do not fatigue. • Conservative use of resistive exercises should be considered, but avoid substitution movement patterns, and do not irritate tender muscle bellies or inflamed nerves.

Table 6.23. Multiple Sclerosis Therapeutic Intervention

Dysfunction or Performance Skill	Symptom	Therapeutic Intervention and Precautions
Motor	• Weakness • Paralysis • Spasticity • Incoordination resulting from decreased proprioception and weakness • Tremors	• Basic self-care, including durable medical equipment and adaptive devices needed. Focus on — *Feeding*—Built-up utensils or universal cuff — *Dressing*—Reacher, sock aid, long shoehorn — *Bathroom mobility*—Tub bench, 3-in-1 commode, versa frames — *Bed mobility*—Bed rail — *Bathing*—Long sponge brush, sitting vs. standing — *Grooming and hygiene*—Long brush or comb, seated with arms supported, electric toothbrush. • Gentle strengthening once exacerbation period is completed. • If spasticity is interfering with function, discuss antispasticity medications with physician. • Balance for self-care. • Avoid fatigue. • Referral for rehabilitation.
Cranial nerve dysfunction	• Optic neuritis—Blurred central vision, faded colors, and blind spots • Diplopia—Horizontal diplopia in lateral gaze (bilateral internuclear ophthalmoplegia resulting from a lesion of the medial longitudinal fasciculus) • Visual loss (resulting from plaque on optic nerve) • Dysphagia	• Referral for neuro-ophthalmologist or neurobehavioral optometrist. • Patching or partial occlusion (see "Vision and Perception" section). • Low vision strategies (see Appendix F). • Swallow evaluation and treatment; precautions as needed (see Chapter 13). • Higher risk for fall because of diplopia.
Sensory	• Numbness • Decreased proprioception	• Sensory precaution education. • Reduce temperature of water to avoid burns. • Do not use moist heat for muscle pain.

Table 6.23. *(continued)*

Dysfunction or Performance Skill	Symptom	Therapeutic Intervention and Precautions
Cerebellar symptoms	• Vertigo • Ataxia and incoordination • Dysmetria • Nystagmus	• Balance and functional mobility. • Basic self-care. • Weighted utensils. • Instruct in precautions for vertigo (see "Precautions for Self-Care With Vestibular Issues" handout in Appendix H).
Bowel and bladder	• Incontinence • Frequency • Urgency • Retention	• May need to work with nursing staff for self-catheterization strategies with decreased coordination. • Instruct in energy and time-saving strategies for clothing management and transfers to the toilet.
Cognition	• Memory • Attention • Safety judgment and impulsivity • Executive dysfunction	• Assess safety judgment for home. • Memory strategies such as writing down questions for health care professional and the answers. • May be impulsive. • Fall risk. • Reduction of environmental distractors.
Speech–language	• Dysarthria • Word-finding deficits	• Recommend speech–language pathology evaluation. • Allow time for the patient to express himself or herself.
Activity tolerance	Fatigues quickly	• Energy conservation and work simplification strategies. • Avoid heat. • Reduce water temperature for shower.
Psychological	• Depression • Anxiety • Irritability • Behavioral issues	• Education regarding the disease especially if treating during the first exacerbation. • Referral for psychology, psychiatry, or both. • Support group resources. • Time allowed for patient to discuss perceived life changes. • Family education.

Note. Created by Judy R. Hamby.

Table 6.24.   Myasthenia Gravis Therapeutic Intervention

Dysfunction or Performance Skill	Symptom	Therapeutic Intervention and Precautions
Motor	• Weakness (proximal more than distal). • Neck flexor weakness is common. • Muscles fatigue with continued activity.	• Weakness can be exacerbated by overactivity, heat, or both. • Active range of motion only during exacerbation, then progress to light resistance exercises. • May have difficulty with ambulation and stair climbing; use rails, durable medical equipment (e.g., cane, walker), or both. • Basic self-care may be affected, necessitating durable medical equipment, adaptive devices and procedures, or both. • Instruct in energy conservation and work simplification strategies. • Referrals — Rehabilitation — Physical therapy.
Visual	• Ptosis or reduced eye closure. • Blurred vision. • Diplopia.	• Patching or partial occlusion if no ptosis (see "Evaluation and Therapeutic Intervention" section). • If the eye will not close, it must be manually closed (tape it closed with gauze). • Higher risk for fall because of diplopia. • May complain of headaches, nausea, and dizziness. • Referrals — Neuro-ophthalmologist — Neurobehavioral optometrist.
Speech	• Dysarthria or slurred speech. • Dysphonia.	— Referral speech–language pathology
Swallow	• Dysphagia.	• Swallow evaluation and treatment; precautions as needed (see Chapter 13).
Breathing	• Crisis may manifest as respiratory distress caused by ineffective cough and weakness of the respiratory muscles and is usually the symptom that necessitates hospital admission.	• Avoid fatigue or overactivity, because it can lead to increased dyspnea and fatigue of respiratory musculature. • May have difficulty coughing to clear secretions.

Table 6.24. (continued)		
Dysfunction or Performance Skill	**Symptom**	**Therapeutic Intervention and Precautions**
	• May need mechanical ventilation. • May have intercostal and diaphragmatic muscle weakness.	

Sources. Bartt and Topel (2007), Bronfin (2005), Moskowitz (1994), *Myasthenia Gravis Fact Sheet* (2008).

nosed (Aybek, Kanaan, & David, 2008; Smith et al., 2007; Teasell & Shapiro, 2002). In those cases, an organic etiology such as MS, myasthenia gravis, or CNS tumor were eventually found.

2. The patient is not intentionally feigning symptoms. Malingering (clear secondary gain) or factitious (voluntary feigning) behavior is not suspected.

3. One or more symptoms are present that suggest a neurological or other medical condition.

4. The symptom significantly affects occupational and social performance or medical status.

5. Symptoms are not limited to sexual dysfunction or pain.

6. Psychological stressors are temporally associated with onset. Conversion disorder generally manifests suddenly, without warning, and in the setting of an extreme psychological stressor. Two primary reasons that a person might manifest a conversion disorder are

• *Primary gain:* Symbolic resolution to avoid conscious awareness of the stressor (American Psychiatric Association, 2000). For instance, if the patient was in an argument, the primary manifestation may be aphasia or paralysis to avoid the awareness of the psychological battle.

• *Secondary gain:* To avoid dealing with an issue, but not intentionally. For example, a soldier may develop a hand paralysis to avoid firing a gun.

In general, symptoms are not anatomically pathway specific but instead manifest according to the patient's understanding of a particular diagnosis; the less educated the patient is, the more erratic the symptoms are. Conversely, the more educated patient will manifest symptoms that are closer to a realistic clinical picture. Symptoms are inconsistent and may include motor or sensory pseudoneurological signs that frequently resemble a stroke or SCI (American Psychiatric Association, 2000; Heruti, Levy, Adunski, & Ohry, 2002).

Motor symptoms may include

• Paralysis of one or more extremities with ataxia or tremor,

• Dystonia and chorea movement patterns (most common),

• Urinary retention or incontinence,

• Speech impairments (e.g., hoarseness, aphonia, dysarthria),

• Swallow deficits or a choking sensation,

• Seizure,

• Bronchospasms, and

• Blepharospasms (i.e., twitching or blinking of the eyelid).

Sensory impairments may include

- Visual deficits (e.g., double vision, blindness),
- Hallucinations,
- Deafness,
- Sensory loss (may follow a stocking–glove distribution with uniform loss of touch, pain, and temperature), and
- Loss of speech (aphasia).

Therapeutic Implications and Precautions

Three approaches should be used concurrently: the behavior modification approach, the psychotherapeutic approach, and the physical approach (Heruti et al., 2002).

The *behavior modification approach* reduces unwanted behaviors by ignoring or reducing attention to them in order to achieve desired behaviors. This is accomplished by rewarding positive versus negative behaviors.

- Treat in private areas so the patient does not see patients with real symptoms that could be worked into his or her own constellation of deficits and symptoms.
- When discussing the diagnosis, information should be vague and should allow for a speedy recovery, such as a "spinal cord concussion" (Heruti et al., 2002, p. 332).
- Communication among team members, especially differences of opinion, should only occur privately, never in front of the patient.

The primary focus of the *psychotherapeutic approach* is to address the initial psychological stressor to alleviate the physical symptoms as the issue is resolved.

The *physical approach* uses a multidisciplinary team that should use generally accepted classical therapeutic interventions that integrate behavioral modification strategies (see Table 6.25 for further details).

- Rehabilitation provides a "culturally accepted intervention or cure to their illness" (Ness, 2007, p. 30). The family should also be involved in this process.

- Systematic progression of functional activities should be emphasized rather than exercises (Oh, Yoo, Yi, & Kwon, 2005).
- Staffing changes should be kept to a minimum to allow for treatment strategy consistency.

Referrals may be made to

- Neuropsychology or psychology,
- Psychiatry, and
- Inpatient rehabilitation;

An interdisciplinary treatment model is the best option (Heruti et al., 2002). The length of stay is generally short, but the patient must be provided with opportunities to recover physical, occupational, and social status in a manner that does not compromise psychological health. Resolution of symptoms can be facilitated via the already existing interdisciplinary model because a mechanism for interdisciplinary communication already exists (Smith et al., 2007). The environment can be more successfully controlled (Oh et al., 2005) to use behavioral modification strategies. Patients should be assigned to a specific diagnostic unit; for example, a patient with stroke symptoms should be assigned to the stroke unit.

Autonomic Nervous System Dysfunction

The following types of ANS dysfunction are specific to neurological clinical care.

Autonomic Neuropathy

Autonomic neuropathy occurs when the nerves that control vital bodily functions are damaged. It primarily presents as hypotension and elevated heart rate with peripheral edema. It can result in dysphagia, loss of bladder control, *gastroparesis* (diarrhea or constipation), and cardiac sympathetic denervation, laying the groundwork for a silent myocardial infarction. This event indicates a change in the severity of neuropathy and is irreversible. Autonomic neuropathy has a mortality rate of 44% after the initial diagnosis (Quattrini & Tesfaye, 2003).

(Text continues on p. 258)

Table 6.25. Conversion Disorder Therapeutic Implications

Client Factor	Process
Psychological	**Evaluation** • Do not tell or even imply to the patient that the symptoms do not actually exist, because the patient has no voluntary control over the symptoms. Simply inform the patient that full recovery is expected and that all tests are negative (Ness, 2007). Avoid confrontation. • A patient needs to feel safe with the therapist; therefore, time spent on building rapport is valuable. • Frequently, the patient appears detached from the physical symptoms (*"la belle indifference"*) with few anxieties associated with the consequences of the deficits (Aybek, Kanaan, & David, 2008; Heruti, Levy, Adunski, & Ohry, 2002; Stone, Zeman, & Sharpe, 2002). • Symptoms do not change with the presence of team members (e.g., the patient's gait pattern does not suddenly worsen when the physical therapist enters). If symptoms worsen or are exaggerated, then another disorder such as factitious disorder would need to be considered (American Psychiatric Association, 2000; Heruti et al., 2002). **Treatment** • The patient easily adopts the patient role or the dependent role. The therapist's role is to assist the patient to move away from the sick role and reestablish healthy occupational performance and roles (Ness, 2007). • Emphasize treatment of the symptoms, not the lack of a specific diagnosis. • Offer a placebo, thus providing the patient with the opportunity to save face. Patients with conversion disorder are very suggestible; therefore, providing the patient with goals for functional improvement with a clinical rationale is the most beneficial approach. For example, tell the patient who is experiencing difficulty walking that the "neuromuscular facilitation of tapping on the quadriceps strengthens the signals to the brain and will allow you to walk to the bathroom." This approach provides the patient with a viable way to save face because dramatic recovery is frequent with the proper intervention. • Remove adaptive devices such as a bedside commode as soon as possible to eliminate suggestions of the sick role that allows the "illness" to be perpetuated. • Encourage the patient to try new strategies and to push through difficulties. • Address stress management strategies. • Goal setting and rewards: — Goals should be concrete with clearly delineated functional expectations. — Suggested functional improvements should also be provided to the patient, such as "You will be able to dress yourself by tomorrow, as quickly as you are improving."

(continued)

Table 6.25. (continued)

Client Factor	Process
	— The patient should be involved in setting the goals and rewards with structuring provided by the therapist.
	— Positive reinforcement can be in the form of rewards such as allowing independence in the room or community passes with the family. For example, allow the patient independent bathroom privileges when mastery of safe and quality functional mobility is demonstrated.
Motor	Deficits can fluctuate and change completely from day to day. For instance, *blepharospasms* (involuntary contraction of the eyelid muscles open or closed or eye blinking) may recover, but the patient may now manifest gait abnormalities.

Evaluation

- Objective testing does not correlate with functional performance. For instance, a manual muscle test may indicate no hand strength, but the patient can reach for a cup of water if thirsty. The limb will often demonstrate "collapsing weakness" (Stone, Zeman, & Sharpe, 2002). The limb falls either with a very light touch or before the therapist has actually touched it during a manual muscle test.

- Spinal Injuries Center Test—Patient is supine and knee is manually flexed. A positive sign is noted when the tester releases the knees and they stay in position. A negative sign is noted if one or both of the legs fall (Smith et al., 2007).

- Hoover's sign—Used in the case of hemiplegia. The patient is supine in the bed, and the therapist puts a hand under each heel. The patient is then asked to actively raise up the "bad" leg. The therapist should feel a downward pressure under the "good" leg. The downward pressure under the good leg will not occur with a conversion disorder (Aybek et al., 2008; Smith et al., 2007; Stone et al., 2002).

- Reflexes are intact, including the bulbocavernosus reflex—A reflexive rectal reflex that is usually absent in spinal cord injury (Smith, et al., 2007).

- Muscle tone is normal. Rectal tone may be diminished because it has a volitional component (Smith et al., 2007).

- Strength in antagonistic muscles may be present. When the patient is attempting to flex the elbow, the extensors are also working, thus preventing flexion.
  - Jerky movements or tremors are exhibited.
  - Slow movements with concurrent exaggerated expressions of effort such as breath holding, painful expression, and tooth grinding are noted.
  - Resistance is felt by the therapist when trying to move a limb into a position.

Table 6.25. **(continued)**

Client Factor	Process

	• A "paralyzed" arm or leg may inadvertently move or move normally when attention is directed elsewhere. For example, during a task such as dressing or when lying down, the patient may move the leg up onto the bed. The patient may not be able to extend the leg, but when putting on pants, the patient stands on one leg.
	
	  — If the "paralyzed" arm is placed above the head, it may stay there for a moment, then fall to the side without hitting the head. Watch the quality of the downward movement.
	
	  — Ipsilateral sternocleidomastoid weakness is common in conversion disorder (Stone et al., 2002).
	
	Gait patterns
	
	• Do not usually follow any known type of gait abnormality, frequently presenting with astasia–abasia (Ness, 2007). This gait pattern presents with unusual incoordination in which the gait disturbance is dramatic, and the patient lurches wildly in various directions and falls only when safe. The patient may walk with the knees flexed, which is more difficult than in the normal manner.
	
	• Patient appears to be "walking on ice" (Aybek et al., 2008).
	
	• Patient may be dragging the entire leg behind him or her while walking (Stone et al., 2002).
	
	• Patients will often avoid a complete fall or injury by "falling" into the bed or grabbing nearby objects or a person to stabilize themselves (Ness, 2007; Stone et al., 2002). They will frequently appear to fail a Romberg test with a large sway pattern, but will grab onto the tester before falling.
	
	Treatment
	
	• Provide progressive challenges in a stepwise manner as patient demonstrates mastery of a skill.
	
	• Provide cues for movement quality vs. quantity, such as "regain control . . . imagine moving your arm correctly."
	
	• Ignore abnormal movement patterns by not commenting on them. Only comment on correct movements or performance.

Sensory	• Glove or stocking distribution with sharply delineated borders. • Patchy sensory loss; does not follow dermatomal patterns. • Inconsistent findings with repeated exams.
Autonomic	• Bowel and bladder control is retained. • No vital sign changes are noted. • Dysphagia is similar for solids and liquids. • No autonomic dysreflexia symptoms are noted in the case of spinal cord injury–type conversion.

Autonomic Dysfunction Syndrome

In *autonomic dysfunction syndrome (ADS)*, the ANS deregulates, causing sympathetic responses to increase significantly. This syndrome is thought to be "a loss of balance between the sympathetic and the parasympathetic nervous systems" (Lemke, 2007, p. 30) and is life threatening.

Autonomic Dysreflexia

Another form of ADS associated with the spinal cord is *autonomic dysreflexia,* which is the response of the ANS to a noxious stimulus that can be a life-threatening complication of SCI. Because it is specific to the SCI population, it is discussed separately (refer to the "Spinal Cord Injuries" section for further information).

Complex Regional Pain Syndrome

Complex regional pain syndrome (CRPS, formally called *reflex sympathetic dystrophy)* is considered a disease of the SNS. The current etiological theory is that the SNS overreacts disproportionately to a noxious stimulus, becoming a continuous sympathetically maintained reflex arc despite elimination of the stimulus. The symptoms may be present in one limb or, in more advanced cases, in multiple limbs, the face and eyes, or both. Occupational therapists do not generally see patients with CRPS as a primary diagnosis but as a comorbidity that may or may not have been diagnosed. However, it is imperative that findings consistent with CRPS be communicated to the medical staff. The treatment of this disorder is complex and time consuming and generally requires a longer duration of intervention than can be addressed in the acute care setting. Refer to Appendix 6.F for further information on symptoms and therapeutic intervention.

Evaluation of and Therapeutic Intervention for Neurological Patients

Because hospital stays are short, evaluation and intervention often occur concurrently. Evaluations for patients with a neurological disease are performed in the same manner as typical acute care evaluations and should be embedded within ADLs. The modality of choice should be ADLs, including functional mobility, because time is so limited. Performance skills that are of particular importance include motor function, cognition, and vision–perception. Neurological evaluations and therapeutic interventions are complex and varied for every patient, but many performance skill deficits are common across diagnostic neurological categories.

Occupation-centered interventions, even at the acute care level, further delineate occupational therapy from other allied health professions. Therapists should address the most important issues during the initial session, such as bed–chair position schedules, splinting needs, obtaining recommended patient equipment before discharge, and instructions for nurses and family regarding transfers, positioning, and feeding. Rehabilitative concepts should enhance strengths and adapt to or remediate functional performance. Judicious application of neuroscience concepts will maximize engagement in occupational endeavors. Client-centered care in a collaborative manner must be the priority focus of any clinician in the environmental context of acute care.

Acute care therapy can facilitate motor recovery in later stages of the continuum of care through appropriate positioning, family education, sensory input, and splinting. Incorporate guided hand-over-hand movement, weight bearing, bilateral usage, and sensory input into all treatment sessions. Provide occupation-centered exercises for the patient with a hemiplegic upper extremity (see Appendix 6.H).

Motor

Ideally, the motor evaluation and intervention should be performed in an upright position, because this position is optimal for function. Issues that should be addressed include

- *Functional ability* of the arms and legs during engagement in functional tasks.
- *Self-protection of the arm:* In all stages of upper-extremity recovery, the therapist

should indicate whether the patient protects the arm appropriately. Lack of self-protection provides a goal for the evaluation and is appropriate for the acute care setting, because injury can cause further complications.

- *Skin integrity* (i.e., reddened area in axilla and palm because of abnormal synergistic tone).
- *Pain:* Location and severity.
- *Tone* (see the Modified Ashworth Scale [Davis, 2001] in Table 6.26): Hypotonic or hypertonic (note whether the tone is flexor or extensor synergistic patterning).
- *Ataxia* (may have normal strength and full ROM but cannot control it effectively). Does not fit into the Modified Ashworth Scale, but may fit with the Brunnstrom levels at approximately Levels 3 or 4 depending on the severity of the dysmetria.
- *Finger-to-nose:* Instruct patient to move finger from his or her own nose to therapist's finger. This motion allows the therapist to assess the quality of the velocity and amplitude of movement.
- *Diadokinesis:* Ability to perform rapidly alternating movement, most commonly evaluated via bilateral pronation or supination.
- *Functional reach and grasp:* Assess the patient's ability to control strength and coordination using a Styrofoam cup. Reach for an empty Styrofoam cup, and raise it up toward the mouth. Assess whether the patient can control the force on the cup as it is grasped and his or her coordination when reaching for and moving the cup. To assess response to treatment and initiate neuromuscular reeducation, incorporate 5 minutes of upper-extremity weight bearing, then repeat the finger-to-nose test and a functional task such as reaching for and using a Styrofoam cup. If successful, then provide instruction to incorporate weight bearing into normal activities (e.g., leaning on the armrest of the chair). This task sets the stage for functional recovery in higher levels of the continuum of care.

Range of Motion and Strength

- Assess premorbid biomechanical limitations such as arthritis, rotator cuff tear, or bursitis.
- Assess proximal and distal ROM and strength, because they often return at different rates.
- ROM should be documented in terms of 0, ¼, ½, ¾, and full versus actual degrees. The degrees may fluctuate significantly on the basis of fatigue, pain, or position. Look at the overall movement of each joint and average the function. Once the clinician is proficient at estimating ROM, a goniometer will not be necessary.
- Do not complete manual muscle testing on a patient with CVA or TBI unless the movement appears near normal. Strength and coordination can fluctuate in neurological patients; therefore, the results of a manual muscle test may not be consistent. However, some physicians may insist on a manual muscle test score, so give an average functional score at the end of the evaluation.
- Provide education on passive ROM (PROM) for the hemiplegic upper extremity for supported shoulder flexion to 90° and external rotation (ER) with scapular mobilization as needed. Self range of motion (SROM) for shoulder flexion and external rotation is not an advantageous therapeutic intervention. No matter how hard the patient tries, the patient will not be able to achieve shoulder flexion above 90° or ER beyond 30° without compromising upper-extremity integrity. Provide these exercises as PROM that the family can perform to ensure that ROM is adequately achieved.
- To improve shoulder ROM, support the hemiplegic or weak arm by holding the humerus approximately 4 inches away from the axilla while maintaining ER. The thumb will also be pointing up. This proximal hold produces greater pain-free flexion at the hemiplegic shoulder than does a distal hold. In a study by Tyson and Chissim (2002), using this hold resulted in a 17.5° improvement in ROM measurements.

(Text continues on p. 263)

Table 6.26. Upper-Extremity Function

Modified Ashworth Scale	Brunnstrom Functional Upper-Extremity Level	Documentation	Acute Care Treatment Issues
0—Flaccid	1—Nonfunctional; total paralysis.	Is patient aware of arm? • Pain • Sensation • PROM • Absence of tone	• Splinting not yet indicated. • Arm positioning (family and nursing education): — Arm up on pillow when seated or in bed — Sling for ambulation only — Elevation to prevent edema. • SROM/PROM program for the family, patient, or both. • Weight bearing incorporated into functional mobility tasks to increase proprioceptive input. • Initiation of bilateral hand-over-hand tasks. • Initiation of weight-bearing strategies.
1—Slight increase in tone at the end of the range	2—Stabilizer-associated reactions signal the emergence of the Brunnstrom stabilizer Level II and can usually be seen with coughing and yawning.	• Flexor or extensor • Ability to bear weight with or without support at elbow and hand	• Splinting not usually indicated yet but if waking for 3 days with hand fisted, then may want to consider splinting. Consider using a resting mitt splint vs. a resting hand splint, because it can more easily be adapted in later levels of the continuum of care. • See other strategies listed earlier.
1+—Slight increase in tone at beginning of the range		• Flexor or extensor • Ability to bear weight with or without support at elbow and hand	• All strategies listed earlier. • Likely can begin gross assist with hand-over-hand tasks.

2—Marked increase in tone through the entire ROM, but arm can easily be passively moved.	3—Gross assist; tone is significant. Patient is usually able to use the hand to grossly grasp an object such as a toothpaste tube while using the other hand to remove lid. Document tasks the patient is able to perform and not perform with the hand, based on an occupational profile; for example, "patient is left handed with left hemiplegia; cannot feed self, but can grasp toothpaste tube to remove lid." 4—Functional assist; patient is able to isolate movement to perform tasks that deviate from limb synergies. Includes touching the small of the back, flexing to 90° with elbow extended, and pronation or supination with elbow at 90°.	• Flexor or extensor • Document tasks patient is able to perform and not perform with affected hand	• Splinting usually indicated. Consider using a resting mitt splint vs. a resting hand splint, because it can more easily be adapted at later levels of the continuum of care. A resting mitt splint places the patient in a reflex-inhibiting position with thumb abducted. • Reflex inhibiting positions would be helpful; that is, arm abducted and externally rotated on a pillow. • Keep a closer watch on skin protection, especially in the palm and axilla. • Gross assist-level activities with increasing independence. • Grasp-and-release and reaching-tasks component skills incorporated into such tasks as brushing teeth and obtaining toilet paper.
3—Tone evident throughout all of ROM, and PROM is difficult	Nonfunctional; may have some gross assist dependent on site of tone (e.g., severe at shoulder, but milder in hand).	• Flexor or extensor	• Also see gross assist level. • May need to aggressively address ROM with either a mobility tech or the family or be integrated into nursing care. • Address pain. • Reflex inhibiting positions recommended.
4—Rigid in flexion and extension	Nonfunctional because of tone.	• Flexor or extensor	• Splinting a must to prevent further permanent deformity. • Discuss with the physician use of antispasticity medications such as Baclofen or Zanaflex.

(continued)

Table 6.26. (continued)

Modified Ashworth Scale	Brunnstrom Functional Upper-Extremity Level	Documentation	Acute Care Treatment Issues
			• Focus all efforts on PROM and tone reduction to prevent joint changes such as heterotopic ossification (especially in traumatic brain injury).
No abnormal tone	5—Nondominant; able to use the hand fairly normally and in isolated movements that are not hindered by any synergistic patterning; may exhibit decreased fine motor coordination.	• Weakness, especially in the intrinsics • Occupational deficits as a result of reduced fine motor coordination • Mild sensory deficits often associated with this level	• Typically, no acute care intervention medically necessary at this level. However, if the patient is very motivated or is unable to pursue outpatient therapy, then provide an intrinsic strengthening home exercise program, including functional tasks handout and resistive exercises (Theraputty or rubber band). • Otherwise screen and recommend outpatient occupational therapy if the patient has a fine motor coordination task especially important to him or her (based on the occupational profile); for example, the patient is a typist or pianist. • Address sensory protection methods.
No abnormal tone	6—Normal; comparable to the unaffected hand. May demonstrate slight incoordination with rapid movements or when tired, but overall back to normal. May have mild intrinsic weakness if complaining of decreased grip when manual muscle testing is 5/5, resulting in very high-level occupational deficits once fatigued, such as playing a piano or typing.	• If this is only deficit, then likely will only screen and not complete a full evaluation	• No acute care intervention is indicated because it is not medically necessary. Engagement in normal activities will likely remediate very mild deficits.

Note. PROM = passive range of motion; ROM = range of motion; SROM = self range of motion.

Source. From Davis, J. (2001, December 17). Improving Upper-Extremity Function in Adult Hemiplegia. *OT Practice, 6,* pp. 8–13. Copyright © 2001 by the American Occupational Therapy Association. Adapted with permission.

Subluxation

- The progression from a mild instability to a rotator cuff tear is not uncommon and can be viewed in the following manner: Instability → Subluxation → Impingement → Rotator cuff tear.

- As motor control returns and spasticity increases, muscle imbalances emerge, and the shoulder girdle malalignment increases. Care must be taken to properly reduce the subluxation to minimize shoulder pathology (Duncan et al., 2005).

- Teach family and nursing proper positioning and precautions. Post written instructions in the patient's room with pictures to illustrate the arm supported in the bed and when up in a chair. Also instruct caregivers to avoid pulling on the arm and support the arm during transfers and mobility.

ROM Precautions

- Must have at least 45° ER before elevating arm. Scaption is optimal to properly align the glenohumeral joint.

- Shoulder should not be passively moved beyond 90° of flexion and abduction unless the scapula is upwardly rotated and the humerus is externally rotated.

- External rotation to 45° ultimately becomes the primary issue with the emergence of flexor synergistic patterning. Without 45° of ER, the patient will not be able to lift the arm.

- Do not use pulleys with unstable shoulders because it will contribute to shoulder tissue injury.

- PROM training for families should include instruction of no PROM past 90° to minimize painful pathologies as synergistic patterning emerges. Families will need education on proper PROM to avoid extreme flexion or abduction of the hemiplegic upper extremity. Maintaining ER of at least 45° is imperative for long-term recovery. If time is available for only one exercise or stretch, choose ER.

Refer to Table 6.26 for information regarding tone management, upper-extremity functional levels, and pertinent therapeutic interventions. (*Note.* The Modified Ashworth Scale and Brunnstrom functional levels have not been formally correlated with each other as implied in Table 6.26; however, because of similar clinical and therapeutic implications, they are presented together for brevity).

Neuroplasticity

Neuroplasticity is the ability of the brain to adapt or change through habituation, learning, and memory to facilitate recovery from injury. In the theory of constraint-induced therapy, the concepts of neuronal unmasking and rerouting skills into redundant sections of the brain are key to plasticity, thus causing anatomical and physiological changes. Neuroplastic changes can occur even in the early stages of acute care intervention because the brain is filled with redundancies that allow therapists to access functions via other routes.

Neuroplasticity applies to more than just constraint-induced upper-extremity exercises. Interventions that can facilitate neuroplasticity can easily be incorporated into intervention during the patient's acute care admission. Examples include using the affected hand to perform part of a sponge bath, self-feeding finger foods, sitting on the edge of the bed, and talking for the patient with aphasia. Functional task completion for cognitive remediation, bringing the affected leg up to don pants versus using a reacher, and instructing family to stand on the patient's affected side to encourage visual attention are other ways to promote neuroplasticity in neurological patients. Implementing therapy in a contextual, goal-directed manner will facilitate the neuronal unmasking through rerouting to the redundant systems.

Sensation

For low-level patients who are minimally conscious or comatose, pain assessment can be performed using nail bed pressure, tugging or pinching the ear, or a sternal rub. An object such as a pen can be used to provide sufficient pressure to elicit a reflexive withdrawal (refer to Chapter 1).

Pathological Reflexes

Although most occupational therapists do not perform reflex testing, a general awareness of pathological reflexes and their implications assists in designing appropriate intervention. *Reflexes* are an involuntary response to a stimulus (Venes, 2005). Abnormal responses indicate signs of upper or lower motor neuron dysfunction. *Upper motor neuron reflexes* usually produce a hyperactive response (i.e., increased tone), and *lower motor neuron reflexes* are hypoactive (see Table 6.27 for more information on reflexes).

Edema

Edema frequently occurs in patients who have reduced movement in a limb and is most prevalent in hypotonic upper extremities with poor sensation (Boomkamp-Koppen et al., 2005) Simple methods for prevention or reduction include elevation, functional use, and ROM. Retrograde massage does not usually reduce the edema in the long term. Edema gloves are not recommended for edematous hands because they lessen sensory input, further hinder already weakened movement and do not allow for functional usage of the hand. "Early recognition of the clinical signs and symptoms of edema of the hand and care for the hand and shoulder are essential to prevent diminishing functioning, delay in the rehabilitation process and the occurrence of shoulder–hand syndrome" (Boomkamp-Koppen, et al., 2005, p. 553). Refer to Chapter 1 for further information.

Splinting

Because Medicare gives a capitated fee for all intervention (medical and therapeutic), hospitals usually absorb the cost of prefabricated and custom splints. Judicious recommendations for splints are important (Lannin, Cusick, McCluskey, & Herbert, 2006). Medically necessary

reasons that might necessitate a splint include increasing tone with the fingers flexed so tightly that palmar skin integrity is at risk, edema, fracture, or nerve palsy. Consider the following:

- What will be the detrimental effects of not providing a splint until the patient is at the next level of the rehabilitation continuum?
- How soon will the patient likely be moving to that next level?
- Splints limit opportunities for normal sensory input.

If a splint is deemed necessary, consider using a volar-based resting mitt splint with wrist in neutral, fingers minimally flexed, and the thumb abducted. This splint allows for a reflex-inhibiting posture for flexor synergistic tone and can be modified later as needed.

Consider scheduling splint wear for nighttime with limited daytime wear (at most 4 hours), for example, splint on from 8:00 p.m. to 8:00 a.m. and from 12:00 p.m. to 4:00 p.m. Coordinate the splint wear schedule to meet the needs of the patient and the nursing staff. This splint schedule allows nurses time to don and doff the splint when they are doing their initial assessments at shift change and during every-4-hour neuro checks.

Cognition

Cognition is frequently the primary factor in determining an appropriate disposition. The most critical cognitive issues to be addressed are attention, working memory, and safety judgment. Several standardized evaluations are available that may be helpful; however, because of constraints they may be difficult to administer. Please see Chapter 1 for a discussion of assessments.

Attention

Attention is a continuum of arousal, alertness, and sensory registration. Clinically, attention manifests in a variety of ways, including (but not limited to) lethargy or hyperactivity, orienting to a stimulus, divided attention, or inability to sustain attention. This deficit area is usually

Table 6.27. **Pathological Reflexes**

Reflex	Stimulus	Normal Response	Abnormal Response
Babinski	Performed by running a blunt object from heel to toes in an arc along the metatarsals.	Flexion of all toes with plantar foot eversion.	Extension of big toe and fanning of other toes; indicative of upper motor neuron damage.
Romberg sign	Patient stands with feet together and eyes closed. Do not perform test if patient cannot maintain balance with eyes open.	Mild sway with no loss of balance.	Inability to maintain balance, indicating a loss of position sense or reduction of peripheral sensation.
Hoffman's sign	Flick the middle-finger nail bed.	No response.	Extension of the distal interphalange with subsequent flexion of the thumb, fingers, or both. Usually present in pyramidal tract lesions.
Doll's eyes	Turn head manually while watching the eyes. May need to hold the eyes open.	While turning the head, the eyes should continue to look at the ceiling.	If the eyes follow the movement of the head, this movement indicates brainstem involvement and a poor prognosis for survival.
Decerebrate posturing (see Figure 6.8)	Observe patient's position.	No abnormal tone.	Jaw clenched, neck extended, and upper and lower limbs internally rotated and extended, indicating neurological impairment of the brainstem from the subthalamus to midpons. Affects respiratory and cardiovascular centers located in the medulla. It is potentially life threatening, and decerebrate is more serious than decorticate. • Patients may progress or regress between decerebrate and decorticate. However, the regression into decerebrate posturing signifies a more life-threatening sequela.
Decorticate posturing (see Figure 6.8)	Observe patient's position.	No abnormal tone.	Upper limbs flex, but lower limbs extend with feet in plantar flexion. Indicates upper motor neuron lesion is above the level of the red nucleus.

Note. Created by Judy R. Hamby.

more prevalent in TBI and CVA patients with right parietal or frontal lobe insults. Attention is the primary skill required for memory and judgment. Gross attention evaluations are generally all that is possible in the acute care setting. Simple strategies might include

- Purposefully distracting the patient during a task by asking a question or initiating a conversation with others in the room. Conversely, remove all environmental distractors from the room to assess whether performance improves.
- Taking the patient on a walk and asking the patient to find his or her way back to his or her room, which will assess the patient's ability to perform a cognitive task in conjunction with the ability to maintain balance.
- Placing many items on the sink to assess whether the patient can attend to the pertinent details involved in choosing the appropriate tools for the job.
- Placing obstacles in the hall where the patient will be walking.
- Increasing alertness by using methods such as a cold washcloth on face, sternal rub, nail bed pressure, moving the bed up and down, or PROM.

Memory

Memory is the ability to recall information. The two types of memory are nondeclarative and declarative. *Nondeclarative,* or *implicit, memory* is more subjective and focused toward motor engrams; learned, emotional responses; and procedural recall. *Declarative,* or *explicit, memory* is the recall of facts, concepts, and events.

Memory involves four separate steps: encoding (greatly affected by attentional skills), consolidation, storage, and retrieval. Ascertaining the patient's ability to recall information and how many steps a patient can recall at any one time is important in assessing working memory for functional tasks such as medication management.

Memory does not need to be evaluated separately; rather, the evaluation can be embedded as part of another evaluation (e.g., upper-extremity motor) or during functional mobility. Refer to Appendix E for further information on memory.

Direction Following

Determining the number of steps the patient can follow and the primary method that elicits a patient's ability to follow directions is critical. The three modalities are *verbal, visual,* and *tactile.* Directions should be provided in the following order to ascertain the modality best suited to the patient (without interference from others in the room):

1. Verbal
2. Visual (demonstration)
3. Tactile (hand over hand)
4. Verbal and visual
5. Verbal and tactile
6. Verbal, visual, and tactile.

Safety Judgment

Safety and judgment should always be noted in the initial evaluation, especially if the patient is being discharged home. Comment on attention to environmental hazards and the patient's ability to anticipate the consequences of actions and ability to make safe decisions. Be explicit in the evaluation about the requirements for a safe environment and the reasons for them. Refer to Appendix M for further information regarding discharge planning. Examples of documentation for safety needs on discharge follow.

- Needs around-the-clock supervision at home to ensure safety because of poor memory and impulsivity.
- Patient safe for performance of BADLs but will need assistance for medications and meal preparation because of decreased memory and inattention to task.
- Patient will require moderate physical assistance and supervision at home because of decreased performance of BADLs, functional mobility, and poor safety judgment.

Vision and Perception

People's ability to accurately see and perceive the world provides the information necessary for them to make accurate motor decisions, protect themselves from hazards, and interact with the environment. *Vision* is the integrity of the ocular system, and *perception* is the analysis of what is seen. In the neurological population, three distinct issues are commonly present: *oculomotor dysfunction, visual deficits,* or *perceptual deficits.*

Ask the patient whether any vision changes such as blurry, double vision or loss of visual field have been noted. Move on to the next performance area if the answer is "no." If functional deficits are noted later, then formally evaluate them.

The following areas should be assessed if functional deficits are noted:

- Visual gaze preference (gross evaluation—Is the patient ignoring one side?)
- Basic ROM in all visual fields, binocularly and monocularly
- Visual field cut (Does the patient seem to be vaguely aware of the impaired visual field, but does not turn head?)
- Visual acuity (tested functionally with clock, TV, employee badge, or get-well card)
- Oculomotor control—Observation of behaviors and physiological symptoms, including
  — Head tilt;
  — Shutting one eye;
  — Squinting;
  — Headaches;
  — Muscle aches;
  — Increased spasticity;
  — Nausea and vomiting;
  — Increased blood pressure, heart rate, and respiration rate with movement; and
  — Decreased cooperation or increased agitation in visually stimulating environments or with increasingly difficult tasks.

If the eye does not close on its own because of a VIIth cranial nerve palsy, the eye must be manually shut at all times; otherwise, the patient can lose sight in that eye because of the high potential for corneal abrasions, infection, and dry eyes. Tape the eye shut if necessary. Never allow a patient to tape his or her eyes open.

Oculomotor Control Deficits

If any of the signs for oculomotor control deficits are present, the patient may have cranial nerve deficits, diplopia, or both (see Table 6.4 regarding cranial nerve testing). The different features of diplopia are

- Horizontal and near-vision diplopia involves IIIrd cranial nerve palsy.
- Horizontal and far-vision diplopia involves VIth cranial nerve palsy.
- Vertical diplopia or rotated diplopia involves IVth cranial nerve palsy (predominantly) or IIIrd cranial nerve palsy (rarely).
- Ptosis involves IIIrd cranial nerve palsy. Do not patch because the ptosis is a natural patch. If the ptosis is partial, then partial occlusion may still be required because diplopia may be present even through a partially opened eye.
- The direction of vision that causes diplopia to be worse indicates the action of the paretic muscle.

Therapeutic intervention for diplopia generally involves patching. The two types of patching techniques are full patching or partial occlusion. However, if the diplopia is the result of increased ICP or anticonvulsant medicine toxicity, patch the eye until the medical issue clears. Do not use partial occlusion.

Patching

Patching has no therapeutic value except when the diplopia is so severe that compensatory strategies are necessary. It does not allow for binocularity in any gaze direction. Patching is compensatory and does not facilitate recovery (Nelms, 2004; Rucker & Tomsak, 2005). It also reduces depth perception, can cause balance difficulties, and can be uncomfortable, especially if the dominant eye is patched.

- Alternate the patch between eyes every couple of hours with an emphasis on the nondominant eye.

- If the patient wears glasses and full patching is desired, tape the entire lens.

Partial Occlusion

Partial occlusion eliminates the field of view that is double while preserving the field of view that is intact.

- Tape, using an opaque tape (e.g., 3M Transpore™ tape) where the diplopia occurs (Rucker & Tomsak, 2005). Unilateral partial occlusion is usually sufficient, but occasionally binasal occlusion produces better results. One side is usually smaller. See Figure 6.10 for examples of partial occlusion.
- Partial occlusion works best for near diplopia.
- If the patient does not wear glasses, try first with safety glasses or lightly tinted sunglasses. If this process works, then ask the family to purchase nonprescription glasses at the drugstore.

Visual Field Cuts

If visual field cuts are present, then educate the patient on scanning strategies, which include scanning in the impaired space first with head turning. Eventually, the patient will reduce this to just eye movements because the head movements may themselves become a distraction.

Gaze Preference

For patients with a significant gaze preference without a field cut or for "pushers" (patients who use their strong arm and leg to push toward the impaired side, causing a severe balance deficit), the following suggestions may be useful:

- Occlude sound visual field and perform tasks (see Figure 6.11).
- Partially occlude vision: Right half-field patching (hemispatial sunglasses) or regular glasses patched in the unaffected space seem to work better than monocular patching (Freeman, 2001).

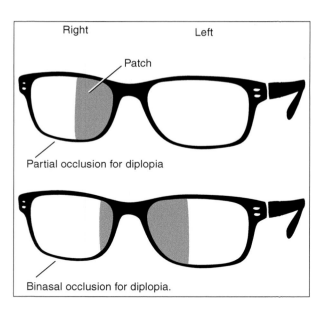

Figure 6.10. Partial occlusion.
Source. Richard Fritzler, Medical Illustrator, Roswell, GA.

Balance and Functional Mobility

The primary motor component skill of functional mobility is static and dynamic sitting and standing balance. This skill must be addressed because it will significantly affect the performance of all tasks. The following progression can be used for evaluation and treatment, but use clinical judgment and start at the highest level possible. If balance is impaired, it is appropriate to write goals to address functional balance and mobility, as long as the goal includes an explicitly stated area of occupation. A functional mobility evaluation should proceed in the following manner:

- *Supported sitting*—Ideally, testing in unsupported positions is the most functional; however, sometimes it is quickly apparent that balance is a significant issue when the patient is slumped over in the bed. A more cautious method of testing is to place a hospital bed into the most upright or full-chair position and observe how well a patient is able to maintain supported sitting and the ability to lean forward and resume midline, upright posture.
- *Unsupported sitting*—If supported sitting is successful, return the bed to a flattened

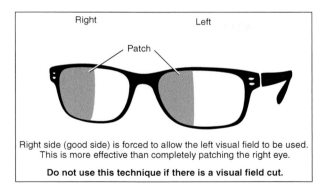

Right

Left

Patch

Right side (good side) is forced to allow the left visual field to be used. This is more effective than completely patching the right eye.

Do not use this technique if there is a visual field cut.

Figure 6.11. Constraint-induced occlusion for left visual inattention.
Source. Richard Fritzler, Medical Illustrator, Roswell, GA.

position and sit the patient on the edge of the bed. Be sure to assess whether the patient is able to sit on the edge of the bed without supporting himself or herself using the arms. If the patient appears to be supporting himself or herself with the arms, request the patient to release support with just one and then both arms. It is acceptable to document information such as "Patient able to sit on edge of the bed with minimal assist; however, requires the support of at least one arm. Therefore, patient requires assistance for bilateral tasks when sitting unsupported." Assessing the patient's ability to maintain balance while engaged in a task is imperative because cognitive demand increases and balance is reduced when the patient is no longer solely focused on maintaining upright sitting.

- *Supported stand (static and dynamic)—* Whether the patient can stand supported determines the most basic ability to perform standing components of BADLs and functional mobility. First, assess whether the patient is able to move the legs against gravity in supine or sitting. If the patient is successful, try marching in place to assess the patient's ability to shift weight and whether the patient can bear weight on both legs. Once basic balance sufficient for mobility is determined, instruct the patient to step away from the bed or chair to ensure he or she is not using the bed to provide stability by leaning his or her legs against

it. Assess the patient without any assistive devices (e.g., walker, cane) to obtain accurate results, but do not compromise patient safety.

- *Unsupported stand (static and dynamic)—* This stand determines the patient's ability to engage in BADLs. Maintain contact with the patient at all times if the patient requires assistance during supported standing. If the patient is unable to stand safely or demonstrates poor insight or judgment (by attempting to get out of bed repeatedly), recommend other safety measures, including identification of the patient as being a high fall risk (usually site-specific patient identifiers) and use of a bed alarm. The patient may also require one-on-one nursing supervision or family involvement. Patients on anticoagulant medication are at a higher risk for internal bleeding, so precautionary fall measures are essential.

- *Transfers and functional mobility—*Begin with side stepping along the edge of the bed. Then, if possible, remove the footboard of the bed and walk around the bed, which will allow the patient to sit quickly if needed. Once the patient's basic mobility with ambulation is assessed, then attempt ambulation to a specific destination, such as the bathroom. Patient success with room mobility may assist in earlier removal of the Foley catheter. If the patient has a hemiparetic leg, transferring to the unaffected side is usually easier. However, the transfer to the affected side must also be evaluated because the patient eventually has to get back into bed. Transferring to the affected side might also be considered a form of constraint-induced therapy, by forcing attention and more weight onto the affected side.

- *Pushers—*Transfer to the affected side, which allows the patient to push in the correct direction.

"The mind can do only what the brain is equipped to do, and so man must find out what kind of brain he has before he can understand his own behavior" (Luce & Segal, 1966).

Conclusion

The therapist's role in the acute care setting is to ascertain the impact of neurological deficits on performance skills by implementing therapy in a contextual, goal-directed manner that will facilitate performance improvement. The context, unique to acute care, also includes the patient's immediate medical needs and issues. The medical issues cannot, at this point in the continuum of care, be relegated to second place behind function because the medical issues define the function. This diverse patient population necessitates that the occupational therapist understand the neurological underpinnings to understand the patient's functional behavior so that efficacious intervention can be provided.

References

Adams, H. P., Jr., del Zoppo, G., Alberts, M. J., Bhatt, D. L., Brass, L., Furlan, A., et al. (2007). Guidelines for the early management of adults with ischemic stroke. *Stroke, 38,* 1655–1711. doi:10.1161/STROKEAHA.107.181486

Adams, H. P., Jr., del Zoppo, G. J., & von Kummer, R. (2006). *Management of stroke: A practical guide for the prevention, evaluation, and treatment of acute stroke* (3rd ed.). West Islip, NY: Professional Communications.

Adler, C. (2006). Spinal cord injury. In H. M. Pendleton & W. Schultz-Krohn (Eds.), *Pedretti's occupational therapy: Practice skills for physical dysfunction* (6th ed., pp. 903–930). St. Louis, MO: Mosby.

Agrawal, A., Timothy, J., & Thapa, A. (2007). Neurogenic fever. *Singapore Medical Journal, 48,* 492–494.

Alberti, A., Paciaroni, M., Caso, V., Venti, M., Palmerini, F., & Agnelli, G. (2008). Early seizures in patients with acute stroke: Frequency, predictive factors, and effect on clinical outcome. *Vascular Health and Risk Management, 4,* 715–720.

American Heart Association. (2009). *Stroke risk factors.* Retrieved June 21, 2009, from www.americanheart.org/presenter.jhtml?identifier=4716

American Psychiatric Association. (1994). *Diagnostic and statistical manual of mental disorders* (4th ed.). Washington, DC: Author.

American Psychiatric Association. (2000). Somatoform disorders: Conversion disorder. In *Diagnostic and statistical manual of mental disorders* (4th ed., text rev., Diagnosis Code 300.11). Washington, DC: Author. Retrieved November 29, 2008, from http://online.statref.com/document.aspx?fxid=37&docid=239

American Spinal Injury Association: International Standards for Neurological Classification of Spinal Cord Injury, revised 2000; Atlanta, GA, Reprinted 2008.

Atkins, M., Clark, D., & Waters, R. (2003). Upper limb orthoses. In V. W. Lin & D. D. Cardenas (Eds.), *Spinal cord medicine: Principles and practice* (pp. 663–674). New York: Demos Medical.

Aybek, S., Kanaan, R. A., & David, A. S. (2008). The neuropsychiatry of conversion disorder. *Current Opinion in Psychiatry, 21,* 275–280.

Barker, E., & Hobdell, R. (1994). Neuromuscular disorders. In E. Barker (Ed.), *Neuroscience nursing* (pp. 591–615). St. Louis, MO: Mosby.

Barron, K. W., & Blair, R. W. (1999). Motor 3: The autonomic nervous system. In H. Cohen (Ed.), *Neuroscience for rehabilitation* (2nd ed., pp. 277–302). Philadelphia: Lippincott Williams & Wilkins.

Bartt, R. E., & Topel, J. L. (2007). Autoimmune and inflammatory disorders. In C. G. Goetz (Ed.), *Textbook of clinical neurology* (3rd ed.). Philadelphia: W. B. Saunders. Retrieved November 4, 2008, from MDConsult database.

Blackman, J. A., Patrick, P. D., Buck, M. L., & Rust, R. S. (2004). Paroxysmal autonomic instability with dystonia after brain injury. *Archives of Neurology, 61,* 321–328.

Bladin, C. F., Alexandov, A. V., Bellavance, A., Bornstein, N., Chambers, B., Coté, R., et al. (2000). Seizures after stroke. *Archives of Neurology, 57,* 1617–1622.

Boomkamp-Koppen, H. G., Visser-Meilly, J. M., Post, M. W., & Prevo, A. J. (August 19, 2005). Post-stroke hand swelling and edema: Prevalence and relationship with impairment and disability. *Clinical Rehabilitation, 19*(5), 552–559.

Broderick, J., Connolly, S., Feldmann, E., Hanley, D., Kase, C., Krieger, D., et al. (2007). Guidelines for the management of spontaneous intracerebral hemorrhage in adults 2007 update. *Stroke, 38,* 2001–2023. doi:10.1161/strokeaha.107.183689

Bronfin, L. (2005). Neuromuscular disorders. In H. H. Zaretsky, E. F. Richter III, & M. G. Eisenberg (Eds.), *Medical aspects of disability: A handbook for the rehabilitation professional* (3rd ed., pp. 382–409). New York: Springer.

Brown, V. (2008, April). *Care of the acute stroke patient.* Lecture presented at Wellstar Stoke Group, Wellstar Cobb Hospital, Austell, Georgia.

Cancer facts and figures 2008 [Monograph]. (2008). Retrieved November 16, 2008, from http://www.cancer.org/acs/groups/content/@nho/documents/document/2008cafffinalsecuredpdf.pdf

Casper, M. L., Nwaise, I. A., Croft, J. B., & Nilasena, D. S. (2008). *2008 atlas of stroke hospitalizations among Medicare beneficiaries.* Atlanta, GA: Centers for Disease Control and Prevention. Retrieved September 18, 2008, from www.cdc.gov/dhdsp/library/stroke_hospitalization_atlas.htm

Davis, J. (2001, December 17). Improving upper-extremity function in adult hemiplegia. *OT Practice, 6,* 8–13. Retrieved August 12, 2008, from http://www.aota.org/Pubs/OTP/1997-2007/Features/2001/f-121701.aspx

Dixon, T. M., Layton, B. S., & Shaw, R. M. (2005). Traumatic brain injury. In H. H. Zaretsky, E. F. Richter III, & M. G. Eisenberg (Eds.), *Medical aspects of disability* (3rd ed., pp. 119–149). New York: Springer.

Duncan, P. W., Zorowitz, R., Bates, B., Choi, J. Y., Glasberg, J. J., Graham, G. D., et al. (2005). Management of adult stroke rehabilitation care: A clinical practice guideline. *Stroke, 36,* 100–143. doi:10.1161/01.str.0000180861.54180.ff

Epilepsy Foundation. (n.d.). *Seizures and syndromes.* Retrieved September 23, 2008, from www.epilepsyfoundation.org/about/types/types/index.cfm

Fernandez, A., Schmidt, J. M., Claassen, J., Pavlicova, M., Huddleston, D., Kreiter, K. T., et al. (2007). Fever after subarachnoid hemorrhage: Risk factors and impact on outcome. *Neurology, 68,* 1013–1019.

Fields, L., Blackshear, C., Mortimer, D., & Wallace, S. (2005). *Guide to the care of the patient with intracranial pressure monitoring* [AANN Clinical Practice Guideline Series]. Retrieved August 5, 2008, from www.aann.org/pubs/guidelines.html

Flaherty, A. W., & Rost, N. S. (2007). *The Massachusetts General Hospital handbook of neurology* (2nd ed.). Philadelphia: Lippincott Williams & Wilkins.

Freeman, E. (2001). Unilateral spatial neglect: New treatment approaches with potential application to occupational therapy. *American Journal of Occupational Therapy, 55,* 401–408.

Frey, L. C. (2003). Epidemiology of posttraumatic epilepsy: A critical review. *Epilepsia, 44*(Suppl. 10), 11–17.

Gerber, C. S. (2005). Understanding and managing coma stimulation: Are we doing everything we can? *Critical Care Nursing Quarterly, 28*(2), 94–108.

Giancino, J. T., & Trott, C. T. (2004). Rehabilitative management of patients with disorders of consciousness. *Journal of Head Trauma Rehabilitation, 19,* 254–265.

Gillett, B. (2007, October 20). *Transient ischemic attack: Evaluation and management.* Lecture presented at WellStar Health System, WellStar Cobb Hospital, Austell, GA.

Gottesman, R. F., Sherman, P. M., Grega, M. A., Yousem, D. M., Borowicz, L. M., Jr., Selnes, O. A., et al. (2006). Watershed strokes after cardiac surgery: Diagnosis, etiology, and outcome. *Stroke, 37,* 2306–2311. doi:10.1161/01.STR.0000236024.68020.3a

Grüner, M. L., & Terhaag, D. (2000). Multimodal early onset stimulation (MEOS) in rehabilitation after brain injury. *Brain Injury, 14*(6), 585–594.

Hagen, C. (1998). *Rancho levels of cognitive functioning: The revised levels* (3rd ed.). Encinitas, CA: Author. Retrieved January 3, 2009, from www.rancho.org/patient_education/cognitive_levels.pdf

Hagen, C., Malkmus, D., & Durham, P. (1979). *Rehabilitation of the head injured adult: Comprehensive physical management.* Downey, CA: Rancho Los Amigos National Rehabilitation Center.

Hallevi, H., Albright, K. C., Aronowski, J., Barreto, A. D., Martin-Schild, S., Khaja, A. M., et al. (2008). Intraventricular hemorrhage: Anatomic relationships and clinical implications. *Neurology, 70,* 848–852.

Hamby, J. R. (2006). Visual and perceptual changes in Parkinson's disease: Impact on motor control and implications for treatment. *Physical Disabilities Special Interest Section Quarterly, 29*(1), 1–4.

Harden, R. N. (2008). *Complex regional pain syndrome: Treatment guidelines.* Retrieved August 30, 2008, from www.rsdsa.org/3/clinical_guidelines/index.html

Hemphill, J. C., III., & Smith, W. S. (2008). Neurologic critical care, including hypoxic-ischemic encephalopathy and subarachnoid hemorrhage. In A. S. Fauci, D. L. Kasper, D. L. Longo, E. Braunwald, S. L. Hauser, J. L. Jameson, et al. (Eds.), *Harrison's principles of internal medicine* (17th ed., pp. 1720–1729). New York: McGraw-Hill. Retrieved November 29, 2008, from STAT!Ref Online Electronic Medical Library database.

Heron, M. P., Hoyert, D. L., Xu, J., Scott, C., & Tejada-Vera, B. (2008). Deaths: Preliminary data for 2006. *National Vital Statistics Reports, 56*(16). Retrieved February 20, 2009, from www.cdc.gov/nchs/data/nvsr/nvsr56/nvsr56_16.pdf

Heruti, R. J., Levy, A., Adunski, A., & Ohry, A. (2002). Conversion motor paralysis disorder: Overview and rehabilitation model. *Spinal Cord, 40,* 327–334.

Honrubia, V. (2000). Quantitative vestibular function tests and the clinical examination. In S. J. Herdman (Ed.), *Vestibular rehabilitation* (2nd ed., pp. 105–171). Philadelphia: F. A. Davis.

Janus, T. J., & Yung, W. A. (2007). Primary neurological tumors. In C. G. Goetz (Ed.), *Textbook of clinical neurology* (3rd ed., pp. 1053–1068). Philadelphia: W. B. Saunders. Retrieved from MDConsult database on November 8, 2008.

Kalmar, K., & Giacino, J. T. (2005). The JFK Coma Recovery Scale—Revised. *Neuropsychological Rehabilitation, 15,* 454–460.

Keshner, E. A. (2007). Postural abnormalities in vestibular disorders. In S. J. Herdman (Ed.), *Vestibular rehabilitation* (3rd ed., pp. 54–75). Philadelphia: F. A. Davis.

Kline, L. B., & Bajandas, F. J. (2004). *Neuroophthalmology* (5th ed.). Thorofare, NJ: Slack.

Lannin, N. A., Cusick, A., McCluskey, A., & Herbert, R. D. (2006). Effects of splinting on wrist contracture after stroke: A randomized controlled trial. *Stroke, 38,* 111–116. doi:10.1161/01.STR.0000251722.77088.12

Lemke, D. M. (2007). Sympathetic storming after severe traumatic brain injury. *Critical Care Nurse, 27*(1), 30–37.

Li, M. (2008). Guillain–Barré syndrome. In F. J. Domino (Ed.), *The 5-minute clinical consult* (16th ed., pp. 528–529). Philadelphia: Lippincott Williams & Wilkins.

Littlejohns, L. (2004). *Correlative neuroanatomy* [DVD]. Placentia, CA: Adventures in Neuroscience & Avant Productions. (Available from American Association of Neuroscience Nurses, 4700 West Lake Avenue, Glenview IL 60025)

Lloyd-Jones, D., Adams, R., Carnethon, M., De Simone, G., Ferguson, B., Flegal, K., et al. (2009). Heart disease and stroke statistics 2009 update: A report from the American Heart Association Statistics Committee and Stroke Statistics Subcommittee. *Circulation, 119,* e21–e181. doi:10.1161/circulationaha.108.191261

Lomen-Hoerth, C. (2004). Characterizations of amyotrophic lateral sclerosis and frontotemporal dementia. *Dementia and Geriatric Cognitive Disorders, 17,* 337–341.

Lowenstein, D. H. (2009). Epilepsy after head injury: An overview. *Epilepsia, 50*(Suppl. 2), 4–9.

Luce, G. G., & Segal, J. (1966). Brain quotes and proverbs. In *Heartquotes: Quotes of the heart.* Retrieved October 5, 2008, from www.heartquotes.net/Brain.html.

Mahanes, D. (2006). Advanced neurologic concepts. In M. Chulay & S. M. Burns (Eds.), *AACN essentials of critical care nursing* (pp. 477–500). New York: McGraw-Hill. Retrieved November 29, 2008, from STAT!Ref Online Electronic Medical Library database.

McGovern-Denk, M., Levine, M., & Casey, P. (2005). Approaching occupation with amyotrophic lateral sclerosis. *Physical Disabilities Special Interest Section Quarterly, 28*(4), 1–4.

Moskowitz, C. (1994). Movement disorders. In E. Barker (Ed.), *Neuroscience nursing* (pp. 536–557). St. Louis, MO: C. V. Mosby.

Myasthenia gravis fact sheet. (2008, July 25). Retrieved November 16, 2008, from www.ninds.nih.gov/disorders/myasthenia_gravis/detail_myasthenia_gravis.htm.

National Cancer Institute. (2008, August 1). *Adult brain tumors treatment (PDQ).* Retrieved November 16, 2008, from www.cancer.gov/cancertopics/pdq/treatment/adultbrain/healthprofessional/allpages.

National Institute of Neurological Disorders and Stroke. (2003, April). *Amyotrophic lateral sclerosis fact sheet* (NIH Publication No. 00–916). Retrieved June 26, 2009, from www.ninds.nih

.gov/disorders/amyotrophiclateralsclerosis/detail _amyotrophiclateralsclerosis.htm.

National Institute of Neurological Disorders and Stroke. (2008a, September 22). *NINDS Miller Fisher syndrome information page.* Retrieved November 15, 2008, from www.ninds.nih.gov/ disorders/miller_fisher/miller_fisher.htm.

National Institute of Neurological Disorders and Stroke. (2008b, July 28). *Traumatic brain injury: Hope through research.* Retrieved August 31, 2008, from www.ninds.nih.gov/disorders/tbi/detail_tbi.htm.

National Institute of Neurological Disorders and Stroke. (2009, May 15). *Transverse myelitis fact sheet* (NIH Publication No. 01–4841). Retrieved June 26, 2009, from www.ninds.nih.gov/disorders/ transversemyelitis/detail_transversemyelitis.htm

National Institute of Neurological Disorders and Stroke. (2010). *NIH Stroke Scale.* Available online at http://www.ninds.nih.gov/doctors/NIH_stroke _scale.pdf

National Spinal Cord Injury Statistical Center. (2009, April). *Spinal cord injury facts and figures at a glance.* Birmingham, AL: Author. Retrieved June 26, 2009, from http://images.main.uab.edu/ spinalcord/pdffiles/FactsApr09.pdf

Nelms, A. C. (2004, December 20). New visions: Collaboration between OTs and optometrists can make a difference in treating clients with visual problems. *OT Practice.* Retrieved May 19, 2005, from http://www.aota.org/Pubs/OTP/1997-2007/ Features/2000/f-071700_1.aspx.

Nervous: Cranial nerves exam. (n.d.). Retrieved March 18, 2008, from www.clinicalexam.com/ pda/n_cranial_nerves_exam.htm

Ness, D. (2007). Physical therapy management for conversion disorder: Case series. *Journal of Neurologic Physical Therapy, 31,* 30–39.

Oh, D. W., Yoo, E. Y., Yi, C. H., & Kwon, O. Y. (2005). Case Report—Physiotherapy strategies for a patient with conversion disorder presenting abnormal gait. *Physiotherapy Research International, 10*(3), 164–168.

Oh, H., & Seo, W. (2003). Sensory stimulation programme to improve recovery in comatose patients. *Journal of Clinical Nursing, 12,* 394–404.

Pelak, V. S. (2004, March). Evaluation of diplopia: An anatomical and systematic approach. *Hospital Physician,* pp. 16–25.

Piper, T. (Ed.). (2008). Watershed. In *Stedman's medical dictionary for the health professions and nursing* (6th ed., p. 1673). Philadelphia: Wolters Kluwer.

Pirko, I., & Noseworthy, J. H. (2007). Demyelinating disorders of the central nervous system. In C. G. Goetz (Ed.), *Textbook of clinical neurology* (3rd ed., pp. 1103–1126). Philadelphia: W. B. Saunders.

Plumb, M., & Bain, P. (2007). *Essential tremor.* New York: Oxford University Press.

Pugh, S., Mathiesen, C., Meighan, M., Summers, D., & Zrelak, P. (2008). *Guide to the care of the hospitalized patient with ischemic stroke* (AANN Clinical Practice Guideline Series; 2nd ed., revised). Retrieved June 24, 2009, http://www .aann.org/pubs/cpg/AANNischemicstroke.pdf

Quattrini, C., & Tesfaye, S. (2003). Understanding the impact of painful diabetic neuropathy. *Diabetes/ Metabolism Research and Reviews, 19*(Suppl. 1), S2–S8.

Rangel-Castillo, L., Gopinath, S., & Robertson, C. S. (2008). Management of intracranial hypertension. *Neurologic Clinics, 22,* 521–541.

Rappaport, M. (2005). The disability rating and coma/ near-coma scales in evaluating severe head injury. *Neuropsychological Rehabilitation, 15,* 442–453.

Redekop, G. J. (2007). Prognostic factors and targets for intervention after subarachnoid hemorrhage [Editorial]. *Stroke, 38,* 2217–2218. doi:10.1161/ STROKEAHA.107.488338

Ringholz, G. M., & Greene, S. R. (2006). The relationship between amyotrophic lateral sclerosis and frontotemporal dementia. *Current Neurology and Neuroscience Reports, 6,* 387–392.

Rosamond, W., Flegal, K., Furie, K., Go, A., Greenlund, K., Haase, N., et al. (2008). Heart disease and stroke statistics—2008 update: A report from the American Heart Association Statistics Committee and Stroke Statistics Subcommittee. *Circulation, 117,* e25–e146. doi:10.1161/circulationaha.107.187998.

Rothstein, J. M., Roy, S. H., & Wolf, S. L. (1998). Neuroanatomy, neurology, and neurological therapy. In *The rehabilitation specialist's handbook* (pp. 233–485). Philadelphia: F. A. Davis.

Rubin, M., & Safdieh, J. E. (2007). *Netter's concise neuroanatomy.* Philadelphia: W. B. Saunders.

Rucker, J. C., & Tomsak, R. L. (2005). Binocular diplopia: A practical approach. *Neurologist, 11,* 98–110.

Sacco, R. L. (2005). Pathogenesis, classification, and epidemiology of cerebrovascular disease. In L. P. Rowland (Ed.), *Merritt's neurology* (11th ed., pp. 275–290). Philadelphia: Lippincott Williams & Wilkins.

Sathornsumetee, S., Rich, J. N., & Reardon, D. A. (2007). Diagnosis and treatment of high-grade astrocytoma. *Neurologic Clinics, 25,* 1111–1139.

Segal, G., Levin, V. A., Steiger, B., & Falk, D. (2005). Functions of the cerebral hemispheres. In *A primer of brain tumors: A patient's reference manual* (Figure 2). Des Plaines, IL: American Brain Tumor Association. Retrieved February 17, 2008, from http://neurosurgery.mgh.harvard.edu/abta/primer.htm#Section8

Sen, J., Belli, A., Albon, H., Morgan, L., Petzold, A., & Kitchen, N. (2003). Triple-H therapy in the management of aneurysmal subarachnoid haemorrhage. *Lancet, 2,* 614–620.

Shields, R. W., & Wilbourn, A. J. (2007). Demyelinating disorders of the peripheral nervous system. In C. G. Goetz (Ed.), *Textbook of clinical neurology* (3rd ed., pp. 1135–1152). Philadelphia: W. B. Saunders.

Smith, H. E., Rynning, R. E., Okafor, C., Zaslavsky, J., Tracy, J. I., Ratliff, J., et al. (2007). Evaluation of neurological deficit without apparent cause: The importance of a multidisciplinary approach. *Journal of Spinal Cord Medicine, 30,* 509–517.

Southam, M., & Schmidt, A. (2006). Disorders of the motor unit. In H. M. Pendleton & W. Schultz-Krohn (Eds.), *Pedretti's occupational therapy: Practice skills for physical dysfunction* (6th ed., pp. 931–949). St. Louis, MO: Mosby.

Stone, J., Zeman, A., & Sharpe, M. (2002). Functional weakness and sensory disturbance. *Journal of Neurology, Neurosurgery, and Psychiatry, 73,* 241–245.

Teasdale, G., & Jennett, B. (1974). Assessment of coma and impaired consciousness: A practical scale. *Lancet, 2,* 81–84.

Teasell, R. W., & Shapiro, A. P. (2002). Case series: Misdiagnosis of conversion disorders. *American Journal of Physical Medicine and Rehabilitation, 81,* 236–240.

Tyson, S. F., & Chissim, C. (2002). The immediate effect of handling technique on range of movement in the hemiplegic shoulder. *Clinical Rehabilitation, 16,* 137–140.

Venes, D. (Ed.). (2005). Reflex. In *Taber's cyclopedic medical dictionary* (20th ed., p. 1864). Philadelphia: F. A. Davis.

Young, P. A., & Young, P. H. (1997). *Basic clinical neuroanatomy.* Baltimore: Lippincott Williams & Wilkins.

Appendix 6.A.

National Institutes of Health (NIH) Stroke Scale

**N I H
STROKE
SCALE**

Patient Identification. ___ ___-___ ___ ___-___ ___ ___

Pt. Date of Birth ___ ___/___ ___/___ ___

Hospital _____(___ ___-___ ___)

Date of Exam ___ ___/___ ___/___ ___

Interval: [ ] Baseline   [ ] 2 hours post treatment   [ ] 24 hours post onset of symptoms ±20 minutes   [ ] 7-10 days
[ ] 3 months   [ ] Other _____(___ ___)

Time: ___ ___:___ ___   [ ]am [ ]pm

Person Administering Scale _____

Administer stroke scale items in the order listed. Record performance in each category after each subscale exam. Do not go back and change scores. Follow directions provided for each exam technique. Scores should reflect what the patient does, not what the clinician thinks the patient can do. The clinician should record answers while administering the exam and work quickly. Except where indicated, the patient should not be coached (i.e., repeated requests to patient to make a special effort).

Instructions	Scale Definition	Score
1a. Level of Consciousness: The investigator must choose a response if a full evaluation is prevented by such obstacles as an endotracheal tube, language barrier, orotracheal trauma/bandages. A 3 is scored only if the patient makes no movement (other than reflexive posturing) in response to noxious stimulation.	0 = **Alert**; keenly responsive. 1 = **Not alert**; but arousable by minor stimulation to obey, answer, or respond. 2 = **Not alert**; requires repeated stimulation to attend, or is obtunded and requires strong or painful stimulation to make movements (not stereotyped). 3 = **Responds** only with reflex motor or autonomic effects or totally unresponsive, flaccid, and areflexic.	_____
1b. LOC Questions: The patient is asked the month and his/her age. The answer must be correct - there is no partial credit for being close. Aphasic and stuporous patients who do not comprehend the questions will score 2. Patients unable to speak because of endotracheal intubation, orotracheal trauma, severe dysarthria from any cause, language barrier, or any other problem not secondary to aphasia are given a 1. It is important that only the initial answer be graded and that the examiner not "help" the patient with verbal or non-verbal cues.	0 = **Answers** both questions correctly. 1 = **Answers** one question correctly. 2 = **Answers** neither question correctly.	_____
1c. LOC Commands: The patient is asked to open and close the eyes and then to grip and release the non-paretic hand. Substitute another one step command if the hands cannot be used. Credit is given if an unequivocal attempt is made but not completed due to weakness. If the patient does not respond to command, the task should be demonstrated to him or her (pantomime), and the result scored (i.e., follows none, one or two commands). Patients with trauma, amputation, or other physical impediments should be given suitable one-step commands. Only the first attempt is scored.	0 = **Performs** both tasks correctly. 1 = **Performs** one task correctly. 2 = **Performs** neither task correctly.	_____
2. Best Gaze: Only horizontal eye movements will be tested. Voluntary or reflexive (oculocephalic) eye movements will be scored, but caloric testing is not done. If the patient has a conjugate deviation of the eyes that can be overcome by voluntary or reflexive activity, the score will be 1. If a patient has an isolated peripheral nerve paresis (CN III, IV or VI), score a 1. Gaze is testable in all aphasic patients. Patients with ocular trauma, bandages, pre-existing blindness, or other disorder of visual acuity or fields should be tested with reflexive movements, and a choice made by the investigator. Establishing eye contact and then moving about the patient from side to side will occasionally clarify the presence of a partial gaze palsy.	0 = **Normal.** 1 = **Partial gaze palsy**; gaze is abnormal in one or both eyes, but forced deviation or total gaze paresis is not present. 2 = **Forced deviation**, or total gaze paresis not overcome by the oculocephalic maneuver.	_____

N I H
STROKE
S C A L E

Patient Identification. ___ ___-___ ___ ___-___ ___ ___

Pt. Date of Birth ___ ___/___ ___/___ ___

Hospital _____(___ ___-___ ___)

Date of Exam ___ ___/___ ___/___ ___

Interval: [ ] Baseline   [ ] 2 hours post treatment   [ ] 24 hours post onset of symptoms ±20 minutes   [ ] 7-10 days
[ ] 3 months   [ ] Other _____(___ ___)

3. Visual: Visual fields (upper and lower quadrants) are tested by confrontation, using finger counting or visual threat, as appropriate. Patients may be encouraged, but if they look at the side of the moving fingers appropriately, this can be scored as normal. If there is unilateral blindness or enucleation, visual fields in the remaining eye are scored. Score 1 only if a clear-cut asymmetry, including quadrantanopia, is found. If patient is blind from any cause, score 3. Double simultaneous stimulation is performed at this point. If there is extinction, patient receives a 1, and the results are used to respond to item 11.	0 = **No visual loss.** 1 = **Partial hemianopia.** 2 = **Complete hemianopia.** 3 = **Bilateral hemianopia** (blind including cortical blindness).	_____
4. Facial Palsy: Ask – or use pantomime to encourage – the patient to show teeth or raise eyebrows and close eyes. Score symmetry of grimace in response to noxious stimuli in the poorly responsive or non-comprehending patient. If facial trauma/bandages, orotracheal tube, tape or other physical barriers obscure the face, these should be removed to the extent possible.	0 = **Normal** symmetrical movements. 1 = **Minor paralysis** (flattened nasolabial fold, asymmetry on smiling). 2 = **Partial paralysis** (total or near-total paralysis of lower face). 3 = **Complete paralysis** of one or both sides (absence of facial movement in the upper and lower face).	_____
5. Motor Arm: The limb is placed in the appropriate position: extend the arms (palms down) 90 degrees (if sitting) or 45 degrees (if supine). Drift is scored if the arm falls before 10 seconds. The aphasic patient is encouraged using urgency in the voice and pantomime, but not noxious stimulation. Each limb is tested in turn, beginning with the non-paretic arm. Only in the case of amputation or joint fusion at the shoulder, the examiner should record the score as untestable (UN), and clearly write the explanation for this choice.	0 = **No drift;** limb holds 90 (or 45) degrees for full 10 seconds. 1 = **Drift;** limb holds 90 (or 45) degrees, but drifts down before full 10 seconds; does not hit bed or other support. 2 = **Some effort against gravity;** limb cannot get to or maintain (if cued) 90 (or 45) degrees, drifts down to bed, but has some effort against gravity. 3 = **No effort against gravity;** limb falls. 4 = **No movement.** UN = **Amputation** or joint fusion, explain: _____ **5a. Left Arm** **5b. Right Arm**	 _____ _____
6. Motor Leg: The limb is placed in the appropriate position: hold the leg at 30 degrees (always tested supine). Drift is scored if the leg falls before 5 seconds. The aphasic patient is encouraged using urgency in the voice and pantomime, but not noxious stimulation. Each limb is tested in turn, beginning with the non-paretic leg. Only in the case of amputation or joint fusion at the hip, the examiner should record the score as untestable (UN), and clearly write the explanation for this choice.	0 = **No drift;** leg holds 30-degree position for full 5 seconds. 1 = **Drift;** leg falls by the end of the 5-second period but does not hit bed. 2 = **Some effort against gravity;** leg falls to bed by 5 seconds, but has some effort against gravity. 3 = **No effort against gravity;** leg falls to bed immediately. 4 = **No movement.** UN = **Amputation** or joint fusion, explain: _____ **6a. Left Leg** **6b. Right Leg**	 _____

N I H
STROKE
S C A L E

Patient Identification. ___ ___-___ ___ ___-___ ___ ___

Pt. Date of Birth ___ ___/___ ___/___ ___

Hospital _____(___ ___-___ ___)

Date of Exam ___ ___/___ ___/___ ___

Interval: [ ] Baseline [ ] 2 hours post treatment [ ] 24 hours post onset of symptoms ±20 minutes [ ] 7-10 days
[ ] 3 months [ ] Other _____(___ ___)

7. Limb Ataxia: This item is aimed at finding evidence of a unilateral cerebellar lesion. Test with eyes open. In case of visual defect, ensure testing is done in intact visual field. The finger-nose-finger and heel-shin tests are performed on both sides, and ataxia is scored only if present out of proportion to weakness. Ataxia is absent in the patient who cannot understand or is paralyzed. Only in the case of amputation or joint fusion, the examiner should record the score as untestable (UN), and clearly write the explanation for this choice. In case of blindness, test by having the patient touch nose from extended arm position.	0 = **Absent.** 1 = **Present in one limb.** 2 = **Present in two limbs.** UN = **Amputation** or joint fusion, explain: _____	_____
8. Sensory: Sensation or grimace to pinprick when tested, or withdrawal from noxious stimulus in the obtunded or aphasic patient. Only sensory loss attributed to stroke is scored as abnormal and the examiner should test as many body areas (arms [not hands], legs, trunk, face) as needed to accurately check for hemisensory loss. A score of 2, "severe or total sensory loss," should only be given when a severe or total loss of sensation can be clearly demonstrated. Stuporous and aphasic patients will, therefore, probably score 1 or 0. The patient with brainstem stroke who has bilateral loss of sensation is scored 2. If the patient does not respond and is quadriplegic, score 2. Patients in a coma (item 1a=3) are automatically given a 2 on this item.	0 = **Normal;** no sensory loss. 1 = **Mild-to-moderate sensory loss;** patient feels pinprick is less sharp or is dull on the affected side; or there is a loss of superficial pain with pinprick, but patient is aware of being touched. 2 = **Severe to total sensory loss;** patient is not aware of being touched in the face, arm, and leg.	_____
9. Best Language: A great deal of information about comprehension will be obtained during the preceding sections of the examination. For this scale item, the patient is asked to describe what is happening in the attached picture, to name the items on the attached naming sheet and to read from the attached list of sentences. Comprehension is judged from responses here, as well as to all of the commands in the preceding general neurological exam. If visual loss interferes with the tests, ask the patient to identify objects placed in the hand, repeat, and produce speech. The intubated patient should be asked to write. The patient in a coma (item 1a=3) will automatically score 3 on this item. The examiner must choose a score for the patient with stupor or limited cooperation, but a score of 3 should be used only if the patient is mute and follows no one-step commands.	0 = **No aphasia;** normal. 1 = **Mild-to-moderate aphasia;** some obvious loss of fluency or facility of comprehension, without significant limitation on ideas expressed or form of expression. Reduction of speech and/or comprehension, however, makes conversation about provided materials difficult or impossible. For example, in conversation about provided materials, examiner can identify picture or naming card content from patient's response. 2 = **Severe aphasia;** all communication is through fragmentary expression; great need for inference, questioning, and guessing by the listener. Range of information that can be exchanged is limited; listener carries burden of communication. Examiner cannot identify materials provided from patient response. 3 = **Mute, global aphasia;** no usable speech or auditory comprehension.	_____
10. Dysarthria: If patient is thought to be normal, an adequate sample of speech must be obtained by asking patient to read or repeat words from the attached list. If the patient has severe aphasia, the clarity of articulation of spontaneous speech can be rated. Only if the patient is intubated or has other physical barriers to producing speech, the examiner should record the score as untestable (UN), and clearly write an explanation for this choice. Do not tell the patient why he or she is being tested.	0 = **Normal.** 1 = **Mild-to-moderate dysarthria;** patient slurs at least some words and, at worst, can be understood with some difficulty. 2 = **Severe dysarthria;** patient's speech is so slurred as to be unintelligible in the absence of or out of proportion to any dysphasia, or is mute/anarthric. UN = **Intubated** or other physical barrier, explain:_____	_____

N I H
STROKE
SCALE

Patient Identification. ___ ___-___ ___ ___-___ ___ ___

Pt. Date of Birth ___ ___/___ ___/___ ___

Hospital _____(___ ___-___ ___)

Date of Exam ___ ___/___ ___/___ ___

Interval: [ ] Baseline   [ ] 2 hours post treatment   [ ] 24 hours post onset of symptoms ±20 minutes   [ ] 7-10 days
 [ ] 3 months   [ ] Other _____(___ ___)

11. Extinction and Inattention (formerly Neglect): Sufficient information to identify neglect may be obtained during the prior testing. If the patient has a severe visual loss preventing visual double simultaneous stimulation, and the cutaneous stimuli are normal, the score is normal. If the patient has aphasia but does appear to attend to both sides, the score is normal. The presence of visual spatial neglect or anosagnosia may also be taken as evidence of abnormality. Since the abnormality is scored only if present, the item is never untestable.	0 = **No abnormality.** 1 = **Visual, tactile, auditory, spatial, or personal inattention** or extinction to bilateral simultaneous stimulation in one of the sensory modalities. 2 = **Profound hemi-inattention or extinction to more than one modality;** does not recognize own hand or orients to only one side of space.	_____

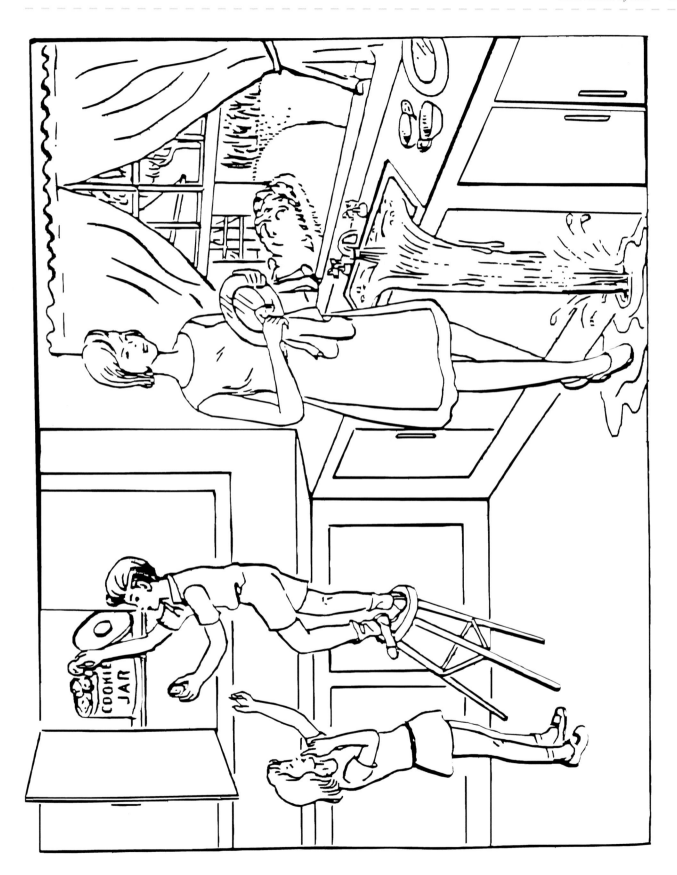

You know how.

Down to earth.

I got home from work.

Near the table in the dining room.

They heard him speak on the radio last night.

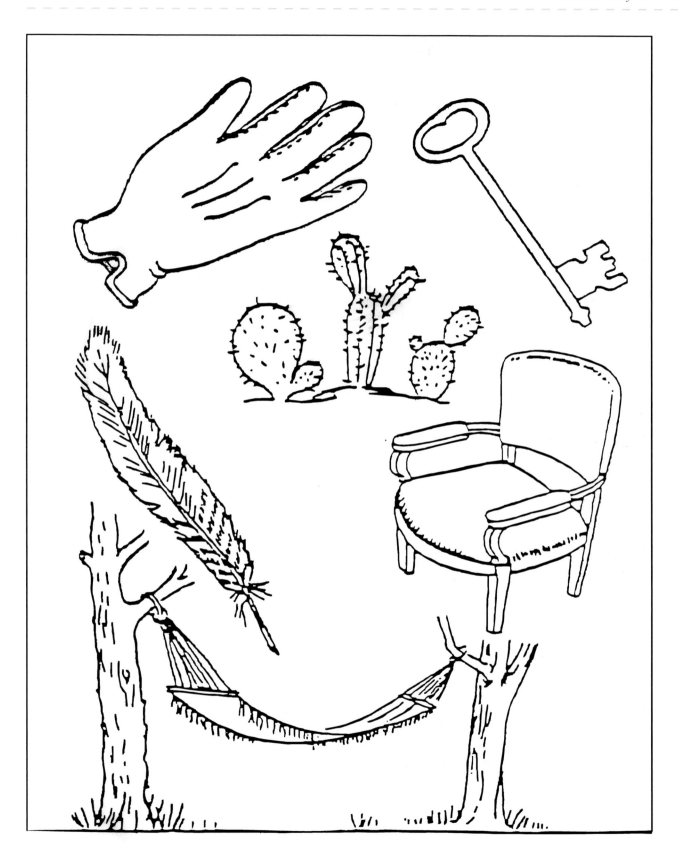

MAMA

TIP – TOP

FIFTY – FIFTY

THANKS

HUCKLEBERRY

BASEBALL PLAYER

Note. CN = cranial nerve.
Source. National Institute of Neurological Disorders and Stroke. (2010). *NIH Stroke Scale.* Available online at http://www.ninds.nih.gov/doctors/NIH_Stroke_Scale.pdf

Appendix 6.B.
Glasgow Coma Scale

Response	Points	Date	Date	Date
Eye opening				
• Spontaneous	4			
• To speech	3			
• To pain	2			
• None	1			
Best motor response				
• Obeys commands	6			
• Localized to pain stimuli	5			
• Withdraws from pain stimuli	4			
• Decorticate flexion	3			
• Decerebrate extension	1			
• None	1			
Verbal response	5			
• Oriented	4			
• Confused conversation	3			
• Inappropriate words	2			
• Incomprehensible sounds	1			
• None				
Score: 3–15 points	Total:			

Note. Head injury classification: severe head injury, Glasgow Coma Scale (GCS) score of ≤8; moderate head injury, GCS score of 9–12; mild head injury, GCS score of 13–15.
Source. Teasdale and Jennett (1974). Adapted with permission.

Appendix 6.C.

Rancho Los Amigos Cognitive Scale–Revised

Date/Time			
Evaluator			
Overall level			
Overall performance			
• Signs of stress (What? When? Where? How long?).			
• Response delay (unable to respond, seconds, minutes).			
• Repetitions of instructions required or patient's questions.			
• Rate of information preferred by patient (slow, chunked, normal).			
• Amount of task, instructions, or questions tolerated by patient.			
• Complexity of steps patient is able to follow verbally (one, two, or three steps). Demonstration (D), verbal (V), tactile (T).			
• "Time out" needed between tasks (unable to continue, seconds, minutes).			
Comments:			
Level I—No response: Total assistance			
• Complete absence of observable change in behavior when presented with visual, auditory, tactile, proprioceptive, vestibular, or painful stimuli.			
Level II—Generalized response: Total assistance			
• Demonstrates generalized reflex response to painful stimuli.			
• Responds to repeated auditory stimuli with increased or decreased activity.			
• Responds to external stimuli with physiological changes generalized, gross body movement, not-purposeful vocalization, or all of these.			
• Responses noted above may be same regardless of type and location of stimulation.			
• Responses may be significantly delayed.			

Level III—Localized response: Total assistance

- Demonstrates withdrawal or vocalization to painful stimuli.

- Turns toward or away from auditory stimuli.

- Blinks when strong light crosses the visual field.

- Follows moving object passed within the visual field.

- Responds to discomfort by pulling tubes or restraints.

- Responds inconsistently to simple commands.

- Responses directly related to type of stimulus.

- May respond to some people (especially family and friends) but not to others.

Level IV—Confused/agitated: Maximal assistance

- Alert and in heightened state of activity.

- Automatic responses to noxious stimuli includes attempts to remove restraints or tubes.

- May perform motor activities such as sitting, reaching, and walking but without any apparent purpose or on another's request.

- Very brief moments of attention to basic familiar persons or activities.

- Absent short-term memory.

- May cry out or scream out of proportion to stimulus even after its removal.

- May exhibit aggressive or flight behavior.

- Mood may swing from euphoric to hostile with no apparent relationship to environmental events.

- Unable to cooperate with treatment efforts.

- Verbalizations are frequently incoherent, inappropriate to activity or environment, or both.

Level V—Confused, inappropriate nonagitated: Maximal assistance

- Alert, not agitated, but may wander randomly or with a vague intention of going home.

- May become agitated in response to external stimulation, lack of environmental structure, or both.

(continued)

• May be oriented to self, but not to place or time.			
• Frequent brief periods, nonpurposeful sustained attention.			
• Severely impaired recent memory, with confusion of past and present in reaction to ongoing activity.			
• Absent goal-directed, problem-solving, self-monitoring behavior.			
• Often demonstrates inappropriate use of objects without external direction.			
• May be able to perform previously learned tasks when structured and cues provided.			
• Unable to learn new information.			
• Able to respond appropriately to simple commands fairly consistently with external structures and cues.			
• Responses to simple commands without external structure are random and nonpurposeful in relation to command.			
• Able to converse on a social, automatic level for brief periods of time when provided external structure and cues.			
• Verbalizations about present events become inappropriate and confabulatory when external structure and cues are not provided.			
Level VI—Confused, appropriate: Moderate assistance			
• Inconsistently oriented to person, time, and place.			
• Able to attend to highly familiar tasks in nondistracting environment for 30 minutes with moderate redirection.			
• Remote memory has more depth and detail than recent memory.			
• Vague recognition of some staff.			
• Able to use assistive memory aid with maximum assistance.			
• Emerging awareness of appropriate response to self, family, and basic needs.			
• Moderate assist to problem-solve barriers to task completion.			
• Shows carryover for relearned familiar tasks (e.g., self-care).			

- Emerging awareness of appropriate response to self, family, and basic needs.

- Shows carryover for relearned familiar tasks (e.g., self-care).

- Maximum assistance for new learning with little or no carryover.

- Unaware of impairments, disabilities, and safety risks.

- Consistently follows simple directions.

- Verbal expressions are appropriate in highly familiar and structured situations.

Level VII—Automatic, appropriate: Minimal assistance for daily living skills

- Consistently oriented to person and place in highly familiar environments. Moderate assistance for orientation to time.

- Able to attend to highly familiar tasks in a nondistracting environment for at least 30 minutes with minimal assist to complete tasks.

- Minimal supervision for new learning.

- Demonstrates carryover of new learning.

- Initiates and carries out steps to complete familiar personal and household routine but has shallow recall of what he or she has been doing.

- Able to monitor accuracy and completeness of each step in routine personal and household ADLs and modify plan with minimal assistance.

- Superficial awareness of his or her condition but unaware of specific impairments and disabilities and the limits they place on his or her ability to safely, accurately, and completely carry out his or her household, community, work, and leisure ADLs.

- Minimal supervision for safety in routine home and community activities.

- Unrealistic planning for the future.

- Limited or absent ability to think about consequences of a decision or action.

- Overestimates abilities.

(continued)

- Limited to absent ability to take others' perspectives.

- Self-focused.

- Limited or absent ability to recognize inappropriate social interaction behavior.

Level VIII—Purposeful, appropriate: Stand-by assistance

- Consistently oriented to person, place, and time.

- Independently attends to and completes familiar tasks for 1 hour in distracting environments.

- Able to recall and integrate past and recent events.

- Uses assistive memory devices to recall daily schedule and to-do lists and record critical information for later use with stand-by assistance.

- Initiates and carries out steps to complete familiar personal, household, community, work, and leisure routines with stand-by assistance and can modify the plan when needed with minimal assistance.

- Requires no assistance once new tasks and activities are learned.

- Aware of and acknowledges impairments and disabilities when they interfere with task completion but requires stand-by assistance to take appropriate corrective action.

- Thinks about consequences of a decision or action with minimal assistance.

- Overestimates or underestimates abilities.

- Acknowledges others' needs and feelings and responds appropriately with minimal assistance.

- Frequently prone to irritability and depression.

- Low frustration tolerance, easily angered.

- Impulsive and self-focused.

- Uncharacteristically dependent or independent

- Able to recognize and acknowledge inappropriate social interaction behavior while it is occurring and takes corrective action with minimal assistance.

Level IX—Purposeful, appropriate: Stand-by assistance on request

• Independently shifts back and forth between tasks and completes them accurately for at least 2 consecutive hours.			
• Uses assistive memory devices to recall daily schedule and to-do lists and record critical information for later use with assistance when requested.			
• Initiates and carries out steps to complete familiar personal, household, work, and leisure tasks independently and unfamiliar personal, household, work, and leisure tasks with assistance when requested.			
• Aware of and acknowledges impairments and disabilities when they interfere with task completion and takes appropriate corrective action, but requires stand-by assistance to anticipate a problem before it occurs and take action to avoid it.			
• Able to think about consequences of decisions or actions with assistance when requested.			
• Accurately estimates abilities but requires stand-by assistance to adjust to task demands.			
• Acknowledges others' needs and feelings and responds appropriately with stand-by assistance.			
• Depression may continue.			
• May be easily irritable.			
• May have low frustration tolerance.			
• Able to self-monitor appropriateness of social interaction with stand-by assistance.			

Level X—Purposeful, appropriate: Modified independent

• Able to handle multiple tasks simultaneously in all environments but may require periodic breaks.			
• Able to independently procure, create, and maintain own assistive memory devices.			
• Independently initiates and carries out steps to complete familiar and unfamiliar personal, household, community, work, and leisure tasks but may require more than usual amount of time or compensatory strategies to complete them.			

(continued)

• Anticipates impact of impairments and disabilities on ability to complete daily living tasks and takes action to avoid problems before they occur, but may require more than usual amount of time, compensatory strategies, or both.			
• Able to independently think about consequences of decisions or actions but may require more than usual amount of time or compensatory strategies to select the appropriate decision or action.			
• Accurately estimates abilities and independently adjusts to task demands.			
• Able to recognize the needs and feelings of others and automatically respond in appropriate manner.			
• Periodic periods of depression may occur.			
• Irritability and low frustration tolerance when sick, fatigued, under emotional stress, or all of these.			
• Social interaction behavior is consistently appropriate.			

Note. ADLs = activities of daily living.
Source. From Hagen, C. (1998). *Rancho Levels of Cognitive Functioning: The Revised Levels* (3rd ed.). Encinitas, CA: Author. Copyright © 1998 by Chris Hagen. Reprinted with permission.

Rancho Los Amigos Cognitive Scale–Original

Rancho Level	Clinical Correlate
I	No response
II	Generalized response
III	Localized response
IV	Confused–agitated
V	Confused–inappropriate
VI	Confused–appropriate
VII	Automatic–inappropriate
VIII	Purposeful and appropriate

Source. From Hagen, C., Malkmus, D., and Durham, P. (1979). *Rehabilitation of the Head Injured Adult: Comprehensive Physical Management* (pp. 87–89). Downey, CA: Professional Staff Association of Rancho Los Amigos National Rehabilitation Center. Copyright © by Rancho Los Amigos National Rehabilitation Center. Reprinted with permission.

Appendix 6.D.

Seizure Documentation

Check all that apply and describe as necessary.

Motor component

Automatisms:

☐ Lip smacking   ☐ Fumbling   ☐ Picking at clothes

☐ Other: _____

_____

Eye deviation (specify direction of gaze):

_____

Jaw clenched

Limb movement (limbs, head, neck, and/or trunk)

☐ Subtle or overt twitching   ☐ Stiffening   ☐ Jerking

Specify limbs:

_____

Progression of seizure

☐ Localized

☐ Spread from one body part to another—Describe progression:

_____

Vital signs/bodily functions

☐ Mouth frothing   ☐ Perspiration   ☐ Incontinence of urine or feces

☐ Respiratory changes (dyspnea, apnea, cyanosis)

Prodromal symptoms and events

☐ Aura (describe):

_____

☐ Describe the events immediately preceding the seizure (in pain from a procedure, exertion, occurred at rest):

_____

Length of seizure: _____ minutes/seconds

Injuries (describe severity and location)

☐ Tongue bitten and bleeding

☐ Bruises:

_____

☐ Dislocated shoulder (right/left)

☐ Broken bones:

_____

☐ Cuts and abrasions:

_____

Postictal phase description

☐ Weakness or paralysis—Right/left, upper extremity, lower extremity, severity:

_____

☐ Speech difficulty (describe):

_____

☐ Pain (where and intensity):

_____

☐ Behavioral changes (lethargy, confused):

_____

☐ Recollection of seizure (none, all, partial)

☐ Did the patient recall the word given at the onset of the seizure? yes/no

☐ No discernible postictal phase

☐ Length of time for recovery: _____

Appendix 6.E.

American Spinal Injury Association Standard Neurological Classification of Spinal Cord Injury

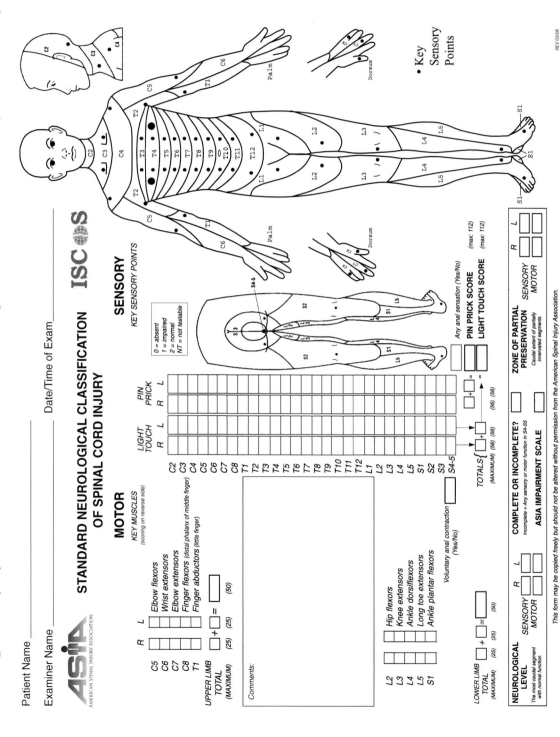

Patient Name _____

Examiner Name _____ Date/Time of Exam _____

STANDARD NEUROLOGICAL CLASSIFICATION OF SPINAL CORD INJURY

ISC⬤S

MOTOR

KEY MUSCLES *(scoring on reverse side)*

R   L
C5 Elbow flexors
C6 Wrist extensors
C7 Elbow extensors
C8 Finger flexors *(distal phalanx of middle finger)*
T1 Finger abductors *(little finger)*

UPPER LIMB TOTAL (MAXIMUM) ☐ (25) + ☐ (25) = ☐ (50)

Comments:

L2 Hip flexors
L3 Knee extensors
L4 Ankle dorsiflexors
L5 Long toe extensors
S1 Ankle plantar flexors

Voluntary anal contraction (Yes/No) ☐

LOWER LIMB TOTAL (MAXIMUM) ☐ (25) + ☐ (25) = ☐ (50)

SENSORY KEY SENSORY POINTS

LIGHT TOUCH   PIN PRICK
R   L   R   L
C2
C3
C4
C5
C6
C7
C8
T1
T2
T3
T4
T5
T6
T7
T8
T9
T10
T11
T12
L1
L2
L3
L4
L5
S1
S2
S3
S4-5

0 = absent
1 = impaired
2 = normal
NT = not testable

TOTALS { ☐ + ☐ (56) (56) = ☐ (MAXIMUM) (112) PIN PRICK SCORE
☐ + ☐ (56) (56) = ☐ (112) LIGHT TOUCH SCORE }

Any anal sensation (Yes/No) ☐

• Key Sensory Points

Palm   Dorsum

NEUROLOGICAL LEVEL
The most caudal segment with normal function
       R   L
SENSORY ☐ ☐
MOTOR ☐ ☐

COMPLETE OR INCOMPLETE?
Incomplete = Any sensory or motor function in S4-S5

ASIA IMPAIRMENT SCALE ☐

ZONE OF PARTIAL PRESERVATION
Caudal extent of partially innervated segments
       R   L
SENSORY ☐ ☐
MOTOR ☐ ☐

This form may be copied freely but should not be altered without permission from the American Spinal Injury Association.

REV 03/06

MUSCLE GRADING

0   total paralysis

1   palpable or visible contraction

2   active movement, full range of motion, gravity eliminated

3   active movement, full range of motion, against gravity

4   active movement, full range of motion, against gravity and provides some resistance

5   active movement, full range of motion, against gravity and provides normal resistance

5* muscle able to exert, in examiner's judgment, sufficient resistance to be considered normal if identifiable inhibiting factors were not present

NT not testable. Patient unable to reliably exert effort or muscle unavailable for testing due to factors such as immobilization, pain on effort or contracture.

ASIA IMPAIRMENT SCALE

☐ **A = Complete:** No motor or sensory function is preserved in the sacral segments S4–S5.

☐ **B = Incomplete:** Sensory but not motor function is preserved below the neurological level and includes the sacral segments S4–S5.

☐ **C = Incomplete:** Motor function is preserved below the neurological level, and more than half of key muscles below the neurological level have a muscle grade less than 3.

☐ **D = Incomplete:** Motor function is preserved below the neurological level, and at least half of key muscles below the neurological level have a muscle grade of 3 or more.

☐ **E = Normal:** Motor and sensory function are normal.

CLINICAL SYNDROMES (OPTIONAL)

☐ Central Cord
☐ Brown–Sequard
☐ Anterior Cord
☐ Conus Medullaris
☐ Cauda Equina

STEPS IN CLASSIFICATION

The following order is recommended in determining the classification of individuals with SCI.

1. Determine sensory levels for right and left sides.

2. Determine motor levels for right and left sides.
   Note: In regions where there is no myotome to test, the motor level is presumed to be the same as the sensory level.

3. Determine the single neurological level.
   This is the lowest segment where motor and sensory function is normal on both sides and is the most cephalad of the sensory and motor levels determined in Steps 1 and 2.

4. Determine whether the injury is Complete or Incomplete (sacral sparing).
   If voluntary anal contraction = No AND all S4–S5 sensory scores = 0 AND any anal sensation = No, then injury is COMPLETE. Otherwise injury is incomplete.

5. Determine ASIA Impairment Scale (AIS) Grade:

   Is injury Complete?   If **YES**, AIS = A   Record ZPP
   (For ZPP record lowest dermatome or myotome on each side with some [non-zero score] preservation)

   NO

   Is injury motor incomplete?   If **NO**, AIS = B
   (Yes = voluntary anal contraction OR motor function more than three levels below the motor level on a given side)

   YES

   Are at least half of the key muscles below the (single) neurological level graded 3 or better?

   NO   YES

   AIS = C   AIS = D

   If sensation and motor function is normal in all segments, AIS = E.
   Note: AIS E is used in follow-up testing when an individual with a documented SCI has recovered normal function. If at initial testing no deficits are found, the individual is neurologically intact; the ASIA Impairment Scale does not apply.

Source. American Spinal Injury Association: International Standards for Neurological Classification of Spinal Cord Injury, revised 2000, Atlanta, GA, Reprinted 2008.

Appendix 6.F.

Complex Regional Pain Syndrome

Symptoms	Medical Intervention	Therapeutic Intervention
Trophic • Skin may change color with activity or while at rest. Colors can range from blue, purple, red, white, and mottled combinations of all the colors. • Brawny skin. • Skin can be dull or shiny. • Hair is sparse and coarse. • Nails may be ridged. Vasomotor • Temperature of extremity may vary widely and suddenly from very cold (usually skin is blue) to very hot (usually skin is red). • Poor tolerance of cold temperatures (especially water). Motor • Muscle atrophy and shortening—May note contractures in advanced cases. • May have dystonia. • Weakness. • Tremors. • Resting position—Usually guarded with fingers flexed or in a lumbrical or half-flexed position with elbow flexed.	Treating Physicians • Neurologists. • Pain specialists. • Orthopedist. Medication • Cymbalta. • Neurontin. Surgical interventions • Ablative sympathectomy. • Sympathetic nerve blocks either at the brachial plexus (for upper extremity) or the lumbar plexus (for lower extremity). • Intrathecal pain pumps (Harden, 2008).	Psychosocial • Be gentle with physical examinations because they may be very painful. • Patients may be leery and fearful of medical professionals if the symptoms have been undiagnosed for a long time. Many patients have already been referred to psychiatry for drug-seeking behaviors and for symptoms being "only in their head." • Patients expect the therapists to minimize the pain and force unrealistic activities. Therapy that sets the stage for future intervention • Weight bearing—May only include placing the hand flat on a smooth warm surface such as his or her own leg or a wooden tabletop. • Functional use—Most patients cannot tolerate using the limb for long periods. Performance of tasks with the affected limb is also what causes the most pain. Helping the patient to understand this conundrum will prove helpful to the rehabilitation process. • Sensory reeducation—Using normal desensitization strategies (e.g., rubbing with different textures, contrast baths, putting hand in dry beans).

(continued)

Appendix 6.F. (*continued*)

Symptoms	Medical Intervention	Therapeutic Intervention
		Contraindications
		• Immobilization is contraindicated and contributes to the disease process. Splinting is contraindicated; however, it may be indicated in some instances (e.g., unstable fractures when patient is not a candidate for surgical intervention) and immobilization is unavoidable.
		• Manual therapy is very painful and should not be attempted in the early stages of intervention.
		• Icing.
		• Heating modalities may decrease pain; however, they must be used with caution because of decreased sensation.
		Discharge recommendations
		• Outpatient therapy with therapist experienced in treating complex regional pain syndrome.
		• Outpatient workup with physician experienced in treating complex regional pain syndrome.
		• Aquatic therapy in a warm pool may reduce pain.

Note. Created by Judy R. Hamby.

Appendix 6.G.

Precautions After Transsphenoidal Adenomectomy (Pituitary Surgery)

Precautions (usually for 4–6 weeks, but check with neurosurgeon):

- Avoid Valsalva maneuvers (holding breath and straining).
- Do not bend or lean forward at the waist.
- No drinking with straws (can increase negative pressure).
- No sneezing through the nose.
- No sniffling.
- Do not pick nose.
- Do not blow nose.

Activities of daily living:

- Sit for all lower-body self-care tasks if they involve leaning over, for example, pulling up pants, putting on socks, or washing feet.
- Do not hold breath and strain when lifting up feet for self-care activities or when on toilet because it increases the pressure at the surgical site.
- Use a reacher to pick up items from the floor.
- Use a long-handled bath sponge to wash feet to avoid bending over.
- Do not lean head back to rinse hair or hold your breath to avoid the water.
- Wipe (vs. brush) teeth gently in the area with the stitches. Can use mouthwash, but swish gently.

Note. Created by Judy R. Hamby.

Appendix 6.H.

Functional Upper-Extremity Activities

Do these activities as often as possible. Use your _____ hand for all checked activities:

☐ Wash your stomach; wash the left/right leg and face.

☐ Eat a roll.

☐ Drink a half-filled cold beverage with a lid.

☐ Brush your hair.

☐ Scratch your nose.

☐ Turn the pages of a book using your whole hand if you cannot yet move your fingers.

☐ Pick up an apple or orange, and put it down gently without dropping it.

☐ Hold a toothbrush with your _____ hand while putting the toothpaste on with the other hand.

☐ Hold a bottle with your _____ hand while taking the lid off with the other hand.

☐ Play cards, holding them with your _____ hand.

☐ Type a letter.

☐ Hold down paper with the _____ hand while writing with your unaffected hand.

☐ Hold an envelope while opening it with the other hand.

☐ Rip pieces of newspaper or paper.

☐ Crunch up pieces of paper.

☐ Pick up coins.

☐ Play the piano.

☐ Wash the table or countertop and dust the furniture.

☐ Rub lotion on your hands, arms, and legs.

☐ Fold towels and washcloths.

☐ Hold a telephone for short periods of time.

Source. Judy R. Hamby

7

Orthopedics and Musculoskeletal Disorders

Debra A. Kerrigan, MS, OTR/L; Kristen Scola, MS, OTR/L; and Sonia Smith, BS, OTR/L

Orthopedics is the branch of medicine that deals with bones, muscles, joints, ligaments, and tendons. Orthopedic diseases and conditions can be the result of congenital and developmental abnormalities, infection, inflammation, arthritis, metabolic dysfunction, tumors, and injury. Orthopedic conditions are often characterized by pain, stiffness, swelling, deformity, altered sensibility, and loss of function. Occupational therapists in the acute care setting help patients with orthopedic conditions to regain their ability to perform important daily occupations through the use of adaptive equipment, environmental adaptations, compensatory strategies, splinting, positioning, and education about managing symptoms. Many orthopedic conditions are treated on an outpatient basis. In this chapter, we focus on those conditions that an occupational therapist would likely encounter in an acute care setting.

The Spine

This section will provide an overview of the human spine, including the diseases, disorders, and conditions likely to be encountered by an occupational therapist in acute care. It will also address precautions and treatment considerations specific to the acute care setting.

Normal Structure and Function

The human spine has three primary functions: (1) to provide support and structure to the head and extremities, (2) to stabilize the body for function and movement, and (3) to protect the spinal cord. The spine is made up of 33 vertebrae that are stacked on top of one another (7 cervical, 12 thoracic, 5 lumbar, 5 sacral, and 4 coccygeal). The body of each vertebra is made up of a large, round portion of bone, and each is attached to a bony ring that is made up of the lamina, pedicles, and the transverse and spinous processes. When stacked on each other, these bony rings create a passageway known as the *vertebral foramen*. The spinal cord passes through the vertebral foramen (see Figure 7.1).

The articular processes (two inferior and two superior) extend from the vertebral body to articulate with the neighboring vertebrae. These articulations are called *facet joints*, which are a type of synovial joint. Between each vertebra is a gelatinous cushion known as the *intervertebral disc*. These discs are made up of an inner soft nucleus and an outer fibrous annulus, act as shock absorbers for the spine, and prevent the vertebral bones from rubbing against one another.

The normal spine has an S-like curve when looking at it from the side. This curve allows for an even distribution of weight. The cervical spine curves slightly inward, the thoracic spine curves outward, and the lumbar spine curves inward. Even though the lower portion of the spine holds most of the body's weight, each segment relies on the strength of the others to function properly.

Conditions, Diseases, and Disorders

Back pain is the most prevalent musculoskeletal cause of physical impairment among adults (Wing, 2001). Approximately 65 million Americans report having a recent episode of acute back pain. More than 16 million adults experience persistent or chronic back pain adversely affecting one or more aspect of their day-to-day functioning (Druss, Olfson, & Pincus, 2002).

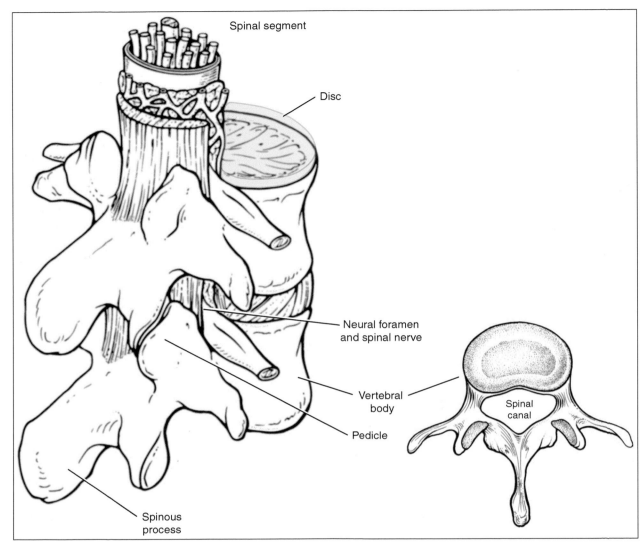

Figure 7.1. Normal vertebrae.
Source. Richard Fritzler, Medical Illustrator, Roswell, GA.

Degenerative Disc Disease

Spinal disease as a result of metastatic or infectious processes is uncommon (Cloyd, Acosta, & Ames, 2008). Most back pain is related to degenerative changes in the structure of the spine, the most common of which is *degenerative disc disease*. As discs age, their water content decreases, the outer fibrous annulus weakens, and their ability to cushion the vertebrae is impaired. In turn, an increased physical load is placed on the facet joints of the spine (Cloyd et al., 2008; Wing, 2001).

Disk Herniations and Bulges

When the disk material extends beyond the intervertebral disk space itself, it is known as a *disk herniation* or *bulge*. The difference between a herniation and a bulge is one of severity of displacement. A disc herniation occurs when less than 50% of the disc's circumference is displaced. A herniation becomes a bulge when more than 50% of the circumference is displaced. These disc displacements cause inflammation, which affects the nerve root, commonly leading to pain that radiates down the person's leg or legs (Barr & Harrast, 2006; see Figure 7.2).

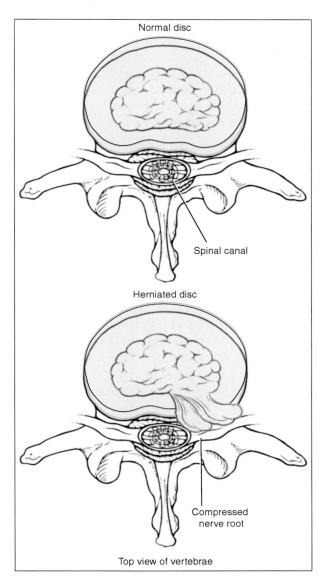

Figure 7.2. Normal vs. herniated disk.
Source. Richard Fritzler, Medical Illustrator, Roswell, GA.

Spinal Stenosis

Another common cause of back pain is *spinal stenosis,* which is a narrowing of the spinal canal. Stenosis occurs most commonly in the cervical and lumbar spine and is typically caused by bulging discs (Cloyd et al., 2008). The narrowing can occur at the center of the spine, in the canals branching off the spine, and/or between the vertebrae. This condition may compress the nerve roots of the spine, leading to increased pain and sensory deficits in the back and in the upper and lower extremities (Wing, 2001).

Spondylolisthesis

Spondylolisthesis is the anterior sliding of one vertebra over another. It can be classified into six etiologies (Barr & Harrast, 2006):

1. *Isthmic spondylolisthesis:* The most prevalent; occurs as a result of a stress fracture at the pars interarticularis;

2. *Dysplastic spondylolisthesis:* Congenital in nature; results from a dysplasia of the facet joints;

3. *Degenerative spondylolisthesis:* Seen in older adults; related to longstanding degenerative changes in the facet joints; most commonly occurs at the 4th or 5th lumbar vertebra;

4. *Pathologic spondylolisthesis:* Disc slippage that results from an infectious process that weakened the integrity of the bone;

5. *Traumatic spondylolisthesis:* Fairly rare; caused by an acute fracture; and

6. *Postsurgical spondylolisthesis:* Results from extensive spinal decompression surgery.

Vertebral Fractures

The five main categories of vertebral fractures follow:

1. *Posterior column fractures* are fractures of the transverse or spinous processes. Fractures of this nature are typically managed conservatively. Conservative treatment typically involves a combination of pain medication, steroidal injections, bracing, and physical therapy, occupational therapy, or both (Prather, Watson, & Gilula, 2007).

2. *Anterior column fractures* are compression fractures that result from flexion injuries. Fractures of this type typically do not affect the spinal cord itself, rarely require surgery, and are often managed conservatively.

3. *Anterior and middle column fractures* are burst fractures and result from a combination of a flexion and compression injury. A burst fracture typically results from an extreme downward force

placed on the vertebrae (e.g., if a person were to fall from a significant height, landing on his or her feet or buttocks). If no neurological deficits result from the fracture, it can likely be treated with several weeks of bracing. If the spinal cord is compressed, then surgery will be required to regain stability (Barr & Harrast, 2006).

4. *Anterior and posterior column fractures* are also known as *chance fractures*. They result from flexion and distraction injuries, most commonly from a seat belt in a high-speed motor vehicle accident (Barr & Harrast, 2006). If no ligamentous damage is present, the fracture will typically be closed reduced, and the patient will be braced in hyperextension for several weeks (Hu, Tribus, Tay, & Carlson, 2003). If surrounding soft tissue has been damaged, then surgery is indicated (Hu et al., 2003).

5. *Osteoporotic compression fractures* result from decreased bone density, either from primary factors such as age, decreased calcium intake, and limited exercise participation or from secondary factors such as oral steroid use, hyperthyroidism, or metastases (Barr & Harrast, 2006). Fractures of this type require surgery only if neurological deficits result or if conservative treatment is not adequately managing the patient's pain (Hu et al., 2003).

Surgical Interventions

This section will provide an overview of common surgical interventions to treat spine disorders, conditions, and diseases.

Laminectomy

A *laminectomy* is a procedure in which the lamina of a particular vertebra is removed. Doing this widens the spinal canal, which in turn decreases the amount of pressure being placed on nearby spinal nerves. If a surgeon locates any bone spurs on the vertebrae that irritate the spinal cord, they are also removed at this time. When a laminectomy is performed on the cervical spine, the risk of facet joint instability increases, allowing the spine to tilt forward. To prevent this tilting, the lamina may not be removed entirely; instead, one side of the lamina is cut and folded backward, allowing the other side of the lamina to open like a hinge, thereby relieving pressure on the spinal cord. Eventually, the cut piece of lamina will grow back, preventing unwanted tilting of the spine.

Diskectomy

A *diskectomy* is the removal of a herniated disc that has been placing excessive pressure on the nerve root. The procedure is performed through an incision down the center of the back over the area of herniation. The surgeon moves the muscles covering the vertebral column to the side and then cuts a small hole in the lamina of the vertebrae. This technique, known as a *laminotomy,* allows the surgeon to better visualize the inside of the spinal canal. Once the herniated disc is located, the surgeon removes as much of the disc as necessary.

After a diskectomy, the muscles of the back are returned to their normal anatomical position around the spine, and the incision is closed with sutures or staples. In some cases, a diskectomy may be combined with a spinal fusion, in which the vertebrae above and below the removed disc are unified into one solid piece.

Spinal Fusion

Spinal fusion surgery eliminates unwanted motion caused by the instability of the vertebrae. With restoration of stability, the patient's mechanical pain is significantly reduced. When a diskectomy or spinal fusion is performed, the surgeon will often use a bone graft to fill in the space left by the removed herniated disc. The bone graft can be an *autograft* (retrieved from the patient's pelvis), an *allograft* (retrieved from cadaver bone), or a *bone graft substitute*, such as *demineralized bone matrix* or *bone morphogenic protein* (Boden, 2006).

Currently, many surgeons are opting for allografts or bone graft substitutes to avoid the pain the patient could experience at the donor site (Boden, 2006). The placement of the bone graft between the two vertebrae will cause the vertebrae to fuse with one another. In addition, the surgeon may place metal plates or screws between the vertebrae to provide additional support to the bones as they heal and grow together.

Spine Precautions

After spinal surgery, it is important that the patient follow general guidelines to protect the surgical site and promote proper healing. These patients should continue to follow these guidelines until the surgeon recommends otherwise. The occupational therapist's role is to educate and train patients and their families in how to incorporate these guidelines into their daily life.

- Avoid bending and twisting the neck and back.

- Avoid picking up or carrying any item weighing more than 10 pounds.

- Cervical patients should avoid reaching for objects above shoulder height, regardless of weight (Pablo, Pradhan, Sueki, Delamarter, & Huffman, 2007).

- Avoid sitting or standing in the same position for longer than 30 minutes (Pablo et al., 2007).

- Patients should not drive until cleared to do so by the physician.

Depending on the physician's orders, patients may be required to wear a brace for additional support in the initial weeks after their surgery.

- If a patient is prescribed to wear a hard collar (e.g., Aspen collar) after a cervical spine surgery, consult the physician regarding the patient's wearing schedule. The surgeon will most commonly require the patient to wear the collar at all times when out of bed to protect the cervical spine and promote healing in the initial days after surgery. In this case, the patient will also be required to wear the collar when showering. He or she will be given a second set of interchangeable pads for the collar, so that the wet pads can be removed after bathing and replaced with the dry pads. Additionally, the surgeon may recommend that the collar only be donned and doffed in the supine position. A family member or caregiver will need to be instructed on how to safely do this for the patient.

- A thoracolumbosacral orthosis is a rigid orthotic that provides support for the lower spine after surgery. The brace is typically custom fit for the patient and, if prescribed, should be worn at all times when the patient is out of bed. Consult the surgeon regarding whether the brace can be donned and doffed in a sitting position or should only be removed when supine.

- Flexible lumbar corsets, abdominal binders, and soft collars are frequently prescribed for patient comfort after surgery. Consult the surgeon for the recommended wearing schedule for these supportive devices.

Occupational Therapy for Clients After Spinal Surgery

Appendix 7.A contains general guidelines for working with postoperative orthopedic patients and strategies for facilitating a safe discharge from the hospital. Occupational therapists also address the following areas when working with patients after spinal surgery or with patients with acute back pain.

Body Mechanics

Proper body mechanics reduces the stress placed on the spine as the body moves or as a person moves an object. To maintain good body mechanics, the patient should avoid any bending, twisting, or arching of the spine in his or her daily activities.

- The log roll technique is recommended for getting in and out of bed. Patients bend their knees, roll themselves to the side with their body moving as one solitary unit, and then use their arms to push their body upright, thus preventing twisting of the spine.

- When picking up objects from the floor, patients should lower themselves by bending at the knees to achieve a squatting position. They should keep the retrieved object close to their body (particularly heavier items) as they return to a standing position, thus keeping the weighted object as close to the body's center of gravity as possible.

- When standing for an extended period of time (e.g., completing grooming tasks at the bathroom sink or preparing a meal at the kitchen counter), patients are recommended to place one foot on a step stool, which puts their pelvis into a posterior tilt, decreasing the strain placed on the lumbar spine.

Functional Mobility

- When going from sitting to standing from a chair, bed, or toilet, patients should use their hip flexors to lower and raise their body, keeping the spine straight while doing so. Patients should avoid sitting in low, soft couches and instead opt for a firm, supportive chair with arms.

- Because toilet seats are particularly low (typically between 15 and 17 inches in height), a patient who has undergone spine surgery may benefit from a commode or raised toilet to decrease pain when transferring on and off the toilet. Additionally, the commode will allow patients to use their arms during the transfer, which is of particular benefit to patients with back pain that radiates to the lower extremities.

- Patients should limit sitting to 20- or 30-minute intervals, broken up by standing or walking for 3–5 minutes, to avoid increased pain and stiffness in the back.

- Walking is an activity that should be encouraged for all spine patients. Brisk walking promotes blood flow to the surgical site and will aid in healing, develop stronger muscles, and increase overall flexibility (Bear-Lehman, 2002).

Activities of Daily Living

- When donning pants, underwear, socks, and shoes, patients are recommended to bring their leg up and cross it over the opposite leg to access their foot as opposed to bending forward. If the patient lacks the flexibility required for this technique, he or she will likely need long-handled adaptive equipment for these tasks (e.g., reacher, sock aid, dressing stick, shoehorn).

- Patients who are unable to stand for prolonged periods of time because of increased back or neck pain should use a tub bench or shower seat when bathing. In addition, a long-handled sponge and/or hand-held shower head will be helpful when patients are washing the lower half of the body by decreasing the need to bend forward to reach their legs and feet.

- Patients may find it helpful to use a toilet aid when performing toilet hygiene. The aid increases the length of their reach, thus decreasing the amount of spinal twisting.

Hip Joint

This section will provide an overview of the hip joint, including the diseases, disorders, and conditions likely to be encountered by an occupational therapist in acute care. It will also address precautions and treatment considerations specific to the acute care setting.

Normal Structure and Function

The hip is the major weight-bearing joint in the body, attaching the largest and strongest bone, the femur, to the pelvis. The *hip* is a multiaxial, synovial ball-and-socket joint with the femoral head being the ball and the acetabulum being the socket (see Figure 7.3). The femoral head is connected to the rest of the femur by a short section of bone called the *femoral neck*. The *greater trochanter* is a small bump of bone that juts out from the top of the femur, near the femoral neck. The greater

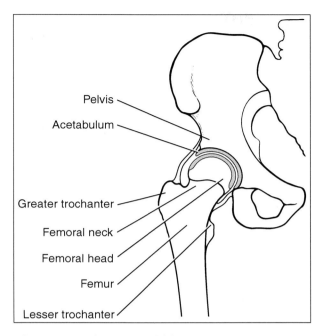

Figure 7.3. The normal hip.
Source. Richard Fritzler, Medical Illustrator, Roswell, GA.

trochanter serves as the attachment site for many of the major hip muscles. The acetabulum and the femoral head are covered in articular cartilage, which reduces friction and absorbs shock, allowing the two bony surfaces to move against each other without causing damage.

A ring of fibrocartilaginous material called the *acetabular labrum* surrounds the acetabulum. The acetabular labrum increases the depth of the acetabulum, thereby increasing the surface and strength of the hip joint. The joint capsule is formed by three strong ligaments that help hold the head of the femur in place and provide the main source of stability for the joint. The *iliotibial band* is a long tendon band that runs alongside the femur from the hip to the knee, providing a connection point for several hip muscles.

The hip allows range of motion (ROM) in all planes. Hip motions include flexion, extension, abduction, adduction, medial (internal) rotation, lateral (external) rotation, and circumduction. The hip joint is designed for stability and for a wide range of movement. After the shoulder joint, the hip is the most moveable

joint in the body. The hip is most stable when a person is bearing weight through it.

Conditions, Diseases, and Disorders

Osteoarthritis (OA) is the most common and problematic joint disease affecting middle-age and older adults (Buckwalter, Saltzman, & Brown, 2004). Detailed information about OA can be found in Appendix 7.B. Other conditions and diseases of the hip include

- *Avascular necrosis:* A bone condition that results from poor blood supply to an area of bone causing bone death. Avascular necrosis is also known as *aseptic necrosis* or *osteonecrosis*. It has been associated with alcoholism, cortisone medications, Cushing's syndrome, radiation exposure, sickle cell disease, pancreatitis, Gaucher disease, and systemic lupus erythematosus.
- *Rheumatoid arthritis:* Refer to the "Musculoskeletal Immunological Disorders" section of this chapter for more information.
- *Hip dysplasia: Hip dysplasia* is a developmental abnormality in which the hip joint is not formed properly. The socket is shallow and the head of the femur is not well rounded, which increases local stresses on the cartilage.
- *Hip fractures:* Refer to the "Hip Fractures" section of this chapter for detailed information on causes, treatment, and prevention of hip fractures.

Patients may elect to undergo hip replacement surgery when conservative treatments (e.g., lifestyle and activity modification, medication, occupational and physical therapy, alternative or complementary treatments) for their hip disease or disorder have failed. Hip arthroplasty is usually performed only after the patient has exhausted the conservative treatments and less invasive surgery (e.g., arthroscopy to trim torn and damaged cartilage and wash out the joint, joint alignment osteotomy, cartilage replacement).

Surgical Interventions

This section provides an overview of common surgical interventions to treat hip disorders, conditions, and diseases.

Hip Arthroplasty

Hip arthroplasty is joint replacement surgery in which all or part of the hip joint is replaced with an artificial device. *Total hip replacement* is also known as *total hip arthroplasty.* Total hip arthroplasty involves three parts:

1. *Stem:* Fits into the femur; usually made of titanium-based or cobalt-chromium-based alloys;

2. *Ball:* Replaces the femoral head; made of cobalt-chromium-based alloys or ceramic materials and polished smooth to allow easy rotation in the hip socket; and

3. *Cup:* Replaces the hip socket; can be made of plastic, metal, ultra-high molecular-weight polyethylene, or a combination of polyethylene backed by metal.

Ceramic-on-ceramic (e.g., ceramic ball, ceramic socket) components are also available. A prosthesis in which the ball and stem are combined into a single component is called a *bipolar prosthesis.* Hip hemiarthroplasty is indicated when only half of the joint needs to be replaced. The component replaced is generally the femoral component (i.e., the ball and stem; see Figure 7.4).

Hip replacements may be *cemented, cementless,* or *hybrid* (a combination of cemented and cementless components). The hybrid approach is common in hip replacement surgery, with the acetabular component being cementless and the femoral component being cemented (American Academy of Orthopaedic Surgeons [AAOS], 2008; Arthritis Foundation, 2009).

Table 7.1 describes the pros and cons of cemented and cementless components.

Posterior (Posterolateral) Hip Replacement

Traditionally, hip replacement surgery is performed using the posterior approach, in which the surgeon makes an incision over the side

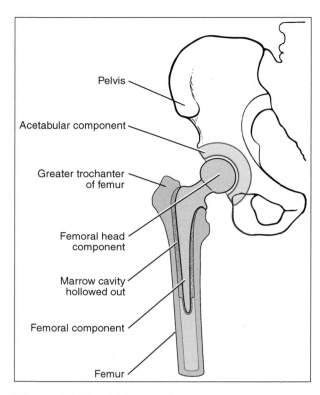

Figure 7.4. Total hip prostheses.
Source. Richard Fritzler, Medical Illustrator, Roswell, GA.

of the hip through the muscles. The hip is accessed in the interval between the gluteus maximus and gluteus medius (Pratt & Gray, 2007). Diseased bone tissue and cartilage are removed, leaving the healthy parts of the joint intact. The acetabular component is implanted, and the femoral component is inserted into the femur. The prosthetic components may be cemented or cementless. The muscles and tendons are replaced, and the surgical incision is closed. Postsurgically, patients are at risk for posterior hip dislocation. Patients must observe posterior hip precautions at least until the scheduled postoperative visit with the orthopedist (see Table 7.2). At the postoperative visit (generally 6 weeks after surgery), the orthopedist may relax the precautions or continue them for another 6 weeks (Pratt & Gray, 2007). The surgeon specifies weight-bearing status (see Table 7.3).

Anterior (Anterolateral) Hip Replacement

Anterolateral hip replacement approaches the hip in the interval between the gluteus

Table 7.1. Cemented vs. Cementless Hip Replacement Components

Features	Cemented	Cementless
Pros	• Full weight bearing immediately after surgery • Faster rehabilitation	• Excellent long-term outcomes • Not subject to cement failures • Easier to revise when component fails
Cons	• Risk of bone resorption causing bone loss around the acetabulum and the femur • Risk of femoral component loosening because of fatigue fractures (cracks) in the cement over time	• Longer healing time because of dependence on new bone growth for stability • Higher incidence of mild thigh pain when large cementless stems are used • Requires protected weight bearing (with walker or crutches) • More expensive implants • More technically demanding to implant
Recommended population	• Older patients • Patients with rheumatoid arthritis • Younger patients with compromised health or poor bone quality or density	• Younger, more active patients • Patients with good bone quality • Patients with juvenile inflammatory arthritis • Patients undergoing more complicated revisions

Sources. American Academy of Orthopaedic Surgeons (2008), Pratt and Gray (2007).

Table 7.2. Hip Replacement Dislocation Precautions

Precaution	Movement Restrictions
Posterior	• No hip flexion beyond 90° • No hip adduction past neutral • No hip internal rotation
Anterior	• No hip extension • No hip external rotation
Trochanteric[a]	• No active hip abduction

[a]Trochanteric precautions may be specified when a trochanteric osteotomy is done in conjunction with hip replacement surgery, which is common in complex hip replacement surgeries and in hip revision surgery.

Table 7.3. Weight-Bearing Precautions

Weight-Bearing Status	Definition
Weight bearing as tolerated (WBAT)	Patient is allowed to put as much weight as he or she can tolerate through the operative extremity, with pain being the limiting factor.
Partial weight bearing (PWB)	Patient is allowed to put up to 50% of his or her body weight on the operative extremity.
Touchdown weight bearing (TDWB)	Patient is not allowed to bear weight on the operative extremity but is allowed to touch his or her toes to the floor to maintain balance.
Non–weight bearing (NWB)	Patient is not allowed to bear any weight on the operative extremity.

medius and tensor fascia lata and carries increased risk of injury to the superior gluteal and femoral nerves. This technique has also been associated with a higher incidence of heterotropic bone formation and greater blood loss (Pratt & Gray, 2007). Because the risk of posterior dislocation is decreased, this approach may be preferable for patients who have significant muscle imbalance or spasticity (e.g., stroke, cerebral palsy; Pratt & Gray, 2007). Patients must observe anterior hip precautions at least until the scheduled postoperative visit with the orthopedist (generally 6 weeks). Weight-bearing status is specified by the surgeon.

Minimally Invasive Hip Replacement

The term *minimally invasive hip replacement* can mean different things to different people. Minimally invasive hip replacement often refers to techniques in which the hip replacement components are implanted through a smaller incision. The hope is that this technique will allow quicker, less painful recovery and quicker return to functional activities. This area is rapidly evolving. The benefits of minimally invasive hip replacement have yet to be proven, and minimally invasive hip replacement may be associated with an increased risk for complications. Lawlor et al. (2005) found no significant benefit in terms of functional transfers, ambulation, or weight bearing in minimally invasive hip replacement versus standard-incision total hip replacement. Minimally invasive hip replacement is also technically more demanding than standard-incision total hip replacement. Minimally invasive hip replacement can be safe and reproducible when done by experienced surgeons on the appropriate patients; however, quality evidence to support expansion of this technique is lacking (Mahmood, Zafar, Majid, Maffulli, & Thompson, 2007).

The anterior approach for minimally invasive total hip arthroplasty is a muscle-sparing technique in which the approach is from the front of the hip. The hip is approached and replaced through a natural interval between muscles. The gluteal muscles that attach to the posterior and lateral pelvis and femur are not disturbed. The use of a specialized orthopedic table facilitates femoral access and reduces the need for secondary incisions. Because muscle attachments and other soft tissues are preserved, risk of hip dislocation is decreased and total hip precautions are not required (Matta, 2007). Anterior mini-invasive hip replacement is not widely used by orthopedic surgeons in the United States because of (1) lack of familiarity, (2) traditional teaching, and (3) the need for specialized equipment and instrumentation (Kreuzer, 2006).

Hip Resurfacing

Hip resurfacing is a newer alternative to total hip replacement in which the femoral head is reshaped and covered with a metal shell with a small stem, thus conserving bone in the femoral head and neck. As in total hip replacement, arthritic bone is removed from the acetabulum and a metal cup is inserted (Snyder & Hanmer, 2006). Hip resurfacing has been in use worldwide since 1997. Two hip resurfacing systems are currently approved by the Food and Drug Administration for use in the United States: the Birmingham Hip Resurfacing system and the Cormet Hip Resurfacing system. Advantages of hip resurfacing include

- Preservation of the femoral head;
- Decreased risk of dislocation because of the ball implant's larger size; and
- Increased likeliness of recovering normal gait compared with total hip replacement.

Current hip resurfacing devices have only been in use for approximately 10 years; therefore, no clinical data regarding longevity and long-term wear exist. Hip resurfacing is appropriate for younger (<age 60), active patients with hip pain resulting from OA, dysplasia, or avascular necrosis and for whom total hip replacement may not be appropriate because of their increased level of physical activity (Snyder & Hanmer, 2006). Patients older than age 60 may be appropriate for hip resurfacing if their bone quality is strong enough to support the implant. Hip precautions are specified by the surgeon on the basis of the surgical approach used.

Revision Total Hip Arthroplasty

Despite the excellent success rate of hip replacement surgery and the many changes in surgical techniques and implant designs, the incidence of *revision total hip arthroplasty* is on the rise (Bozic et al., 2009). Total hip arthroplasty may fail for several reasons, including (1) mechanical loosening, (2) dislocation, (3) implant failure, (4) periprosthetic fracture, and (5) infection. Bozic et al. (2009) found that hip instability and dislocation and mechanical loosening are the most common reasons for

revision total hip arthroplasty in the United States. During hip revision surgery, part or all of the old prosthesis is removed and replaced with new components. As in primary total hip arthroplasty, the surgeon will specify the hip precautions and weight-bearing precautions on the basis of the surgical approach and which components were replaced.

Girdlestone Procedure

Historically, hip resection arthroplasty, also known as a *Girdlestone procedure*, was commonly performed after failure of a primary total hip arthroplasty. However, with advancements in hip revision surgery, Girdlestone procedures are no longer commonly performed. Girdlestone procedures are now considered a last resort or salvage procedure when (1) infection has occurred after total hip arthroplasty, (2) a failed hip replacement cannot be revised, or (3) total hip arthroplasty is not a viable option for a painful hip that is affecting quality of life.

In a Girdlestone procedure, the head of the femur is removed. Although pain is alleviated, the limb is shortened, the hip is stiff, and an assistive device is required for walking. In some cases, a Girdlestone can be converted to a total hip replacement.

Hip Precautions

The risk of dislocation is based on the surgical approach. Precautions are generally followed for 3–6 months, as directed by the surgeon. Table 7.2 specifies the dislocation precautions for each surgical approach. Weight-bearing status is determined by the surgeon on the basis of his or her preference and whether the femoral component is cemented or uncemented. Complex revision surgeries, those requiring extensive bone grafting, or those with intra-operative complications may require a more restrictive weight-bearing status. Refer to Table 7.3 for common weight-bearing terms.

Hip Fractures

Hip fractures are a serious medical problem among older adults. Approximately 345,000 older men and women are hospitalized each year for hip fractures, with the number of hip fractures expected to exceed 500,000 by 2040 (Born, 2009; Centers for Disease and Prevention [CDC] Injury Center, 2008). According to the CDC Injury Center, more than 90% of hip fractures are caused by falls. These populations are at an increased risk for sustaining a hip fracture (CDC Injury Center, 2008):

- Older adults (adults ages 85 or older are at a 10%–15% greater risk for sustaining hip fractures than those ages 60–65)
- Women (approximately 76% of all hip fractures occur in women)
- People with osteoporosis.

Hip fractures are costly to the health care system. The CDC Injury Center (2008) has estimated that hospital stays for patients with hip fractures are approximately 1 week long. They have also estimated that 25% of adults living independently before their hip fracture require at least 1 year in a nursing home to recover after their injury. Approximately 20% of adults who sustain a hip fracture die within 1 year of their injury. Common causes of falls leading to hip fractures include

- Decreased strength with age
- Decreased balance with age
- Home environment hazards (e.g., clutter, poor lighting)
- Medication side effects (e.g., drowsiness, lethargy, dizziness)
- Impaired vision
- Dementia (Born, 2009; CDC Injury Center, 2008).

Treatment for a hip fracture usually consists of reducing the fracture and holding it in place with an internal device while the bone heals. This type of surgery is known as *open reduction internal fixation (ORIF)*. The devices used to hold the bones in place vary with the type of fracture. Some hip fractures may require a partial hip replacement (hemiarthroplasty). Table 7.4 lists the most common types of hip fractures and the most common surgical techniques used to repair them. The surgeon will determine the amount of weight the patient may place on the operated leg on the basis of the type of fracture and the type of repair.

In some rare cases, a hip fracture may not be treated surgically. Patients who may not be a candidate for surgical repair of a hip fracture include those

- Who are too ill to undergo any form of anesthesia;
- Who were bedridden or nonambulatory before the injury and are not in much pain; and
- Whose fracture is considered stable and does not require surgical repair. These patients are monitored closely for displacement over time.

The Pelvis

This section will provide an overview of the pelvis, including the diseases, disorders, and conditions likely to be encountered by an occupational therapist in acute care. It will also address precautions and treatment considerations specific to the acute care setting.

Normal Structure and Function

The pelvis is the ringlike structure of bones at the lower end of the trunk that provides the transition between the trunk and the lower limbs, as depicted in Figure 7.5. The mature bony pelvis is formed by four bones:

- *Two hip bones:* Each hip bone is a large, irregularly shaped bone that develops from the fusion during puberty of three bones: (1) the *ilium*—the superior, broad, flaring (fan-shaped) portion of the hip bone; (2) the *ischium*—the body of the ischium helps form the acetabular portion of the hip joint; and (3) the *pubis*—the lower, posterior part of the hip bone; the superior ramus of the pubis helps to form the acetabular portion of the hip joint;
- *The sacrum:* A spade-shaped bone formed by the fusion of five originally separate sacral vertebrae; and
- *The coccyx:* Formed by the fusion of four originally separate coccygeal vertebrae. The coccyx is also called the *tail bone.*

Table 7.4. Common Hip Fractures and Surgical Repairs

Fracture Type	Surgical Repair	Comments
Intracapsular (nondisplaced fracture or displaced fracture in a younger patient)	• Percutaneous pinning[a] • Compression hip screw[b]	Femoral neck fractures are especially common in people older than age 60 and in women.
Intracapsular (displaced fracture in an older patient)	• Total hip replacement[c] • Hemiarthroplasty[c]	Likelihood that head of the femur is damaged or that blood supply to the femoral head is damaged is increased. Older patients fare better when some of the hip components are replaced.
Intertrochanteric	• Compression hip screw • Intramedullary nail (IM nail)[d]	Decision on which device to use is based on surgeon preference and experience. In both cases, a large lag screw is placed into the head and neck.
Subtrochanteric	• Intramedullary nail with large lag screw • Plate and screw	Surgeon may add locking screws at the lower end of the nail near the knee.

[a]*Percutaneous pinning*: Multiple individual screws are used to fix the fracture.

[b]*Compression hip screw*: A single larger screw that slides within the barrel of a plate.

[c]Refer to the "Hip Arthroplasty" section of this chapter for an explanation of total hip replacement and hemiarthroplasty.

[d]*Intramedullary nail*: Long nail placed directly into the marrow canal of the bone through an opening made at the top of the greater trochanter.

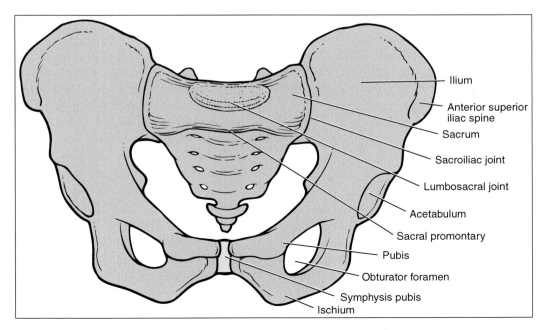

Figure 7.5. The normal pelvis.
Source. Richard Fritzler, Medical Illustrator, Roswell, GA.

The main functions of the pelvis are to

- Support the spinal column;
- Protect the abdominal organs;
- Transfer weight of the upper body to the lower limbs; and
- Withstand compression and other forces from its support of body weight.

Pelvic Fractures

Pelvic fractures are rare, representing 3% of all skeletal fractures (Crawford Mechem, 2008). Pelvic fractures can vary greatly in severity and are classified as follows:

- *Stable:* One breakpoint in the pelvic ring; minimal hemorrhage; pelvic bones remain in place
- *Unstable:* Two or more breakpoints in pelvic ring; moderate to severe hemorrhage; pelvis is unstable
- *Open:* Open skin wound present in the lower abdomen
- *Closed:* No open skin wound.

The most common form of pelvic fracture results from high-impact accidents such as a motor vehicle accident or falling from a great height. These fractures can be life threatening because of shock, internal bleeding, and damage to internal organs. Emergency treatment is focused on stabilizing the patient. External fixators are generally used to stabilize the pelvic region and allow the surgeons to address internal injuries to the organs, blood supply, and nerves. Further surgical repair with plates and screws may be necessary in some cases. Chronic pain and physical disabilities may result from the internal injuries associated with the traumatic fracture.

Older people and people with osteoporosis may sustain pelvic fractures spontaneously or after minor falls. These fractures are generally stable and are treated nonsurgically with pain medication and blood thinners to prevent blood clots. Patients will need to ambulate with an assistive device for protective weight bearing. It can take up to 3 months for pelvic fractures to heal. Less commonly,

pelvic fractures can occur in young athletes. These fractures are generally stable and are also treated nonsurgically.

The Knee Joint

This section provides an overview of the knee joint, including the diseases, disorders, and conditions likely to be encountered by an occupational therapist in acute care. It also addresses treatment recommendations and considerations specific to the knee joint and lower extremities fractures in the acute care setting.

Normal Structure and Function

The human *knee*, which is often thought of as a simple hinge joint, is actually a double condyloid joint, made up of three articulations that allow for flexion, extension, and medial and lateral rotation (Rybski, 2004). Between the lateral and medial condyles of the femur and the lateral and medial condyles of the tibia are two articulations; these articulations are known as the *inferior* and *superior tibiofemoral joints*. The third articulation of the knee joint occurs between the patella bone and the femur. Normal knee ROM in a healthy joint is 130° of flexion and 0° to –10° of extension (see Figure 7.6).

Ligaments

The stability of the knee joint is provided by its two collateral ligaments and two cruciate ligaments. The *anterior cruciate ligament* crosses from the lateral femoral condyle to its insertion site on the medial tibial spine. This ligament serves to restrain anterior subluxation of the tibia relative to the femur. The *posterior cruciate ligament* crosses from the medial femoral condyle to the posterior aspect of the tibia. The posterior cruciate ligament prevents posterior subluxation of the tibia on the femur.

On either side of the knee joint are the medial and lateral collateral ligaments. The *medial collateral ligament* runs from the medial aspect of the tibia to the medial aspect of the femur. It stabilizes the knee against valgus (toward the body's midline) and rotational stresses. The *lateral collateral ligament* runs from the lateral

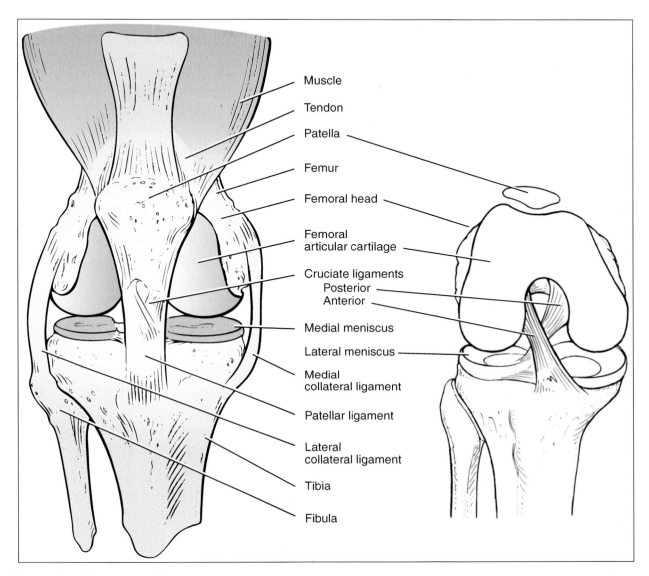

Figure 7.6. The normal knee.
Source. Richard Fritzler, Medical Illustrator, Roswell, GA.

femoral condyle and attaches at the head of the fibula. It is the main stabilizer against varus stress (away from the body's midline) and also resists external rotation.

Menisci

The knee joint is also supported by the medial and lateral menisci. The menisci are two semi-lunar cartilaginous discs, which act as the shock absorbers for the joint. The menisci also allow for a smooth and stable articulation between the tibial and femoral surfaces and aid in the distribution of synovial fluid, the lubricator of the knee joint.

Indications for Knee Replacement Surgery

OA in the knee joint is a result of the deterioration of the menisci of the knees resulting from age-related changes, repetitive trauma, or obesity (Pottenger, 2003; Skinner, Zhou, & Weinstein, 2006). As the cartilage deteriorates, the articulation between the tibia and femur is no longer smooth as a result of bone-on-bone contact. When the bones rub together, pain increases, as does inflammation in the tendons, ligaments, and synovial lining of the joint (National Institute of Arthritis and

Musculoskeletal and Skin Diseases [NIAMS], 2006; Pottenger, 2003). Additionally, the friction caused by bone-on-bone contact can cause the formation of bone spurs. Buildup of these spurs can in turn limit ROM in the knee (NIAMS, 2006). In the United States alone, more than 13.5 million adults report having knee joint pain, swelling, and stiffness associated with OA, half of whom are older than age 65 (American Academy of Orthopedic Surgeons [AAOS], 2007a).

The knee cartilage that wears away because of arthritis cannot be regenerated. Therefore, in patients with areas of full-thickness loss of cartilage and chronic pain, which limits their ability to walk even short distances, knee arthroplasty may be a potential remedy (Pottenger, 2003). OA accounts for roughly 65% of knee replacements annually (Rolston et al., 2007). Other causes of cartilage destruction include rheumatoid arthritis, hemophilia, crystal deposition diseases, idiopathic or steroid-induced avascular necrosis, bone dysplasia, and bone cancer.

Typically, before undergoing an elective knee arthroplasty, a patient should have exhausted all other medical treatment options, which include the use of oral analgesics and NSAIDs, cortisone injections, physical therapy for muscle strengthening and conditioning, and the use of joint protection techniques in the patient's daily routine (Pottenger, 2003).

A common procedure that can precede a total knee replacement is knee arthroscopy. *Knee arthroscopy* is a minimally invasive procedure in which a small scope is inserted into the knee. The scope projects a picture of the knee's interior to a television. If the damage to the knee is not extensive, the surgeon can insert surgical instruments through this small incision in the knee to debride or repair damaged tissues.

Total Knee Arthroplasty

An *arthroplasty* is a surgery in which one or more of the articular surfaces of a joint are replaced by a synthetic prosthesis (see Figure 7.7). The prosthetic is typically made of metal or high-density polyethylene (Pottenger, 2003). The prosthesis may be either cemented

to the bone or cementless. The cementless prostheses are typically made of a type of porous metal, with the anticipation that the new bone will grow into the prosthesis (Lonner, 2003). The prosthetic knee is made up of these three components:

1. The tibial component (to replace the top of the tibia);
2. The femoral component (to replace the two femoral condyles and the patellar groove); and
3. The patellar component (to replace the bottom surface of the kneecap).

In 2005, approximately 534,000 knee replacements were performed in the United States (DeFrances, Lucas, Buie, & Golosinskiy, 2008). In the past, patients between ages 60–75 years were considered the "typical" patient to undergo knee arthroplasty (NIAMS, 2006). However, in the past 20 years, the age range has broadened to include patients older than age 75, as well as patients in their 40s and 50s (NIAMS, 2006). This trend may in part be the result of older adults living longer and younger adults having a more active lifestyle.

If only the medial or the lateral side of the knee joint is affected by OA, then a unicompartmental (or partial) knee replacement can be performed. A unicompartmental knee replacement occurs when only one side of the knee is replaced by a specialized prosthesis and the ligaments and cartilage of the unaffected side of the knee remain intact and unaffected by the surgery (Lonner, 2003). The advantage of unicompartmental surgery is that it involves a smaller surgical cut, less blood loss, and less tissue damage, and patients may experience a faster recovery time (National Institutes of Health [NIH], 2008). When both sides (medial and lateral) of a patient's knee are affected by arthritis, then a total knee replacement is performed (Lonner, 2003). Unicompartmental knee surgery accounts for only 8% of knee replacement surgeries in the United States. However, the number of unicompartmental knee surgeries being performed yearly is increasing at a faster rate than that of total knee replacements (Riddle, Jiranek, & McGlynn, 2008). Between

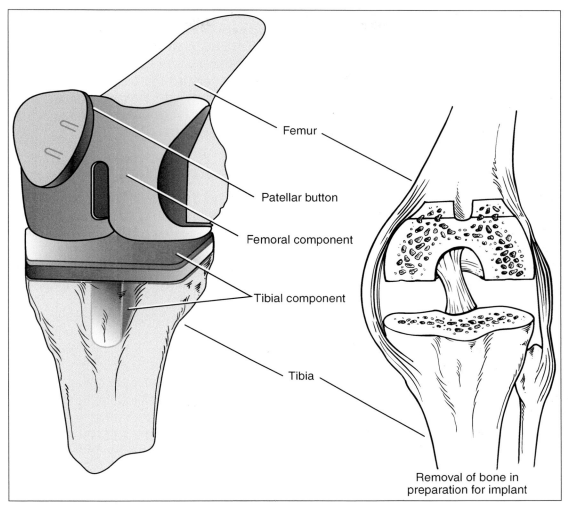

Figure 7.7. Total knee prosthesis.
Source. Richard Fritzler, Medical Illustrator, Roswell, GA.

1994 and 2005, the number of unicompartmental knee replacements grew at a rate of 35%, and the number of total knee replacements increased only 9% (Riddle et al., 2008).

Surgical Technique

Although knee surgeries vary from patient to patient, the average knee replacement takes about 2 hours. Generally, all surgeons use prophylactic antibiotics and anticoagulation medication before surgery to prevent infection and thromboembolic complications, respectively (Malik, Chougle, Pradhan, Gambhir, & Porter, 2005). While undergoing surgery, the patient may be under general anesthesia, in which the patient is unconscious during the surgery,

or awake with spinal or epidural anesthesia. *Spinal* and *epidural anesthesia* are two types of regional anesthesia that temporarily block feeling in the lower part of the body (Martin, 2007).

The size of the incision required to perform this surgery ranges between 6 and 12 inches (Martin, 2007). The first portion of the surgery is dedicated to removing the damaged bone and cartilage from the tibia and femur. Next, the surgeon performs an osteotomy of the distal tibia and the distal femur, removing the anterior and posterior femoral condyles, and also shaves off the articular surface of the patella (Cacanindin, Wong, & Ries, 2007). Once this process is complete, the surgeon inserts the femoral and tibial components into the shaft of the femur and tibia. Finally, the patellar component is adhered to the posterior portion of the patella (Cacanindin et al., 2007).

After the surgery is completed, the patient will be allowed to bear weight through his or her operated leg as tolerated and will not have any restrictions regarding knee ROM. If for some reason a complication occurred during the surgery, for example, a fracture of the femur when placing the prosthetic, the surgeon may request that the patient bear less weight on his or her extremity to allow for healing. Intra-operative fractures such as this are rare, occurring at a rate of 0.6% (Su, DeWal, & Di Cesare, 2004). For complete descriptions of weight-bearing precautions, refer to Table 7.3.

Continuous Passive Motion Machine

Depending on the facility and the surgeon's preference, continuous passive motion machines may be part of the postoperative protocol for the knee replacement patient. Research has shown that use of the continuous passive motion machine allows for improved postoperative knee flexion, reduction of adhesion formation, and the promotion of wound healing (Cacanindin et al., 2007). Although the physical therapist's role is to determine the schedule and ROM settings for the patient, it is important that the occupational therapist be able to apply and remove the machine correctly and also take the continuous passive motion schedule into account when planning treatment sessions for the day.

Knee Revision Surgery

Despite the excellent success rate of knee replacement surgery, approximately 10% of implants fail, requiring a second procedure or revision (Younger, 2007). During a knee revision surgery, part or all of the old prosthesis is removed and replaced with new components (Younger, 2007). In the remaining 90% of knee replacement patients, the prosthesis will last between 10 and 20 years (Younger, 2007).

Hardware fails for a variety of reasons, including perioperative fracture, loosening, infection, or patient-related factors such as age, activity level, and obesity (Younger, 2007). Unless otherwise specified by the physician, intervention for a patient with knee revision surgery is the same as that for a patient undergoing a primary knee replacement.

Lower Leg Fractures

Lower leg fractures, such as ankle fractures and proximal tibia or fibula fractures, are commonly treated on an outpatient basis and are therefore not always seen by the acute care occupational therapist. However, if a patient is older, has multiple comorbidities, or is having pain control difficulties, he or she may be admitted to the hospital for observation overnight. In this case, the patient would have the opportunity to be seen by the occupational therapist for ADL and functional mobility training before returning home.

Lower leg fractures may be treated nonsurgically (casting or splinting) if they are stable or nondisplaced or by surgical means (ORIF or external fixation) if the fracture is unstable, displaced, or comminuted (Crist, 2007). The orthopedic surgeon will determine weight-bearing and movement restrictions. A patient with a lower leg fracture will most commonly not be allowed to bear weight on the affected leg for a minimum of 6 weeks to allow optimal healing (Crist, 2007), after which the patient will gradually be allowed to progress the amount of weight placed on the lower extremity. Additionally, if a proximal tibia or fibula fracture involves the articulation of the knee joint, the patient may be placed in an immobilizing brace and have additional ROM restrictions.

Occupational Therapy for Clients With Lower-Body Surgeries and Fractures

Appendix 7.A contains general guidelines for working with postoperative orthopedic patients and strategies for facilitating a safe discharge from the hospital. When working with patients after lower-extremity joint replacement surgery or with lower-extremity fractures, the occupational therapist will also address the following areas.

Dressing and Bathing

Patients who have undergone a total hip replacement, hip resurfacing, total knee replacement, or lower-extremity ORIF will either require the use of or benefit from long-handled adaptive equipment for dressing and bathing.

- For the patient with posterior hip precautions, this equipment (e.g., reacher, sock aid, dressing stick, shoehorn, sponge) will be necessary to maintain precautions while dressing, undressing, and bathing.

- Patients with anterior hip precautions or those who have undergone a total knee replacement or ORIF or have had nonsurgical treatment of their fracture may benefit from the use of long-handled equipment to facilitate independence and reduce pain and stress while performing lower-body ADLs.

- Patients with weight-bearing restrictions may need to be taught alternative dressing and undressing techniques if they are not able to maintain their weight-bearing precautions while putting on their pants or donning their shoes.

- Shower seats or tub transfer benches may be recommended for patients who have weight-bearing restrictions or who have posterior hip precautions, depending on their home bathroom setup.

- Patients with posterior hip precautions who have a tub–shower combination in their home may need a tub bench to safely get in and out of their bathtub without exceeding 90° of hip flexion.

- Patients who are not permitted to put full weight on one of their lower extremities will need a tub bench or seat to ensure safety and prevent falls while showering.

Toileting

Patients with posterior hip precautions will need a commode or raised toilet seat to maintain hip precautions. Additionally, these patients should be taught to perform toilet hygiene in a standing position to prevent bending at the hip beyond 90°.

Other patients may benefit from the increased height and arms of a commode or raised toilet seat to facilitate ease of and reduce pain during toilet transfers. For example, a patient who has had a knee replacement may not be able to comfortably transfer on and off a standard height toilet because of the amount of flexion required of the operative knee.

Patients with lower-extremity fractures (e.g., hip, pelvis, tibial plateau) who have restricted weight bearing may be limited in ambulation distance and may need to use a bedside commode for toileting.

Functional Mobility

- Patients with posterior hip precautions will need to be taught how to transfer in and out of bed without internally rotating or adducting their operative leg.

- Patients on anterior hip precautions will need to be taught how to transfer in and out of bed without externally rotating the operative leg.

- Patients with trochanteric precautions should be taught to transfer out of bed on their nonoperative side to avoid active abduction of the operative hip. Caregivers and family members can be taught to passively abduct the operative hip if the patient must transfer out of bed on the operative side.

- People who have undergone knee replacement surgery or who have a lower-extremity fracture will likely not have movement restrictions dictating how they get in and out of bed. In general, it is best to have these patients get in and out of bed on their operative side to decrease the distance they have to move their operative leg.

- Furniture risers and bed transfer rails may be useful for patients having difficulty transferring in and out of bed.

- Patients with anterior or posterior hip precautions should be cautious of turning the operative leg inward or outward when turning around in tight spaces with their assistive device (e.g., in the bathroom). Instead, they should take very small steps, keeping their toes facing forward.

- Patients with posterior hip precautions must be cautious when getting in and out of a car. Typically, higher cars, such as trucks or SUVs, will be easier to get in and out of than a sports vehicle, which is lower to the ground. When getting into the passenger seat of a vehicle, it is important that the seat be pushed back as far as it can go and in a reclined position to allow the patient to bring the operative leg into the car and to decrease the amount of flexion required at the hip when sitting in the car.

Sleeping

Patients should be educated about the use of pillows to maintain hip precautions in different sleeping positions. Patient handouts that demonstrate safe sleeping positions for posterior hip precautions are available at http://nih.kramesonline.com/HealthSheets/3,S,82359.

Patients with anterior hip precautions should not sleep on their stomachs and should place pillows on the lateral side of their operative leg to prevent external rotation.

Sexual Activity

Occupational therapists should be prepared to address any questions a patient may have about safe positions to maintain hip precautions during sexual intercourse. Patient handouts addressing safe sexual intercourse after hip surgery are available at http://nih.kramesonline.com/HealthSheets/3,S,40019.

Patient, Family, and Caregiver Education

Occupational therapists should be prepared to address any questions a patient may have about managing at home, such as meal preparation, housekeeping, child care, and pet care.

Patients who have fallen are at an increased risk for another fall. Patients and caregivers should be educated about fall prevention and home safety. Free fall prevention and home safety checklist brochures and posters are available from the CDC at www.cdc.gov/HomeandRecreationalSafety/Falls/index-pr.html.

The Shoulder

This section will provide an overview of the shoulder, including the diseases, disorders, and conditions likely to be encountered by an occupational therapist in acute care. It will also address precautions and treatment considerations specific to the acute care setting.

Normal Structure and Function

The shoulder is the most mobile and unstable joint in the body. It consists of three bones—the scapula, the humerus, and the clavicle—and four articulations:

1. *Glenohumeral joint:* The articulation of the head of the humerus in the glenoid fossa of the scapula. This joint is a ball-and-socket joint that allows for excessive motion and accounts for the joint's decreased stability. The glenoid fossa is deepened by a fibrocartilaginous ring called the *glenoid labrum.* The glenoid labrum is formed by the biceps tendon (superiorly) and the inferior glenoid ligament (inferiorly). The glenoid labrum contributes little to joint stability. The glenohumeral joint is reinforced by these ligaments:

   - The *coracohumeral ligament,* which extends from the coracoid process of the scapula to the greater tubercle of the humerus, provides strong thickening of the joint capsule and helps support the weight of the upper limb;

- The *inferior glenohumeral ligament complex,* which is made up of the anterior band (restrains humeral head interiorly when in 90° of abduction), the posterior band (restrains humeral head posteriorly when in 90° of abduction), and the inferior band (keeps humeral head from subluxing inferiorly); and
- The *transverse humeral ligament,* which spans the gap between the humeral tubercles.

The major stabilizers of the glenohumeral joint consist of

- The tendon of the long head of the biceps brachii muscle, which secures the head of the humerus against the glenoid cavity, and
- The rotator cuff, which is made up of the tendons of the subscapularis, supraspinatus, infraspinatus, and teres minor muscles and, in addition to stability, provide mobility and strength to the shoulder, allowing elevation and rotation of the arm.

2. *Acromioclavicular joint:* A diarthrodial (synovial) joint made up of the articulation of the medial edge of the acromion with the acromial (lateral) end of the clavical.

3. *Sternoclavicular joint:* A saddle joint formed by the articulation of the medial end of the clavicle with the sternum.

4. *Scapulothoracic joint:* Not a true joint; formed by the articulation of the scapula with the posterior thorax. This articulation allows shoulder motion beyond the 120° offered by the glenohumeral joint.

Conditions, Diseases, and Disorders

Shoulder problems are commonly treated on an outpatient basis and are therefore not frequently seen by the acute care occupational therapist. However, if a patient is older, has mul-

tiple comorbidities, or is having pain control difficulties, he or she may be admitted to the hospital overnight for observation. In this case, the patient would have the opportunity to be seen by the occupational therapist for ADL and therapeutic exercise training before returning home. In this section, we discuss the shoulder conditions most likely to be encountered by the acute care occupational therapist.

Rotator Cuff Repair

Rotator cuff injuries can occur as the result of two different pathological processes:

1. *Degeneration:* With age, tissues change, minute tears develop, and scarring and calcification occur, commonly near the insertion of the supraspinatus muscle.

2. *Trauma:* The rotator cuff, usually the supraspinatus, tears as a result of lifting against heavy resistance or when protecting oneself from falling (e.g., falling on outstretched hand).

Pain, weakness, and loss of ROM may occur when one of the tendons of the rotator cuff tears. However, not all rotator cuff tears cause pain or decreased function. Conservative treatment for a rotator cuff tear includes

- Activity modification and rest
- Heat or cold
- NSAIDs
- Cortisone injections
- Electrical stimulation
- Ultrasound
- Exercises to improve ROM, strength, and function.

Surgical repair may be indicated when the tear is associated with weakness or loss of function and the patient has not responded to conservative treatments. The goal of the surgical repair is to heal the torn tendon back to the humeral head from where it was torn (AAOS, 2007b). The choice of surgical technique is based on surgeon preference and experience. The most common surgical techniques include

- *Arthroscopic repair:* This technique uses multiple small incisions and arthroscopic technology.

- *Open repair:* An incision (usually several centimeters long) is made over the shoulder, and the deltoid muscle is detached. It is often combined with *acromioplasty* (i.e., the removal of bone spurs from under the acromion).

- *Mini-open repair:* This technique is a smaller version of the open repair that uses a 3- to 5-centimeter incision and incorporating arthroscopic removal of bone spurs. It eliminates the need to detach the deltoid muscle.

Occupational therapy treatment in this first phase of postoperative treatment is focused on

- Patient education to protect the surgical site and healing structures;

- ADLs while maintaining ROM precautions; and

- Therapeutic exercise within the surgical guidelines.

Therapeutic exercises are typically initiated Postoperative Day 0 or 1 and include active ROM of joints distal to the surgical site. Pendulums may or may not be allowed, based on surgeon preference and the complexity of the repair. Passive ROM (PROM) of the shoulder is initiated within the patient's tolerance and generally includes shoulder flexion, abduction, and external rotation to 0° (Ghilarducci & Maxey, 2007). Patients are generally required to wear a sling at all times. On the basis of surgeon preference, they may be allowed to remove the sling for hygiene and exercise.

Proximal Humerus Fractures

Proximal humerus fractures are generally treated conservatively with immobilization in a splint, sling, or both. Severe proximal humerus fractures may be treated with an ORIF or shoulder replacement surgery.

Shoulder Replacement (Total Shoulder Arthroplasty)

OA and severe shoulder (proximal humerus) fractures are the most common reasons for patients to undergo shoulder replacement surgery. Occupational therapy treatment in this first phase of postoperative treatment is focused on

- Patient education to protect the surgical site and healing structures;

- ADLs while maintaining ROM precautions; and

- Therapeutic exercise within the surgical guidelines.

Therapeutic exercises are typically initiated Postoperative Day 0 or 1 and include active ROM of joints distal to the surgical site, pendulums, and PROM of the shoulder (Sebelski & Guanache, 2007). Some surgeons may allow patients to perform self-assisted ROM exercises of the operative shoulder. Slings are generally prescribed for patient comfort and are encouraged until the follow-up visit with the surgeon.

Occupational Therapy for Patients With Upper-Extremity Fractures and Surgery

In addition to the general guidelines for working with the orthopedic patient (Appendix 7.A), the occupational therapist will address the following areas.

Dressing and Bathing

- Patients may benefit from instruction in one-handed techniques for bathing, dressing, and hygiene.

- Patients may benefit from adaptive equipment (e.g., long shoehorn, elastic laces) to facilitate independence with dressing and undressing.

- Patients should follow physician guidelines for when showering is allowed. Patients should be instructed in how to keep affected areas dry while showering.

- Patients with shoulder ROM restrictions should

  — Be instructed in how to don and doff their sling.

— Be instructed in how to perform lower-body ADLs while their affected arm is in the sling.

— Wear front-opening shirts. Patients should don shirts by standing with their knees and waist slightly bent and the elbow extended, slipping the shirt sleeve over the affected arm first and then slipping the unaffected arm into its sleeve. The elbow, wrist, and hand of the affected arm can be used to help fasten the buttons. The procedure is reversed for doffing the shirt. Patients with limited ROM in their nonoperative extremity may benefit from using a dressing stick to aid in upper-body dressing.

— Use only the unaffected arm for bathing. The same position used for dressing and undressing can be used to wash, dry, and apply deodorant under the affected arm.

Toileting

Patients may have difficulty performing toilet hygiene with their nondominant hand. The use of toilet aids and premoistened wipes may be helpful.

Functional Mobility

- A physical therapy consult may be indicated if the patient's gait becomes unsteady after injury or surgery or if the patient previously ambulated with an assistive device and is not able to continue with that device.

Sleeping

- Patients should be instructed in the use of pillows to maintain the shoulder in a comfortable position for sleeping.

- Patients with forearm or wrist injuries or surgery should be instructed in the use of pillows to elevate their operative arm to prevent edema.

Discharge Considerations

- Family and caregivers may need to be instructed in how to perform PROM exercises.

- A referral for home occupational therapy may be indicated if

— The patient is unable to perform the prescribed exercises;

— The patient does not have a family member or caregiver who can perform prescribed PROM exercises; or

— The patient requires additional training or practice to facilitate greater independence with ADLs.

Rib Fractures

The most common cause of a fractured rib is a direct blow to the chest. Although the most common mechanism of rib fracture for adults is a motor vehicle accident, older people are more likely to sustain rib fractures from a fall. Patients whose bones are weak (e.g., from cancer or osteoporosis) can fracture a rib from coughing hard (Doty & Sinert, 2008). Rib fractures generally take at least 6 weeks to heal. Patients are treated with rest, ice to the affected area, and pain medications. Because it can be painful to take deep breaths, patients with rib fractures are at risk for hypoventilation, atelectasis, and pneumonia.

In the acute care setting, occupational therapists can teach patients with rib fractures

- To use a pillow or folded blanket as a splint to reduce pain while coughing or deep breathing;

- Modified techniques to reduce pain during ADLs, including the use of adaptive equipment if needed;

- Energy conservation and pacing; and

- Fall prevention and home safety.

Gout

Gout is an inflammatory type of arthritis that typically affects the synovial capsule of joints. Over the years, gout has been known as *metabolic arthritis, acute gout arthritis, visceral gout, transitory gout,* or *migratory gout.* It is a metabolic disease associated with an unusually high level of uric acid in the body, which is known as *hyperuricemia*. Hyperuricemia can be the result of overproduction or underexcretion of uric acid, or sometimes both.

The onset of gout is typically acute, frequently nocturnal, and usually monarticular. Although the metatarsophalangeal joint of the great toe is the most susceptible joint (*podagra*), other commonly affected joints, in decreasing order, are the instep or forefoot, the ankle, the knee, the wrist, and the fingers (Harris, Siegel, & Alloway, 1999). Instances of gout have also been reported on the heel and on the rim of the ears, the hand, and the olecranon. Although gout is usually monarticular, it can be polyarticular (i.e., more than one joint affected during the same gout attack). *Polyarticular gout* is usually *asymmetric*, meaning the joints affected on each side of the body are not identical.

Most cases of primary gout are idiopathic. Gout is commonly precipitated by

- Excess alcohol (particularly beer);
- Purine-rich foods (e.g., red meat, seafood);
- Medication changes that affect urate metabolism; and
- Fasting before medical procedures.

Acute care patients may suffer an attack of gout because of dietary changes, fluid intake, or medications that lead to rapid reductions or increases in the serum urate level during their hospitalization (Hellman & Imboden, 2009). The four stages of gout are provided in Table 7.5.

Prevalence

More than 2 million Americans have suffered at least one attack of gout (Gout & Uric Acid Education Society, n.d.). About 90% of patients with primary gout are men, usually older than age 30. In women, the onset of gout is typically after menopause. Additionally, certain ethnicities, such as African and Pacific Islander, have an increased likelihood of developing gout (Hellman & Imboden, 2009).

Diagnosis and Medical Treatment

An acute onset of gout is often confused with cellulitis. Physicians use laboratory tests, imaging, and diagnostic procedures to diagnose gout. Laboratory tests detect (1) elevated serum uric acid levels, (2) increased white blood cell counts, and (3) elevated urine uric

Table 7.5. **Characteristics of Gout on the Basis of Gout Stage**

Stage	Characteristics
Asymptomatic hyperuricemia	• Increased urate levels in the blood • No visible signs or symptoms
Acute gout or gouty arthritis	• Symptomatic gout urate crystals within the joint(s) • Sudden and intense pain • Involved joint is swollen and tender and the overlying skin is tense, warm, and dusky red
Interval or intercritical gout	• Chronic recurrent episodes of gout with an asymptomatic period between acute episodes.
Chronic tophaceous gout	• Deforming polyarthritis of upper and lower extremities that mimics rheumatoid arthritis

acid levels. Early stages of the disease show no radiographic changes. Chronic gout may appear as punched-out erosions ("rat-bite") in X-rays of articular cartilage and subchondral bone (Hellman & Imboden, 2009; *Nurse's Quick Check*, 2009). Currently, the only way to accurately diagnose gout is through a site withdrawal of synovial or tophaceous fluid through arthrocentesis, which will show monosodium needlelike urate crystals.

Asymptomatic gout is not treated. Treatment for acute symptomatic gout consists of pharmacological treatment of the arthritis with NSAIDs and corticosteroids. Joint aspiration may be performed before corticosteroids are given. Long-term management of gout includes (1) lifestyle modifications, such as dietary changes to reduce purine intake, losing weight, and reduction of alcohol intake; (2) avoidance of hyperuricemic medications; (3) an assistive device for walking during acute episodes with increased joint inflammation; and (4) colchicine medication to help prevent another attack. *Pseudogout,* also known as *calcium pyrophosphate dehydrate,* is caused by crystals from calcium salts that cause pain and swelling similar to gout. Pseudogout is more likely to occur in the knee, wrist, and ankle.

Musculoskeletal Immunological Disorders

The acute care therapist may encounter several common musculoskeletal immunological disorders, which include rheumatoid arthritis, systemic lupus erythematosus, fibromyalgia, scleroderma, and ankylosing spondylitis. Although these disorders are generally treated on an outpatient basis and will generally be a comorbidity rather than the reason for an acute admission, the presence of these disorders may interfere with occupational performance during an acute care admission. It is important to have a good understanding of these disorders, the medical approach to them, their long-term prognosis, and how they may interfere with occupational performance. Table 7.6 outlines the characteristics of each disorder, prevalence and risk factors, and current medical treatment.

Occupational Therapy for Patients With Acute Gout and Musculoskeletal Immunological Disorders

In the acute care setting, patients can experience inflammatory, painful joint conditions that may interfere with occupational performance. Occupational therapists may use a combination of activity modification, joint protection techniques, and patient–caregiver education to promote functional independence and protection of the inflamed or painful joint(s). It is not crucial to measure ROM or strength in patients with acute painful conditions because

- ROM and strength testing may produce false results;
- ROM and strength testing can exacerbate the pain and inflammation; and
- Increased pain from ROM and strength testing can lead to poor rapport with the patient who is already in pain.

The occupational therapist should assess the patient for

- Pain,
- Skin integrity,
- Sensory disturbances,
- Presence of or propensity for deformities,
- Knowledge of the disease,
- Dysphagia (in patients with rheumatoid arthritis in the cervical joints or scleroderma),
- Activity tolerance,
- Depression,
- Cognitive impairments,
- Visual perceptual impairments,
- Edema.

In the acute care setting, occupational therapists should ensure that the patient's call bell is adequate for the patient's level of grasp. They may need to modify the bed rails or trapeze to facilitate bed mobility. Platform walkers or

(*Text continues on p. 328*)

Table 7.6. **Characteristics and Treatment of Common Musculoskeletal Immunological Disorders**

Disorder	Characteristics and Description	Prevalence and Risk Factors	Medical Treatment
Rheumatoid arthritis (RA)	• Chronic systemic inflammatory disorder. • Causes synovitis of multiple joints, generally symmetric. • Most commonly affects wrist, metacarpophalangeal and proximal interphalangeal joints of fingers, knees, ankles, and metatarsophalangeal joints. Any diarthrodial joint may be affected. • Can affect the neck (supporting ligaments of the atlanto-axial joint). • Can cause synovial cysts, ruptured tendons, and entrapment syndromes (particularly carpal tunnel syndrome). • Diagnosed when 4 of 7 American College of Rheumatology criteria are met (Rindfleisch & Muller, 2005): (1) morning stiffness in and around joints lasting at least 30–60 minutes before maximal improvement; (2) soft tissue swelling of ≥3 joint areas observed by a physician; (3) swelling of the proximal interphalangeal, metacarpophalangeal, or wrist joints; (4) symmetric swelling; (5) rheumatoid nodules; (6) presence of rheumatoid factor; and (7) radiographic erosions or periarticular osteopenia in hand or wrist joints. • Clinical course is marked by expontaneous remissions and relapses. • Other symptoms may include dryness of the mouth, eyes, and other mucous membranes; palmar erythema; pulmonary fibrosis; and small vessel vasculitis.	• More common in women than in men (female:male ratio 3:1) • Peak onset in the 4th or 5th decade for women and the 6th to 8th decade for men (Hellman & Imboden, 2009) • Affects 1.3 million Americans	• Disease-modifying antirheumatic drugs • Nonsteroidal anti-inflammatory drugs • Corticosteroids • Occupational and physical therapy • Surgery: Tenosynovectomy, repair of ruptured tendons, arthrodesis, osteotomy, joint reconstruction or total joint arthroplasty in advanced cases

Disorder	Description	Prevalence	Treatment
Systemic lupus erythematosus (SLE)	• Inflammatory, autoimmune disorder. • Can affect multiple organ systems. • Clinical course is marked by expontaneous remissions and relapses. • Systemic features include fever, anorexia, malaise, and weight loss. • Joint symptoms with or without active synovitis occur in >90% of cases (early manifestation). • Ocular manifestations include conjunctivitis, photophobia, transient or permanent monocular blindness, and blurring vision. • Characteristic "butterfly" rash. • Neurologic complications including psychosis, cognitive impairment, seizures, and strokes. • Diagnosed when 4 of 11 American College of Rheumatology criteria are met (Hellman & Imboden, 2009): facial rash, discoid or malar rash, sun sensitivity, oral ulcers, arthritis, serositis, kidney disease, neurologic complications (e.g., seizures, psychosis, peripheral and cranial neuropathies, transverse myelitis, stroke), hematologic disorders, immunologic abnormalities, and positive antinuclear antibody.	• Prevalence includes gender, race, and genetic inheritance • About 85% of patients are women • Gender differences are equalized among older adults • Affects all ages, with peak incidence in young adulthood • 1:1,000 White women vs. 1:250 Black women	• Immunosuppressive drugs • Corticosteroids • Nonsteroidal anti-inflammatory medications • Occupational and physical therapy • Dialysis or kidney transplant for renal failure • Education and emotional support
Fibromyalgia	• One of the most common rheumatic syndromes. • Chronic pain and stiffness involving entire body. • Even minor exertion aggravates pain and increases fatigue. • Unknown cause. • Aberrant perception of pain stimuli, sleep disorder, depression, and viral infection have been proposed as causes. • Can be a rare complication of hypothyroidism, rheumatoid arthritis or, in men, sleep apnea. • Not progressive.	Most frequent in women ages 20–50	• No effective pharmacologic treatment • Occupational and physical therapy • Patient education • Reassure patient that symptoms are the result of a disease and are not psychosomatic

(continued)

Table 7.6. (*continued*)

Disorder	Characteristics and Description	Prevalence and Risk Factors	Medical Treatment
Scleroderma	• Rare, chronic disease. • Characterized by diffuse fibrosis of the skin and internal organs. • Two forms: Limited (80% of cases) and diffuse (20%). • Characteristics of limited scleroderma: — Raynaud's phenomenon — Antinuclear antibodies — Esophageal motility disorder — Sclerodactyly and telangiectasia — Hardening of skin in face and hands — Susceptible to digital ischemia leading to finger loss and to life-threatening pulmonary hypertension. • Characteristics of diffuse scleroderma: — Raynaud's phenomenon — Skin changes involving the trunk and proximal extremities — Polyarthralgia — Weight loss — Malaise — Renal failure or interstitial lung disease — Dysphagia.	• Female:male ratio ranges from 3:1 to 8:1; higher in child-bearing years • Symptoms usually appear in the 30s–50s	• Treatment is symptomatic and focuses on the organ systems involved • In general, better outcome with limited scleroderma
Ankylosing spondylitis	• Chronic inflammatory disease of the joints of the axial skeleton. • Usually occurs as a primary disorder, but may occur secondary to psoriatic arthritis, reactive arthritis (Reiter's syndrome), or inflammatory bowel syndrome.	• Affects ≥0.5 million people in the United States (Spondylitis Association of America [SAA], 2008)	• Disease-modifying anti-rheumatic drugs • Nonsteroidal anti-inflammatory medicines

- For a reliable diagnosis, the patient must meet Criterion 7 and any one of Criteria 1–5, or any 5 of Criteria 1–6 if Criterion 7 is not met:
  1. Axial skeleton stiffness for at least 3 months that is relieved by exercises
  2. Lumbar pain that persists at rest
  3. Thoracic cage pain of ≥3 months duration that persists at rest
  4. Past or current iritis
  5. Decreased lumbar range of motion
  6. Decreased chest expansion (age related)
  7. Bilateral, symmetrical sacroiliitis demonstrated by radiographic studies.

- More prevalent than multiple sclerosis, cystic fibrosis, and amyotrophic lateral sclerosis combined (SAA, 2008)
- More prevalent in men than women
- Onset commonly occurs between the ages 17 and 35

- Corticosteroids not used because they have a minimal impact on disease and can worsen osteopenia
- Exercise
- Thermal modalities
- Education about maintaining posture
- Surgery: Total hip arthroplasty or spinal wedge osteotomy for severe spinal involvement

hemi walkers may be necessary for patients who are not able to maintain their grasp on a standard or rolling walker. Patients should be encouraged to be out of bed and to participate in activity as tolerated.

Occupational therapists may teach the patient

- To keep the affected joint elevated to facilitate venous return and reduce edema;
- Joint protection and body mechanic techniques, including the use of adaptive equipment and larger muscles during ADLs, instrumental ADLs, and leisure activities and avoiding sustained positions;
- To maintain skin integrity by inspecting skin and wearing appropriate footwear;
- To reduce edema via positioning and active ROM;
- Energy conservation and work simplification techniques;
- Relaxation and breathing techniques to help reduce and cope with pain;
- One-handed techniques;
- How to perform functional transfers without putting pressure through the affected joint; and
- Use of flexible rather than rigid sock aids.

Joint protection and activity modification techniques may include

- Splinting according to the patient's needs to prevent, correct, or minimize deformities;
- Bed cradles to reduce pressure from bed linens on affected joints;
- Postsurgical shoes to shift weight off the affected big toe of patients with gout;
- Using partial weight bearing during functional mobility and standing activities;
- Built-up utensils for self-feeding; and
- Bed mobility without putting pressure on the inflamed joint.

Occupational therapists may also educate the patient about

- The disease, including symptoms, treatments, and side effects of medication;
- Initiating and progressing gentle ROM exercises of the affected joint, within the patient's pain tolerance;
- The importance of following dietary guidelines to reduce the risk of future gout attacks;
- Lifestyle modifications, including losing weight if needed;
- Lifelong exercise to maintain joint mobility and strength;
- Availability of community services and disease-specific organizations, such as the Arthritis Foundation, Gout and Uric Acid Education Society, Lupus Foundation of America, the Scleroderma Foundation, and the Spondylitis Association of America; and
- The availability of complementary and alternative treatments such as yoga, tai chi, hydrotherapy, and acupuncture. Patients should be encouraged to consult with their physician before starting any new treatment to ensure that it will not cause damage or interfere with medical treatment.

References

American Academy of Orthopaedic Surgeons. (2007a). *Knee osteoarthritis statistics.* Retrieved February 2, 2009, from http://orthoinfo.aaos.org/topic.cfm?topic=A00399

American Academy of Orthopaedic Surgeons. (2007b). *Rotator cuff tears and treatment options.* Retrieved May 3, 2009, from http://orthoinfo.aaos.org/topic.cfm?topic=A00406

American Academy of Orthopaedic Surgeons. (2008). *Your orthopedic connection.* Retrieved October 10, 2008, from http://orthoinfo.aaos.org

Arthritis Foundation (2009). *Surgery center.* Retrieved February 2, 2009, from www.arthritis.org/types-replacement-parts.php

Barr, K., & Harrast, M. (2006). Low back pain. In R. Braddom (Ed.), *Physical medicine and rehabilitation* (3rd ed., pp. 883–928). St Louis, MO: Elsevier.

Bear-Lehman, J. (2002). Orthopedic conditions. In C. Trombly & M. Radomski (Eds.), *Occupational therapy for physical dysfunction* (5th ed., pp.909–925). Philadelphia: Lippincott Williams & Wilkins.

Boden, S. (2006). Bone graft substitutes for lumbar spine fusion surgery. *Spine Health*. Retrieved May 24, 2009, from www.spine-health.com/treatment/spinal-fusion/bone-graft-substitutes-lumbar-spine-fusion-surgery

Born, C. T. (2009). *Hip fractures*. Retrieved May 19, 2009, from http://orthoinfo.aaos.org/topic.cfm? topic =A00392

Bozic, K. J., Kurtz, S. M., Lau, E., Ong, K., Vail, T. P., & Berry, D. J. (2009). The epidemiology of revision total hip arthroplasty in the United States. *Journal of Bone and Joint Surgery*, 91, 128–133.

Buckwalter, J. A., Saltzman, C., & Brown, T. (2004). The impact of osteoarthritis: Implications for research. *Clinical Orthopedics and Related Research, 427*(Suppl.), S6–S15.

Cacanindin, N., Wong, J., & Ries, M. (2007). Total knee arthroplasty. In L. Maxey & J. Magnusson (Eds.), *Rehabilitation for the postsurgical orthopedic patient* (2nd ed., pp. 398–401). St. Louis, MO: Mosby.

Centers for Disease Control and Prevention. (2005). *Catheter-associated urinary tract infections*. Retrieved March 31, 2009, from http://www.cdc.gov/ncidod/dhqp/dpac_uti_pc.html

Centers for Disease Control and Prevention. (2008). *Surgical site infections*. Retrieved March 31, 2009, from http://www.cdc.gov/ncidod/dhqp/FAQ_SSI.html

Centers for Disease Control and Prevention, Injury Center. (2008, June 10). *Hip fractures among older adults*. Retrieved October 7, 2008, from www.cdc.gov/ncipc/factsheets/adulthipfx.htm

Clark, B. (2000). Rheumatology: 9. Physical and occupational therapy in the management of arthritis. *Canadian Medical Association Journal, 163*, 999–1005.

Cloyd, J., Acosta, F., & Ames, C. (2008). Complications and outcomes of lumbar spine surgery in elderly people: A review of the literature. *Journal of the American Geriatrics Society*, 56, 1318–1327.

Crawford Mechem, C. (2008). *Fracture, pelvic*. Retrieved November 16, 2008, from www.emedicine.com/emerg/TOPIC203.HTM

Crist, B. (2007). *Ankle fractures*. Retrieved March 31, 2009, from http://orthoinfo.aaos.org/topic.cfm? topic=A00391

DeFrances, C., Lucas, C., Buie, C., & Golosinskiy, A. (2008, July 30). 2006 national hospital discharge survey. *National Health Statistics Reports, 5*. Retrieved May 24, 2009, from www.cdc.gov/nchs/data/nhsr/nhsr005.pdf

Doty, C. I., & Sinert, R. (2008). *Fracture, rib*. Retrieved April 15, 2009, from http://emedicine.medscape.com/article/825981-overview

Druss, B., Olfson, M., & Pincus, H. A. (2002). The most expensive medical conditions in America. *Health Affairs, 21*, 105–111.

Ghilarducci, M., & Maxey, L. (2007). Rotator cuff repair and rehabilitation. In L. Maxey & J. Magnusson (Eds.), *Rehabilitation for the postsurgical orthopedic patient* (2nd ed., pp. 65–88). St. Louis, MO: Mosby.

Gout & Uric Acid Education Society. (n.d.) *About gout: FAQs*. Retrieved April 1, 2009, from http://gouteducation.org/patient/faqs/

Harris, M. D., Siegel, L. B., & Alloway, J. A. (1999). Gout and hyperuricemia. *American Family Physician, 59*. Retrieved April 1, 2009, from www.aafp.org/afp/990215ap/925.html

Hellman, D. B., & Imboden, J. B. (2009). Musculoskeletal immunologic disorders. In S. J. McPhee & M. A. Papdakis (Eds.), *2009 current medical diagnosis and treatment* (pp. 708–765). New York: McGraw-Hill.

Hu, S., Tribus, C., Tay, B., & Carlson, G. (2003). Disorders, diseases, and injuries of the spine. In H. Skinner (Ed.), *Current diagnosis and treatment in orthopedics* (3rd ed., p. 285). New York: McGraw-Hill.

Kreuzer, S. (2006). *Anterior approach: Hip replacement surgery*. Retrieved April 15, 2009, from www.anteriorhip.net

Lawlor, M., Humphreys, P., Morrow, E., Ogonda, L., Bennet, D., Elliott, D., et al. (2005). Comparison of early postoperative functional levels following total hip replacement using minimally invasive versus standard incisions: A prospective randomized blinded trial. *Clinical Rehabilitation, 19*, 465–474.

Lonner, J. (2003). A 57-year-old man with osteo-arthritis of the knee. *JAMA, 289,* 1016–1025.

Mahmood, A., Zafar, M., Majid, I., Maffulli, N., & Thompson, J. (2007). Minimally invasive hip arthroplasty: A quantitative review of the literature. *British Medical Bulletin, 84,* 37–48.

Malik, M., Chougle, A., Pradhan, N., Gambhir, A., & Porter, M. (2005). Primary total knee replacement: A comparison of a nationally agreed guide to best practice and current surgical technique as determined by the North West Regional Arthroplasty Register. *Annals of the Royal College of Surgeons of England, 87,* 117–121.

Martin, G. (2007). *Patient information: Total knee replacement (arthroplasty).* Retrieved January 5, 2009, from www.uptodate.com/patients/content/topic.do?topicKey=bone_joi/2365

Matta, J. M. (2007). New approaches in total hip replacement: The anterior approach for mini-invasive total hip arthroplasty. In L. Maxey & J. Magnusson (Eds.), *Rehabilitation for the post-surgical orthopedic patient* (2nd ed., pp. 525–530). St. Louis, MO: Mosby.

Murkherjee, S. (2008). *Ileus.* Retrieved March 31, 2009, from http://emedicine.medscape.com/article/178948-overview

National Institute of Arthritis and Musculoskeletal and Skin Diseases. (2006). *Knee problems.* Available online at www.niams.nih.gov/Health_Info/Knee_Problems/default.asp

National Institutes of Health. (2008). *Unicom-partmental knee arthroplasty.* Retrieved May 24, 2009, from www.nlm.nih.gov/medlineplus/ency/article/007256.htm

Nazon, D., Abergel, G., & Hatem, C. (2003). Critical care in orthopedic and spine surgery. *Critical Care Clinics, 19,* 33–53.

Nurses Quick Check: Diseases (2nd ed.). (2009). Philadelphia: Lippincott Williams & Wilkins.

Pablo, V., Pradhan, B., Sueki, D., Delamarter, R., & Huffman, J. (2007). Anterior cervical discectomy and fusion. In L. Maxey & J. Magnusson (Eds.), *Rehabilitation for the postsurgical orthopedic patient* (2nd ed., pp. 217–279). St. Louis, MO: Mosby.

Pottenger, L. (2003). Orthopedic problems with aging. In C. Cassel, R. Leipzig, H. G. Cohen, E. Larson, & D. Meier (Eds.), *Geriatric medicine: An evidence-based approach* (4th ed., pp. 651–655). New York: Springer.

Prather, H., Watson, J., & Gilula, L. (2007). Non-operative management of osteoporotic vertebral compression fractures. *Injury, 38,* 133–155.

Pratt, E., & Gray, P. A. (2007). Total hip arthroplasty. In L. Maxey & J. Magnusson (Eds.), *Rehabilitation for the postsurgical orthopedic patient* (2nd ed., pp. 525–530). St. Louis, MO: Elsevier.

Riddle, D., Jiranek, W., & McGlynn, F. (2008). Yearly incidence of unicompartmental knee arthroplasty in the United States. *Journal of Arthroplasty, 23,* 408–412.

Rindfleisch, J. A., & Muller, D. (2005). Diagnosis and management of rheumatoid arthritis. *American Family Physician, 72,* 1037–1050. Retrieved April 1, 2009, from www.aafp.org/afp/20050915/1037.html

Rolston, L., Bresch, J., Engh, G., Franz, A., Kreuzer, S., Nadaud M., et al. (2007). Bicompartmental knee arthroplasty: A bone-sparing, ligament-sparing, and minimally invasive alternative for active patients. *Orthopedics, 30,* 70–73.

Rybski, M. (2004). *Kinesiology for occupational therapy.* Thorofare, NJ: Slack.

Sebelski, C. A., & Guanache, C. A. (2007). Total shoulder arthroplasty. In L. Maxey & J. Magnusson (Eds.), *Rehabilitation for the postsurgical ortho-pedic patient* (2nd ed., pp. 113–135). St. Louis, MO: Mosby.

Skinner, J., Zhou, W., & Weinstein, J. (2006) The influence of income and race on total knee arthroplasty in the United States. *Journal of Bone and Joint Surgery, 88,* 2159–2166.

Snyder, D. C., & Hanmer, A. (2006). *Massachusetts surgeons introduce unique alternative to total hip replacement.* Retrieved February 16, 2009, from www.bostonhipresurfacing.com

Spondylosis Association of America. (2008). *Anky-losing spondylitis.* Retrieved April 4, 2009, from www.spondylitis.org/about/as.aspx

Srikanth, V., Fryer, J., Zhai, G., Winzenberg, T. M., Hosmer, D., & Jones, G. (2005). A meta-analysis of sex differences prevalence, incidence and severity of osteoarthritis. *OsteoArthritis and Cartilage, 13,* 769–781.

Su, E., DeWal, H., & Di Cesare, P. (2004). Periprosthetic femoral fractures above total knee replacements. *Journal of American Academy of Orthopedic Surgery, 12*(1), 12–20.

Wing, P. (2001). Rheumatology: 13. Minimizing disability in patients with low back pain. *Canadian Medical Association Journal, 164,* 1459–1468.

Younger, T. (2007). *Joint revision surgery: When do I need it?* Retrieved February 18, 2009, from http://orthoinfo.aaos.org/topic.cfm?topic=A00510

Appendix 7.A.

General Guidelines for Working With the Orthopedic Patient

The primary roles of the occupational therapist working with the orthopedic patient are to educate and train the patient in the use of alternative techniques to perform activities of daily living (ADLs) and to work with the patient and family to modify their home environment to optimize the patient's level of functioning and safety on discharge (Clark, 2000). In the acute care setting, many factors may affect a patient's recovery, ability to participate in occupational therapy, and discharge plan. These guidelines will help the acute care occupational therapist effectively treat the orthopedic patient.

Clarification of Orders

Before evaluating the orthopedic patient, the occupational therapist should check the physician's orders to determine whether any weight-bearing or range of motion (ROM) precautions or restrictions need to be followed and whether any splints, braces, or slings are needed.

Coordination of Services

In the busy acute care environment, it is important to plan and schedule occupational therapy evaluation and treatment time around other interventions. Occupational therapists should

- Check with the unit coordinator or patient's nurse to determine whether the patient is scheduled to be off the floor for any tests or procedures.
- Check the patient's medical record or with the patient's nurse to determine when the patient last received pain medication and is due for his or her next dose. Ideally, it is best to see patients when their pain is well controlled. Patients will not perform optimally if they are in pain and are due for or have just received pain medication.
- Coordinate with the patient's physical therapist to plan treatment times and goals for each discipline. For example, it may work best for the physical therapist to see a patient first and leave the patient sitting in the chair for an occupational therapy ADL training session. In other cases, it may work best for the occupational therapist to see the patient first and leave the patient dressed in preparation for stair training with the physical therapist.
- Check with the patient's case manager or discharge planner to determine whether completed occupational therapy notes are needed to initiate screens for a rehabilitation facility.

Lab Values

Appendix P provides common lab values and the parameters for which treatment is contraindicated or needs to be modified. *Hematocrit (HCT)* is the lab value of most concern when working with an orthopedic patient. Patients with a HCT lower than 25 are likely to receive a blood transfusion. Occupational therapy should be deferred or conducted at bed level. Patients with HCT between 25–30 may or may not be transfused depending on several factors, such as age, vital signs, cardiac history, and the presence of orthostatic symptoms. It is important to carefully monitor the patient for signs and symptoms of orthostatic hypotension during occupational therapy evaluation and treatment. It is also important to consider that patients with a low HCT may fatigue easily, and treatment plans may need to be modified. In addition to checking HCT levels, occupational therapists should also check potassium levels (especially in patients with a cardiac history) and glucose levels (especially in patients with a history of diabetes) when determining whether occupational therapy treatment is appropriate for a patient.

Orthostatic Hypotension

Orthostatic hypotension is a condition in which a patient experiences a sudden drop in systolic blood pressure (usually ≥20 mm Hg) when assuming a standing position. This is usually accompanied by a heart rate of 20 beats per minute or more. Patients may experience light-headedness, dizziness, nausea, diaphoresis, or fainting. In the postsurgical patient, orthostatic hypotension can be caused by

- A low HCT
- Dehydration
- The wearing off of anesthesia
- Certain narcotic pain medications
- Certain blood pressure medications.

Occupational therapists should monitor vital signs closely and observe the patient for any signs or symptoms of orthostatic hypotension. Baseline vital signs should be taken before initiating occupational therapy treatment and compared with vital signs taken with each position change (e.g., supine to sit and sit to stand). Patients may experience signs or symptoms of orthostatic hypotension when transitioning from supine to sitting. If the symptoms resolve, it is appropriate to proceed with out-of-bed activity. Patients who experience orthostatic hypotension should be returned to supine, with the head of the bed flat to facilitate return of blood flow to the head. In extreme cases, the bed can be placed in the *Trendelenburg position* (head lower than the feet on an inclined plane) until the symptoms resolve. When symptoms have resolved, the patient should be encouraged to keep the head of the bed raised as much as possible, drink plenty of fluids, perform ankle pumps before standing, and stand up slowly rather than quickly. The patient's nurse should also be notified. The medical team may choose to order a blood transfusion (if the patient's HCT is low) or a fluid bolus (if the patient is dehydrated). Persistent orthostatic hypotension may necessitate a change in pain or blood pressure medications.

Occupational therapists may sometimes observe a drop in the patient's blood pressure without the patient experiencing any signs or symptoms of orthostatic hypotension. The occupational therapist may choose to leave the patient sitting up in a chair while continuing to monitor vital signs. If the vital signs stabilize, the patient may remain sitting up in the chair, with instructions to ring the call bell if he or she begins to feel light-headed, dizzy, or nauseated. However, if the systolic blood pressure continues to trend down, the patient should be returned to bed regardless of whether he or she is experiencing any symptoms.

Pain Management

The primary method for managing pain in the orthopedic patient is pain medication. The choice of medication varies with facility and physician preference. The following medications are commonly used to treat postsurgical pain:

- Oxycodone
- Morphine
- Hydromorphone
- Vicodin
- Percocet.

Refer to Appendix B for more information about these medications.

When patients are receiving their pain medications orally, occupational therapists should plan to see them during the medication's effective period. Some patients may be receiving their medication through a patient-controlled analgesic pump. Occupational therapists should inform the patient what time they plan to see them and encourage them to use the patient-controlled analgesic pump before the scheduled treatment time.

Occupational therapists should be aware of the potential side effects of narcotic pain medications such as dizziness, light-headedness, nausea, and orthostatic hypotension. Treatment may need to be modified if the patient is experiencing any of these symptoms. Nursing and the medical team should be notified if the patient's ability to participate in occupational therapy is hindered by medication side effects.

Older adults may be particularly sensitive to narcotic pain medications. Hence, they may be receiving only non-narcotic pain medications, and pain may limit their ability to participate in occupational therapy. Older adults who are taking narcotic pain medications may experience confusion or delirium. Acute mental status changes should be reported to the patient's nurse.

Occupational therapists can be effective in helping patients manage their pain by

- Providing ice packs to the affected area;
- Positioning affected limbs or joints for comfort;
- Teaching deep or relaxation breathing; and
- Encouraging patients to take pain medication on schedule even if they are not experiencing pain at rest.

Refer to Appendix J for more information regarding pain management in the acute care setting.

Postoperative Complications

All surgeries pose a risk of complication. Postoperative complications in the orthopedic patient occur at a relatively low rate and are largely related to a patient's age and comorbidities. Although the occupational therapist does not play a direct role in treating these complications, the acute care occupational therapist should be able to recognize the symptoms of these complications and relay the pertinent information to the other health care providers.

Deep Vein Thrombosis

Postsurgical patients are at increased risk for developing a blood clot or deep vein thrombosis (DVT). The following methods are generally used to reduce risk of DVT:

- *Anticoagulation medication (e.g., Coumadin):* Patients on anticoagulants are at a greater risk for bleeding if they fall or cut themselves. It is important to assess a patient for fall risk and to educate the patient and his or her family about home safety to prevent falls.
- *Intermittent pneumatic compression (IPC) devices (e.g., Venodyne boots):* IPC devices squeeze the calf muscles to promote blood circulation and prevent blood clots. Occupational therapists should be sure to apply the patient's IPC devices when they return the patient to bed.
- *Elastic stockings (e.g., thromboembolic deterrents):* Elastic stockings are prescribed on the basis of surgeon preference. Many surgeons prefer to have their orthopedic patients wear elastic stockings at home during the day (they may be removed at night) until the follow-up postoperative visit. Occupational therapists should instruct the patient on how to apply and remove the elastic stockings, using adaptive equipment if necessary. Patients who are unable to don or doff elastic stockings independently may need a family member or caregiver to assist them at home. Patients should be instructed to don the elastic stockings as soon as they awake, before they are up and about for the day.

Edema and Compartment Syndrome

Swelling is common with fractures and after surgical procedures. Occupational therapists can educate patients who have nonoperable fractures or who are postsurgery to control edema by keeping the affected limb elevated and by performing active ROM of the unaffected joints.

Excessive bleeding and swelling can lead to muscle and nerve ischemia, resulting in an unusually painful, swollen, or tense limb, which is called *compartment syndrome*. Muscle groups in the arms, hands, legs, and feet, along with their corresponding blood vessels, nerves, and the fascia covering them, are called a *compartment*. The lack of blood flow to the muscles and nerves can cause cell death within hours, leading to permanent disability or death.

Compartment syndrome is a medical emergency. When a patient complains of pain that is out of proportion to the original problem, pain that is not relieved by medication, decreased mobility of the digits, or paresthesias, the occupational therapist should report these symptoms to the doctor immediately. The doctor will assess the patient for compartment syndrome. Dressings, splints, or casts may be removed to relieve pressure. A *fasciotomy* (surgical decompression) may be performed to relieve pressure in the threatened compartment.

Pulmonary Complications

Pulmonary complications such as pneumonia or *atelectasis* (a collapse of the alveoli) can arise because of decreased deep breathing in the initial days after surgery. Discomfort after an operation can make it hard to take deep breaths or to cough to clear mucus out of the lungs. Additionally, the lungs may take a few days to recover from anesthesia and regain their optimal functioning. Patients with baseline chronic obstructive pulmonary disease are much more likely to have postoperative pulmonary complications, occurring at a rate of nearly 70% (Nazon, Abergel, & Hatem, 2003). Deep breathing exercises or the use of an incentive spirometer and out-of-bed activity should be encouraged to aid in clearing out the patient's lungs.

Urinary Retention

Urinary retention occurs when a patient is unable to empty his or her bladder as a result of anesthesia. Typically, patients will have a catheter inserted to empty the bladder until they have regained their bladder control.

Urinary Tract Infection

The urinary tract is the most common site of infection in acute care hospital settings (Centers for Disease Control and Prevention [CDC], 2005). Nearly two-thirds of these infections are a result of urinary catheterization (CDC, 2005). Some common symptoms of urinary tract infection include urinary frequency, pain with urination, hematuria, low-grade fever, and abdominal pain. In the older patient, a urinary tract infection will often present itself as a change in mental status, a general ill feeling, or an increased tendency to fall.

Surgical Infection

Surgical infection can occur when bacteria enter the site of the surgery. These infections are dangerous because they can easily travel to nearby tissue and organs through the bloodstream. Infections can be treated with antibiotics, irrigation and debridement of the wound, or drainage of any abscesses. Surgical site infections occur in less than 1% of all orthopedic surgeries (CDC, 2008). Some common signs of a surgical infection are an incision that is red, swollen, or warm; fever; chills; and swollen lymph nodes.

Paralytic Ileus

A *paralytic ileus* is a hypomotility of the gastrointestinal tract. In the setting of orthopedic surgery, they typically occur as a result of narcotic pain medications. Some common symptoms of an ileus are decreased bowel sounds, a distended abdomen, nausea, and vomiting. Typically, the digestive system will regain normal function within 1–2 days (Mukherjee, 2008).

Discharge Planning

Given that patients are generally discharged from the acute care setting on Postoperative Day 3 or 4, another role of the occupational therapist is to help determine discharge disposition. Patients may be discharged home with or without services or transferred to a short-term rehabilitation facility (skilled nursing facility or acute inpatient rehabilitation facility). Good communication with the patient's case manager or discharge planner and physical therapist is important because the patient's health insurance, facility requirements, and physical therapy needs can affect discharge disposition options.

Discharge planning begins with the occupational therapy evaluation and continues throughout the patient's stay. During the initial evaluation, the therapist gathers information about the patient's supports (e.g., who the patient lives with, who is available to help after discharge), living situation (e.g., house vs. apartment, location of bedrooms and bathrooms), bathroom setup (e.g., tub vs. shower stall, toilet height, grab bars), durable medical equipment (e.g., commode, shower seat), prior level of function (e.g., was the patient receiving assistance with any ADLs or instrumental activities of daily living [IADLs] before admission), patient goals (e.g., preference for home vs. rehabilitation facility, which ADLs and IADLs the patient needs to perform independently), and current level of functioning.

The occupational therapist will make a discharge recommendation based on the patient's evaluation, goals, and progress toward goals. The discharge recommendation includes

- Disposition (e.g., skilled nursing facility, acute rehabilitation facility, home)
- Services (e.g., level of supervision, home occupational therapy, home health aide)
- Durable medical equipment (e.g., commode, shower seat)
- Adaptive equipment (e.g., sock aid, reacher, shoehorn, dressing stick).

The occupational therapist is responsible for ensuring that the patient has the information he or she needs to procure any recommended equipment that is not issued by the facility.

Appendix 7.B.

Osteoarthritis

Osteoarthritis (OA) is a degenerative joint disease in which articular cartilage is progressively lost. When the cartilage is damaged, the normally smooth movement of the joint is replaced by painful friction. As the disease progresses, the cartilage may disappear, causing bone to rub on bone. Bony spurs usually form around the joint.

Worldwide, OA affects 10% of people older than age 60 (Buckwalter, Saltzman, & Brown, 2004). OA affects people of all ethnic backgrounds and in all geographic locations. Although OA affects both men and women, it is more common in women (Buckwalter et al., 2004; Srikanth et al., 2005). Although a gender difference is not apparent in the prevalence of hip OA, women have a higher prevalence of knee and hand OA, and men younger than age 55 appear to be at higher risk for cervical spine degeneration (Srikanth et al., 2005). OA can be classified as primary or secondary. Table 7.B.1 describes the characteristics of primary and secondary osteoarthritis.

Physicians use radiographic imaging, physical examination, and patient report of symptoms to diagnose OA. Radiographic imaging shows joint space narrowing, thinning or erosion of the bone, excess fluid in the joint, osteophytes, or bony sclerosis. During the physical examination, the

Table 7.B.1. Primary and Secondary Osteoarthritis (OA)

Characteristics	Primary OA	Secondary OA
Joints affected	• Most common in hand, foot, knee, spine, and hip joints • Rarely occurs in ankle, wrist, elbow, or shoulder	• Occurs in ankle, wrist, elbow, and shoulder at least as often as the foot, knee, spine, and hip joints
Cause	• No known cause of joint degeneration	• Joint injury • Joint dysplasia • Joint infection • Aseptic necrosis • Neuropathic arthropathy • Hemophilia
Risk factors (Buckwalter, Saltzman, & Brown, 2004)	• The percentage of people with OA in one or more joints increases with age: 15–44, <5%; 45–64, 25%–30%; ≥65, 60%–90% • Genetic predisposition • Obesity • Greater bone density • Joint laxity • Excessive repetitive joint loading (e.g., physically demanding jobs, high-impact sports)	• Joint injury: Meniscal, ligament, and joint capsule tears; dislocations; and intra-articular fractures • Age—Increased risk of posttraumatic OA with older age at time of injury • Hip dysplasia

doctor looks for pain or restricted motion with the affected joint in various positions; *crepitus* (i.e., creaking or grinding noises that indicate bone-on-bone friction); muscle atrophy; and signs of injury to muscles, tendons, and ligaments.

Symptoms of OA may range from mild to severe, depending on how much the disease has progressed. Symptoms may include

- Morning discomfort or stiffness
- Increased pain with activity that goes away with rest
- Joint swelling
- Grating of the joint with motion
- Joint pain in rainy weather
- Pain that is not relieved with rest (severe cases).

OA has no cure. Treatment for OA aims to

- Reduce pain and other symptoms;
- Improve the ability to perform daily activities; and
- Slow the progression of the disease.

Nonsurgical treatment for OA usually consists of a combination of the following elements:

- Lifestyle modification, which includes weight reduction and switching to lower-impact activities (e.g., bicycling or swimming instead of running);
- Occupational therapy for (1) education about joint protection and modification of tasks to eliminate or reduce stress on affected joints, (2) recommendations about equipment and devices to perform daily activities more comfortably, and (3) splints and positioning devices to stabilize joints and reduce pain;
- Physical therapy for (1) exercises to improve strength and flexibility, (2) pain management techniques, and (3) training in the use of supportive devices (e.g., cane or walker); and
- Medication; a combination of medications tailored to the individual patient's specific needs may include (1) analgesics to reduce pain without reducing inflammation; (2) topical analgesics applied directly over the painful area; (3) NSAIDs to reduce inflammation, swelling, and pain (e.g., aspirin, ibuprofen, naproxen); (3) COX-2 inhibitors to reduce pain and inflammation (e.g., Celebrex, Vioxx); (4) corticosteroids (anti-inflammatory agents that are injected directly into the joint); and (e) viscosupplements, which are specifically for the knee joint and involve the injection of hyaluronic acid directly into the joint.

Some patients choose to use over-the-counter supplements to relieve OA pain. These supplements include glucosamine and chondroitin sulfate. They should be used with caution because they can cause side effects and may interfere with other medications. Other alternative or complementary treatments commonly used for OA include acupuncture and chiropractic care. Up-to-date information about the risks and effectiveness of alternative and complementary OA treatments can be found on the American Academy of Orthopaedic Surgeons Web site at www.aaos.org/ or the Arthritis Foundation Disease Center at www.arthritis.org/disease-center.php.

Joint surgery may be indicated in later stages of the disease or when nonsurgical treatments are no longer effective. Refer to the joint-specific sections of this chapter for more information about surgical options for specific joints. Although OA is generally not the primary diagnosis for an acute hospitalization, it is often a comorbidity that may affect occupational performance. In addition, OA is the most common diagnosis leading to acute care admissions for joint replacement surgery.

8

The Endocrine System

Suzanne E. Holm, MA, OTR, BCPR

The endocrine system is essential for basic life function and homeostasis. This system, essential for metabolism, immune system function, reproduction, water–electrolyte regulation, and body size, relies on and communicates through the actions of hormones. *Endocrine glands* produce and secrete hormones, which directly enter the bloodstream in response to specific stimuli. Hormones are chemical messengers; they act as catalysts for chemical changes by influencing target cells through binding to specific receptors that may include other endocrine glands, organs, or body tissues. In contrast, *exocrine glands,* such as salivary and sweat glands, secrete products directly into ducts, onto the body surface, or into body cavities.

The endocrine system controls many aspects of human physiology and works in concert with the nervous system to regulate homeostasis and body metabolism. Deleterious consequences from endocrine dysfunction or disease can result in permanent damage to the skeletal system, kidneys, immune system, liver, gastrointestinal system, heart, and circulatory system. Endocrine disorders, including diabetes mellitus, diabetes insipidus, hyperthyroidism, and adrenal insufficiency, may also result in long-term and potentially fatal neurological complications (Simpson, 2005).

Although the incidence of endocrine disease ranges from illnesses that are quite rare to those that are more widespread, the trend overall is upward shifting, especially for diseases such as hypothyroidism and pituitary gland dysfunction. Hypothyroidism is now present in as many as 20% of women and 8% of men (Laurberg, Andersen, Bulow Pedersen, & Carle, 2005). A 2004 study (Ezzat et al., 2004) found a more than 16% incidence of pituitary gland tumors. Endocrine diseases, often chronic, are increasing as a result of multiple factors, including a rise in obesity, sedentary lifestyles, the aging population, and consumption of highly processed foods (Kim & Popkin, 2006).

Occupational therapists are likely to encounter many clients, especially those with sedentary lifestyles, who have or are at risk for the more familiar endocrine and endocrine-related diseases, such as diabetes mellitus, hypertension, and osteoporosis, in the acute care setting. The Centers for Disease Control and Prevention (CDC) National Health and Nutrition Examination Survey (2008a) found that more than 65% of U.S. adults are overweight or obese, which increases the risk for development of diabetes, hypertension, osteoarthritis, stroke, and some types of cancer. More than 8% of the U.S. population have diabetes and 60% have hypertension; 55% of people age 50 and older have osteoporosis (CDC, 2008a, 2008b). Autoimmune diseases and central nervous system impairment both have strong endocrine components. Therefore, although an endocrinological disease process may not be the specific reason for a hospital admission, the endocrine system remains susceptible to disruption, and underlying endocrine dysfunction may already exist.

Because of the endocrine system's complexities and intricacies, this chapter will provide an overview of the basics of the primary endocrine system glands and related key hormones with a summary of some of the more common acute and chronic effects of endocrine disease.

Normal Structure and Function

The endocrine system relies on hormones to control homeostasis. Hormones regulate many parts of the body, including human growth and development, metabolism, reproduction, and the capacity for handling stress. The endocrine system also plays a major role in regulating the body's glucose control, water balance, and electrolyte function. The body must increase its metabolism when energy demands increase. Finally, the endocrine system's regulation process to ensure homeostasis is conducted primarily through a negative feedback system to maintain hormone levels within a specified range. Regulation is critical because too much or too little of a hormone can be detrimental to the body.

Hormones

Hormones are chemical messengers that are released by the various endocrine glands in the body into the bloodstream. Hormones are essential in regulating homeostasis in body organs, tissues, and cells. In addition to hormone-secreting glands, research has also discovered hormone secretion from adipose tissue and the heart, liver, and kidneys, including atrial natriuretic peptide, which is produced in the heart to release sodium in the urine, and erythropoietin, which is released from the kidneys to increase the volume of red blood cells (Alvidrez & Kravitz, 2008).

Hormones differ in their chemical composition and how they affect their target cells. Hormones can be classified as either nonsteroid hormones or steroid hormones. *Nonsteroid hormones* include amine hormones, such as epinephrine and thyroxine, which are derived from amino acids. *Peptide* or *protein hormones*, like vasopressin and insulin, are formed by peptide bonds between multiple amino acids. Large peptide hormones are called *proteins*. Both amine and peptide hormones are water soluble and are transported within blood plasma, but do not enter the cell. These nonsteroid hormones bind to plasma membrane receptors and generate a chemical signal inside the target cell. The rates of metabolism of circulating hormones vary, but amine and peptide hormones typically require only a short time (minutes) to exert their function.

Steroid hormones, which include cortisol and sex hormones, are made from cholesterol and are able to pass through the plasma membrane. However, steroid hormones must be bound to plasma proteins to be transported to their target tissue. This protein binding complicates the activity of steroid hormones, delaying the time to stimulate a biological response (Robergs & Kravitz, 2005).

Role in Glucose Metabolism and Water–Electrolyte Regulation

The body requires glucose for muscle function and fuel. Plasma, or blood glucose, is regulated by the hormones glucagon, epinephrine, norepinephrine, and cortisol. In a normal state, these hormones increase the breakdown of glycogen (i.e., *glycogenolysis*) and are involved in the making of additional glucose (i.e., *glycogenesis*), both of which are required during increased activity demands, and the hormone insulin facilitates the transport of glucose into muscles, adipose tissue, and the liver (Wilmore, Costill, & Kenney, 2008).

The kidneys and intestines have primary roles in water balance and electrolyte regulation. Two hormones, the antidiuretic hormone (ADH, or vasopressin) and aldosterone, act on the kidneys. ADH promotes water conservation, especially during exercise and sweating, to minimize dehydration. Aldosterone works by reabsorbing and retaining sodium, which then retains more fluid. When sodium is retained in the body, potassium is excreted. Increased ADH action is stimulated by decreased plasma sodium, decreased blood volume, a decline in blood pressure, and increased potassium (Wilmore et al., 2008).

The endocrine system's role in fluid homeostasis also affects electrolyte levels in the body. *Electrolytes*, including sodium, calcium, potassium, and chloride, are minerals that control fluid levels, acid–base balance (pH), nerve conduction, blood clotting, and muscle contraction. Refer to Appendix P for additional information on electrolyte levels and clinical implications.

Negative Feedback System

Regulation of the endocrine system is obtained through a negative feedback system so that hormone levels are maintained within a specific range. An example of a simple negative feedback system involves the parathyroid gland and regulation of blood calcium levels. If blood calcium levels are low, the parathyroid gland increases secretion of parathyroid hormone (PTH). PTH stimulates the release of calcium from the bones and increases the calcium uptake from the kidneys through the ascending loop of Henle, distal tubule, and collecting tubule to increase plasma calcium levels. Alternatively, if blood calcium levels are too high, PTH release is withheld to ensure homeostasis.

An example of a complex negative feedback mechanism is what is known as the *hypothalamic–pituitary–adrenal axis,* which describes the interconnection among the hypothalamus, the pituitary gland, and the adrenal glands. When the body experiences a stressful, short-term event (i.e., fight-or-flight response), the hypothalamus is stimulated to release corticotrophin-releasing factor (CRF) from the hypothalamus. CRF triggers the anterior pituitary gland to release adrenocorticotropic hormone (ACTH). ACTH stimulates the adrenal gland cortex to release cortisol into the bloodstream. Increased cortisol levels allow the person to address the stressful event by increasing blood pressure, blood glucose levels, and the metabolism of fat, protein, and carbohydrates. The ACTH levels in the bloodstream provide feedback to the hypothalamus to control the release or inhibition of further CRF.

If high levels of cortisol remain in the bloodstream, the release of additional CRF is inhibited, therefore restricting release of extra ACTH and cortisol. Alternatively, if inadequate levels of plasma cortisol continue, then CRF triggers ACTH to release more cortisol. The side effects of chronic cortisol release or dysfunction is discussed further in the "Adrenal Gland Dysfunction" and "Steroid-Induced Side Effects and Endocrine Myopathies" sections of this chapter.

Endocrine Anatomy and Physiology

Figure 8.1 shows the location of the primary endocrine system glands.

Pituitary Gland

The *pituitary gland* is located just below the brain within the sphenoid bone and is just posterior to the hypothalamus. The pituitary gland is referred to as the *master gland* because of its control over the activities of most other endocrine glands. The pituitary gland is strongly influenced by the hypothalamus, and the functional relationship between the pituitary gland and the hypothalamus is referred to as the *hypothalamo–pituitary axis.*

The pituitary is divided into anterior and posterior sections, which each synthesize hormones differently. Hormones released by the pituitary gland are referred to as *neuroendocrine hormones.* Neuroendocrine hormones are regulated by the hypothalamus, which is discussed next, and influence the body's nervous system through both neural and hormonal pathways.

The anterior pituitary releases six neuroendocrine hormones. Each hormone has an effect on the individual target glands.

1. *ACTH* acts on the adrenal glands to stimulate production of cortisol for maintenance of blood pressure and blood glucose levels.

2. *Growth hormone (GH)* stimulates growth of bones and muscles and regulates protein and fat metabolism. GH is also known as *somatotropin.*

3. *Thyroid-stimulating hormone (TSH)* acts on the thyroid gland to stimulate the production of thyroxin. Thyroid hormones regulate the body's metabolism, energy, growth, development, and nervous system activity.

4. *Follicle-stimulating hormone (FSH)* promotes growth of ovaries and the secretion of estrogen in women and the development of seminiferous tubules for spermatazoa production in men.

5. *Lutenizing hormone (LH)* induces ovulation along with FSH, stimulates the production of estrogens, and further develops the corpus luteum and secretion of progesterone after ovulation in women. It also

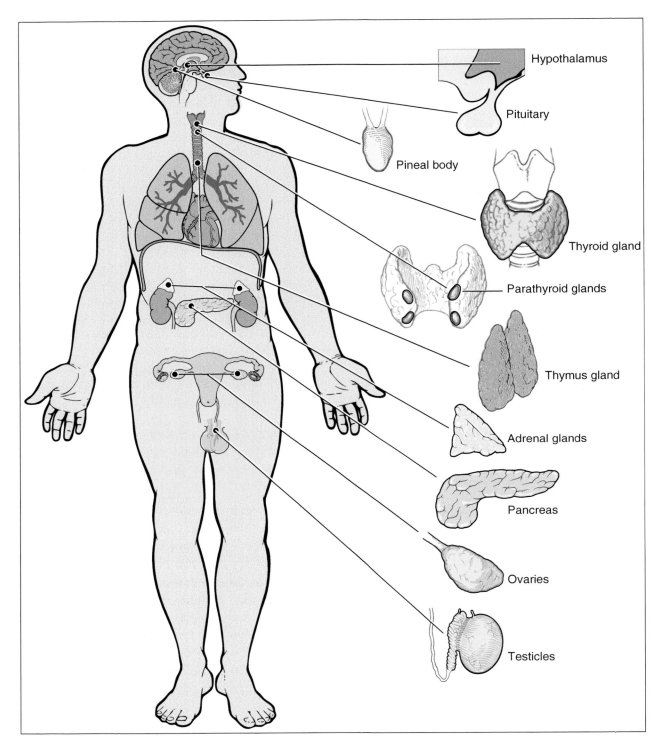

Figure 8.1. The primary endocrine system glands.
Source. Richard Fritzler, Medical Illustrator, Roswell, GA.

facilitates secretion of testosterone by the testes in men.

6. *Prolactin hormone* stimulates milk production in the mammary glands and affects sex hormone levels.

Hormones synthesized in the posterior pituitary include vasopressin and oxytocin. These hormones are produced in the neurons originating from the hypothalamus.

- ADH, or vasopressin, acts on the kidneys to regulate water balance by facilitating resorption of water into the blood and reducing the volume of urine formed.

- Oxytocin affects milk flow and uterine contractions and acts on the nucleus accumbens and amygdala, where it enhances maternal behavior. Oxytocin also plays a role in social memory, anxiety, and stress coping (Neumann, 2008).

Hypothalamus

The *hypothalamus* is located within the brain, below the thalamus, and functions in controlling hunger, thirst, blood pressure, heart rate, temperature, circadian rhythms, sexual functions, and emotions. Cells from the hypothalamus influence the secretion of hormones from the pituitary gland. The hypothalamus serves as the major link between the endocrine and nervous systems, and its specialized hormones are produced by neurons. These neuroendocrine hormones regulate body homeostasis by being released into the blood vessels that connect the hypothalamus and the pituitary gland. These hormones have either stimulating or inhibitory effects on the pituitary and include

- *Corticotropin-releasing hormone,* which stimulates the release of ACTH to control metabolism, sodium, and water regulation;

- *Thyrotropin-releasing hormone,* which stimulates the release of TSH;

- *Growth hormone-releasing hormone,* which stimulates the release of GH;

- *Gonadotropin-releasing hormone,* which stimulates the release of LH and FSH;

- *Somatostatin,* which inhibits the release of GH and TSH; and

- *Dopamine,* which inhibits the release of prolactin. Dopamine usually functions as a neurotransmitter.

Thyroid Glands

The thyroid glands are the largest in the traditional endocrine system. These butterfly-shaped glands are located in the front of the neck, wrapping around the trachea. The thyroid secretes amine thyroid hormones thyroxine (T4) and tri-iodothyronine (T3), which regulate the body's metabolism by controlling temperature, growth, nervous system development, and neuronal activity. T4 and T3 can increase the body's metabolic rate by 60%–100% and enhance glycolysis, gluconeogenesis, and glucose uptake (Wilmore et al., 2008). *Glycolysis* is the breakdown of glucose to release energy for metabolic needs. *Gluconeogenesis* is the formation of glucose.

Thyroid hormone concentrations are regulated by TSH from the anterior pituitary. The thyroid also releases the peptide hormone thyrocalcitonin, also known as *calcitonin*. Calcitonin lowers calcium concentration levels in the blood by inhibiting calcium release from the bone and plays a role in protecting the skeleton from excess resorption of calcium.

Parathyroid Glands

The four parathyroid glands are located in the neck behind the thyroid. These glands secrete the peptide PTH that causes the kidneys to increase calcium resorption and promote phosphate excretion through a negative feedback system. Calcium metabolism is integral in a functioning nervous and muscular system. This regulation involves the kidney, intestines, and skeletal system. If serum calcium levels decrease, the parathyroid glands secrete more PTH, which causes the skeletal system to release calcium into the bloodstream. PTH also stimulates the conversion of Vitamin D into a more active form that enhances blood calcium levels by increasing absorption of calcium by the gastrointestinal tract.

Adrenal Glands

The two adrenal glands, located on the superior aspects of the kidneys, are composed of both an inner layer known as the *medulla* and an *outer cortex*. The hormones secreted by the adrenal glands are very different in their effects on the body and are based on the originating source of the hormones (i.e., medulla or cortex). The inner medulla secretes adrenaline and noradrenaline (i.e., epinephrine and norepinephrine).

Epinephrine and norepinephrine are referred to as *catecholamines* because they are produced in the adrenal medulla. *Epinephrine* is secreted in response to sympathetic nervous system activation (i.e., flight-or-fight response) affecting cardiac muscle, smooth muscle, and organs. Epinephrine increases the heart rate, accelerates breathing, slows digestion, increases blood pressure, and raises blood glucose levels through the conversion of stored fat and protein in response to a stress event. *Norepinephrine* causes vasoconstriction, increases heart rate and blood pressure, and increases blood glucose levels.

The outer cortex of the adrenal glands secretes steroid hormones, also known as *corticosteroids*. The three major types of corticosteroids are categorized as mineralocorticoids, glucocorticoids, or gonadocorticoids (i.e., sex hormones). *Mineralocorticoids*, such as aldosterone, regulate electrolyte and water balance by promoting sodium absorption and excretion of potassium by the kidneys. This balance of sodium and potassium plays an important role in maintaining blood pressure. *Glucocorticoids* help the body adapt in stressful situations and help to maintain plasma glucose homeostasis. Glucocorticoids, like cortisol, increase glucose synthesis and glycogen formation, mobilize fat and protein for energy needs and cellular repair, reduce inflammation, and suppress the immune response. *Gonadocorticoids* (i.e., androgens and estrogens) assist in the development of male and female sex characteristics.

Pancreas

The *pancreas* is located slightly below and behind the stomach and functions as both an exocrine organ and an endocrine gland. It is primarily an exocrine organ because most pancreatic cells produce digestive enzymes to aid in the digestive process. However, the pancreas also functions as an endocrine gland and secretes the two main hormones, *insulin*

and *glucagon*. These hormones, with opposing function, aid in glucose homeostasis. Specifically, the pancreatic beta cells produce insulin, which reduces plasma glucose levels. The alpha cells in the Islets of Langerhans produce glucagon to increase plasma glucose levels.

Insulin is the only hormone that lowers the amount of glucose circulating in the blood. When blood glucose levels elevate, especially after a meal, the pancreas responds by producing insulin. Pancreatic insulin production is affected not only by postprandial peaks (i.e., after meal ingestion) but also in relation to diurnal cycles and other mechanisms to maintain a basal level of insulin. Insulin facilitates the transport of glucose into muscle cells, promotes glycogenesis, and has a role in protein and fat metabolism for energy needs. Insulin stimulates the liver to store glucose as glycogen, promotes synthesis of fatty acids (i.e., lipogenesis), and inhibits the breakdown of fat in adipose tissue. These actions decrease the concentration of blood glucose and enable it to be used for energy needs.

The pancreas secretes glucagon, however, when blood sugar levels are low. Glucagon has the opposite effect of insulin and raises blood glucose levels by breaking down glycogen, which is stored in the liver and in lipids and proteins, into glucose. Glucagon also increases gluconeogenesis, which increases plasma glucose levels.

In addition to insulin and glucagon, the pancreas also produces the hormones somatostatin and pancreatic polypeptide. *Somatostatin*, which is also released by the hypothalamus, slows the absorption of food and inhibits insulin production when released by the pancreas. *Pancreatic polypeptide* has a role in regulation of pancreatic enzyme production and appetite reduction.

Thymus Gland

The *thymus gland* is located in the thoracic cavity below the neck and behind the sternum. The thymus is typically large in children, and its cortex begins to shrink during puberty, gradually being replaced by fibrous and adipose tissue. The thymus secretes the peptide hormone thymosin, and some other thymic hormones, that are essential in the development and maintenance of a normal immune system and immune response. Thymosin stimulates lymphocyte formation and development of *T-cells* (i.e., cells that develop or mature in the thymus gland). These T-cells, also known as *T-lymphocytes,* eventually travel to the lymph nodes where they help the immune system protect the body against infections as white blood cells.

Because the thymus gland shrinks with age, a correlating drop in thymus gland hormone activity occurs with aging, as do possible alterations in effective immune function. Research by Napolitano et al. (2008) has found that the use of growth hormone (GH) treatment improved T-cell recovery in adults infected with HIV-1 by augmenting the adult thymus gland's role in immunity.

Pineal Gland

The *pineal gland* is located in the diencephalon of the brain and is responsible for secretion of melatonin, an amine hormone. *Melatonin* slows the production of FSH and LH by the pituitary gland. Melatonin has a significant role in the regulation of circadian rhythms, sleep, mood, and aging. Calcification of the pineal gland typically begins before puberty with diminished melatonin production over the lifespan. This reduction in melatonin may play a role in the reduced quality and quantity of sleep and the onset of depression sometimes seen with aging (Zhdanova & Tucci, 2003).

Reiter et al. (2003) cited numerous studies supporting the use of synthetic melatonin as an antioxidant to stimulate the immune system, minimize the severity of tissue damage resulting from brain ischemia, reduce chronic degenerative central nervous system changes in Alzheimer's and Parkinson's disease, and improve pharmacological efficacy of certain drugs.

Reproductive Glands

The *ovaries* in females and the *testes* in males are the primary reproductive organs. These organs are responsible for producing the sperm and ova but are considered endocrine glands. LH and FSH from the anterior pituitary stimulate the gonads. Specifically, LH stimulates

the testes to produce steroid hormones called *androgens.* One of these hormones, *testosterone,* is responsible for the growth and development of the male reproductive structures and secondary sex characteristics. In females, LH stimulates ovaries to produce *estrogens* (estradiol, estrone, estriol) and *progesterone,* the female sex hormones. FSH controls gamete (egg or sperm) production. The development and function of the reproductive organs and sex characteristics, therefore, is dependent on these steroid hormones.

Endocrine Diseases and Treatment

The endocrine system is complex in both anatomy and physiology, and although this chapter discusses rare endocrine diseases, it does not address all endocrine-related issues. Instead, it focuses on the principal endocrine glands, key hormones, and health effects of major hormonal imbalances and subsequent syndromes or disease processes.

Disorders of the Pituitary and Pancreas

Diabetes insipidus and diabetes mellitus are separate medical conditions resulting from distinct areas of dysfunction within the body, the pituitary gland or the pancreas. The kidneys are unable to conserve fluid and maintain hydration with diabetes insipidus. The pancreas is unable to produce insulin or make enough insulin in order to metabolize glucose with diabetes mellitus. Although both types of diabetes may result in similar symptoms that include excessive urination and excessive thirst, each condition is treated independently.

Diabetes Insipidus

Diabetes insipidus (DI), which is considered a rare condition, is caused by a lack of response to ADH, or vasopressin. The two types of DI are *central diabetes insipidus* and *nephrogenic diabetes insipidus.* With central DI, ADH is lacking or is produced in insufficient levels. Disruption of the posterior pituitary gland, from which ADH is released, may be the result of brain injury, stroke, nephrogenic abnormalities, or tumors or from certain drugs such as lithium. Normally, ADH controls the kidneys to conserve water and minimize urine output so that dehydration does not occur. Central DI results in both excessive thirst (i.e., *polydipsia*) and urine production (i.e., *polyuria*). People with central DI experience fatigue and are at risk for dehydration, which can result in both low blood pressure and shock.

Nephrogenic diabetes insipidus is the result of kidney disease that makes the kidneys unable to respond to ADH even though enough ADH is in the system. The kidneys are unable, therefore, to conserve water. The symptoms are the same as in central DI and include polyuria and polydipsia; however, the cause of and the treatment for each disease are different.

Treatment of central diabetes insipidus includes use of vasopressin (e.g., desmopressin) to control polydipsia, polyuria, and dehydration; diuretics (e.g., chlorthiazide); ADH-releasing drugs (e.g., chlorpropamide, carbamazepine, clofibrate); and prostaglandin inhibitors (e.g., indomethacin) that also treat polyuria (Chapman, 2006). Nephrogenic diabetes insipidus can be treated with anti-inflammatory medication (e.g., indomethacin) and diuretics (e.g., amiloride, hydrochlorothiazide). Although no specific pharmacological protocol exists, emphasis is on restriction of fluid intake or diuretics to minimize urine dilution (Armstrong & Tashjian, 2008).

Additional disorders of the pituitary include acromegaly and gigantism, which are beyond the scope of this section. Addison's disease and Cushing's disease may be the result of pituitary gland dysfunction or adrenal gland disorders and are covered in the "Adrenal Gland Dysfunction" section.

Diabetes Mellitus Types 1 and 2

Diabetes mellitus is a disease in which glucose is insufficiently metabolized. Abnormal glucose metabolism results in high glucose levels in the blood (i.e., *hyperglycemia*) and urine (i.e., *glycosuria*) because of an absolute lack of insulin or lack of insulin action to lower blood sugars. Insulin enables the body to move sugar from the bloodstream into the tissues to be used for

energy. When glucose is insufficient, the body uses proteins and fat for energy. (Diabetes as the result of drug or chemical treatment or gestational diabetes mellitus are beyond the scope of this chapter.)

Type 1 diabetes is the result of an absolute deficiency of insulin secretion. An autoimmune process destroys the pancreatic beta cells, resulting in the body's inability to regulate blood glucose. Insulin is not produced or released into the bloodstream, and amino acids and lipids are not able to store glucose. This form of diabetes accounts for 5%–10% of all diagnosed cases, and some viral illnesses are hypothesized to trigger an autoimmune response in people who are genetically predisposed to Type 1 diabetes (Shu, Myers, & Shoelson, 2008). Type 1 diabetes was previously referred to as *insulin-dependent diabetes mellitus* and *juvenile diabetes*.

Type 2 diabetes results when the body is resistant to the effect of insulin or the beta cells produce insulin but in insufficient amounts. As the body's need for insulin rises, the pancreas is unable to produce it; therefore, the tissues do not absorb glucose, and it stays in the bloodstream. Because glucose is not available for use, the body also begins to burn protein and fat. Type 2 diabetes accounts for 90%–95% of all cases, and obesity is the most important risk factor for its development (Shu et al., 2008). Type 2 diabetes mellitus has been referred to as *non–insulin-dependent diabetes mellitus* and is associated with insulin resistance, family history, sedentary lifestyle, aging, and some ethnicities. Table 8.1 compares the signs and symptoms of diabetes insipidus and diabetes mellitus.

Prediabetes is a condition in which fasting blood glucose levels are higher than normal (>100 milligrams/deciliter) but not high enough to be considered as having Type 2 diabetes mellitus (>126 milligrams/deciliter). Making significant lifestyle changes by adding moderate-intensity physical activity for 30–60 minutes a day, reducing weight by 5%–10%, and incorporating healthy eating (e.g., calorie restriction, increased fiber, limiting carbohydrates) has been shown to reduce the conversion of prediabetes to Type 2 diabetes (Garber et al., 2008).

Complications resulting from either insufficient or excessive blood glucose levels can

Table 8.1. **Signs and Symptoms of Diabetes Insipidus and Diabetes Mellitus**

Systemic Presentation	Diabetes Insipidus	Diabetes Mellitus	
		Type 1	**Type 2**
Onset	Wide age range	Abrupt onset, <age 30	Gradual onset, usually >age 30
Metabolism and weight	Fatigue, dehydration, sudden weight loss	Fatigue, weight loss with overeating	Fatigue, weight loss with overeating
Psychological status	Lethargy, irritability, restlessness, confusion	Emotional lability, irritability	Emotional lability, irritability
Cardiovascular	Tachycardia, hypotension	Orthostatic hypotension, arrhythmias	Strongly associated with hypertension, heart disease, and stroke
Musculoskeletal	Weakness, hyperreflexia, spasticity	Weakness, muscle cramps, muscle wasting	Paresthesias, sensory neuropathy, myopathy
Skin, hair, and nails	Dry mouth, inability to sweat, decreased skin turgor	Delayed healing, prone to infections	Dry skin, delayed healing, prone to infections
Other	Abrupt polydipsia, polyuria, nocturia	Polydipsia, polyuria, nausea, vomiting, visual changes	Visual changes, gastroparesis

develop into life-threatening conditions. *Hyperglycemia*, or abnormally high blood sugar of more than 200 milligrams per deciliter, may be the result of not taking enough insulin, overeating, lack of exercise, too-strenuous exercise, illness, infection, or stress. Symptoms include polyuria, polydipsia, dry mouth, diminished appetite, fatigue, and drowsiness. Untreated hyperglycemia can result in ketoacidosis (primarily with Type 1 diabetes) or hyperosmolar hyperglycemic state (i.e., nonketotic hyperosmolar syndrome) for those with Type 2 diabetes or prediabetes. Hyperosmolar hyperglycemic state is associated with severe dehydration and a blood sugar level of 600 milligrams per deciliter or more and can develop over the course of days or weeks (Sergot & Nelson, 2008).

When insulin is insufficient to maintain adequate blood sugar levels, the body will resort to using fat for basic metabolism and energy needs. This process may result in *ketoacidosis*, a severe buildup of ketones and acids in the bloodstream resulting in metabolic acidosis. *Ketones* are by-products of fat metabolism. Diabetic ketoacidosis, associated with dehydration and hyperglycemia, is a serious medical emergency that can be life threatening. Symptoms can include loss of appetite, headache, shortness of breath, nausea, vomiting, dry mouth, and fruity-smelling breath.

Hypoglycemia, or abnormally low blood sugar below 70 milligrams per deciliter, can result from too much exogenous insulin, eating too little food, excessive alcohol intake, or exercising without sufficient glucose in the bloodstream. Symptoms can include hunger, perspiration, weakness, tremors, anxiety, irritability, headache, or sleepiness. Hypoglycemia can lead to coma or convulsions if not treated.

The increasing incidence of diabetes mellitus, especially Type 2 and prediabetes, requires the occupational therapist to be aware of possible long-term health complications. Complications associated with diabetes include both large-vessel diseases, such as myocardial infarction, stroke, and peripheral vascular disease, and small vessel diseases, such as neuropathy, retinopathy, and nephropathy. Additional health issues include atherosclerosis, gastroparesis, depression, and reduced wound healing. Garber et al. (2008) also stated that good glycemic control can reduce both microvascular and neuropathic complications and minimize the risk for macrovascular disease.

Treatment of Type 1 diabetes must include insulin administration by injection or a pump and careful self-monitoring of blood glucose to ensure the correct dosage of insulin (Triplitt, Reasner, & Isley, 2005). Different types of insulin are used on the basis of how long the insulin remains active and how quickly it begins to work. Ultra-rapid-acting insulins include lispro (e.g., Humalog), aspart (e.g., Novolog), and glulisine (e.g., Apidra); short-acting insulins include regular human insulin (e.g., Humulin R, Novolin R); intermediate-acting insulin includes NPH human insulin (Novolin N, Humulin N); and long-acting insulins include detemir (e.g., Levemir) and glargine (e.g., Lantus; Shu et al., 2008). Typically, both short- and long-acting insulins are used together.

Additionally, a balanced diet and regular exercise will assist in glycemic control. Specifically, exercise lasting longer than 30 minutes increases the body's sensitivity to insulin (so the body requires less insulin) and increases plasma glucagon to maintain adequate concentrations (Wilmore et al., 2008).

Type 2 diabetes treatment includes a balanced diet with reduction of carbohydrates, saturated and trans fats, and cholesterol intake, weight control, and exercise, including both resistance training and aerobic exercise. In some cases, a good control of diet, weight loss, and exercise may normalize blood sugars and minimize the need for oral hypoglycemic drugs (Crandall et al., 2008). Oral hypoglycemic medications used for glycemic control include sulfonylureas to increase insulin secretion; biguanides (e.g., metformin) to enhance insulin sensitivity in hepatic and peripheral tissues; alpha-glucosidase inhibitors (e.g., acarbose and miglitol) to delay absorption of glucose from the intestine; and thiazolidinediones to increase muscle, liver, and fat tissue sensitivity to insulin (Triplitt et al., 2005). In severe cases, Type 2 diabetes may be treated with insulin.

Thyroid Disease

The thyroid gland assists in control of body metabolism, calcium homeostasis, and how responsive the body should be to other hormones. Therefore, any dysfunction of the thyroid will result in the body's inability to regulate basic metabolic activity.

Hypothyroidism

Hypothyroidism is the failure of the thyroid gland to secrete TH or to secrete enough TH. Symptoms may include pervasive fatigue, drowsiness, and cold intolerance with dry or itchy skin, constipation, forgetfulness, and personality changes. Associated fluid retention and decreased metabolism contribute to weight gain. Hypothyroidism may imitate Parkinson's disease or dementia in older adults and is a known side effect for those on lithium therapy (Porter, 2006).

Hashimoto's thyroiditis, also known as an *autoimmune thyroiditis,* is a type of hypothyroidism that is characterized by the production of autoantibodies and immune cells that can damage thyroid cells and compromise their ability to make thyroid hormone. A *goiter,* or an enlarged thyroid, can be caused by multiple factors, including lack of iodine in the diet, excess TSH, or an autoimmune process causing an inflammatory reaction.

Treatment for hypothyroidism aims to restore normal thyroid hormone concentration through the use of natural or synthetic thyroid preparations and to suppress TSH from the pituitary gland. Natural thyroid preparations (e.g., Thyroid USP, thyroglobulin) and synthetic preparations (e.g., levothyroxine, liothyronine, liotrix) are frequently used to treat hypothyroidism (Talbert, 2005).

Hyperthyroidism and Graves' Disease

Hyperthyroidism can result from excessive amounts of thyroid hormone. Excessive thyroid hormone may result in anxiety, irritability, tremors, weight loss, increased and irregular heart rate, muscle weakness, goiter, low tolerance for heat, and accelerated loss of calcium from bones.

Graves' disease is an autoimmune dysfunction that results in thyroid enlargement and hyperthyroidism. Additional symptoms of Graves' disease include swelling of the muscles and tissues around the eyes that can result in orbital prominence, discomfort, or diplopia. Table 8.2 compares the signs and symptoms of hypothyroidism and hyperthyroidism.

Treatment for hyperthyroidism includes surgical thyroidectomy, antithyroid medicine, and radioactive iodine, which all work to eliminate excess thyroid hormone and complications from hyperthyroidism. Pharmacological therapy includes thiourea drugs (e.g., propylthiouracil and methimazole, both of which inhibit the biosynthesis of thyroid hormone); iodides that block thyroid hormone release, inhibit thyroid hormone synthesis, and decrease vascularity of the gland; adrenergic blockers (e.g., beta blockers, propranolol) to treat symptoms such as tremor and anxiety; and radioactive iodine (e.g., sodium iodide 131) to disrupt hormone synthesis (Talbert, 2005).

Adrenal Gland Dysfunction

The *adrenal glands,* through interaction with the hypothalamus and pituitary gland, assist in regulating kidney function through fluid and electrolyte balance, control stress-related hormones, and manage glucose levels. Although disorders of the adrenal glands are considered rare, if left untreated, they can be life threatening.

Cushing's Syndrome and Cushing's Disease

Cushing's syndrome, also know as *hypercortisolism,* is a rare condition resulting from excess cortisol production or from prolonged

Table 8.2. Thyroid Disease Signs and Symptoms

Systemic Presentation	Hypothyroidism	Hyperthyroidism
Metabolism and weight	Fatigue, lethargy, cold intolerance, weight gain	Fatigue, heat intolerance, sweating, weight loss, increased appetite
Psychological status	Depression, irritability, memory impairment	Nervousness, agitation, insomnia
Cardiovascular	Bradycardia, poor peripheral circulation	Palpitations, chest pain, hypertension, tachycardia
Musculoskeletal	Limb weakness, cramps, joint pain, stiffness, neuropathy	Weakness, tremors, proximal muscle wasting, myopathy
Skin, hair, and nails	Dry, rough skin; coarse, thinning hair; thin, brittle nails	Warm, moist skin; hair loss
Other	Decreased libido; constipation; puffy eyes; goiter	Protruding eyeballs, diplopia; dyspnea; gastrointestinal motility; goiter

corticosteroid or glucocorticoid administration. *Cushing's disease* is a type of Cushing's syndrome caused by excess ACTH production from the pituitary gland. Typically, a pituitary adenoma (i.e., tumor of the pituitary gland) stimulates the adrenal glands to secrete too much cortisol. In both cases, excess cortisol results in a progressive loss of protein and peripheral fat, muscle weakness with proximal myopathy, and loss of bone mass.

People with Cushing's syndrome frequently present with reduced insulin sensitivity, elevated blood glucose, easy bruising, diminished white blood cell counts, central obesity, rounded face, abdominal striae, hypertension, and hirsutism. Arnaldi et al. (2003) reported that people may also experience neuropsychological and sleep disturbances, depression, irritability, and cognitive impairments.

Treatment for Cushing's syndrome includes surgical resection of tumors, irradiation of the pituitary, and pharmacology. Pharmacotherapy can include steroidogenic inhibition used to block steroid synthesis (e.g., metyrapone, aminoglutethimide, ketoconazole), adrenolytic agents that inhibit adrenal enzymes (e.g., mitotane), neuromodulators of ACTH release (e.g., cyproheptadine, bromocriptine, valproic acid, ritanserin, octreotide), and glucocorticoid-receptor blocking agents (e.g., mifepristone, or RU-486; Gums & Tovar, 2005).

Adrenal Insufficiency and Addison's Disease

Adrenal insufficiency is caused by an insufficient production of adrenocortical hormones (i.e., cortisol and aldosterone) of the adrenal gland cortex. *Primary adrenal insufficiency,* or *Addison's disease,* results when the adrenal glands are unable to produce cortisol, aldosterone, or both. Secondary adrenal insufficiency occurs when the pituitary gland or hypothalamus is unable to adequately stimulate the production of adrenocorticotropic hormone.

Inadequate cortisol results in weakness; fatigue; vague abdominal pain, sometimes with nausea and vomiting; weight loss; low blood pressure; dizziness; and fainting. Specifically with Addison's disease, hyperpigmentation of the skin and a craving for salt may also be present. People with inadequate cortisol levels typically respond poorly to physical stress such as injury, anesthesia, surgery, or other medical illnesses. Acute adrenocortical insufficiency, or adrenal crisis, can develop as the result of sepsis or surgical stress. Characterized by extreme weakness, low blood pressure, dehydration, and shock, adrenal crisis may be life threatening.

Treatment of adrenal insufficiency requires correction of electrolyte and metabolic deficits, and pharmacology addresses cortisol deficits through the use of glucocorticoid steroids and mineralocorticoids, especially hydrocortisone, prednisone, and cortisone (Gums & Tovar, 2005).

Aldosteronism and Conn's Syndrome

Aldosteronism is an overproduction of aldosterone that is usually caused by benign tumors of the adrenal gland or overactive adrenal glands that result in sodium retention and potassium loss. *Conn's syndrome* (a type of hyperaldosteronism) is characterized by hypertension and water retention by the kidneys resulting in hypokalemia. People with Conn's syndrome typically experience fatigue, muscle weakness or cramps, headaches, polydipsia, and polyuria. Signs and symptoms of adrenal gland diseases are compared in Table 8.3.

Treatment for aldosteronism requires medication or intervention to control blood pressure and hypertension and correct hypokalemia. With Conn's syndrome, surgical removal of the adrenal gland (i.e., adrenalectomy) may be indicated.

Parathyroid Diseases

The *parathyroid glands* regulate the amount of calcium in the blood, which controls the nervous system, muscular effectiveness, and skeletal strength. Elevated blood calcium (*hypercalcemia*) has negative effects on the body's major organs and systems; hyperparathyroidism is a leading cause of hypercalcemia.

Hypoparathyroidism

Hypoparathyroidism is very rare and is usually the result of damage or removal of the para thyroid or thyroid glands from surgery. Decreased activity of PTH leads to reduced

Table 8.3. Adrenal Gland Diseases Signs and Symptoms				
Systemic Presentation	**Cushing's Syndrome (Hypercortisolism)**	**Addison's Disease (Hypocortisolism)**	**Conn's Syndrome (Hyperaldosteronism)**
Metabolism and weight	Chronic fatigue, weight gain, central obesity, increased appetite	Chronic fatigue, weight loss, lack of appetite, anorexia	Chronic fatigue
Psychological status	Irritability or euphoria; decreased concentration and memory; depression	Irritability, depression, apathy, anhedonia	Headaches
Cardiovascular	Hypertension	Hypotension	Hypertension
Musculoskeletal	Fatty hump between shoulders, weakness, osteopenia, corticosteroid myopathy	Weakness, decreased exercise tolerance, myopathy	Weakness, intermittent paralysis, paresthesias
Skin, hair, and nails	Rounded face, striations, thin skin, hirsutism, impaired wound healing	Hyperpigmentation; craving for salty food	No symptoms noted
Other	Polydipsia, polyuria	Constipation or diarrhea, vomiting, nausea	Polydipsia, polyuria

levels of calcium (i.e., *hypocalcemia*) and increased levels of phosphorus (i.e., *hyperphosphatemia*) that affect cardiac, intestinal, and musculoskeletal systems. Symptoms of hypoparathyroidism can include laryngospasm (i.e., laryngeal spasm), neuromuscular irritability (e.g., paresthesias, muscle cramps, tetany, muscle spasms), cardiac arrhythmias, syncope, and seizures.

Treatment of hypoparathyroidism initially includes intravenous calcium until serum calcium levels are stabilized, and then intervention includes oral dietary modification (foods high in calcium), vitamin D, and additional calcium supplements (e.g., calcium carbonate, calcium citrate, calcium gluconate, calcitriol; Gonzalez-Campoy, 2007).

Hyperparathyroidism

Hyperparathyroidism results from the parathyroid glands secreting too much PTH, resulting in elevated levels of plasma calcium. High levels of calcium in the blood cause excess calcium to be released from the bones into the bloodstream, ultimately resulting in reduced bone density that contributes to the development of osteopenia or osteoporosis. *Primary hyperparathyroidism* is usually the result of a parathyroid adenoma or tumor. Symptoms may include a loss of energy, general malaise, kidney stones, decreased concentration, depression, bone pain, and difficulty sleeping. *Secondary hyperparathyroidism* is caused by hypocalcemia or resistance to parathyroid hormone and may result from chronic kidney disease, preventing vitamin D conversion and allowing increased PTH concentrations. The signs and symptoms of hypoparathyroidism and hyperparathyroidism are compared in Table 8.4.

Treatment for hyperparathyroidism focuses on minimizing calcium resorption from bone. Pharmacology includes bisphosphonates, to improve bone mineral density; calcimimetics, to normalize serum calcium and prevent calcium reabsorption; and dietary modification

Table 8.4. Parathyroid Disease Signs and Symptoms

Systemic Presentation	Hypoparathyroidism	Hyperparathyroidism
Metabolism and weight	Lethargy	Fatigue, loss of appetite, anorexia
Psychological status	Anxiety or depression, irritability	Confusion, loss of memory, personality changes, lability, depression
Cardiovascular	No symptoms noted	Hypertension, dysrhythmias
Musculoskeletal	Cramps, paresthesias, tetany	Proximal muscle weakness, myopathy, osteoporosis, osteopenia
Skin, hair, and nails	Dry, coarse skin; alopecia; vitiligo	Itchy, dry skin
Other	Dysphagia, laryngospasm, weakened tooth enamel	Polydipsia, polyuria, nausea, vomiting, kidney stones, pancreatitis

(low in calcium and high in vitamin D; Kim, 2008). A parathyroidectomy may also be indicated.

Obesity and Metabolic Syndrome

Researchers have established an association between obesity and endocrine disease. Over the past decade, adipose tissue has become regarded as an endocrine organ through the identification of *adipokines*, bioactive peptides produced by adipose tissue that play a role in immunity, insulin sensitivity, blood pressure, and homeostasis (Ronti, Lupattelli, & Mannarino, 2006). *Obesity*, as viewed by the American Association of Clinical Endocrinologists "is, in part, an endocrine and metabolic disorder that is clearly associated with several endocrine and metabolic comorbidities that require ongoing medical management, including Type 2 diabetes mellitus, hypertension, dyslipidemia, and gout" (Dickey et al., 1998, p. 300).

Metabolic syndrome refers to a cluster of risk factors that can predispose one to cardiovascular disease, stroke, or diabetes and is strongly associated with obesity and inactivity. Metabolic syndrome has also been referred to as *syndrome X* or *insulin resistance syndrome,* and various clinical criteria define the syndrome's characteristics. Metabolic syndrome's main features, as defined by the National Cholesterol Education Program's Adult Treatment Panel III report (Grundy, Brewer, Cleeman, Smith, & Lenfant, 2004), include abdominal obesity, dyslipidemia, elevated blood pressure, insulin resistance, glucose intolerance, indication of a proinflammatory state, and indication of a prothrombotic state. A *proinflammatory state* refers to elevated levels of C-reactive protein, and a *prothrombotic state* indicates increased plasma plasminogen activator inhibitor and fibrogen levels (Grundy et al., 2004).

Because of the multiple medical and psychological complications that can arise from obesity that limit participation in occupational performance areas and patterns, occupational therapists can be instrumental in recommending intervention strategies for long-term health and wellness practices (Clark, Reingold, & Salles-Jordan, 2007). Occupational therapists can also have a role in identifying and promoting healthy lifestyle changes to people at risk for metabolic syndrome owing to its strong association with obesity and reduced physical activity.

Neuroendocrine Dysfunction

Acute illness, neurological disease, or trauma may result in the development of endocrine disease. Research has focused on endocrine function during critical illness, especially in the areas of hypothalamic–pituitary–adrenal axis control, the role of blood glucose regulation, and the actions of vasopressin (Annane et al., 2004, 2006; Marik et al., 2008).

Neuroendocrine dysfunction is associated with traumatic brain injury (TBI). Research has focused on pituitary and hypothalamic dysfunction resulting from head trauma or subarachnoid hemorrhages. Research by Tanriverdi et al. (2006) has indicated that the most common pituitary dysfunction after TBI is growth hormone deficiency, with more than 50% of people 12 months after TBI having at least one anterior pituitary hormone deficiency. Studies on endocrine dysfunction resulting from TBI have cited these neuroendocrine disease processes:

- Posttraumatic hypopituitarism (Tanriverdi et al., 2006);
- Diabetes insipidus and syndrome of inappropriate secretion of antidiuretic hormone (Agham et al., 2004; Behan, Phillips, Thompson, & Agha, 2008);
- Glucocorticoid deficiency resulting in lethargy, muscle fatigue, and poor exercise capacity (Agha & Thompson, 2006);
- GH deficiencies and low cortisol levels that compromise overall health, well-being, and rehabilitation potential (Lieberman, Oberoi, Gilkison, Masel, & Urban, 2001); and
- Deficiencies in thyroid hormones resulting in anergia (i.e., lack of energy), muscle weakness, and neuropsychiatric disorders (Tanriverdi et al., 2006).

Steroid-Induced Side Effects and Endocrine Myopathies

Many endocrine diseases are treated through the use of steroids, which have well-documented side effects with long-term use. Steroid treatment can include both corticosteroids and glucocorticoid therapies. Corticosteroids are synthetic hormones generally used to decrease inflammation by blocking the production of substances that trigger inflammatory reactions. Glucocorticoid therapy is frequently used for anti-inflammatory and immunosuppressive purposes and may also be used in the treatment of some rheumatologic conditions (Mahajan & Tandon, 2005).

Side effects of general steroid use can include behavior changes, weight gain, hypertension, skin atrophy, impaired wound healing, decreased immune responsiveness, skin infections, hyperglycemia, and depression. Steroids can impair function of white blood cells, which results in increased susceptibility to infection. Long-term use of steroid therapy can result in additional systemic disease processes like osteoporosis, diabetes mellitus, or Cushing's syndrome. Myopathy, or weakening or atrophy of skeletal muscles, can be a sign and symptom of both endocrine disease and the use of chronic steroid treatment.

Modifying treatment or discontinuing steroid treatment also has potential side effects including adrenal insufficiency or cortisol deficiency resulting from hypothalamic–pituitary–adrenal axis suppression, recurring underlying disease process, and steroid withdrawal symptoms (Hopkins & Leinung, 2005; Igaz, Rácz, Tóth, Gláz, & Tulassay, 2007).

Endocrine Disruptors

Natural and synthetic chemicals are present in everyday life. Some chemicals, known as *endocrine-disrupting chemicals (EDCs)*, have been shown to affect reproductive, neurological, and immunological function. Other EDCs have been linked with cancer-causing properties.

Reiter et al. (1998) and Daston, Cook, and Kavlock (2003) have acknowledged that most research has evaluated EDCs in relation to reproductive development and carcinogenetic effects in lab animals, not in humans. In 1996, the Environmental Protection Agency developed the Endocrine Disruptor Screening and Testing Advisory Committee, now known as the Endocrine Disruptor Screening Program (2007). This program screens pesticide chemicals and environmental contaminants for their potential to affect the endocrine systems of humans and wildlife. Research on the initial and long-term effects of EDCs on humans continues to be investigated.

Role of Occupational Therapy

The *Occupational Therapy Practice Framework: Domain and Process 2nd Edition* (2nd ed; American Occupational Therapy Association, 2008) includes metabolic and endocrine systems under client factors and body functions, stating, "Occupational therapy practitioners have knowledge of these body functions and understand broadly the interaction that occurs between these functions to support health and participation in life through engagement in occupation" (p. 636).

Occupational Therapy Practice and Endocrine Disease

The *Framework* outlines an evaluation and intervention strategy with regard to a client's areas of occupation (e.g., activities of daily living [ADLs], instrumental activities of daily living [IADLs]), client factors (e.g., values, body functions, body structures), activity demands (e.g., social demands, sequence, timing), performance skills (e.g., motor, sensory, cognition), performance patterns (e.g., habits, routines, roles), and contexts (e.g., cultural, temporal). Endocrine disease impairs energy levels and engagement in functional activity, frequently increases stress while limiting effective coping mechanisms, and plays a role in metabolic dysfunction.

In the acute care setting, physical signs of endocrine impairment or disability may not always be evident. Endocrine dysfunction, which can be linked to obesity, a sedentary lifestyle, limited endurance, low activity tolerance, and lowered energy levels, will eventually result in occupational performance deficits. The therapist's role with the client is to establish realistic expectations regarding participation in occupational performance areas, skills, and patterns. The occupational therapist's role may include education to increase the client's awareness and understanding of the disease process, development of compensatory strategies for performance deficits, and recommendations for engagement in a wellness program to optimize occupational functioning.

Endocrine disease may not be the primary reason for which the client has been hospitalized, but it can influence the recovery process, prognosis, and long-term outcome, increasing the complexity of the healing process. A client admitted to acute care for management of a hip fracture resulting from a fall who did not have any previously identified risk factors might be further evaluated for underlying hyperthyroidism or osteoporosis. If a client's past medical history includes a concomitant history of long-standing uncontrolled diabetes, then the therapist needs to be aware that this client is at an increased risk for additional complications such as small vessel disease, atherosclerosis, and impaired immune function. Uncontrolled cardiovascular risk factors and diabetes can also result in delayed wound healing, diabetic neuropathy, or stroke.

Cognitive, social, and emotional regulation skills are another area of concern for the occupational therapist. Diabetes mellitus, hypoglycemia, thyroid disorders, parathyroid disorders, and adrenal disorders are some endocrine diseases associated with psychiatric symptoms and syndromes (Levenson, 2006). The signs and symptoms of chronic endocrine impairments may include anxiety, depression, and irritability. Clients may also present with decreased attention, concentration, poor memory, and a reduced ability to compensate for cognitive deficits.

Intervention

Clients with endocrine dysfunction will benefit from occupational therapy intervention that addresses health management and maintenance through occupation-based intervention, purposeful activity, and preparatory methods.

Education and Consultation on Health Management and Maintenance

Client education should focus on how to increase physical activity and reduce the effects of deconditioning and limited activity tolerance through the use of exercise. Exercise programs that include weight-loading or resistive physical activity and incorporate moderate aerobic activity are of the greatest benefit to most people. The advantage of exercise is that it can address many deficits resulting from chronic disease and conditions. "It [exercises] restores hypothalamic sensitivity, improves glucose tolerance, reduces insulin levels and enhances growth hormone secretion" (Dean, 2008, "Approaches to Improve Age-Related Alterations in the Energy Homeostat," para. 1). However, people with endocrine diseases should seek medical advice and follow specific guidelines (e.g., exercise restrictions if fasting blood glucose is >300 milligrams per deciliter or <100 milligrams per deciliter) before initiation of a routine exercise program.

Specifically, occupational therapists should plan health activities for both the mind and the body. For example, the incorporation of activities that release endorphins, like yoga, tai chi, and qigong may slow down the release of stress-related hormones, boost the immune system, and improve glucose metabolism (Yeh et al., 2007). Over the long term, improved energy levels and flexibility may result in more efficient and satisfying ADLs. Consultation on wellness and lifestyle factors can improve quality of life and minimize additional health issues. Education on smoking and alcohol cessation, relevant diet modifications, and sleep preparation and participation may improve quality of life.

Modification of Activity Demands and Task Simplification

Many endocrine diseases diminish overall body metabolism, resulting in lethargy, inactivity, and weakness. Education on relevant energy conservation techniques and ADL or IADL modifications will enhance the client's participation in self-chosen occupations by assisting him or her in task prioritization and activity pacing. Refer to Appendix D on energy conservation strategies for more information.

Awareness of Cognitive and Behavioral Changes

Education to increase the person's awareness of common cognitive and behavioral issues associated with specific endocrine diseases, especially with neuroendocrine syndromes, may improve the integration and effectiveness of compensatory strategies. Occupational therapists may incorporate the use of cognitive screening tools to objectify deficits in the areas of attention, concentration, working memory, and executive functioning. Identification of cognitive impairments may better assist the client's incorporation of compensatory strategies. Similarly, education on behavioral changes associated with specific endocrine diseases (e.g., anxiety and depression are linked with both hypothyroidism and hyperthyroidism) may aid the client in seeking additional external support through counseling or pharmacology. Additionally, endocrine disease intervention can be addressed through the provision of external community resources and referrals.

Education and Specialty Support

Ideally, an endocrinologist should follow people with endocrine dysfunction. However, this specialized area lacks medical support, with practitioners available to fill only 50% of the needed positions (Stewart, 2008). To supplement education resources and support, the Power of Prevention (POP) organization was developed by the American Association of Clinical Endocrinologists and the American College of Endocrinology. Therapists can refer patients to the POP Web site, where the focus is on promoting healthy lives for those with endocrine disorders and diseases (see www.powerof prevention.com/e_health.php).

Specifically for diabetes management, clients can consult with a certified diabetes educator. A certified diabetes educator is a health care professional trained and certified to educate people with diabetes in the skills needed to attain and maintain health through specialized diabetes education, suggestions for glucose control, and recommendations for a healthy lifestyle.

Mental Well-Being

People with endocrine diseases frequently have issues related to depression and anxiety. Referrals to therapists who can educate clients in effective coping strategies to minimize the effects of chronic stress are recommended.

Social Support

In addition to one-on-one education, referrals to external group education sessions can provide encouragement and disease management strategies. Group sessions can help minimize fear and anxiety by providing a neutral platform from which people with endocrine disease can express their needs and share their concerns. Groups can provide information on symptom management, research, and treatments. Online groups can also provide support and education.

References

Agha, A., & Thompson, C. J. (2006). Anterior pituitary dysfunction following traumatic brain injury (TBI). *Clinical Endocrinology, 64,* 481–488.

Agham, A., Thorton, E., O'Kelly, P., Tormey, W., Phillips, J., & Thompson, C. J. (2004). Posterior pituitary dysfunction after traumatic brain injury. *Journal of Clinical Endocrinology and Metabolism, 89,* 5987–5992.

Alvidrez, L. M., & Kravitz, L. (2008). Hormonal responses to resistance exercise variables. *IDEA Fitness Journal, 5*(3), 23–25.

American Occupational Therapy Association. (2008). Occupational therapy practice framework: Domain and process (2nd ed.). *American Journal of Occupational Therapy, 62,* 625–683.

Annane, D., Bellissant, E., Bollaert, P. E., Breigel, J., Keh, D., & Kupfer, Y. (2004). Corticosteroids for severe sepsis and septic shock: A systematic review and meta-analysis. *British Medical Journal, 329,* 480. Retrieved July 28, 2008, from www.pubmedcentral.nih.gov/articlerender.fcgi?tool=pubmed&pubmedid=15289273

Annane, D., Maxime, V., Ibrahim, F., Alvarez, J. C., Abe, E., & Boudou, P. (2006). Diagnosis of adrenal insufficiency in severe sepsis and septic shock. *American Journal of Respiratory and Critical Care Medicine, 174,* 1319–1326.

Armstrong, E. J., & Tashjian, A. H., Jr. (2008). Pharmacology of the hypothalamus and pituitary gland. In D. E. Golan, A. H. Tashjian, E. J. Armstrong, & A. W. Armstrong (Eds.), *Principles of pharmacology: The pathophysiologic basis of drug therapy* (2nd ed., pp. 469–482). Baltimore: Lippincott Williams & Wilkins.

Arnaldi, G., Angeli, A., Atkinson, A. B., Bertagna, X., Cavagnini, F., & Chrousos, G. P. (2003). Diagnosis and complications of Cushing's syndrome: A consensus statement. *Journal of Clinical Endocrinology and Metabolism, 88,* 5593–5602.

Behan, L. A., Phillips, J., Thompson, C. J., & Agha, A. (2008). Neuroendocrine disorders after traumatic brain injury. *Journal of Neurology, Neurosurgery, and Psychiatry, 79,* 753–759.

Centers for Disease Control and Prevention. (2008a). *National Health and Nutrition Examination Survey for prevalence of overweight and obesity among adults: United States, 1999–2002.* Retrieved October 4, 2010, from www.cdc.gov/nchs/data/hestat/obese/obese99.htm

Centers for Disease Control and Prevention. (2008b). *Number of people with diabetes increases to 24 million* [Press release]. Retrieved July 28, 2008, from www.cdc.gov/media/pressrel/2008/r080624.htm

Chapman, M. (2006). Central diabetes insipidus. From M. H. Beers (Ed.), *The Merck manual of diagnosis and therapy* (18th ed.). Whitehouse Station, NJ: Merck. Retrieved August 1, 2008, from www.merck.com/mmpe/sec12/ch151/ch151h.html

Clark, F., Reingold, F. S., & Salles-Jordan, K. (2007). Obesity and occupational therapy [Position paper]. *American Journal of Occupational Therapy, 61,* 701–703.

Crandall, J. P., Knowler, W. C., Kahn, S. E., Marrero, D., Florez, J. C., Bray, G. A., et al. [Diabetes Prevention Program Research Group]. (2008). The prevention of Type 2 diabetes. *Nature Clinical Practice Endocrinology and Metabolism, 4,* 382–393. Retrieved June 21, 2009, from www.pubmedcentral.nih.gov/articlerender.fcgi?tool=pubmed&pubmedid=18493227

Daston, G. P., Cook, J. C., & Kavlock, R. J. (2003). Uncertainties for endocrine disrupters: Our view on progress. *Toxicological Sciences, 74,* 245–252.

Dean, W. (2008). *Neuroendocrine theory of aging, Chapter 3, Part 1.* Retrieved June 28, 2008, from www.vrp.com/articles.aspx?page=LIST&ProdID=253&qid=&zTYPE=2

Dickey, R. A., Bartuska, D. G., Bray, G. W., Callaway, C. W., Davidson, E. T., Feld, S., et al. [AACE/ACE Obesity Task Force]. (1998). AACE/ACE position statement on the prevention, diagnosis, and treatment of obesity. *Endocrine Practice, 4,* 297–349.

Endocrine Disruptor Screening Program. (2007). Retrieved February 8, 2009, from www.epa.gov/scipoly/oscpendo/index.htm

Ezzat, S., Asa, S. L., Couldwell, W. T., Barr, C. E., Dodge, W. E., Vance, M. L., et al. (2004). The prevalence of pituitary adenomas. *Cancer, 101,* 613–619.

Garber, A. J., Handelsman, Y., Einhorn, D., Bergman, D. A., Bloomgarden, Z. T., Fonseca, V., et al. (2008). Diagnosis and management of prediabetes in the continuum of hyperglycemia—When do the risks of diabetes begin? A consensus statement from the American College of Endocrinology and the American Association of Clinical Endocrinologists. *Endocrine Practice, 14,* 934–946. Retrieved June 21, 2009, from www.aace.com/pub/pdf/guidelines/prediabetesConsensus.pdf

Gonzalez-Campoy, J. M. (2007). Hypoparathyroidism. *eMedicine.* Retrieved August 1, 2008, from www.emedicine.com/med/topic1131.htm

Grundy, S. M., Brewer, H. B., Jr., Cleeman, J. I., Smith, S. C., Jr., & Lenfant, C. (2004). Definition of metabolic syndrome: Report of the National Heart, Lung, and Blood Institute/American Heart Association conference on scientific issues related to definition. *Circulation, 109,* 433–438. Retrieved June 28, 2009, from http://circ.ahajournals.org/cgi/reprint/109/3/433

Gums, J. G., & Tovar, J. M. (2005). Adrenal gland disorders. In J. T. Dipiro, R. L. Talbert, G. C. Yee, G. R. Matzke, B. G. Wells, & L. M. Posey (Eds.), *Pharmacotherapy: A pathophysiologic approach* (6th ed., pp. 1391–1406). New York: McGraw-Hill.

Hopkins, R. L., & Leinung, M. C. (2005). Exogenous Cushing's syndrome and glucocorticoid withdrawal. *Endocrinology and Metabolism Clinics of North America, 34,* 371–384.

Igaz, P., Rácz, K., Tóth, M., Gláz, E., & Tulassay, Z. (2007). Treatment of iatrogenic Cushing syndrome: Questions of glucocorticoid withdrawal. *Orvosi Hetilap, 148,* 195–202.

Kim, L. (2008). Hyperparathyroidism. *eMedicine.* Retrieved August 1, 2008, from www.emedicine.com/med/topic3200.htm

Kim, S., & Popkin, B. M. (2006). Commentary: Understanding the epidemiology of overweight and obesity—A real global public health concern. *International Journal of Epidemiology, 25,* 60–67.

Laurberg, P., Andersen, S., Bulow Pedersen, I., & Carle, A. (2005). Hypothyroidism in the elderly: Pathophysiology, diagnosis and treatment. *Drugs and Aging, 22*(1), 23–38.

Levenson, J. L. (2006). Psychiatric issues in endocrinology. *Primary Psychiatry, 13*(4), 27–30.

Lieberman, S. A, Oberoi, A. L., Gilkison, C. R., Masel, B. E., & Urban, R. J. (2001). Prevalence of neuroendocrine dysfunction in patients recovering from traumatic brain injury. *Journal of Clinical Endocrinology and Metabolism, 86,* 2752–2756.

Mahajan, A., & Tandon, V. R. (2005). Corticosteroids in rheumatology: Friends or foes. *Journal of Indian Academy of Clinical Medicine, 6,* 275–280.

Marik, P. E., Pastores, S. M., Annane, D., Meduri, G. U., Sprung, C. L., Arlt, W., et al. (2008). Recommendations for the diagnosis and management of corticosteroid insufficiency in critically ill adult patients: Consensus statements from an international task force by the American College of Critical Care Medicine. *Critical Care Medicine, 36,* 1937–1949.

Napolitano, L., Schmidt, D., Gotway, M. B., Ameli, N., Filbert, E. L., Ng, M. M., et al. (2008). Growth hormone enhances thymic function in HIV-1-infected adults. *Journal of Clinical Investigation, 118,* 1085–1098.

Neumann, I. D. (2008). Brain oxytocin: A key regulator of emotional and social behaviours in both females and males. *Journal of Neuroendocrinology, 20,* 858–865.

Porter, R. S. (2006). Hypothyroidism. From M. H. Beers (Ed.), *The Merck manual of diagnosis and therapy* (18th ed.). Whitehouse Station, NJ: Merck. Retrieved June 17, 2008, from http://www.merck.com/mmpe/index.html

Reiter, L. W., DeRosa, C., Kavlock, R. J., Lucier, G., Mac, M. J., Melnick, R. L., et al. (1998). The U.S. federal framework for research on endocrine disruptors and an analysis of research programs supported during fiscal year 1996. *Environmental Health Perspective, 106,* 105–113.

Reiter, R. J., Tan, D., Mayo, J. C., Sainz, R. M., Leon, J., & Czarnocki, Z. (2003). Melatonin as an antioxidant: Biochemical mechanisms and pathophysiological implications in humans. *Acta Biochimica Polonica, 50,* 1129–1146.

Robergs, R. A., & Kravitz, L. (2005). The role of cortisol in concurrent training. *IDEA Fitness Journal, 2*(9), 20–23.

Ronti, T., Lupattelli, G., & Mannarino, E. (2006). The endocrine function of adipose tissue: An update. *Clinical Endocrinology, 64,* 355–365. Retrieved June 21, 2009, from doi: 10.1111/j.1365-2265.2006.02474.x

Sergot, P. B., & Nelson, L. S. (2008). Hyperosmolar hyperglycemic state. *eMedicine.* Retrieved June 28, 2009, from http://emedicine.medscape.com/article/766804-overview

Shu, A. D., Myers, M. G., Jr., & Shoelson, S. E. (2008). Pharmacology of endocrine pancreas. In D. E. Golan, A. H. Tashjian, E. J. Armstrong, & A. W. Armstrong (Eds.), *Principles of pharmacology: The pathophysiologic basis of drug therapy* (2nd ed., pp. 524–541). Baltimore: Lippincott Williams & Wilkins.

Simpson, E. P. (2005). Neurologic complications of systemic disease: Endocrine system. In G. A. Thibodeau & K. T. Patton (Eds.), *Anatomy and physiology* (5th ed., pp. 484–527). St. Louis, MO: Mosby.

Stewart, A. F. (2008). The United States endocrinology workforce: A supply–demand mismatch. *Journal of Clinical Endocrinology and Metabolism, 93,* 1164–1166.

Talbert, R. A. (2005). Thyroid disorders. In J. T. Dipiro, R. L. Talbert, G. C. Yee, G. R. Matzke, B. G. Wells, & L. M. Posey (Eds.), *Pharmacotherapy: A pathophysiologic approach* (6th ed., pp. 1369–1390). New York: McGraw-Hill.

Tanriverdi, F., Senyurek, H., Unluhizarci, K., Selcuklu, A., Casanueva, F. F., & Kelestimur, F. (2006). High risk of hypopituitarism after traumatic brain injury: A prospective investigation of anterior pituitary function in the acute phase and 12 months after trauma. *Journal of Clinical Endocrinology and Metabolism, 91,* 2105–2111.

Triplitt, C. L., Reasner, C. A., & Isley, W. L. (2005). Diabetes mellitus. In J. T. Dipiro, R. L. Talbert, G. C. Yee, G. R. Matzke, B. G. Wells, & L. M. Posey (Eds.), *Pharmacotherapy: A pathophysiologic approach* (6th ed., pp. 133–1368). New York: McGraw-Hill.

Wilmore, J. H., Costill, D., & Kenney, W. L. (2008). *Physiology of sport and exercise* (4th ed.). Champaign, IL: Human Kinetics.

Yeh, S. H., Chuang, H., Lin, L. W., Hsiao, C. Y., Wang, P. W., & Yang, K. D. (2007). Tai chi chuan exercise decreases A1C levels along with increase of regulatory T-cells and decrease of cytotoxic T-cell population in type 2 diabetic patients. *Diabetes Care, 30,* 716–718.

Zhdanova, I. V., & Tucci, V. (2003). Melatonin, circadian rhythms, and sleep. *Current Treatment Options in Neurology, 5,* 225–229. Retrieved June 21, 2009, from www.springerlink.com/content/7217587222716ggt

9

The Gastrointestinal System

Helene Smith-Gabai, OTD, OTR/L, BCPR

Most people are consciously aware of their gastrointestinal (GI) system on a daily basis. Eating, digestion, and defecation, unlike other body functions, are part of people's daily lives, with physical and psychological ramifications. Organic and psychological issues can also have a marked effect on the digestive process, causing GI symptoms and disorders. Therapists working with patients with GI disorders need to take a holistic approach because this system has a strong mind–body connection.

According to a Centers for Disease Control and Prevention national hospital report (Pitts, Niska, Xu, & Burt, 2008), in 2006 emergency room visits for digestive disorders totaled more than 7 million. GI problems may be related to the organs of the GI tract itself or a sign of a systemic disorder. Many minor GI problems may be corrected by simple diet and lifestyle modifications. However, even relatively minor symptoms can be indicative of a more serious underlying disorder (Friedman, McQuaid, & Grendell, 2003). The GI system, which provides nutrients for body processes essential to life, has a profound effect on people's health and sense of well-being. Appendices 9.A and 9.B list nutritional, mineral, and trace element, deficiencies and their impact on body systems; Appendix 9.C gives common hospital diets; and Appendix 9.D describes enteral and parenteral modes of nutrition delivery.

Normal Structure and Function

Each part of the GI system plays a role in the digestion and absorption of nutrients that keep the body functioning efficiently. The four main functions of the GI system are ingestion, digestion, absorption, and elimination (Hughes, 2005; see Figure 9.1). Muscles, hormones, and nerves control motility of food through the GI system. Food is pushed through each portion of the GI tract to the next by wavelike muscular contractions called *peristalsis*.

Ingestion, Digestion, Absorption, and Elimination

The ingestion and digestion process begins in the oral cavity. Food entering the mouth is broken down by chewing and mixes with saliva, forming into a cohesive ball for swallowing called a *bolus*. The reflexive phase of the swallowing process begins with the pharynx and continues through the esophagus and into the stomach where acids further break down food (refer to Chapter 13 for details on the swallowing process and information on swallowing disorders).

Enzymes and acids in the stomach break down foods and destroy bacteria found in food. From the stomach, the digested food (*chyme*) travels through the pyloric sphincter into the small intestine (duodenum, jejunum, and ileum). Here, other secretions from the GI system mix with the digested food and absorption of nutrients, water, and electrolytes takes place. Throughout the upper GI tract, food is progressively broken down into smaller absorbable molecules of glucose, amino acids, fatty acids, and glycerol and converted into a form the body can use as fuel. Appendix 9.C lists common hospital diets modified by consistency and nutrients specific to patients' needs.

In the lower GI system, the large intestine and colon further absorb water and electrolytes. The ileum of the small intestine passes material on to the large intestine through the ileocecal valve. Material then travels from the cecum to the colon and rectum. Elimination occurs when undigested material passes through the anus.

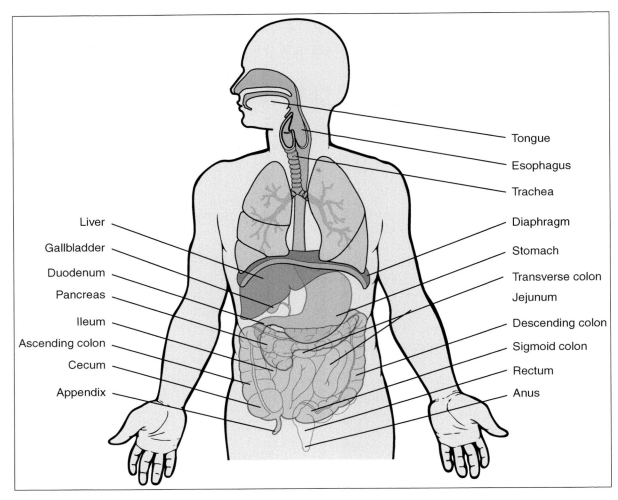

Figure 9.1. The gastrointestinal tract.
Source. Richard Fritzler, Medical Illustrator, Roswell, GA.

Layers of the GI Tract

The GI tract has four main layers that run the length of the *alimentary canal,* or *GI tract.* They include mucous, submucosa, muscularis, and serosa (listed from the innermost to outermost layers). Depending on the location in the GI tract, the function of the *mucous membrane* is either protective or involved in secretion and absorption. In certain areas, the mucous layer folds on itself, increasing surface area. The stomach also has a specialized mucosa for acid and enzyme production. The *submucosa* contains blood and lymph vessels and nerves, attaching the muscularis to the mucous layer. *Muscularis* is a smooth muscle layer responsible for peristalsis through the GI tract. The *serous* layer is connective tissue that anchors the GI tract to the mesentery.

Accessory Organs

The solid accessory organs that aid in digestion include the liver, gallbladder, pancreas, and spleen. The accessory organs are not involved in physical digestion but produce secretions responsible for chemical digestion. The accessory organs perform the following functions:

- The pancreas produces insulin, which regulates blood glucose levels. The pancreas also produces various enzymes, which break down carbohydrates, fats, and proteins so they can be absorbed through the walls of the intestines.

- The hepatobiliary system consists of the liver, bile ducts, and gallbladder. Figure 9.2 illustrates the hepatobiliary system.

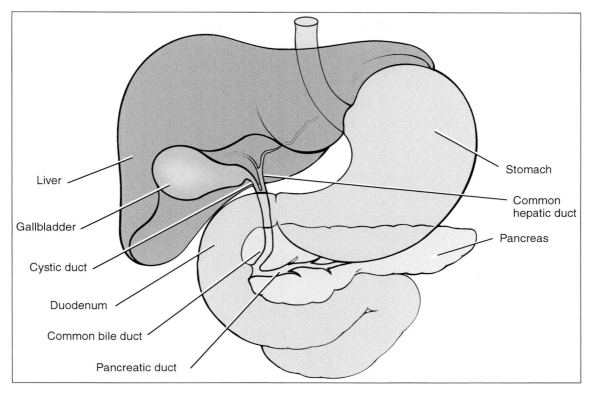

Figure 9.2. The hepatobiliary system.
Source. Richard Fritzler, Medical Illustrator, Roswell, GA.

— *Liver:* The liver is the largest organ in the body; it removes germs and bacteria from blood, aids the body's immune system, filters toxins (e.g., alcohol, drugs, tobacco), and produces bile, which helps absorb fats. The liver actually performs more than 100 different functions in the body.

— *Bile ducts and gallbladder:* Bile ducts carry bile from the liver to the gallbladder, where excess bile is stored between meals. When food enters the stomach, the gallbladder releases bile through the common bile duct and into the duodenum. Bile digests, emulsifies, and aids in the absorption of fats. Most of the salts in bile are reabsorbed and reused.

• The spleen is occasionally listed as a GI accessory organ. The spleen aids in clearing bacteria from the body and is part of the lymphatic system but has no direct role in digestion.

Vascular and Nervous System Input

The vascular and nervous systems also play an important part in digestion.

• Digested nutrients absorbed in the intestines cross the mucosa into the bloodstream, where the vascular system transports them throughout the body. Blood is supplied to the GI system through the inferior and superior mesenteric, rectal, and internal iliac arteries.

• The nervous system stimulates release of secretions and hormones for digestion and chemicals that assist with motility. The enteric nervous system, a division of the autonomic nervous system and the vagus nerve, is involved in signaling the central nervous system to coordinate digestion and regulate food intake and energy expenditure (Grundy & Schemann, 2007). Close communication between the central and enteric nervous systems is important for maintenance of homeostasis and normal functioning. For example, a thyroid disorder may slow digestion, resulting in constipation and bloating, or speed up emptying, resulting in diarrhea (Rosenthal, 1998).

GI Diseases and Disorders

Many factors such as stress, depression, infection, toxins, and congenital defects affect how the GI system functions. Abdominal pains, changes in bowel habits, nausea, vomiting,

Table 9.1. Common Gastrointestinal (GI) Diagnostic Tests

Test	Description
Barium enema	Barium sulfate is a type of contrast inserted as an enema into the rectal area, allowing an X-ray picture of the large intestines; used to detect colon cancer, polyps, and inflammatory bowel diseases.
Barium swallow	A barium swallow uses a videofluoroscopy or moving X-ray to detect structural and physiologic abnormalities in the upper digestive tract, usually from the pharynx through the esophagus and stomach. It is different from a modified barium swallow test, also known as a videofluoroscopic swallow study, which also uses fluoroscopy, but examines oral, pharyngeal, and esophageal function for patients with dysphagia. This test assesses for the presence of aspiration but also assesses the use of food textures and swallowing techniques that optimize safe swallowing.
Colonoscopy	Endoscopic examination of the colon, used for detecting the presence of polyps, colon cancer, and inflammatory bowel disease.
EGD	In an EGD, a flexible endoscope is placed down the throat to study the lining of the esophagus, stomach, or small intestine (upper duodenum). An EGD is used to detect causes of pain, abnormalities, and swallowing difficulties and sources of GI bleeds and to examine for presence of tumors, ulcers, or inflammation. A biopsy may also be performed during an EGD.
Endoscopic retrograde cholangiopancreatography	Performed by inserting a flexible fiberoptic scope through the patient's mouth and down through the esophagus, stomach, and duodenum. As a treatment modality, it is used for stone extraction, stent placement, and other procedures associated with the gallbladder and pancreas.
Esophageal pH monitoring	A probe is inserted and a recorder is attached to measure the pH of the esophagus. This esophageal monitor is generally an ambulatory device worn up to 24 hours that provides information on GI reflux while the patient is in different positions (e.g., upright, supine).
KUB	This abdominal X-ray is used to detect GI disorders and to ensure proper placement of nasogastric tubes.

Table 9.1.   (continued)

Test	Description
Liver function tests	A variety of blood tests that evaluate the overall liver and biliary systems. They include serum albumin, prothrombin time, and liver enzymes that are markers for liver disease (e.g., alanine aminotransferase, aspartate aminotransferase, gammaglutamyltranspeptidase, alkaline phosphatase). Liver function tests are more indicative of liver damage than overall liver function. Refer to Appendix P for more information.
Manometry	A catheter is placed in the esophagus; it provides information on lower esophageal sphincter pressure, sphincter relaxation, and esophageal peristalsis. This test is typically recommended before antireflux surgery.
Upper GI series	X-ray used to detect disorders of the esophagus, stomach, and duodenum. A swallowed barium solution makes these organs more visible on the X-ray and shows how the digestive system is functioning.

Note. EGD = esophagogastroduodenscopy; KUB = kidneys, ureter, and bladder.

diarrhea, jaundice, or blood in the stool are symptoms that may prompt a patient to seek medical attention. GI disorders may be the result of problems with motility, absorption, obstruction, inflammation, or hemorrhage. Refer to Table 9.1 for a list of diagnostic tests specific to GI disorders.

Common GI symptoms or manifestations may be normal, innocuous, or symptomatic of disorder. Commonly experienced GI symptoms are

- *Nausea:* The sensation of stomach queasiness. Causes may be physical or psychological.

- *Vomiting:* The forcible emptying of stomach contents, often preceded by feelings of nausea. Receptors in the medulla (i.e., the vomiting center) and GI tract can trigger a vomiting response as a protective mechanism. Several causes of nausea and vomiting are listed in Table 9.2.

- *Diarrhea:* Unusually frequent, loose, or watery stool. Diarrhea may be acute or chronic. Common causes of diarrhea are viruses, bacteria, side effects of medication, or lactose intolerance. Chronic diarrhea

may also be symptomatic of inflammatory diseases or malabsorptive disorders.

- *Constipation:* Three or fewer bowel movements per week or excessive straining with defecation. Constipation is common in hospitalized patients and is a common complaint among older adults. Constipation is associated with a sedentary lifestyle, a low-fiber diet, or regular ingestion of constipating medications (e.g., pain relievers, medications for high blood pressure; Friedman et al., 2003).

- *Burping and belching:* Generally caused by swallowed air and commonly seen in patients with gastroesophageal reflux disease (GERD). The body normally absorbs the oxygen in swallowed air, but not the nitrogen (78% of air). Chewing gum, smoking, eating quickly, and drinking carbonated beverages can contribute to burping, which in turn can lead to bloating, abdominal discomfort, and flatus (Friedman et al., 2003).

- *Flatus:* Gas is produced in the stomach and intestines when food is broken down. Swallowed air and gas that are not absorbed in

Table 9.2.　Causes of Nausea and Vomiting

Infection	Gastroenteritis
	Food poisoning
	Infections outside the GI tract (e.g., bladder or kidney infection)
Motility disorders	Pseudo-obstruction
	Amyloidosis
	Pancreatic cancer with obstruction
	Paraneoplastic syndromes
	Gastroparesis
	Ileus
Mechanical obstruction	Hernia
	Adhesions
	Volvulus (twisting of the intestines)
	Small tumors
	Crohn's disease with stricture
	Gastric outlet obstruction
	Chronic peptic ulcer disease
Inflammation	Pancreatitis
	Crohn's disease
	Ulcerative colitis
	Cholecystitis
	Appendicitis
	Diverticulitis
	Viral hepatitis
Hormonal and metabolic disorders	Diabetes
	Hyperthyroidism
	Addison's disease
Central nervous system	Motion sickness
	Labyrinthitis
	Migraines
	Increased intracranial pressure
	Meningitis
	Encephalitis
	Central nervous system tumors
	Seizures
	Head trauma
	Multiple sclerosis

Systemic conditions	Kidney failure
	Myocardial infarction
	Pregnancy
Psychiatric disorders	Bulimia
	Anorexia nervosa
	Anxiety
	Depression
Medication	Chemotherapy drugs
	Anesthetic agents
	Nonsteroidal anti-inflammatory drugs
	Antibiotics
	Narcotics
	Digoxin
Miscellaneous	Radiation therapy
	Alcohol intoxication

Table 9.2.   *(continued)*

Sources. From Friedman, McQuaid, & Grendell (2003); Gastrointestinal system (2007); Porter & Gyawali (2010).
Note. GI = gastrointestinal.

the intestines are expelled from the body as flatus, which is composed of hydrogen, carbon dioxide, and methane. Flatus may be more pronounced with diseases of malabsorption.

- *Bowel sounds:* Heard when food moves through the intestines. Reduced or absent bowel sounds may indicate that the intestines are not working properly because of an obstruction, ileus, or constipation. Hyperactive bowel sounds may be present with irritable bowel diseases such as Crohn's disease and ulcerative colitis.

Disorders of the Esophagus

Peristalsis propels food, liquids, and saliva through the *esophagus,* a long muscular tube that runs from the pharynx to the stomach. This section reviews the esophageal disorders of gastroestophageal reflux, Barret's esophagus, esophageal cancer, and esophageal varices.

Gastroesophageal Reflux

GERD, commonly referred to as *heartburn* or *indigestion,* affects more than 40% of Americans (Hanahan, 2007; Todd, Corsnitz, Ray, & Nassar, 2002). Approximately $8–$10 billion are spent annually to treat GERD (Forister, Taliferro, Ramos, & Blessing, 2002; Hanahan, 2007), including $4–$5 billion per year for antacids (Richter, 2008). Diagnosed by frequency and severity of symptoms, GERD is rarely a primary diagnosis for hospital admission but is a common comorbidity with implications for quality of life. Ingestion of aspirin or nonsteroidal anti-inflammatory drugs (NSAIDs), obesity, pregnancy, and prolonged nasogastric intubation may lead to the development of GERD.

Etiology. During swallowing, the lower esophageal sphincter (LES) normally relaxes to allow food into the stomach. This relaxation of the LES lasts less than 10 seconds and is typically an effective antireflux barrier. When the LES is weak or inappropriately relaxes, contents from the stomach leak back into the esophagus, causing sensations of discomfort and acid reflux. Esophageal injury occurs when refluxed acids and enzymes damage the esophageal mucosa. Large hiatal hernias can also affect the functioning of the LES by displacing it. A hiatal hernia occurs when an upper portion of the stomach protrudes through an opening in the diaphragm (the diaphragmatic hiatus) and into the chest, allowing easier reflux into the esophagus. Treatment for hiatal hernias includes minimizing activities that increase intra-abdominal pressure (e.g., coughing, straining, bending), surgical repair, or treatment approaches used in addressing GERD.

Treatment. Treatment for GERD may include lifestyle modifications, medication, surgery, or a combination of these treatments.

- Lifestyle modifications for GERD include losing weight if obese, eating smaller meals (less acid production), sitting up during and after meals (avoid reclining after a meal), avoidance of bedtime snacks (not eating within 3 hours of bedtime), and increased fluid intake. Recommendations also include sleeping on the left side of the body with the head of the bed elevated, thereby using gravity to decrease reflux (Forister et al., 2002). People with GERD also traditionally avoid items they feel exacerbate GERD symptoms, such as caffeine, chocolate, peppermint, citrus fruits, tomato products, peppers, spicy foods, high-fat foods, alcohol, and cigarettes (Hanahan, 2007; Rayhorn, Argel, & Demchak, 2003). Patients with GERD should also avoid positions that increase intra-abdominal pressure, including coughing, bending, wearing tight clothing, or engaging in vigorous exercises ("Gastrointestinal System," 2007).

- Medications for GERD consist of over-the-counter antacids, histamine 2 blockers (e.g., Zantac, Tagamet), or proton pump inhibitors (e.g., Prevacid, Prilosec, Nexium, Protonix). These drugs reduce and suppress acid secretions and therefore minimize damage to the esophagus. Proton pump inhibitors have become a mainstay of GERD treatment because they are beneficial in healing esophagitis and ulcers (Hanahan, 2007).

- Surgical intervention for treating GERD may include laparoscopic Nissen fundoplication. In this type of surgery, the fundus of the stomach is wrapped around the lower part of the esophagus, thereby creating an external esophageal sphincter that prevents food from flowing back into the esophagus. Fundoplication has been a successful approach, with more than 85% of patients reporting relief of GERD symptoms (Friedman et al., 2003).

Barrett's Esophagus

If GERD is untreated, it can lead to Barrett's esophagus, a condition that affects 700,000 Americans each year (Fichandler & Malone, 2006). *Barrett's esophagus* is a precancerous condition in which columnar epithelial metaplasia replaces normal epithelium, thus narrowing and damaging the lining of the esophagus. Although chronic GERD is believed to be the predominant cause of Barrett's esophagus, smoking and alcohol are also considered risk factors. It is important to closely monitor and treat this condition because patients with Barrett's esophagus are at a much greater risk for developing esophageal cancer (Friedman et al., 2003; Paz & Nicoloro, 2009).

Initially, treatment of Barrett's esophagus is similar to treatment of GERD: medication and lifestyle modification. However, when cancerous changes occur, the lining of the esophagus or the lower esophagus is removed. Endoscopic approaches including photodynamic therapy, ablation, or mucosal resection to remove or destroy the Barrett's lining allow normal regrowth of cells ("What Is Esophagectomy?" 2006). An *esophagectomy* (i.e., Ivor-Lewis) is a surgical procedure in which a portion of the esophagus is removed and a section of the stomach (or intestines) is attached to the healthy remaining part of the esophagus, maintaining a structurally intact passage for food. An advantage of an esophagectomy is that it eliminates the risk of esophageal adenocarcinoma, which has a poor prognosis.

Esophageal Cancer

Esophageal cancers can include squamous cell carcinoma or the rarer adenocarcinoma (which is usually located in the lower third of the esophagus). The etiology of this type of adenocarcinoma is unknown; however, risk factors may include heavy cigarette smoking, alcohol use, previous head and neck tumors, diets rich in nitrosamines (e.g., fried bacon, cured meat, beer), achalasia, or stricture ("Gastrointestinal Disorders," 2006). This cancer metastasizes early through the lymphatic system to nearby organs (refer to Chapter 11 for more information on cancers of the GI tract).

With esophageal tumor obstruction, an *esophagostomy* (artificial opening into the esophagus) with a drainage stoma or spit fistula may be performed. A *spit fistula* is an external pouch or esophageal drainage stoma attached to a hole in the throat. Secretions such as saliva, or anything taken by mouth, drains into the pouch and thereby eliminates the risk of aspiration into the lungs. It also allows patients to have the sensation of eating or drinking even though what they swallow never enters the stomach.

Esophageal Varices

Portal hypertension may cause esophageal blood vessels to dilate, resulting in *esophageal varices* (enlarged veins). This condition is serious because it can lead to blood vessel rupture and hemorrhage. Refer to the "Portal Hypertension and Variceal Bleeding" section in this chapter for additional information on this condition.

Disorders of the Stomach

The stomach mixes ingested food it receives from the esophagus with acids for digestion, and passes it along to the small intestines. This section briefly reviews gastritis, peptic ulcer disease, gastroparesis, dumping syndrome, and stomach cancer.

Gastritis

Gastritis is an inflammation of the lining of the stomach and mucosa with symptoms and treatment similar to those of GERD. Causes of acute gastritis include eating spicy foods, caffeine, alcohol, aspirin, NSAIDs, corticosteroids, trauma, renal or liver failure, or physi-

ological stress ("Gastrointestinal Disorders," 2006; Paz & Nicoloro, 2009). Chronic gastritis is common among older adults and is associated with pernicious anemia and *Helicobacter pylori* infection.

Treatment for gastritis includes medications such as antibiotics, antacids, proton pump inhibitors, histamine antagonists, and prostoglandins and avoidance of caffeine, spicy foods, and aspirin ("Gastrointestinal Disorders," 2006). Treatment may also consist of letting the stomach rest with the use of a nasogastric tubing for pressure relief, eating nothing by mouth (*nil per os*, or NPO), and receiving IV hydration and parenteral nutrition (Fichandler & Malone, 2006). Refer to Appendix 9.D for a description of enteral and parenteral modes of nutrition delivery.

Peptic Ulcer Disease

Peptic ulcer disease occurs in approximately 10% of the population. This condition is the result of an imbalance in stomach secretions and mucosa, causing epithelium erosions, and is associated with *H. pylori* bacteria and use of NSAIDs (Paz & Nicoloro, 2009). Although peptic ulcers can occur in the stomach, approximately 80% occur in the duodenum ("Gastrointestinal System," 2007). Symptoms of peptic ulcers include abdominal pain, nausea with or without vomiting, and burping. Peptic ulcers can lead to epithelium erosions, perforation, bleeding, or obstruction. Treatment usually consists of antibiotics, anti-ulcer medications, avoidance of alcohol and caffeine, not eating before bedtime, and eating smaller meals.

Gastroparesis and Dumping Syndrome

Gastroparesis is a motility disorder in which food is delayed in moving from the stomach to the intestines. Gastroparesis is associated with damage to the vagus nerve and may be a result of gastric bypass surgery, diabetes, hypothyroidism, anorexia, Parkinson's disease, scleroderma, or amyloidosis. It is typically treated through diet and medication.

Rapid gastric emptying, or *dumping syndrome*, is the opposite of gastroparesis and occurs when undigested food passes too quickly from the stomach to the intestines. This condition is also commonly associated with gastric bypass surgery, gastric resection, gallbladder surgery, or the consumption of excess sugars. Dumping syndrome can result in hypoglycemia, abdominal discomfort, nausea, and diarrhea. Treatment includes diet modification, eating smaller and more frequent meals high in protein and low in simple carbohydrates, and avoidance of fluid intake during meals (Gould, 2006).

Stomach Cancer

Diets high in smoked foods and preservatives, heredity, blood type A, chronic gastritis, and polyps are all associated with stomach cancer (Gould, 2006). *Gastric cancer,* or *adenocarcinoma,* is treated surgically by tumor and lymph node resection. Surgical gastrectomy may be partial, in which the intestines are attached to the remaining stomach, or total, in which the intestines are attached to the esophagus. The extent of surgery depends on the location and size of the tumor (Conroy, Uwer, & Deblock, 2007). Gastric cancer is initially asymptomatic until the disease is well advanced. Without early detection, mortality is high. More than 21,000 new cases of stomach cancer were diagnosed in the United States in 2007 with more than 50% mortality (Goodman, 2009). Refer to Chapter 11 for more information.

Disorders of the Intestines and Bowel

Digested and liquefied food from the stomach passes into the small intestine for further digestion and absorption. The large intestine is involved in water reabsorption, maintenance of fluid balance, and elimination of solid waste material. Disorders of the intestines and bowel can involve inflammation, motility, and malabsorption.

Irritable Bowel Syndrome

Irritable bowel syndrome (IBS) is often confused with inflammatory bowel disease (IBD), but they are two different conditions. IBS, commonly known as *spastic colon,* affects approximately 20 million Americans (Fichandler & Malone, 2006). Its symptoms are abdominal cramping or spasms, nausea, bloating, diarrhea, or constipation. The colon functions abnormally without presence of inflammation. IBS is attributed to a heightened sensitivity of the colon to certain foods (e.g., coffee, fruits, vegetables), hormonal changes, laxative abuse, or emotional stress ("Gastrointestinal Disorders," 2006; "Gastrointestinal System," 2007; Fichandler & Malone, 2006). Treatment typically consists of changing dietary habits (i.e., the BRAT diet: *b*ananas, *r*ice, *t*ea, *a*nd *t*oast), increasing dietary fiber, avoiding trigger foods, engaging in exercise, reducing stress, and using medication to stabilize colon motility (e.g., laxatives, antidiarrheal medications, fiber supplements; Fichandler & Malone, 2006).

Inflammatory Bowel Disease

In contrast to IBS, *IBD* is a chronic inflammatory condition marked by periods of exacerbation and remission. Approximately 1 million Americans have IBD (Rayhorn & Rayhorn, 2002a). The two most common chronic inflammatory diseases are Crohn's disease (CD) and ulcerative colitis (UC; see Table 9.3). The exact cause of these diseases is unknown. However, infection, genetics, the environment, or an autoimmune response may play a part in the development of these diseases.

IBD can involve other organs in the body, with extraintestinal symptoms affecting the musculoskeletal system (e.g., arthritis, ankylosing spondylitis), the eyes (e.g., ocular lesions), blood (e.g., increased risk of thrombosis and hypercoagulability), or skin conditions (Rayhorn & Rayhorn, 2002a, 2002b; Stein, 2004). Approximately 30% of patients with IBD have an extraintestinal manifestation (Rayhorn & Rayhorn, 2002b).

Symptoms of IBD generally include diarrhea, abdominal discomfort, fatigue, weight loss, malnutrition, and malabsorption. Treatment for IBD focuses on symptom relief, including anti-inflammatory, antimicrobial, antidiarrheal, and immunomodulator medications; psychosocial support; and maintaining adequate nutrition, fluids, and electrolytes. Although patients with

Table 9.3. Inflammatory Bowel Disease: Comparison of Crohn's Disease and Ulcerative Colitis

Presentation	Crohn's Disease	Ulcerative Colitis
Distribution of disease	Can occur anywhere along the GI tract, predominantly in terminal ileum	Only affects colon
Clinical course	Remissions and exacerbations	Remissions and exacerbations
Family history	20%–25%	20%
Gender	Equal in men and women	Equal in men and women
Inflammation	Can extend through all layers of the bowel	Affects only mucosal lining
Clinical manifestations	• Diarrhea • Weight loss • Abdominal pain • Mild skin rash • Mild to moderate joint pain	• Diarrhea • Weight loss • Rectal bleeding • Mild skin rash • Mild to moderate joint pain
Fissures and fistulas	Common	Absent
Granulomas	Typical	Uncommon
Narrowed lumen or obstruction	Typical	Uncommon
Cancer risk	Mildly increased	Increased
Medication	• 5-aminosalicylates • Steroids • Immunosuppressants	• 5-aminosalicylates • Suppositories • Biologic agents (IV)
Surgery	• Resection and anastomosis • Not a cure for disease; palliative • Temporary colostomy	• Removal of colon is cure • Loop or permanent ileostomy

Source. From Goodman, C. C. (2009). The Gastrointestinal System. In C. C. Goodman & K. S. Fuller (Eds.), *Pathology: Implications for the Physical Therapist* (3rd ed., p. 853). St. Louis, MO: W. B. Saunders. Copyright © 2009 by W. B. Saunders. Adapted with permission.

Note. GI = gastrointestinal.

IBD lead productive lives, the nature of these diseases and their symptoms can have a profound effect on quality of life, body image, and self-esteem (Berndtsson, Lindholm, & Ekman, 2005).

Crohn's Disease

CD may occur anywhere from the mouth to the anus but is most commonly found in the terminal ileum (Geraghty & Desser, 2006; Stein, 2004; Veronesi, 2003). Unlike colitis, the entire thickness of the bowel wall can be affected in CD, with the appearance of skip lesions (patchy ulcerations). Patients with CD are also at risk for small bowel obstruction, fistulas, anal fissures, and perianal abscesses. Fistulas are abnormal connections or tunnels between two different loops of intestines or between the intestines and another organ (e.g., bladder, vagina, or even out to the skin). Fistulas are treated with antibiotics or immunosuppressants or are surgically repaired.

Initial pharmacological treatment for CD and UC are similar, including anti-inflammatory 5-aminosalicylates. Medication for more extensive disease may include corticosteroids, immune modulating agents, or biological response modifiers (Rayhorn & Rayhorn, 2002a). Steroids are used when 5-aminosalicylic drugs are ineffective; however, serious adverse side effects are associated with long-term steroid use. Surgery is warranted when conservative treatment is ineffective. Approximately 70% to 80% of patients with CD will require at least one surgical procedure because of obstruction or stricture (Rayhorn & Rayhorn, 2002a; Veronesi, 2003). With surgical resection, diseased portions of the intestines are removed, and the healthy ends are *anastomosed,* or joined together. An *ileostomy* (temporary or permanent) may also be performed, in which waste products are drained into a pouch through a hole in the abdomen.

CD has no cure. Even with surgery, the disease is still present and may reappear at any time. In addition, patients may subsequently require additional resections, leading to short bowel syndrome and reliance on total parenteral nutrition (TPN). Tobacco exacerbates CD, and patients should be educated on smoking cessation and limiting exposure to it (Pardi, Loftus, & Camilleri, 2002).

Ulcerative Colitis

UC is also a chronic condition marked by exacerbations and remissions, but it only affects the mucosa, or inner lining, of the rectum and colon. Symptoms may include abdominal pain, bloody stools, fecal urgency, malaise, and weight loss (Berndtsson et al., 2005). UC can lead to fluid and electrolyte imbalances, dehydration, anemia, obstruction, perforation, or toxic megacolon ("Gastrointestinal System," 2007).

Although typically treated with medication, the only definitive cure for colitis is a *colectomy (proctocolectomy),* or surgical removal of the colon. Approximately 25%–50% of patients with UC require surgery (Fichandler & Malone, 2006). However, a colectomy does not resolve any extraintestinal manifestations of this disease (Rayhorn & Rayhorn, 2002b).

A colectomy may necessitate an ileostomy for drainage of small intestine contents. In this ostomy procedure, the ileum is connected to an external appliance through a stoma or hole in the abdominal wall. Stool empties into an ostomy or plastic bag, which is emptied several times a day as needed. Another type of ileostomy is the continent ileostomy (see Figure 9.3), in which a pouch is fashioned internally with the presence of only a valve pulled through the stoma; there is no external ostomy bag. The patient accesses or catheterizes the pouch several times a day by inserting a tube through the valve in the stoma (Doughty, 2008).

When the anal canal and sphincter are spared, an internal ileal pouch can be connected to the patient's own sphincter (instead of through a stoma). One of the benefits of this procedure is that the patient defecates more normally. Either type of ileostomy carries the risk of infection, problems with the stoma, inflammation of the pouching system (pouchitis), obstruction, or incontinence (Doughty, 2008; Stein, 2004). Pouchitis occurs in 40% of patients, resulting in fecal incontinence, cramping, bleeding, and increased frequency.

In the acute care setting, a specialized wound, ostomy, and continence nurse (WOCN) typically assists patients with ostomy care. However, if the patient is being discharged home and the WOCN is unable to instruct the patient in independent ostomy care (e.g., because of a functional limitation), the occupational therapist may be consulted to help problem solve how the patient can successfully perform this self-care activity.

With a hemicolectomy, only a part of the colon is removed. Because fluid absorption differs in the different parts of the colon, patients undergoing a right hemicolectomy are more prone to diarrhea than are patients with other types of hemicolectomies (Stein, 2004). Patients with UC are also at an increased risk

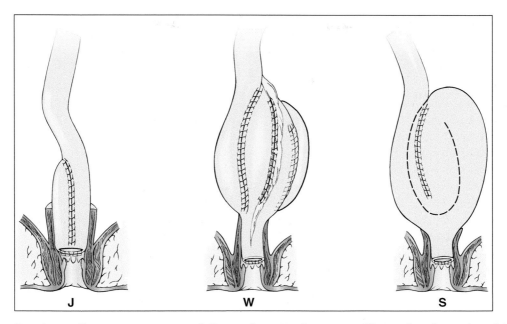

Figure 9.3. Continent ileostomy: J, W, and S pouches. Each name reflects the shape in which the ileum is cut and joined together to make the pouch. A W pouch is a larger pouch, as it is several sections sewn together.
Source. Richard Fritzler, Medical Illustrator, Roswell, GA.

of developing colorectal cancer. Colorectal cancer is one of the most common types of cancer after lung and breast cancer. Refer to Chapter 11 for more information on colorectal cancer. A permanent colostomy may be fashioned for low rectal cancers (Doughty, 2008).

Short Bowel Syndrome (Short Gut Syndrome)

In the United States, approximately 10,000 patients have *short bowel syndrome* (Nauth et al., 2004). This condition typically results from bowel resection surgery in which more than 50% of the small intestine is removed or less than 200 centimeters of small intestine remain (Buchman, 2006; Nauth et al., 2004). Surgical resection of the small intestine may be the result of CD, adhesions, clots, ischemia, or trauma. Consequences may include malabsorption, malnutrition with weight loss, dumping syndrome, diarrhea, or choleithiasis (Broadbent, Heaney, & Weyman, 2006). With short bowel syndrome, the colon must take on the role of digestion by absorbing sodium, water, some amino acids, and energy (Buchman, 2006). Treatment usually consists of TPN and hydration.

Small Bowel Obstruction

The three main causes of *small bowel obstruction (SBO)* are intrinsic, extrinsic, and intraluminal lesions.

Intrinsic lesions include benign and malignant tumors, ischemia, hematomas, or inflammatory lesions resulting from CD. *Extrinsic lesions* can include adhesions, hernias, tumors, or abscesses. *Intraluminal lesions* may be the result of gallstones, blockage from feces, tumors, or foreign objects (Geraghty & Desser, 2006; Waldman, 2001). *Postoperative ileus* (also referred to as *functional obstruction*) is a common cause of nonmechanical obstruction. However, of all causes of SBO, postsurgical adhesions are the most common, accounting for approximately 30% of all intestinal obstructions (Vakil, Kaira, Raul, Paljor, & Joseph, 2007). If SBO is left untreated, perforation or ischemia from compromised circulation may occur (Geraghty & Desser, 2006). Most patients admitted with SBO require surgical intervention. Symptoms of SBO may include abdominal distension, pain, vomiting, and the inability to pass flatus.

With obstruction, the GI tract initially tries to compensate by increasing the force of peristalsis. Eventually this process slows down, and secretions and swallowed air accumulate, leading to distension. In addition, the blood supply to the bowel may be compromised, and normal intestinal bacterial flora builds up, causing further problems with absorption, with an increased risk of systemic infection or sepsis (Waldman, 2001). Occluded blood flow from the obstruction can cause intestinal ischemia, which can lead to necrosis, peritonitis, perforation, and death.

Partial SBO has been treated with nasogastric tube decompression or suctioning and IV fluid replacement. Complete bowel obstruction is treated surgically through stenting, resection, lysis of adhesions, bypass of obstruction, or decompression with an ileostomy (Waldman, 2001). A temporary colostomy may also be used to decompress the obstructed colon (Doughty, 2008). The different types of SBOs are listed in Table 9.4.

Paralytic Ileus

Paralytic ileus is a disruption in the GI tract's normal motility and is present to some degree after any abdominal surgery. Paralytic ileus usually resolves by itself after a few days. Ileus is marked by the absence of bowel sounds and can be caused by medications, infection, mesenteric ischemia, or complications from surgery (Juhn, Eltz, & Stacy, 2008). Prolonged postoperative ileus is associated with distension, bloating, nausea, vomiting, inability or delayed ability to pass flatus, and inability to tolerate oral intake, thereby affecting nutritional status and wound healing. Postoperative ileus may lead to bowel or blood vessel obstruction, hypokalemia, or infection (Juhn et al., 2008).

Treatment consists of bowel rest with nasogastric tube decompression. Prophylactic use of nasogastric decompression after abdominal surgery should be selective because no evidence exists that it speeds recovery or increases patient comfort (Nelson, Edwards, & Tse, 2007). Fast-track programs include early oral feedings, laxatives, and early mobilization. The passage of flatus marks the return of bowel function.

Table 9.4. Small Bowel Obstructions

Test	Cause
Neurogenic	Adynamic (paralytic) ileus is a sympathetic nervous system response to manipulation of the intestines during abdominal surgery. Causes include nonsurgical trauma, myocardial infarction, vascular insufficiency, chemotherapy, and hypokalemia.
Mechanical	Adhesions, volvulus (a section of twisted bowel), hernia, diverticulitis, tumor, gallstones, intussusception (a section of bowel that moves into another section), stenosis, constipation, and Hirschsprung's disease (congenital megacolon).
Vascular	Complete or partial occlusion of the arterial blood supply to the intestines. 50% of acute mesenteric ischemias are secondary to superior mesenteric artery occlusion from a thrombus or embolus and are a surgical emergency. Mortality is 75% if diagnosis is delayed.
Pseudo-obstruction	Abdominal malignancy, myocardial infarction, cerebrovascular accident, renal failure, or chest infection (Ogilvie's syndrome).

Sources. Hughes (2005), "Trouble Down Under" (2005).

Diverticular Disease

Diverticula are small pockets that project through the wall of the colon and are primarily seen in the sigmoid and distal descending colon, areas in which the colon wall is weakened. According to a 1998 report by the American Gastroenterological Association, approximately 2.2 million people in the United States have diverticular disease (Kang, Melville, & Maxwell, 2004). The prevalence of this disease significantly increases with age and is rarely seen in people younger than age 40. Diverticular disease is also linked to a low-fiber diet and is a risk factor for lower GI bleeding. Aspirin and NSAIDs also increase the risk of bleeding.

Most people with diverticulosis are asymptomatic or have few symptoms. However, complications such as infection or inflammation carry the risk of peritonitis, colon perforation, fistulation, abscess, obstruction or stricture formation, or septicemia (Kang et al., 2004; "Gastrointestinal System," 2007). Diverticular disease is usually treated medically through diet modification, medication, and exercise. Foods high in fiber are encouraged; however, foods that may get trapped in the diverticulum (e.g., nuts, popcorn, seeds) are discouraged. In some cases, surgery is warranted to drain pus or address perforation, necrosis, or obstruction (i.e., colon resection).

Gastrointestinal Bleeds

Gastrointestinal bleeds (*GIBs*) are disorders that can occur anywhere along the GI tract and are classified as either upper or lower GI bleeds (UGIBs or LGIBs, respectively), depending on the source or location of the bleeding. *UGIBs* occur in the GI tract above the duodenojejunal junction, whereas *LGIBs* occur below.

Signs of GIBs may include vomiting blood or bloody stools. Black tarry stools referred to as *melena* may occur with a UGIB. Stool has this appearance after blood has contact with hydrochloric acid during the digestive process (Lehrer, 2009). Signs of LGIB may include the appearance of maroon or bright red blood in the stool.

Treatment for GIBs includes close monitoring of vital signs, replacement of fluid or blood products, nasogastric tube suctioning, medication, or surgery. Medically, the focus is to stop the acute bleeding and minimize risk of rebleeding (Friedman et al., 2003). In many cases, GIBs resolve spontaneously.

Notify medical and nursing staff if the following signs of GIB occur:

- Rapid respiration, tachycardia, or thready pulse;
- Cold, clammy skin;
- Pallor;
- Systolic blood pressure below 100 and orthostatic hypotension;
- Complaints of dizziness, nausea, thirst, restlessness, or confusion;
- Hematemesis (vomiting blood);
- Melena or hematochezia (blood in the stool, bright red or black and tarry; if noted in the toilet, do not flush, but notify medical staff); or
- Complaints of abdominal pain.

Disorders of the Accessory Organs of Digestion

Disorders in this section include the pancreas, gallbladder, bile ducts, and liver. These organs produce secretions (e.g., bile, enzymes) that assist with the digestive process.

Pancreas

The pancreas is both an endocrine and exocrine gland. Anatomically, the stomach rests on the body of the pancreas, and the spleen rests on its tail. The head of the pancreas joins the common bile duct and empties pancreatic juices into the duodenum for digestion. Of these secretions, amylase helps digest starches, trypsin helps digest protein, and lipase digests triglycerides. The Islets of Langerhans contain beta cells that produce insulin and alpha cells that produce glucagon (refer to Chapter 8 for more information).

Pancreatitis. *Pancreatitis* is an autodigestion inflammatory condition classified as acute or chronic, edematous, or necrotizing ("Gastrointestinal System," 2007; Phillips,

2006). *Acute edematous pancreatitis* causes swelling and is not as serious as *necrotizing pancreatitis,* which causes cell death and can lead to multisystem organ failure. Acute pancreatitis is idiopathic or caused by obstruction (e.g., gallstones, tumors, lesions), stenosis, infections (e.g., viruses, bacteria, parasites), toxins (e.g., alcohol abuse), or trauma from a procedure (Phillips, 2006). Other causes include viruses such as measles, mumps, rubella, Epstein-Barr, or cytomegalovirus; biliary tract disease; and endocrine or metabolic disorders.

Chronic pancreatitis results in progressive episodes of inflammation that lead to permanent structural changes in the pancreas. It is generally attributed to heavy alcohol consumption over a long period of time. With damage to the pancreas, ability to digest and absorb nutrients is affected, and malnutrition can occur. Diabetes may be caused by damage to Islets of Langerhans cells. Pancreatitis may also lead to portal and splenic vein thrombosis, pseudocysts, biliary obstruction, and respiratory failure ("Gastrointestinal System," 2007).

Symptoms of pancreatitis include nausea, vomiting, abdominal pain, malaise, and low-grade fever. Other symptoms include mild jaundice, tachycardia, tachypnea, hypotension, and abdominal distension (Phillips, 2006). Medical treatment includes replacement of fluids and electrolytes, nutritional support, pain management, and in some cases surgical debridement of the necrotized and infected tissue. Patients are often NPO to rest the pancreas and prevent release of pancreatic enzymes into the digestive system. Nasogastric suctioning may be used to prevent vomiting. Therapists should note that sitting up and leaning forward are positions that are more comfortable for patients; walking and lying supine exacerbate pain and discomfort.

Pancreatic Cancer. *Pancreatic cancer* is the fourth leading cause of cancer-related death and has a 5-year survival rate of 1%–4% (Muir, 2004). Most pancreatic cancers are adenocarcinomas arising from exocrine cells. Of the cancers, 70% are located in the head of the pancreas, 10% in the body, and 15% in the tail (Goodman & Peterson, 2009). Risk factors

include obesity, tobacco, high-fat diets, and chronic pancreatitis. Red meat, processed meats, and adult-onset diabetes mellitus are also linked to increased risk for pancreatic cancer (Goodman & Peterson, 2009).

Pancreatic cancer can metastasize to the lungs, liver, or adrenal glands. Surgical resection with a pancreaticoduodenectomy (Whipple procedure) is the only cure. However, surgical resection is only appropriate for a very small percentage of patients (15%–20%; Conroy et al., 2007; Goodman & Peterson, 2009). Radiation and chemotherapy are also treatment approaches; however, palliative care is the predominant approach for symptom relief and improved quality of life (Conroy et al., 2007). Mortality is approximately 100% with locally advanced and metastatic pancreatic cancer (Goodman & Peterson, 2009) and is usually terminal within 1 year of diagnosis ("Gastrointestinal Disorders," 2006). Patients with pancreatic cancer often deal with anorexia, depression, fatigue, and pain, which are common symptoms of an inoperable disease process (Conroy et al., 2007).

Gallbladder

There are two main disorders related to the gallbladder, cholelithiasis and cholecystitis. Although bile is produced in the liver, it is stored until needed in the gallbladder. Bile is released into the duodenum in response to food entering the intestines, where it helps digest and absorb dietary fats and vitamins from the intestines. However, bile that has a high concentration of cholesterol or has a deficit in bile salts may result in the formation of gallstones (Gould, 2006). *Cholelithiasis* (formation of gallstones) is one of the most common disorders of the GI tract.

Stones form in the gallbladder, but symptoms do not occur until these stones block bile ducts. Risk factors for cholelithiasis include age (incidence increases with age), genetics (e.g., sickle cell anemia), obesity, diabetes mellitus, rheumatoid arthritis, liver disease, rapid weight loss (i.e., after gastric bypass surgery), pregnancy, TPN, or certain drugs such as oral contraceptives (Goodman & Peterson, 2009).

Cholecystitis is a condition in which gallstones block the cystic duct, causing inflammation and distension of the gallbladder. Complications of cholecystitis may include perforation, gangrene, empyema, cholangitis, hepatitis, pancreatitis, or gallstone ileus ("Gastrointestinal System," 2007). Treatment approaches include a laparoscopic cholecystectomy, percutaneous transhepatic cholecystostomy, or lithotripsy (i.e., ultrasound used to break up stones). More than 500,000 people undergo a cholecystectomy (removal of the gallbladder) every year secondary to gallbladder disease and associated pain. With a cholecystectomy, bile drains from the liver directly into the intestines, eliminating future stone formation. After a laparoscopic cholecystecomy, activity or exercise are usually not restricted because this procedure is minimally invasive (Goodman & Peterson, 2009).

Biliary Ducts

Disorders of the biliary ducts can be due to inflammation, infection, cancer, scarring, or obstruction. The two conditions reviewed in this section are cholangitis and primary sclerosing cholangitis.

Cholangitis. *Cholangitis* is an inflammation of the bile duct. Infection can occur when the common bile duct is obstructed (e.g., stones, pancreatic cancer). Symptoms consist of Charcot's triad of fever, jaundice, and right upper-quadrant pain, which is noted in 50%–100% of patients with cholangitis (Goodman & Peterson, 2009). Acute cholangitis requires biliary drainage and can be a life-threatening condition (Muir, 2004). Biliary peritonitis occurs when a perforation occurs in the duodenum or gallbladder, resulting in bile leaking into the abdominal cavity.

Treatment for cholangitis depends on the grade of the disease. Grade I, or mild, disease is treated with antibiotics and laparoscopic cholecystectomy. Treatment for Grade II disease consists of antibiotics, biliary drainage, and then open or laparoscopic cholecystectomy. Grade III disease requires intensive care support and urgent endoscopic or percutaneous transhepatic biliary drainage (Goodman & Peterson, 2009).

Primary Sclerosing Cholangitis. *Primary sclerosing cholangitis* is a progressive disease that affects the intra- and extrahepatic biliary ducts. The etiology is unknown but may be linked to toxins or an immune system reaction. In primary sclerosing cholangitis, chronic inflammation and scarring of the bile ducts leads to the development of liver disease and liver failure. Of patients with sclerosing cholangitis, 80% also have an IBD, especially UC, but only 5% of patients with UC have sclerosing cholangitis (Goodman & Peterson, 2009). In the early stages of the disease, patients are usually asymptomatic. With disease progression, pruritus (itching), fatigue, fever, abdominal pain, chills, diarrhea, anorexia, and jaundice may develop. Treatment for sclerosing cholangitis focuses on symptom management; transplantation is the only cure.

Liver

The liver, the largest internal organ, plays a crucial role in maintaining health. Venous return from the stomach, intestines, pancreas, and spleen all pass through the liver. In addition, many important bodily functions are carried out in the liver, including storage of vitamins, fats, sugar, and iron. The liver also produces albumin (a water-soluble protein produced in the liver that helps maintain normal blood volume and blood pressure), converts and excretes bilirubin, and metabolizes nutrients and hormones. The liver also filters toxins (e.g., drugs, alcohol, tobacco) from the body and produces clotting factors. "The liver is a 'workhorse' for metabolic activity" (Klein & Rubin, 2002, p. 303). Therefore, hepatic dysfunction can have a profound effect on other organ systems and overall health and well-being.

Liver injury is most commonly attributed to diseases such as hepatitis and cirrhosis; however, drugs, chemicals and solvents, or certain herbal remedies can also lead to hepatotoxicity. Common drugs include acetaminophen, aspirin, and oral contraceptives. Herbal supplements such as chaparral, comfrey, germander, Jin Bu Huan, mistletoe, nutmeg, ragwort, sassafras, senna, and tansy may cause liver toxicity in people with underlying liver disease (Goodman & Peterson, 2009). Liver transplantation may be the only recourse for long-term survival of patients with liver failure and end-stage liver disease. Living donor liver transplantation is possible because the liver can regenerate itself (refer to Chapter 14 for more information).

Symptoms of Liver Dysfunction. Signs and symptoms of liver disease are similar to those of other GI disorders, including nausea, vomiting, abdominal pain, fatigue, loss of appetite or anorexia, weight loss, and bleeding. However, patients with liver disorder may also have the additional symptoms of pruritus (intense itching), peripheral edema, varices, splenomegaly, or petichia (refer to Table 9.5 for a list of liver disease manifestations).

The most common symptoms of liver disease include

- *Jaundice:* Bile pigment is formed as an end product of heme breakdown. When the liver cannot metabolize or excrete unconjugated bilirubin, it accumulates in the blood, which manifests as yellowing of the eyes (sclera), nails, and skin, known as

Table 9.5.   Characteristics of Hepatic Dysfunction

Signs and Symptoms	Pathophysiology
Fatigue, weight loss	• Hepatic metabolic dysfunction • Portal hypertension
Ascites and peripheral edema	• Portal hypertension • Elevated aldosterone and antidiuretic hormone • Decreased albumin • Lymphatic obstruction
Esophageal varices	• Portal hypertension and collateral circulation
Splenomegaly	• Portal hypertension
Anemia	• Splenomegaly • Decreased absorption and storage of iron and Vitamin B12 • Malabsorption • Bleeding
Pruritus	• Biliary obstruction causing deposition of bile salts in tissue
Jaundice	• Bilirubin that is not excreted into bile • Biliary obstruction, stricture • Decreased production of bile
Hepatic encephalopathy	• Metabolic dysfunction resulting in ammonia buildup
Increased bleeding, purpura	• Decreased absorption of Vitamin K • Decreased production of clotting factors • Thrombocytopenia
Leukopenia, thrombocytopenia	• Splenomegaly

Source. From Gould, B. E. (2006). Digestive System Disorders. In *Pathophysiology for the Health Professions* (3rd ed., p. 464). St. Louis, MO: W. B. Saunders. Copyright © 2006 by W. B. Saunders. Adapted with permission.

Table 9.6. Serum Bilirubin Levels

Value	Associated Manifestation
0.1–1.0 mg/dl	Normal
2–3 mg/dl	Eyes appear yellow.
5–6 mg/dl	Skin appears yellow, urine is darker, and stools are lighter.

Source. Goodman & Peterson (2009).

jaundice. Urine has a dark tea color, and stool has a light color (bile is what gives stool its brown appearance). Bile deposits in the skin may also cause pruritus, and if bile cannot reach the gallbladder for storage (as in cirrhosis), it may result in gallstones. Elevated bilirubin levels may also result in nausea and anorexia. Serum bilirubin levels and associated changes are listed in Table 9.6. Strenuous exercise should be avoided by people with jaundice because rest promotes healing (Goodman & Peterson, 2009). Treatment focuses on addressing the underlying cause of the jaundice.

- *Bruising:* Bruising occurs because proteins necessary for blood clotting are no longer produced by the liver, resulting in coagulopathy. Patients may have prolonged bleeding times with increased prothrombin time (PT) and partial thromboplastin time values (PPT), which necessitates caution by therapists when handling patients, including engagement in resistive exercises or even use of gait belts (Goodman & Peterson, 2009). Therapists should monitor patient safety and educate patients on fall prevention.

- *Hepatic encephalopathy:* Hepatic encephalopathy can manifest as changes in mental status, decreased safety awareness, and sleep disturbances. Hepatic encephalopathy has been associated with an accumulation of ammonia in the bloodstream. Ammonia is normally excreted in the urine after it is metabolized in the liver. However, when this process is compromised, ammonia travels to the brain, causing mental status changes. Refer to Table 9.7 for stages of hepatic encephalopathy and associated changes. Treatment for hepatic encephalopathy focuses on addressing the underlying cause.

- *Ascites:* Fluid builds up in the peritoneal cavity surrounding the intestines, leading to increased abdominal girth. When the liver no longer produces albumin, fluid builds up in the peritoneal cavity, resulting in ascites, anasarca (generalized edema), or lower-extremity edema. Ascites may also displace patients' center of gravity, resulting in decreased balance, or press on the diaphragm, resulting in complaints of dyspnea on exertion. Cirrhosis is present in 85% of patients with ascites (Heidelbaugh & Sherbondy, 2006).

Additionally, patients with liver dysfunction may have impaired glucose production or decreased Vitamin D absorption. Low blood sugar may result in decreased energy, and impaired Vitamin D absorption may result in osteoporosis with increased risk of pathologic or compression fractures (Lee & Moinzadeh, 2009). Treatment for liver disease includes dietary modification, nutritional support, symptom relief, minimizing liver metabolic demands, surgical intervention, or all of these.

Cirrhosis. Cirrhosis is responsible for more than 25,000 deaths annually and is the 12th leading cause of death in the United States (Fichandler & Malone, 2006; Goodman & Peterson, 2009; Gould, 2006). With cirrhosis, fibrous scar tissue and regenerating nodules replace normal liver tissue, resulting in restricted portal circulation and disruption of normal liver function.

Cirrhosis has many causes. It is most commonly associated with chronic alcohol abuse, as in alcoholic liver disease (ALD) and chronic hepatitis. Other causes of cirrhosis include autoimmune diseases (e.g., sarcoidosis), sclerosing cholangitis, right-sided heart failure,

Table 9.7.   Stages of Hepatic Encephalopathy

Stage I (Prodromal)	Stage II (Impending)	Stage III (Arousal)	Stage IV (Comatose)
Slight personality changes Slight tremor Bilateral numbness/ tingling Muscular incoordination Apraxia	Tremor progresses to asterixis Resistance to passive movement Myoclonus Lethargy Unusual behavior (abusive, violent, noisy) Apraxia Sleep disorders Slow or slurred speech	Hyperventilation Marked confusion Inchoherent speech Asterixis (liver flap) Muscle rigidity Hyporeactive deep tendon reflexes Sleeping most of the time	No asterixis Positive Babinski's reflex Oclocephalic (doll's eye) reflex Decerebrate posturing Dilated pupils Lack of response to stimuli

Source. From Goodman, C. C., & Peterson, C. (2009). The Hepatic, Pancreatic, and Biliary Systems. In C. C. Goodman & K. S. Fuller (Eds.), *Pathology: Implications for the Physical Therapist* (3rd ed., p. 889). St. Louis, MO: W. B. Saunders. Copyright © 2009 by W. B. Saunders. Reprinted with permission.

alpha-1 antitrypsin deficiency, blocked bile ducts, Wilson's disease, or hemochromatosis ("Gastrointestinal Disorders," 2006). *Wilson's disease* and *hemochromatosis* are genetic disorders that result in an accumulation of metals in the liver (e.g., copper, iron) that damage the liver.

ALD is considered a lifestyle disease, with hospital costs estimated at $600 million to $1.8 billion annually (Tsukamoto, 2007). Lifestyle factors related to ALD include alcohol consumption, smoking, drugs, obesity, high-fat diets, and malnutrition. Comorbid risk factors include viral hepatitis, diabetes, iron disorders, sleep apnea, and genetics (Tsukamoto, 2007). ALD is also a risk factor for hepatocellular carcinoma. Alcohol is responsible for approximately 40% of deaths from cirrhosis, and alcohol-related liver disease accounts for 30% of hepatocellular carcinoma cases (Goodman & Peterson, 2009).

Men can develop ALD by consuming 6–8 alcoholic beverages a day for more than 5 years; however, women may need to consume only 3–4 drinks a day over the same period of time to develop ALD (Goodman & Peterson, 2009). Heavy alcohol consumption also leads to fatty liver disease, alcoholic hepatitis, or an enlarged liver or spleen.

As liver function fails, symptoms of cirrhosis may include fatigue, weight loss, weakness, pruritus, jaundice, coagulopathy, loss of ability to metabolize drugs, and hypoalbuminemia (Goodman & Peterson, 2009). Common complications of cirrhosis include ascites and lower-extremity edema, spontaneous bacterial peritonitis, bleeding varices, portal hypertension, hepatorenal syndrome, and hepatic encephalopathy (Heidelbaugh & Sherbondy, 2006).

Spontaneous bacterial peritonitis, a serious complication of cirrhosis, is an infection of ascitic fluid and generally has a poor prognosis, with a mortality rate of 40%–79% (Bandy, 2009). Symptoms of peritonitis may include fever, pain, nausea, vomiting, bloating, tachycardia, hypotension, and diminished bowel sounds. Another complication of cirrhosis is hepatic encephalopathy. Mental status changes may manifest as changes in reaction time, difficulty concentrating, or personality changes (e.g., confusion, forgetfulness). Although hepatic encephalopathy is considered reversible, it can lead to coma and death.

Portal hypertension, another complication of cirrhosis, occurs because of changes in resistance to portal flow with increased pressure in the portal vein. Variceal bleeding, ascites, and encephalopathy predominantly result from portal hypertension (Blei, 2007). Additional symptoms of cirrhosis include bruising easily, acute renal failure, and hepatopulmonary syndrome.

Treatment in the early stages of cirrhosis focuses on treating the underlying cause, reducing complications, and preventing disease progression, which usually entails use of diuretics, restriction of sodium, and total alcohol abstinence (Heidelbaugh & Sherbondy, 2006). Additional therapies include transjugular intrahepatic portosystemic shunt (TIPS), banding, and sclerotherapy.

Cirrhosis is irreversible in advanced stages; if the patient does not respond to conventional treatment, then liver transplantation is indicated. A MELD score (model for end-stage disease) is used in predicting survival of patients with end-stage liver disease and is one criterion for placement on a transplantation list. Refer to Chapter 14 for more information on liver transplantation.

Portal Hypertension and Variceal Bleeding.
Vasoconstriction from cirrhotic changes contributes to increased resistance to blood flow. Consequently, portal vein pressure increases, resulting in esophageal varices, ascites, and portal hypertension. Most of the blood supply to the liver is from the venous system, not the arteries. Collateral veins to the esophagus become dilated because of a back flow of blood from the liver. These dilated blood vessels now have a high pressure with the risk of rupture. Variceal rebleeding is associated with a high mortality rate and is defined as the occurrence of new hematemesis or melena at least 1 day after an acute episode (Ferguson & Hayes,

2006). The aim of medical management for portal hypertension and variceal bleeding is prevention of rebleeding. The several treatment approaches include sclerotherapy, variceal band ligation, surgery, and medication (Blei, 2007; Ferguson & Hayes, 2006). Nonselective beta blockers are also sometimes used to treat portal hypertension (Blei, 2007; Goodman & Peterson, 2009).

Another treatment approach is TIPS (see Figure 9.4). This nonsurgical radiological intervention reduces pressure in the liver by diverting blood around it. This procedure addresses variceal bleeding, prevents rebleeding, and is used when refractory ascites is present (Bureau, 2006). In a TIPS procedure, a catheter is inserted into the jugular vein and threaded into the veins of the liver. A connection or pathway is made between the portal vein and a hepatic vein. This new shunt or channel is kept open with a stent. The greatest risk of rebleeding is 48–72 hours after the procedure, with more than half occurring within the first 10 days (Heidelbaugh & Sherbondy, 2006). TIPS increases the risk of hepatic encephalopathy and stent dysfunction. With TIPS, ammonia metabolization is now bypassed in the liver and instead travels to the brain, contributing to encephalopathy. Stents can also occlude, but the incidence has decreased with the use of covered stents.

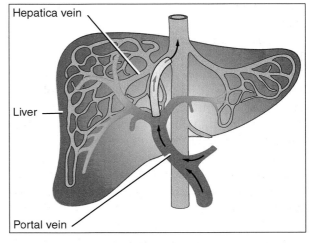

Figure 9.4. Transjugular intrahepatic portocaval shunt.
Source. Richard Fritzler, Medical Illustrator, Roswell, GA.

Hepatitis

Hepatitis is an acute or chronic inflammatory condition caused by viruses, toxins, drugs, or alcohol abuse. Although hepatitis has seven different types, in the United States the most common forms are hepatitis B (43%), hepatitis A (32%), and hepatitis C (21%; Holcomb, 2002). Approximately 500,000 Americans are infected with some type of hepatitis each year, with 15,000 dying from complications (Goodman & Peterson, 2009). Vaccinations are available for hepatitis A and B but not for hepatitis C.

Symptoms for all forms of hepatitis are similar and include fever, fatigue, jaundice, right upper-quadrant pain, weight loss, nausea, and diarrhea. The goal of treatment for hepatitis B and C is viral clearance with interferon and prevention of cirrhosis and hepatocellular carcinoma (Cainelli, 2008). As with any liver disease, rest is important in minimizing energy demands on the liver.

Approximately 125,000–200,000 new cases of *hepatitis A* occur each year, with 99% of patients fully recovering (Holcomb, 2002). Hepatitis A is spread though the fecal–oral route. Most at risk are people who work in institutions such as hospitals and prisons, IV drug users, people with chronic hepatitis B and C, and people who live in areas with poor sanitation and contaminated food and water. Hepatitis A can also "occur through shared use of oral utensils such as straws, silverware, and toothbrushes" (Goodman & Peterson, 2009, p. 893). Hepatitis A has no treatment, and it usually resolves on its own with a few weeks of bedrest.

Hepatitis B is spread through blood and body fluids and can be transmitted through sexual activity or IV drug use and perinatally. Hepatitis B is 10 times more contagious than hepatitis C and 100 times more contagious than HIV (Goodman & Peterson, 2009). If treated early, 90%–95% of patients recover.

Approximately 170 million people worldwide are infected with *hepatitis C,* including 3.2 million Americans (Rustgi, 2007). Most patients with hepatitis C develop chronic hepatitis and cirrhosis, although this process may take 20–30 years (Holcomb, 2002; Rustgi, 2007). Hepatitis C is spread through IV drug use, blood transfusions before 1992 (when blood bank screening began), and receiving clotting factors before 1987. Hepatitis C infection is also associated with body piercing, tattoos, acupuncture, having multiple sex partners, and health care workers exposed to infected needle sticks. Patients undergoing hemodialysis are also at increased risk because they have a vascular access that may come in contact with equipment, devices, supplies, or surfaces that are contaminated (Goodman & Peterson, 2009; Rustgi, 2007). Hepatitis C is also commonly found in older adults, especially those older than age 80 (Cainelli, 2008).

Hepatitis C also has a greater incidence in the population than HIV (Rustgi, 2007). However, if a patient is infected with both hepatitis C and AIDS, cirrhosis may develop more quickly and twice as often (Goodman & Peterson, 2009). More so than alcohol abuse, hepatitis C is the leading cause of liver cirrhosis. Hepatitis C can also progress to end-stage liver disease and hepatocellular carcinoma, requiring transplantation as the best treatment option.

Nonalcoholic steatohepatitis (NASH) is a type of hepatitis in which inflammation and fat buildup in the liver causes tissue scarring, leading to hepatocellular injury (Yan, Durazo, Tong, & Hong, 2007). NASH is similar to ALD but is unrelated to alcohol consumption. NASH is associated with diabetes, obesity, and high cholesterol and is linked to insulin resistance. NASH is generally asymptomatic unless cirrhosis develops. NASH has no specific treatment. Patients are encouraged to make lifestyle modifications such as losing weight if they are obese and controlling diabetes if they are diabetic. NASH may replace hepatitis C as the main diagnosis requiring liver transplantation (Yan et al., 2007).

Nonalcoholic Fatty Liver Disease.

Nonalcoholic fatty liver disease (NFLD) is another liver disorder unrelated to significant amounts of alcohol consumption. NFLD occurs with fat buildup in the liver cells that exceeds 5% of the weight of the liver (Angulo, 2007). NFLD is primarily associated with metabolic syndrome, obesity, and diabetes mellitus (Angulo, 2007; Fitzgerald, 2007; Sublett, 2007). NFLD is present in approximately 20% of the general population; however, the risk increases with the presence of risk factors such as obesity and diabetes mellitus, which are on the rise in the United States (Angulo, 2007; Fitzgerald, 2007; Yan et al., 2007).

Approximately 75% of patients with Type 2 diabetes have some degree of NFLD present (Sublett, 2007). NFLD may also be secondary to bariatric surgery, rapid weight loss in people who are obese, and hepatotoxic medications (Sublett, 2007). As many as 75% of NFLD patients have hepatomegaly (Yan et al., 2007). Symptoms of NFLD include fatigue, malaise, and right upper-quadrant discomfort.

NFLD can progress to *steatosis* (accumulation of fat in liver cells), NASH, cirrhosis, or hepatocellular carcinoma (Yan et al., 2007). Without inflammation, NFLD is a relatively benign disorder. Treatment for NFLD focuses on addressing lifestyle modifications for underlying causes (e.g., obesity, diabetes), or transplantation may be indicated. Rapid weight loss is not recommended because it can exacerbate NFLD (Fitzgerald, 2007).

Primary Biliary Cirrhosis. *Primary biliary cirrhosis* is an autoimmune-based progressive disease involving the small bile ducts of the liver. This disease is irreversible and leads to liver failure. Patients may initially be asymptomatic but can develop pruritus, osteoporosis, portal hypertension, steatorrhea, and extreme fatigue. Primary biliary cirrhosis is treated with medication (e.g., ursodeoxycholic acid); however, transplantation may be indicated with advanced disease.

Occupational Therapy Approach

Occupational therapists can play an important role in the care of patients with GI disorders because of their holistic approach to patient care. Occupational therapists have an appreciation of how occupational selection and performance affects the mind, body, and spirit. Food and digestive system function play a key role in people's sense of well-being on both an emotional and a physical level. Symptoms of GI disorder are the most commonly and pervasively experienced over all body systems.

With GI dysfunction or disruption, patients' body structures and function may no longer be healthy and normal, resulting in diminished areas of performance skills, performance patterns, and even future roles. For example, a person's sense of self-worth and engagement in work or leisure activities can be negatively influenced by leakage or the daily care associated with an ileostomy. Eating takes on a new meaning if the patient is limited to certain food types or consistencies or is restricted from eating and receives nutrition through TPN. Moreover, even basic mobility for the GI patient in an acute care setting may be difficult and precarious because of IV poles, drainage bulbs, or a rectal tube.

Occupational therapists are often consulted to address the sequelae of GI disorders such as deconditioning, poor activity tolerance, and limitations in performance of basic activities of daily living. Patients may be weak from disease, poor nutritional status, or a surgical procedure. In addition, patients often have difficulty performing self-care skills because of incisional pain or discomfort, ascites, extremity edema, or the presence of multiple lines and drainage bulbs. Patients may also have nasogastric feeding or suctioning tubes, which make even the simple tasks of brushing teeth or washing the face more challenging.

The following guidelines and precautions may assist therapists working with the GI patient:

- Patients may have difficulty performing lower-body activities of daily living (ADLs) because of *anasarca* (generalized edema), lower-extremity edema, ascites, or discomfort from abdominal incisions.

- Patients with ascites may have an altered center of gravity that can affect their balance during mobility and transfers.

- After abdominal surgery, resistive exercise or lifting are often restricted; verify parameters with medical staff.

- After abdominal surgery, early mobilization may minimize the risk of paralytic ileus and pulmonary complications.

- Be careful working around feeding tubes, especially nasogastric tubes during light hygiene and grooming activities.
- Observe whether patients are NPO or have swallowing precautions or whether ice chips are permissible.
- Be aware of whether patients are on strict fluid intake and output monitoring. Input and output may be important, depending on the patient's condition (i.e., volume overload) or whether patients are being monitored for response to certain medications (i.e., diuretics). Check first before giving patients fluids or discarding urine.
- Make sure the head of the bed is elevated (preferably to 90°) during mealtimes to minimize risk of aspiration. Encourage eating meals sitting up in a chair when possible.
- To minimize the risk of aspiration, set feeding pumps on hold or detach the nasogastric tube from the pump if patients need to lay flat for repositioning in bed. Keep the head of the bed at greater than 30°. Always consult with medical staff first because patients may require a particular schedule of nutritional intake or the line may need to be flushed.
- Monitor for location of incisions, bulbs, drains, and ostomy bags or other external appliances when handling patients or applying a gait belt.
- Patients with liver disease may bruise easily or bleed spontaneously, so be careful with handling techniques. Check PT, PPT, and international normalized ratio levels before working with patients.
- Avoid Valsalva effects (buildup of intrathoracic or intra-abdominal pressure) with patients who have portal hypertension or varices.
- Patients with active liver disease often experience extreme fatigue and weakness and should not be overexerted. Modify activities to decrease metabolic demands on the liver. Balance activity with rest and reinforce energy conservation strategies.

- Therapists should use caution when handling patients with liver disease, including engagement in resistive exercises or even use of gait belts (Goodman & Peterson, 2009). Therapists should monitor patient safety and educate patients on fall prevention.
- Patients with GERD should avoid positions that increase intra-abdominal pressure, including coughing, bending, wearing tight clothing, or engaging in vigorous exercise ("Gastrointestinal System," 2007).
- Patients with GERD should sit up and not recline during and after meals to minimize reflux.
- When working with patients with pancreatitis, therapists should note that sitting up and leaning forward are more comfortable for patients; walking and lying supine exacerbate pain and discomfort.
- If working with patients with hepatitis, therapists should be vaccinated and observe standard precautions. Refer to Chapter 12 for information on personal protection and standard precautions.

In general, occupational therapy intervention for GI disorders focuses on improving endurance through engagement in ADLs, exercise, education in energy conservation strategies, and stress management. Therapists can also analyze and modify activity demands through

- Positioning, by propping the lower extremities on a stool for lower-body dressing;
- Adaptive equipment, such as using a long-handled reacher or sock aid for lower-body dressing; and
- Durable medical equipment recommendations, such as the use of a raised toilet seat or bath chair.

GI function is an important aspect of people's daily lives and sense of well-being. By addressing symptoms of GI disease and disorder, occupational therapy can be instrumental in maximizing independence in performance of desired occupations and improving quality of life.

References

Angulo, P. (2007). Obesity and nonalcoholic fatty liver disease. *Nutrition Reviews, 65*(Suppl. 1), S57–S63.

Bandy, S. M., (2009, December 2). Spontaneous bacterial peritonitis. *eMedicine.* Retrieved August 20, 2010, from http://emedicine.medscape.com/article/789105-overview

Berndtsson, I., Lindholm, E., & Ekman, I. (2005). Thirty years of experience living with a continent ileostomy: Bad restrooms—not my reservoir—decide my life. *Journal of Wound, Ostomy, and Continence Nursing, 32,* 321–326.

Blei, A. T. (2007). Portal hypertension and its complications. *Current Opinion in Gastroenterology, 23,* 275–282.

Broadbent, A. M., Heaney, A., & Weyman, K. (2006). A review of short bowel syndrome and palliation: A case report and medication guideline. *Journal of Palliative Medicine, 9,* 1481–1491.

Buchman, A. L. (2006). Etiology and initial management of short bowel syndrome. *Gastroenterology, 130*(2, Suppl. 1), S3–S4.

Bureau, C. (2006). Covered stents for TIPS: Are all problems solved? *European Journal of Gastroenterology and Hepatology, 18,* 581–583.

Cainelli, F. (2008). Hepatitis C virus infection in the elderly: Epidemiology, natural history and management. *Drugs and Aging, 25*(1), 9–18.

Conroy, T., Uwer, L., & Deblock, M. (2007). Health-related quality-of-life assessment in gastrointestinal cancer: Are results relevant for clinical practice? *Current Opinion in Oncology, 19,* 401–406.

Doughty, D. (2008). History of ostomy surgery. *Journal of Wound, Ostomy, and Continence Nursing, 35*(1), 34–38.

Feldman, M., Friedman, L. S., & Sleisenger, M. H. (2002). *Sleisenger and Fordtran's gastrointestinal and liver disease: Pathophysiology/diagnosis/management* (7th ed., Vol. 1). Philadelphia: W. B. Saunders.

Ferguson, J. W., & Hayes, P. C. (2006). Transjugular intrahepatic portosystemic shunt in the prevention of rebleeding in oesophageal varices. *European Journal of Gastroenterology and Hepatology, 18*(1), 1167–1171.

Fichandler, D., & Malone, D. J. (2006). Gastrointestinal diseases and disorders. In D. J. Malone &

K. L. B. Lindsay (Eds.), *Physical therapy in acute care: A clinician's guide* (pp. 425–476). Thorofare, NJ: Slack.

Fitzgerald, M. (2007). Nonalcoholic fatty liver disease. *Nurse Practitioner, 32*(2), 24–25.

Forister, J. G., Taliferro, M., Ramos, B., & Blessing, J. D. (2002). Diagnosing and managing gastroesophageal disease. *Physician Assistant, 26*(12), 17–23.

Friedman, S., McQuaid, K., & Grendell, J. (2003). *Current diagnosis and treatment in gastroenterology* (2nd ed.). New York: Lange Medical Books.

Gastrointestinal disorders. (2006). In J. Munden (Ed.), *Atlas of pathophysiology* (2nd ed., pp. 160–211). Philadelphia: Lippincott Williams & Wilkins.

Gastrointestinal system. (2007). In J. Munden (Ed.), *Professional guide to pathophysiology* (2nd ed., pp. 353–405). Philadelphia: Lippincott Williams & Wilkins.

Geraghty, P., & Desser, T. S. (2006). MDCT of the small bowel. *Applied Radiology, 35*(9), 11–23.

Goodman, C. C. (2009). The gastrointestinal system. In C. C. Goodman & K. S. Fuller (Eds.), *Pathology: Implications for the physical therapist* (3rd ed., pp. 828–880). St. Louis, MO: W. B. Saunders.

Goodman, C. C., & Peterson, C. (2009). The hepatic, pancreatic, and biliary systems. In C. C. Goodman & K. S. Fuller (Eds.), *Pathology: Implications for the physical therapist* (3rd ed., pp. 881–926). St. Louis, MO: W. B. Saunders.

Gould, B. E. (2006). Digestive system disorders. In *Pathophysiology for the health professions* (3rd ed., pp. 422–491). St. Louis, MO: W. B. Saunders.

Grundy, D., & Schemann, M. (2007). Enteric nervous system. *Current Opinion in Gastroenterology, 23,* 121–126.

Hanahan, A. (2007). Feel the burn: Gastroesophageal reflux disease. *Maryland Nurse, 8*(4), 22.

Heidelbaugh, J. J., & Sherbondy, M. (2006). Cirrhosis and chronic liver failure: Part II. Complications and treatment. *American Family Physician, 74,* 767–776.

Holcomb, S. S. (2002). Hepatitis, Part 1: Which types are trouble? *Nursing, 12*(6), 32cc31–32cc34.

Hughes, E. (2005). Caring for the patient with an intestinal obstruction. *Nursing Standard, 19*(47), 56–64.

Juhn, G., Eltz, D. R., & Stacy, K. A. (2008). *Intestinal obstruction.* Retrieved December 21, 2008, from www.nlm.nih.gov/medlineplus/ency/article/000260.htm

Kang, J.-Y., Melville, D., & Maxwell, J. D. (2004). Epidemiology and management of diverticular disease of the colon. *Drugs and Aging, 21,* 211–228.

Klein, S., & Rubin, D. C. (2002). Enteral and parenteral nutrition. In M. Feldman, L. S. Friedman, & M. H. Sleisenger (Eds.), *Gastrointestinal and liver disease: Pathophysiology/diagnosis/management* (7th ed., Vol. 1, pp. 287–309). Philadelphia: W. B. Saunders.

Lee, J., & Moinzadeh, L. (2009). Organ transplantation. In J. C. Paz & M. P. West (Eds.), *Acute care handbook for physical therapists* (3d ed., p. 409). St. Louis, MO: W. B. Saunders.

Lehrer, J. K. (2009). *Bloody or tarry stools.* Retrieved May 18, 2008, from www.nlm.nih.gov/medlineplus/ency/article/003130.htm

Muir, C. A. (2004). Acute ascending cholangitis. *Clinical Journal of Oncology Nursing, 8,* 157–160.

Nauth, J., Chang, C., Mobarhan, S., Sparks, S., Borton, M., & Svoboda, S. (2004). A therapeutic approach to wean total parenteral nutrition in the management of short bowel syndrome: Three cases using nocturnal enteral rehydration. *Nutrition Reviews, 62,* 221–231.

Nelson, R., Edwards, S., & Tse, B. (2007). Prophylactic nasogastric decompression after abdominal surgery. *Cochrane Database of Systematic Reviews, 2007,* CD004929.

Pardi, D. S., Loftus, E. V., Jr., & Camilleri, M. (2002). Therapy in practice: Treatment of inflammatory bowel disease in the elderly. *Drugs and Aging, 19,* 355–363.

Paz, J. C., & Nicoloro, D. (2009). Gastrointestinal system. In J. C. Paz & M. P. West (Eds.), *Acute care handbook for physical therapists* (3rd ed., pp. 297–325). St. Louis, MO: W. B. Saunders.

Phillips, R. A. (2006). Acute pancreatitis: Inflammation gone wild. *Nursing Made Incredibly Easy, 6,* 18–28.

Pitts, S. R., Niska, R. W., Xu, J., & Burt, C. W. (2008, August 6). National Hospital Ambulatory Medical Care Survey: 2006 emergency department summary. *National Health Statistics Reports, 7.* Retrieved December 11, 2008, from www.cdc.gov/nchs/data/nhsr/nhsr007.pdf

Porter, R. F., & Gyawali, C. P. (2010). *Nausea and vomiting.* Retrieved August 20, 2010, from http://www.acg.gi.org/patients/gihealth/nausea.asp

Rayhorn, N., Argel, N., & Demchak, K. (2003). Understanding gastroesophageal reflux disease. *Nursing, 33*(10), 36–42.

Rayhorn, N., & Rayhorn, D. J. (2002a). An in-depth look at inflammatory bowel disease. *Nursing, 32*(7), 37–43.

Rayhorn, N., & Rayhorn, D. J. (2002b). Inflammatory bowel disease: Symptoms in the bowel and beyond. *Nurse Practitioner, 27*(11), 13–27.

Richter, J. E. (2008). Approach to the patient with gastroesophageal reflux disease. In T. Yamada (Ed.), *Principles of clinical gastroenterology* (pp. 83–98). Oxford, England: Wiley.

Rosenthal, M. S. (1998). *The gastro-intestinal sourcebook.* Los Angeles: Lowell House.

Rustgi, V. K. (2007). The epidemiology of hepatitis C infection in the United States. *Journal of Gastroenterology, 42,* 513–521.

Stein, P. (2004). Home study program: Ulcerative colitis—Diagnosis and surgical treatment. *AORN Journal, 80,* 242–262.

Sublett, L. (2007). Deconstructing nonalcoholic fatty liver disease. *Nurse Practitioner, 32*(8), 12–17.

Todd, S., Corsnitz, D., Ray, S., & Nassar, J. (2002). Outpatient laparoscopic nissen fundoplication. *AORN Journal, 75,* 955–956, 959, 961, 963–964, 967–968, 970–971, 973–974, 976–983, 985–986.

Trouble down under: Understanding small bowel obstruction. (2005). *Nursing, 35*(7), 32–36.

Tsukamoto, H. (2007). Conceptual importance of identifying alcoholic liver disease as a lifestyle disease. *Journal of Gastroenterology, 42,* 603–609.

Vakil, R., Kaira, S., Raul, S., Paljor, Y., & Joseph, S. (2007). Role of water-soluble contrast study in adhesive small bowel obstruction: A randomized controlled study. *Indian Journal of Surgery, 69*(2), 47–51.

Veronesi, J. (2003). Inflammatory bowel disease. *RN, 66*(6), 38–45.

Waldman, A. R. (2001). Bowel obstruction. *Clinical Journal of Oncology Nursing, 5,* 281–282.

What is esophagectomy? (2006). Retrieved May 11, 2008, from www.barrettsinfo.com/content/8a _what_is_esophagectomy.htm

Yan, E., Durazo, F., Tong, M., & Hong, K. (2007). Nonalcoholic fatty liver disease: Pathogenesis, identification, progression, and management. *Nutrition Reviews, 65,* 376–382.

Appendix 9.A.

Signs and Symptoms of Nutritional Deficiency

Organ System	Systems or Sign	Possible Nutrient Deficiency
Skin	Pallor	Iron, folate, Vitamin B12, Vitamins A and C
	Dermatitis	Zinc, Vitamin A, niacin, riboflavin, essential fatty acids
	Perifollicular petechiae	Vitamin C
	Bruising, purpura	Vitamins C and K
Hair	Easily plucked, alopecia	Protein, zinc, biotin
	Corkscrew hairs, coiled hair	Vitamins A and C
Eyes	Night blindness, keratomalacia, photophobia	Vitamin A
	Conjunctival inflammation	Vitamin A, riboflavin
Mouth	Glossitis	Riboflavin, niacin, folate, Vitamin B12
	Bleeding or receding gums	Vitamins A, C, and K; folate
	Burning or sore mouth/tongue	Vitamin B12 and C; folate, niacin
	Tetany	Calcium, magnesium
Neurologic	Paresthesias	Thiamine, phyridoxine
	Loss of reflexes, wrist drop, foot drop, loss of vibratory and position sense	Vitamin B12 and E
	Dementia, disorientation	Niacin, Vitamin B12
	Ophthalmoplegia	Thiamine

Source. Feldman, M., Friedman, L. S., & Sleisenger, M. H. (2002). *Sleisenger and Fordtran's gastrointestinal and liver disease: Pathophysiology/diagnosis/management* (7th ed., Vol. 1, p. 272). Philadelphia: W. B. Saunders. Copyright © 2002 by W. B. Saunders. Adapted with permission.

Appendix 9.B.

Signs and Symptoms of Mineral and Trace Element Deficiencies

Mineral	Sign and Symptoms of Deficiency
Sodium	Hypovolemia, weakness
Potassium	Weakness, paresthesias, arrhythmias
Magnesium	Weakness, twitching, tetany, arrhythmias, hypocalcemia
Calcium	Osteomalacia, tetany, arrhythmias
Phosphorus	Weakness, fatigue, leukocyte and platelet dysfunction, hemolytic anemia, cardiac failure, decreased oxygenation
Chromium	Glucose intolerance, peripheral neuropathy, encephalopathy
Copper	Anemia, neutropenia, osteoporosis, diarrhea
Iodine	Hypothyroidism, goiter
Iron	Microcytic hypochromic anemia
Manganese	Hypercholesterolemia, dementia, dermatitis
Selenium	Cardiomyopathy, muscle weakness
Zinc	Growth retardation, delayed sexual maturation, hypogonadism, alopecia, acro-orificial skin lesions, diarrhea, mental status changes

Source. Feldman, M., Friedman, L. S., & Sleisenger, M. H. (2002). *Sleisenger and Fordtran's gastrointestinal and liver disease: Pathophysiology/diagnosis/management* (7th ed., Vol. 1, p. 269). Philadelphia: W. B. Saunders. Copyright © 2002 by W. B. Saunders. Adapted with permission.

Appendix 9.C.

Common Hospital Diets, Modified by Nutrients and Consistency

Diet	Consistency and Nutrients
Clear liquid	Includes clear juices, broth, gelatin desserts, and popsicles
Full liquid	Cream soups, milk, and ice cream
Pureed	Foods blended to baby food consistency; often ordered for patients with dysphagia
Mechanical soft	Ground meat with gravy, soft-cooked vegetables, canned fruit; may be ordered for patients with poor dentition
Selected soft	Contains meat, fruit, and vegetables chopped into bite-sized pieces; often ordered for patients with dysphagia
Soft	Regular textured food but no fresh fruits or vegetables
Low sodium	Sodium restricted to <2,000 mg/day
Low fat	All forms of fat restricted to <50 g/day
Low protein	Protein restricted to <60 g/day (vitamin and mineral supplements may be required to ensure adequate nutrition)
High fiber	Daily fiber intake of >20 g/day (additional fluid may be required to ensure soft stools)
Low fiber	Contains mostly eggs, tender meats, milk, rice, white bread, cooked vegetables, strained juices, and canned or cooked fruit; no raw vegetables, nuts, or seeds

Source. Klein, S., & Rubin, D. C. (2002). Enteral and parenteral nutrition. In M. Feldman, L. S. Friedman, & M. H. Sleisenger (Eds.), *Gastrointestinal and liver disease: Pathophysiology/diagnosis/management* (7th ed., Vol. 1, pp. 288). Philadelphia: W. B. Saunders. Adapted with permission.

Appendix 9.D.

Enteral and Parenteral Nutrition

Patients with gastrointestinal (GI) disease often have difficulty with malnutrition and malabsorption, compromising their health and healing. Enteral and parenteral nutrition are often used to supplement or meet the nutritional needs of patients with GI disorders or significant multiorgan disease. In addition, parenteral feeding may allow the bowel to rest while preventing malnutrition.

Enteral Nutrition

Enteral nutrition is delivered through a feeding tube directly into the GI tract (stomach or small intestine). It has fewer associated complications than parenteral nutrition and is therefore preferable. The patient must have a functioning GI tract.

Enteral nutrition has several delivery modes (type of access depends on the anticipated duration, risk of aspiration, patient preference, gut motility, and clinical prognosis):

- Nasogastric tube, which is used for short-term nutritional support (<4 weeks);
- Nasoduodenal tube;
- Nasojejunal tube;
- Percutaneous endoscopic gastronomy tube, which is for patients generally requiring more than 4 weeks of nutrition support and can be continuous or intermittent (usually 4–6 feedings per day administered over 30–40 minutes).
  - Associated mortality is 0.5%.
  - Major complications are peristomal leakage, peritonitis, necrotizing fascitis, and gastric hemorrhage in 1% of patients.
  - Minor complications are wound infections, stomal leaks, tube migration, aspiration, gastrocolic fistula, ileus, and fever (in 8% of patients).
- Jejunostomy (continuous rather than intermittent feedings are preferable to avoid dumping symptoms)
- Pharyngostomy
- Esophagostomy.

Complications of enteral nutrition can be

- Mechanical (tube misplacement, tube occlusion);
- Metabolic (fluid and electrolyte imbalance, e.g., hypokalemia, hyponatremia, hyperglycemia, or hypophospatemia);
- Gastrointestinal side effects (intestinal intolerance: nausea, vomiting, diarrhea, or abdominal pain); or
- Pulmonary (aspiration from secretions and refluxed tube feedings):
  - The head of the bed should be elevated to more than 30° during feedings to minimize risk of aspiration and
  - Therapists should set feeding pumps on hold if patients are to lie flat during bed repositioning. In addition, therapists should consult with nursing before detaching a percutaneous endoscopic gastronomy tube (from the feeding pump) when planning out-of-bed activities.

Parenteral Nutrition (Total Parenteral Nutrition)

Parenteral nutrition is used when enteral feeding is contraindicated or inadequate, such as with persistent vomiting, nausea, diarrhea, extreme abdominal pain, ileus, GI ischemia, severe malabsorption, or mechanical obstruction. It may be used in the short term for cancer patients undergoing chemotherapy.

Parenteral nutrition is accessed through the vascular system (central or peripheral vein) and supplies all basic nutrients (fluid, protein, carbohydrates, fats, minerals, vitamins, and trace elements). It requires careful monitoring.

Complications can be

- Mechanical (insertion or incorrect placement of catheter can cause damage to local structures, pneumothorax, hemothorax, brachial plexus injury, thoracic duct injury, or subclavian or carotid artery puncture);

- Vascular (air embolism with catheter insertion or catheter occlusion from thrombus);

- Infection (risk of line sepsis; can be life threatening);

- Metabolic (inaccurate nutrition is provided; an excess or deficiency of required nutrients can lead to fluid overload, hyperglycemia, hyperammonemia, renal stones, or pancreatitis); metabolic bone disease (e.g., osteomalacia, osteopenia) is also a risk with prolonged parenteral nutrition (>3 months); and

- Gastrointestinal (hepatic abnormalities; risk for steatosis, steatohepatitis, cholestasis, fibrosis, cirrhosis, cholelithiasis, or gallbladder sludge, as a result of gastric stasis).

Source. Klein and Rubin (2002).

10
The Genitourinary System

Sharon K. Hennigan, MA, OTR/L, CHT

Occupational therapists in the acute hospital setting assess how people's medical conditions affect their physical, mental, and emotional abilities to participate in daily occupations. Occupational therapists as team members deliver health care services to people with multiple medical conditions (e.g., cardiopulmonary diseases, orthopedic surgeries, neurological conditions) that may affect or be affected by the function of the genitourinary system (GU) and who may possibly have an undiagnosed GU condition.

The GU system's primary function is to cleanse the body of its wastes. The medical signs and symptoms of a problem within this system are difficult to diagnosis because they may be vague or indicative of other issues in the entire body. Health care staff monitor signs and symptoms that reflect changes in the GU system's ability to rid the body of its wastes. The medical status of the GU system can affect a person's physical and cognitive status. These problems can result in a reduced capacity to participate in daily occupational roles and activities. A person's decreased ability to perform daily tasks leads to the need for occupational therapists to assess, educate, and assist the person in regaining independence in performing these necessary tasks.

Genitourinary Structure and Function

The *genitourinary system* is made up of the reproductive and urinary organs (see Figure 10.1). These organs are grouped together because of their proximity and common use of pathways. The female reproductive organs are the *vagina, uterus, ovaries,* and *fallopian tubes.*

The male reproductive organs are the *testicles, prostate,* and *penis.* The urinary organs are the *kidneys, bladder, ureters,* and *urethra.* The urinary system is responsible for disposing of the body's wastes and by-products.

Kidneys

The *kidneys'* primary function is to remove metabolic wastes from the blood system. They produce *urine,* which is the discarded waste product of metabolism from every cell in the body. The kidneys filter these wastes through the excretory organs and the urinary system.

The two kidneys are located just below the ribs in the lower back region. The back muscles on each side of the vertebral column, along with the lower ribs, protect the kidneys. Each kidney is surrounded by fibrous tissue that forms a firm and smooth covering to the organ. When this layer is removed, the kidney is found to be smooth and a deep-red color. Kidney tissue is dense but easily lacerated with force. A vertical section of the kidney shows the components that perform its function.

Structures enter into and leave each kidney through the *hilum,* which contains the vessels, nerves, and ureter. These structures enter into the kidney at its central cavity, called the *sinus.* The excretory duct, the *ureter,* eventually branches into the *infundibula.* The renal artery supplies blood to the kidney and branches into arterioles that eventually terminate into several clumps of capillaries called *glomerulus.* The glomerulus' function is to filter the blood and remove the fluid and waste molecules such as urea and glucose.

Renal veins arise from three sources within the kidney and exit the kidney at the hilum, which opens into the inferior vena cava vessel. The *lymphatics* consist of superficial and deep structures that terminate in the lumbar glands.

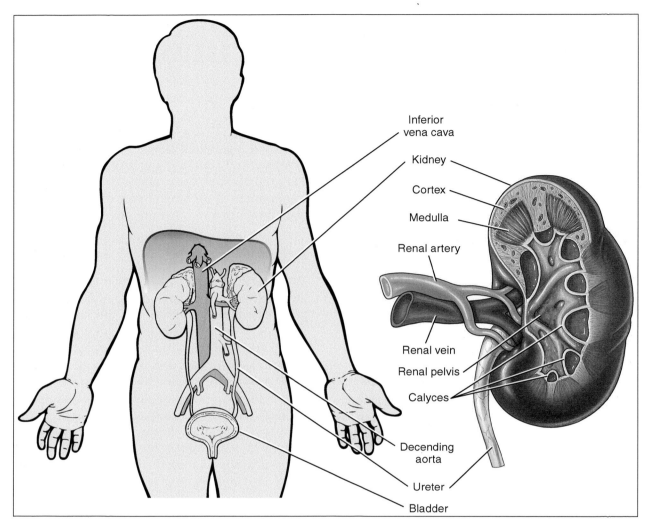

Figure 10.1. Genitourinary system.
Source. Richard Fritzler, Medical Illustrator, Roswell, GA.

The approximately 15 nerves of the kidney are small, and they accompany the renal artery and its branches (Gray, 1974).

Components of Urine

Excretion is the process of moving materials from inside a cell to outside. The kidneys' primary function is to remove the metabolic wastes produced by the cells that are deposited into the bloodstream. The components of urine are nitrogenous compounds. These compounds include urea, creatinine, ammonia, and uric acid. *Urea* results from amino acid metabolism, and *creatinine* is a compound that results from muscle metabolism. *Ammonia,* another nitrogenous compound, results from bacteria that

break down proteins, and *uric acid* consists of broken-down nucleotides. This high concentration of compounds attracts water. The water moves from the collecting ducts into the medulla of the kidney, where the capillaries absorb and return the water to the blood. The fluid and solutes that remain in the tubules of the nephron become urine.

Ureters

The *ureters* are two tubes that move the urine into the bladder. Small branches or tubes begin within the kidney, forming a pouch called the *renal pelvis,* then pass through the hilum of the kidney as the ureter, and eventually connect to the bladder. After the kidney creates the urine concentrate, this concentrate moves from the ascending loop of Henle to a collecting duct. Minute amounts of urine drop into the collecting ducts of the kidney's nephrons to the renal pelvis. The renal pelvis moves the urine into a ureter, which connects directly to the bladder. The ureter is composed of three coats: fibrous, muscular, and mucous. The *fibrous coat* is the outer layer of tissue covering the ureter. The *muscular layer* contracts in waves, moving the urine from the kidney to the bladder. The *mucous layer* lines the inside of the ureter (Gray, 1974).

Bladder

The *bladder* is a musculo-membranous sac located in the pelvis, and it is the reservoir for the urine. In males, the bladder is behind the pubic bones and in front of the rectum. It is larger in its vertical diameter than in its horizontal diameter. The bladder in females is situated in front of the uterus and vagina and is larger in its horizontal diameter than in its vertical diameter. The female bladder's capacity is greater than the male bladder's capacity. The bladder is held in place by ligaments, which are formed by the recto-vesical fascia and the peritoneum (Gray, 1974). The neck or cervix of the bladder is the beginning point of the urethra.

Male Urethra. The *male urethra* extends from the neck of the bladder to the meatus urinarius at the end of the penis. The urethra is divided lengthwise into three sections: prostatic, membranous, and spongy. The *prostatic section* is the widest, and it passes through the prostate gland to the membranous section. The *membranous section* is the smallest. It is surrounded by the compressor urethrae muscle. The longest section of the urethra is the *spongy section*, which begins at the terminal end of the membranous section and extends to the meatus urinarius.

Female Urethra. The *female urethra* is approximately 1.5 inches long and very narrow. It extends from the neck of the bladder to the meatus urinarius. It sits directly in front of the vaginal opening and behind the glans clitoridis.

Prostate Gland

The *prostate gland* is located below the neck of the male bladder and around the beginning of the urethra. It is a firm, partly glandular and partly muscular body. It is situated in the pelvic cavity and rests on the rectum (Gray, 1974).

Genitourinary Diseases and Disorders

Occupational therapists should be familiar with the diseases and disorders of the GU system. A reduced capacity of the GU system to process and rid the body of its wastes will directly affect the function of the body's other systems. The changes throughout the body may be reflected in the person's reduced physical capacity to perform self-care tasks or a decreased cognitive capacity to engage in these activities with health care providers. Occupational therapists should monitor for physical and cognitive changes while working with their patients, as these change may reflect the onset of functional changes within the GU system.

Renal Diseases

Kidney failure can exist for a long period of time, with a person losing as much as 75% of normal kidney function before symptoms are noted and correctly diagnosed. This reduced capacity may be because of the kidney's large reserve capability. As kidney function decreases, the associated symptoms may be interpreted as depression or fatigue or attributed to other life issues or medical problems. As a result, the person's kidney function may be at 25%–30% of normal function when kidney disease is first identified and treated.

The warning signs of kidney and urinary tract conditions include

- High blood pressure;
- Protein in the urine;
- Blood in the urine;
- Elevated or abnormal levels of creatinine;
- Abnormal blood urea nitrogen (BUN) blood values;
- Glomerular filtration rate (GFR; a blood creatinine test) less than 90 milliliters per minute/1.73^2 (normal rates are above 60 milliliters per minute/1.73^2);

- More frequent urination, particularly at night;
- Difficult or painful urination;
- Puffiness around the eyes;
- Swelling of the hands and feet (National Kidney Foundation, 2009).

Acute Renal Failure

Acute renal failure (ARF) occurs when renal function decreases over hours to days, resulting in a retention of nitrogenous wastes. The primary laboratory marker for ARF is an increase in serum creatinine, which occurs because of decreased kidney function. *Azotemia* is an increase in urea levels resulting from renal insufficiency. *Uremia* is a condition resulting from renal failure in which the increase in urea and creatinine levels may lead to nausea, vomiting, malaise, and an altered sensory system (Fichandler & Malone, 2006).

ARF may also lead to disruption of function in other body systems. For example, gastrointestinal issues may include anorexia, nausea, vomiting, diarrhea, constipation, or uremic breath. Central nervous system symptoms can include headache, sleepiness, irritability, confusion, seizures, or coma. The cardiovascular system may experience hypotension and, as this disease progresses, hypertension, fluid overload, heart failure, or systemic edema ("Renal Failure," 2004).

The primary causes of ARF are categorized as prerenal, intrinsic, or postrenal:

- *Prerenal:* Results in diminished blood flow to the kidneys. Decreased blood flow may occur from shock, embolism, heart failure, arrhythmias, hypovolemia, autoimmune conditions, and blood disorders. Symptoms may include hypotension, dry mucous membranes, oliguria, or anuria (Fichandler & Malone, 2006).
- *Intrinsic:* Results in damage directly to the kidneys and is associated with tissue ischemia, toxins, and vascular and systemic disorders (Fichandler & Malone, 2006).
- *Postrenal:* Results when urine outflow is obstructed. This condition may be the

result of benign prostatic hyperplasis (BPH), tumors, clots, kidney stones, or edema caused by catheterization (Paz, 2009).

The medical treatment goal is to identify and treat the reversible primary causes of ARF. Additionally, the person's diet and fluids are closely monitored and modified as needed. Electrolytes are regularly tracked to detect *hyperkalemia,* which is the kidneys' inability to extract excessive amounts of potassium. Treatments for ARF may include dialysis, hypertonic glucose, insulin infusion, and intravenous calcium ("Renal Failure," 2004; Paz, 2009).

Chronic Renal Disease and Chronic Renal Failure

Chronic renal disease (CRD) affects 1 in 9 adults; however, most people are unaware of the condition because they are asymptomatic (Watnick & Morrison, 2007). *Chronic renal failure (CRF)* may be caused by severe or prolonged hypertension, diabetes mellitus, glomerulopathies, obstructive uropathy, and hereditary or congenital renal diseases or disorders (Fichandler & Malone, 2006). This condition is typically irreversible and leads to a gradual decline in renal function. If the condition is left unchecked, uremic toxins build up and produce fatal physiological changes in all major organ systems. Survival of this condition is dependent on dialysis or a kidney transplant.

CRD creates changes in all major body systems, as outlined in Table 10.1. The medical treatment goal for CRD is to correct symptoms, minimize complications, and slow the progression of the disease. Most people with CRD are placed on a low-protein diet, which reduces the amount of end-products produced during protein metabolism that the kidneys cannot excrete. Foods high in potassium (e.g., potatoes, tomatoes, bananas, oranges) and high in phosphorous (e.g., dairy products, dried beans, cola, peanut butter) are usually avoided because they can affect cardiac function and weaken bones. Excess sodium is also avoided because it may lead to water retention, resulting in high blood

Table 10.1. **Signs and Symptoms of Chronic Kidney Disease, by Body System**

Body System	Signs and Symptoms
Cardiovascular system	• Hypertension, arrhythmias, uremic pericarditis, heart failure, peripheral edema.
Respiratory system	• Susceptibility to edema, pulmonary edema, pleuritic pain, uremic pleuritis, uremic lung, dyspnea from heart failure.
Gastrointestinal system	• Stomatitis, gum ulceration and bleeding, esophagitis, gastritis, duodenal ulcers, lesions on the bowels, uremic colitis, pancreatitis. • Other signs include a metal taste in the mouth, an ammonia smell to breath, anorexia, nausea, vomiting.
Cutaneous system	• Skin yellowish or bronze, dry or scaly. • Severe itching; ecchymoses; thin, brittle fingernails; dry, brittle hair that may change color or fall out.
Neurological system	• Restless leg syndrome (i.e., pain, burning, itching in the legs and feet), which may lead to foot drop. • Muscle cramps, twitches, shortened memory and attention span, drowsiness, irritability, confusion, seizures, coma.
Endocrine system	• Decreased libido, infertility, amenorrhea or cessation of menses, impotence, decreased sperm production. • Impaired carbohydrate metabolism, causing increase in blood glucose levels similar to diabetes mellitus.
Skeletal system	Calcium–phosphorus imbalance; parathyroid hormone imbalance that leads to bone and muscle pain; skeletal demineralization; pathologic fractures; calcifications in the brain, eyes, gums, joints, myocardium, blood vessels.
Renal and urological systems	• Hypotension, dry mouth, loss of skin turgor, listlessness, fatigue, nausea. • Decreased capacity of kidneys to excrete sodium, leading to sodium retention and overload. • Potassium buildup in muscles, creating muscle irritability and weakness. • Fluid overload and metabolic acidosis. • Decreased urine output.

pressure, congestive heart failure, or pulmonary edema. Patients on dialysis limit foods high in potassium and sodium content; however, their diets are high in protein. This diet prevents ketoacidosis and a negative nitrogen balance that can result in catabolism and tissue atrophy ("Renal Failure," 2004).

End-Stage Renal Disease

End-stage renal disease (ESRD) is characterized by a GFR of less than 20% of normal ("Chronic Renal Failure," 2005). With ESRD, the kidneys completely fail to work, resulting in a chronic buildup of wastes and toxins in the body and an inability to regulate electrolytes and hormones. The most common cause of ESRD is diabetes mellitus (Patel, 2008). If left untreated, renal failure results in uremia or azotemia, which can be fatal. Symptoms of ESRD include

- Changes in mental status,
- Impaired sensation of hands and feet,
- Decreased urine output,
- Nausea,
- Vomiting,
- Headache,
- Easy bruising or bleeding, and
- Fatigue (Patel, 2008).

This condition necessitates dialysis, which removes these toxins and wastes, a function the kidneys can no longer perform. The only cure for ESRD is kidney transplantation.

Dialysis

Three types of dialysis may be performed for people with ARF, CRD, and ESRD. These treatments are *hemodialysis (HD)*, *peritoneal dialysis (PD)*, and *continuous renal replacement therapy (CRRT)*. All types of dialysis control most symptoms noted with these conditions. However, maintenance dialysis may produce complications, which include protein wasting and dialysis dementia, necessitating a kidney transplant.

- HD requires the placement of an arterio-vascular fistula in the arm (i.e., an artery and vein are connected under this site to form a vascular access for dialysis; see Figure 10.2). A thrill or vibration may be felt over the arteriovascular fistula site as blood circulates. The person is connected to a hemodialysis machine. The blood is passed out of the body, wastes are cleansed through the machine, and the cleansed blood is returned to the body. This treatment may take between 4–5 hours. HD carries a risk of hypotension, bone disease, pruritus, and insomnia.

- PD requires a surgical procedure in which a special tube is placed into the lower abdomen (see Figure 10.3). *Dialysate* is a solution introduced through this tube that absorbs body wastes and toxins. The physician determines the length of time (dwell time) the solution remains in the abdominal area and the required number of sessions per day. This process usually requires four sessions per day with 4–6 hours of dwell time (National Kidney and Urologic Diseases Information Clearinghouse, 2006). The solution is then drained, measured, and discharged, and clean dialysate is placed in the abdominal area again for the prescribed period of time. This process of exchange takes approximately 30–40 minutes. An advantage of PD is that it can be performed at home. However, the risk of infection is always present, specifically peritonitis because the PD catheter is placed in the peritoneum.

- CRRT is a specialized treatment used with patients with ARF and patients in critical condition in the intensive care unit. These patients require fluid removal to help correct electrolyte imbalances. CRRT requires a central venous access with a double lumen catheter. The catheter is connected to the filter circuit on the CRRT machine located next to the patient's hospital bed. The patient's blood is removed, cleansed, and returned to the patient via the lumen catheter. The CRRT functions as the kidneys and may be operated 24 hours a day, depending on the patient's needs (Langford, Slivar, Tucker, & Bourbonnais, 2008).

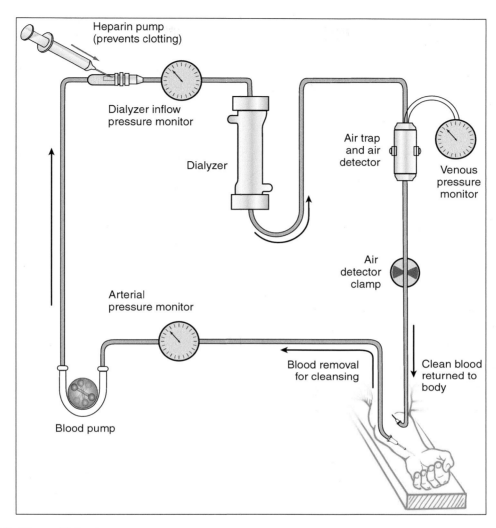

Figure 10.2. Hemodialysis.
Source. Richard Fritzler, Medical Illustrator, Roswell, GA.

Bladder

The function of the bladder, ureters and urethra are to store and eliminate urine from the body. Various infections to these structures create pain and inflammation reducing the person's ability to effectively void. *Urinary incontinence* is a leakage of urine and does affect a person's hygiene, as well as a reluctance to engage in social interactions with family and friends. If the symptoms and conditions are left unaddressed, it may begin a cycle of repeated infections and related conditions that reduce the function of the structures and affect the person's general health and social activities.

Urinary Tract Infections

Urinary tract infections (UTIs) are common conditions that account for approximately 10 million medical office visits per year (National Kidney Foundation, 2009). *Escherichia coli* and coliform bacteria are responsible for uncomplicated UTIs, which are resolved quickly with the use of oral antibiotics. Unresolved UTIs occur when the urinary tract is never cleansed during the initial treatment. These UTIs may result from noncompliance with medication, mixed infections, bacteria resistance to treatment, and renal insufficiency. *Reinfections* are infections with different bacteria that occur after successful

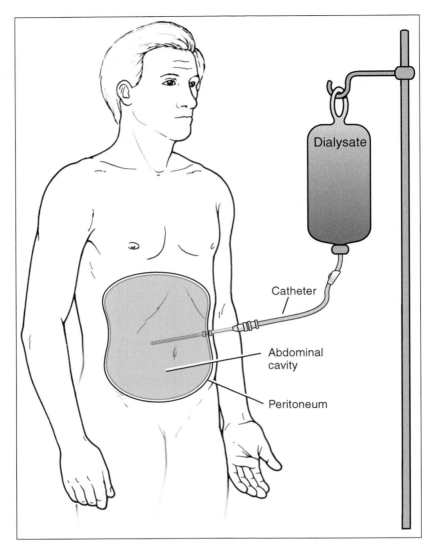

Dialysate

Catheter

Abdominal
cavity

Peritoneum

Figure 10.3. Peritoneal dialysis.
Source. Richard Fritzler, Medical Illustrator, Roswell, GA.

treatment for a prior infection. Ascending infection from the urethra is the most common route. Women are at risk for UTI because the female urethra is short, which facilitates the infection's ascent into the bladder (National Kidney Foundation, 2009; Stoller, Kane, & Carroll, 2007).

People who have had more than 3 episodes of UTI in a year are candidates for prophylactic treatment. A thorough evaluation of the urinary tract system is performed before initiating prophylactic treatment. Selected medications need to be successful at eliminating pathogenic bacteria and not cause bacteria resistance (Stoller et al., 2007).

Hematuria

Hematuria is the presence of blood in the urine. The presence of blood when voiding may help to define the source of the problem. Blood observed at the beginning of the urinary stream may imply an anterior urethral source. Blood observed at the end of the urinary stream may imply a bladder neck or prostatic urethral source. Blood observed throughout the urinary stream may imply a bladder or upper tract source. Associated symptoms occurring with these observations and an understanding of other medical conditions and related drug management help to determine the cause. If hematuria persists after treatment, further medical evaluation is warranted (Stoller et al., 2007).

Acute Cystitis

Acute cystitis is a bladder infection caused by bacteria that travel through the urethra to the bladder. The primary symptoms of this infection include complaints of frequency of urination, urgency to urinate, and discomfort or pain during urination. A urinalysis test is performed to assess for pyuria and bacteria in the urine.

In women, acute cystitis is differentiated from pelvic inflammatory disease by a pelvic exam and urinalysis. In men, urethritis and prostastis are differentiated with a physical exam. Cystitis is rare in men and may suggest other pathological processes that require further evaluation (Stoller et al., 2007).

Urinary Incontinence

Urinary incontinence is common in older people. It results from a decrease in function of the involuntary smooth muscle of the bladder and the voluntary skeletal muscle of the sphincter, permitting leakage of urine from the sphincter. The various classifications of urinary incontinence are total incontinence, stress incontinence, urge incontinence, overflow incontinence, functional incontinence, and enuresis (Fichandler & Malone, 2006; Paz, 2009; Stoller et al., 2007).

- *Total incontinence:* A person loses urine at all times and in all positions. The sphincter is unable to function, possibly as a result of surgery, nerve damage, or cancer.

- *Stress incontinence:* Loss of urine occurs during activities that increase abdominal pressure, such as coughing, sneezing, lifting, or exercising, caused by a laxity in the pelvic floor muscles or as a result of pelvic surgery.

- *Urge incontinence:* This type of incontinence involves a strong, unexpected urge to void followed by the uncontrolled loss of urine. It is unrelated to position and activities. Inflammatory conditions or neurogenic disorders of the bladder are associated with this type of incontinence.

- *Overflow incontinence:* The bladder is chronically distended; the intravesical pressure exceeds the outlet resistance, permitting urine to dribble.

- *Functional incontinence:* This incontinence is caused by a physical condition that prevents accessing a bathroom in time (e.g., limited mobility, poor vision), difficulty positioning to use the toilet, and difficulty removing clothing (e.g., impaired coordination). It may also be an unwillingness to urinate because of psychological or emotional issues (e.g., anger, anxiety, depression, dementia, refusing to use certain bathrooms).

- *Enuresis:* Involuntary voiding during sleep may result from an obstructive or neurological disease of the lower urinary tract or dysfunctional voiding.

An older person may have transient causes of incontinence; once these causes are treated, bladder control may be restored. One transient cause of incontinence is delirium. This problem may occur in a person who has a decreased sensory system and hence the inability to perceive the urge to urinate. Infections are another transient cause of incontinence. Infections may facilitate a person's urge to urinate. Medications such as diuretics, anticholinergics, psychotropics, opioid analgesics, beta blockers, beta agonists, and calcium channel blockers may increase urine production and the need to urinate. Stool impaction is a common cause of incontinence in people who are hospitalized or have reduced mobility.

Patients with voiding issues and incontinence may use a urinary catheter. The purpose of a catheter is to relieve urinary retention, restore bladder muscle tone, obtain cultures, monitor urine output, or treat underlying bladder conditions. Associated symptoms that may occur with catheter use include

- Pain,
- Leakage,
- Bladder spasms,
- Kidney stone formation,
- Increased risk of UTIs,

- Skin breakdown, and
- Trauma to the urethra and surrounding structures (Ramakrishnan & Mold, 2005).

According to Ramakrishnan and Mold (2005) and Paz (2009), the various types of catheters include the following:

- *Indwelling catheter:* This catheter may be urethral or subrapubic. Urethral catherization uses a sterile, lubricated catheter placed into the urethra. It drains urine freely from the bladder into a drainage bag. A *Foley catheter* uses a balloon to keep the catheter within the urethra and is the most common catheter. A *subrapubic catheter* is placed through the abdominal wall, situated above the pubic bones, and placed into the bladder. This catheter is used with patients who have sustained a high spinal cord injury.
- *Condom catheter:* This catheter is used with male patients who are able to spontaneously void. It fits over the penis and is held in place by Velcro. This type of catheter is more comfortable for the patient and is associated with less risk of infections.
- *Self-catheterization:* The patient intermittently catheterizes himself or herself to drain urine from the bladder. The patient needs to be able to spontaneously void. This catheterization has less risk of infection, bladder spasm, or stone formation.

Bladder Cancer

Bladder cancer is the second most common cancer of the urological system. Risk factors accounting for 60% of these cancers include cigarette smoking and exposure to industrial dyes and chemicals (Stoller et al., 2007). Primary symptoms of bladder cancer are hematuria and irritative voiding; however, these patients are not uncommonly asymptomatic. Laboratory work, imaging, and biopsies are used to evaluate and diagnose bladder cancers.

Treatment choices for bladder cancer include intravesical chemotherapy, cystectomy, radiation, and chemotherapy. Intravesical chemotherapy uses chemotherapeutic agents delivered directly into the bladder by a urethral catheter. This treatment is used to eliminate the existing disease or to reduce the recurrence of disease after a complete transurethral resection. The initial treatment duration is 6–12 weeks and may be followed with a maintenance regimen.

The grade of the lesions and depth of infiltration of the disease determines the type of surgical intervention. A partial cystectomy may be used with single lesions. Radical cystectomy is used when the cancer invades other components of the system and requires the removal of the bladder, prostate, seminal vesicles, and surrounding fat for men and removal of the uterus, cervix, urethra, anterior vaginal vault, and ovaries for women. Additionally, pelvic lymph nodes are removed with this procedure. The urinary tract is reconstructed using a conduit of the small or large intestine. Recent developments in urinary diversion have reduced the use of an external appliance, giving people undergoing this procedure improved quality of life.

Radiation is used by delivering an external beam to the lesion site for 6–8 weeks. Bladder, bowel, and rectal complications arise from this treatment, including recurrence of the cancer. Chemotherapy is recommended in cases in which the disease has metastasized, for people who have undergone a radical cystectomy, or in combination with radiation therapy.

Prostate Gland

The purpose of the prostate gland is to produce seminal fluids that provide nutrients and assist with the mobility of the sperm. It is located below the neck of the bladder and around the urethra. The prostate gland changes with age and these changes can affect the function of the bladder, ureters, and urethra. Conditions of the prostate gland can affect the person's ability to void, affecting the general health and social activities of the person.

Benign Prostatic Hyperplasia

Benign prostatic hyperplasia (BPH) is the most common benign tumor in men and its incidence increases with age. Approximately 20% of men ages 41–50, 50% of men ages 51–60, and more than 90% of men older than age 80 present with this disorder (Stoller et al., 2007). The primary symptom of this condition is difficulty with voiding. Risk factors are unclear but may be related to genetics and race. The etiology of BPH is also unclear but appears to have multiple factors and may be under the control of the endocrine system ("Recent Evidence Suggests," 2004; Stoller et al., 2007).

The pathology of BPH is an increase in cell numbers. Microscopic studies reveal a nodular growth that consists of varying amounts of stroma and epithelium. The symptoms of BPH are obstructive and irritative complaints with voiding by the person. Obstructive symptoms may be hesitancy and decreased force of the urine stream. The bladder does not feel completely empty. Other obstructive symptoms include urinating a second time within 2 hours, known as *double voiding*; straining to urinate; and postvoid dribbling. Irritative symptoms may include a sense of urgency to void, frequency of voiding, and increased voiding at bedtime, known as *nocturia*.

Laboratory studies include a urinalysis to rule out infection or hematuria, serum creatinine to assess renal function, and a serum prostate-specific antigen (PSA) test. *PSA* is a blood test that assesses the amount of an immunogenic glycoprotein produced by the prostate gland. A PSA of 3 nanograms per milliliter is considered the upper level of normal for the screen. An annual screen is recommended for men beginning at age 40 (Stoller et al., 2007).

The conventional surgical therapy for BPH is *transurethral resection of the prostate (TURP)*. Most of these procedures are performed endoscopically, using a spinal anesthetic that requires a longer hospital stay. The risk factors for TURP include retrograde ejaculation, impotence, and urinary incontinence. Complications from the procedure include bleeding, urethral stricture or bladder neck contracture, perforation of the prostate capsule, and transurethral resection syndrome, which results from the hypotonic solution absorbed by the body during the surgical procedure. This problem may occur in surgical procedures that are longer than 90 minutes. The symptoms of this syndrome are nausea, vomiting, confusion, hypertension, increased heart rate, and changes in vision (Stoller et al., 2007).

Laser therapy is an alternative to TURP. Its advantages are minimal blood loss and the ability to treat patients who are on anticoagulation therapies. The disadvantages of laser therapy are longer catheterization times, patient complaints of frequent irritative voiding and the lack of pathology tissue to assess after the procedure. Large, randomized studies that compare TURP, laser therapy, and other treatments for BPH are lacking.

Prostate Cancer

According to the Prostate Cancer Foundation (2010), one in six men will develop *prostate cancer*. The foundation estimates that more than 218,000 men will be diagnosed with prostate cancer, and 32,000 men will die from it (Prostate Cancer Foundation, 2010). The disease's clinical incidence does not match its prevalence as noted at autopsy, where more than 40% of men older than age 50 were found to have prostate carcinoma (Stoller et al., 2007).

This cancer is small and remains contained within the prostate gland. Most prostate cancers arise in the tissue around the prostate gland. Pathologists use the Gleason grading system (Stoller et al., 2007), which is based on architectural rather than histologic criteria. This system applies a grade based on the architectural pattern of the cancerous glands occupying the largest area of the specimen. The grade assesses tumor volume, stage, and prognosis (Stoller et al., 2007).

The patterns of prostate cancer progression are well defined. Small and differentiated cancers are usually confined within the prostate. Poorly differentiated cancers may metastasize to regional lymph nodes or bone (Stoller et al., 2007; refer to Chapter 11 in this volume for more information).

The prostate gland can appear normal during a physical examination. Symptoms associated with prostate cancer are obstructive voiding, urinary retention, and neurological symptoms. The PSA serum screen is the most common diagnostic assessment for prostate cancer. PSA is a glycoprotein produced in the prostate cells. Initial and repeated testing with the PSA screen may be useful in detecting and staging prostate cancer, assessing responses to treatment, and detecting a recurrence of the disease (Prostate Cancer Foundation, 2009; Stoller et al., 2007).

Treatment of prostate cancer is based on tumor grade and stage and the person's age and health. Radiation therapy and radical prostatectomy appear to result in the best survival rate for this cancer. *Radiation therapy* uses a variety of techniques that range from an external beam to transperineal implantation of radioisotopes. *Radical prostatectomy* removes the prostate, seminal vesicles, and the ampullae of the vas deferens. Another treatment choice is *cryosurgery.* This procedure destroys tissue by freezing the prostate with liquid nitrogen. Cryosurgery is less invasive than radical prostatectomy and works well for a localized tumor.

The term *surveillance* is used to describe the medical management of people with very low volume and low-grade tumors that do not progress and require only medical management. Surveillance management is used to recognize and separate two groups of patients, those who show no signs of tumor progression and those with tumors that are changing and require intervention. Patients with low-volume or low-grade cancer undergo regular PSA screens, rectal exams, and periodic biopsies.

Genitourinary Diagnostic Tests

A variety of diagnostic tools are used to screen and assess for diseases and disorders of the GU system. It is helpful for occupational therapists to have a working knowledge of the purpose of the common diagnostic tests and the possible findings diagnosticians are seeking when administering these tests. Understanding the test findings can assist occupational therapists during the occupational therapy evaluation. The test findings of the GU system can be used to assess and explore performance issues during self-care tasks and therapy can be directed to modifications or permanent changes in how the person will continue to perform self-care tasks once discharged from the hospital.

Urinalysis

A *urinalysis* is conducted on urine collected midstream during voiding. It is examined within an hour of collection and includes a dipstick examination, followed by microscopic study if findings are in question. The dipstick test assesses for protein, urine pH, hemoglobin, glucose, and ketones, along with other items. Studying the urine under a microscope allows the examiner to assess for formed elements such as crystals, cells, or organisms (Stoller et al., 2007). The urinalysis assesses for *proteinuria*, or excessive protein that is excreted through the urine. A finding of 150–160 milligrams within 24 hours is considered excessive in adults.

Proteinuria is accompanied by other abnormal findings in the urinalysis such as elevated BUN and serum creatinine levels. *Creatinine* is the by-product of muscle metabolism. It is produced at a constant rate, filtered by the glomerulus, and cleared by renal excretion. When renal function is normal, creatinine production and renal excretion are the same (Watnick & Morrison, 2007). A 24-hour urine sample is collected to assess the level of creatinine in a day. Refer to Appendix P for additional diagnostic descriptions.

Approximately 30%–70% of urea is reabsorbed in the nephron. Reabsorption of urea is low in a well-hydrated adult. However, dehydration increases reabsorption of urea, resulting in an increased BUN reading. The ratio of BUN to creatinine is assessed; in adults, it should be 10:1. If a person is dehydrated, the ratio may increase to 20:1.

Radionuclide Studies

Radionuclide studies provide a measurement of the GFR. A dye is injected intravenously, filtered by the glomerulus, and used to study the GFR. The purpose of this study is to assess the function and flow of the kidneys and each kidney's contribution to the renal system.

Intravenous Urographies

An *intravenous pyelogram* is used to evaluate the kidneys, ureters, and bladder. This study may be used to assess renal size and shape, presence of kidney stones, and kidney function. It is being replaced by computed tomography scans because they are less invasive to the system.

Kidneys, Ureters, and Bladder X-Ray

A *kidney, ureters, and bladder abdominal X-ray* is used in diagnosing tumors, kidney stones, and some gastrointestinal disorders or ensuring correct placement of feeding tubes. The intravenous pyelogram is superior in examining the kidneys, ureters, and bladder.

Cystoscopy

In a *cystoscopy*, a fiberoptic scope is inserted into the bladder and urethra to examine causes of hematuria, dysuria, urinary incontinence, urinary retention or urgency, UTIs, tumors, or stones.

Other Diagnostic Studies

Other diagnostic studies include ultrasound, computed tomography scans, and MRIs. These studies are used to study the size of the kidneys, renal cortex, medulla, pyramids, and urinary tract. They are also used to assess for obstructions and renal lesions, screen for polycystic kidney disease, and assess for residual urine in the bladder with voiding.

Occupational Therapy Considerations

A person entering the acute hospital setting may have little to no choice or voice in the matter, experiencing an abrupt change in his or her physical and mental abilities (e.g., stroke, heart attack) or being admitted for a deteriorating chronic condition (e.g., renal disease). The entrance into the hospital changes the person's daily occupations from roles and activities he or she controls and enjoys to focusing on life-sustaining tasks that he or she may have little to no control in directing.

The acute hospital setting can be a very hectic, fast-paced environment. The occupational therapist is communicating with multiple health care providers to determine each assigned patient's medical status so as to administer occupational therapy interventions that are safe and effective. A patient may be overwhelmed, attempting to digest the information provided by the various health care providers. Occupational therapy can provide a sense of purpose and control over these situations by including the patient's personal goals in the selection of these treatments and related-tasks.

Occupational Therapy Intervention

Occupational therapy intervention in this setting does focus on the person's ability to safely perform self-care tasks and light household activities. The therapy sessions are short due to the patient's reduced physical or cognitive status. Each therapy session provides the opportunity to assess changes and improvements in the person's self-care performance. Therapy interventions with this patient population does include education and practice in energy conservation, rest breaks and pacing techniques, safety and environmental awareness when practicing self-care tasks, and the safe use of adaptive and mobility equipment.

The initial therapy session may begin with the therapist assisting the patient by performing more of the steps to complete a self-care task. As the patient's strength and endurance improves, the patient assumes control of these steps, with the therapist providing feedback on rest breaks and pacing techniques, how to incorporate the use of the adaptive or mobility equipment into the task, and reviewing safety issues and concerns.

After Surgery and Radiation Treatment

As the occupational therapist develops the treatment plan, he or she needs to understand the medical treatments and their possible effects on the patient's abilities to participate in therapy. A person who has undergone radiation, surgery, or both will present with generalized fatigue and weakness. The patient may lack the functional strength and mobility to easily perform normal self-care tasks. Occupational therapy intervention can include educating the person on energy conservation techniques. Practicing these techniques allows the person to understand his or her endurance to complete activities and how to pace the tasks to remain safe (e.g., reducing the possibility of falls). Allowing the person to choose a self-care task to practice provides him or her with choice and control in resuming the process of managing his or her health and autonomy.

After Urinary Tract Reconstruction

Someone who has undergone removal of the bladder with a urinary tract reconstruction and placement of an ostomy requires assistance in performing self-care tasks and other daily activities. The occupational therapist teams with nursing to assist the patient in understanding how to care for the ostomy and continue to participate in daily activities. The patient may feel overwhelmed by learning how to care for and incorporate this device into self-care tasks and frustrated, angry, or scared by the change in his or her self-image. Occupational therapy can reduce the patient's anxiety, offer support, and improve confidence by breaking down and practicing the steps needed to complete bathing and dressing tasks.

Urinary Tract Infections

A patient with a UTI may not be able to participate in therapy until the disease is under control. The therapist should note the patient's complaints of pain, fever, or nausea because these symptoms may indicate the onset or recurrence of a UTI. The patient may also exhibit an altered mental status. Changes noted in the patient's mental status, when combined with other symptoms, may indicate a UTI. The presence of these signs and symptoms should be reported to the medical staff.

When the patient begins therapy, he or she may exhibit decreased strength and endurance, necessitating shorter therapy sessions. A patient with a Foley catheter should be positioned so the collection bag is below waist level to prevent urine from backing up into the catheter tubing, thereby reducing the possibility of an infection. In addition, blood noted in urine

or fecal matter during toileting tasks should also be reported to the nursing staff.

Addressing Incontinence

A patient who has undergone radiation may experience incontinence for approximately 2 months after the radiation treatment ends. This side effect, along with other medical conditions, may necessitate the need to wear adult diapers. The patient, caregiver, or both will need education on caring for skin to prevent skin breakdown. Nursing staff generally provide most of this education and training. Occupational therapists partner with nursing staff to help the patient and caregiver practice new habits of checking the skin and addressing skin changes during bathing and toileting tasks.

Functional incontinence is another problem experienced by patients in the acute hospital setting. Patients demonstrate decreased mobility, coordination, and strength that restricts their ability to move from the bed to the toilet, remove lower-extremity garments, and position themselves on the toilet. Occupational therapists may recommend a bedside commode for the hospital room and for home to reduce the amount of walking necessary to reach the toilet. Clothing options are discussed with the patient to improve his or her ability to don and doff lower-extremity clothing and undergarments. Adult diapers may be a solution to reduce cleanup after leakage. Lighting, especially at night, can improve the patient's mobility and safety. Signage from the primary living areas to the bathrooms can reduce confusion for patients and assist them in quickly locating these areas in their homes.

Patients on Dialysis

Confirm the physician's orders in the medical chart regarding activity levels that may occur during dialysis treatments. Check with the nursing staff on the status of a patient undergoing PD or CRRT before initiating therapy. These two types of dialysis treatments may restrict the patient's physical ability to participate during an occupational therapy session. It may be possible to provide therapy during a PD treatment; however, the session may be limited to bed activities. Therapy during a CRRT session is very unlikely because the patient may be critically ill and unable to physically participate or mentally focus on activities.

Therapists should be aware that hemodialysis is fatiguing for most patients. Therapy may be scheduled on non–dialysis treatment days or before the dialysis treatment. If therapy is provided after the dialysis treatment, monitor the patient's vital signs and energy level. The therapy session may be shortened if the patient's endurance level decreases.

Throughout the therapy session, monitor the patient's vital signs because he or she may experience dehydration, electrolyte imbalances, and hypotension as a result of the dialysis treatment. Bedside therapy is appropriate during dialysis; however, functional mobility is generally contraindicated during the dialysis treatment. Blood pressure should not be taken from the arm in which the AV fistula is created. Avoid activities and movements that can occlude blood flow at the AV fistula site. Patients receiving dialysis treatments benefit from education and practice on energy conservation techniques (refer to Appendix D for suggestions).

Monitoring Dietary Requirements During Occupational Therapy Sessions

Occupational therapists should be sensitive to all patients' diet requirements. Check with the nursing staff and confirm patients' diet requirements in their charts. Use this information when performing meal and eating activities with the patients. Do not assume a patient may have fluids or water during a therapy session. Intake and output (often referred to as *I&O*) are routinely monitored for most patients. During toileting tasks, urine may need to be collected, measured, and recorded in the chart. Check with nursing on any questions about collecting and recording the urine for a specific patient before toileting tasks.

References

Chronic renal failure. (2005). In *Pathophysiology: A 2 in 1 reference for nurses* (pp. 533–538). Philadelphia: Lippincott Williams & Wilkins.

Fichandler, D., & Malone, D. J. (2006). Genitourinary diseases and disorders. In D. J. Malone & K. L. B. Lindsay (Eds.), *Physical therapy in acute care: A clinician's guide* (pp. 477–502). Thorofare, NJ: Slack.

Follin, S. A., & Lenker, D. P. (Eds.). (2004). Renal failure, chronic. In *Handbook of diseases* (3rd ed., pp. 714–719). Philadelphia; Lippincott Williams & Wilkins.

Gray, H. (1974). The urinary organs. In T. Pickering Pick & R. Howden (Eds.), *Gray's anatomy* (pp. 985–1014). Philadelphia: Running Press.

Langford, S., Slivar, S., Tucker, S., & Bourbonnais, F. (2008). Exploring CRRT practices in ICU: A survey of Canadian hospitals. *Canadian Association of Critical Care Nurses, 19*, 18–23.

National Kidney and Urologic Diseases Information Clearinghouse. (2006). *Treatment methods for kidney failure: Peritoneal dialysis.* Bethesda, MD: National Institute of Diabetes and Digestive and Kidney Diseases. Retrieved May 31, 2009, from http://kidney.niddk.nih.gov/kudiseases/pubs/peritoneal/#how

National Kidney Foundation. (2009). *Warning signs of kidney and urinary tract diseases.* Retrieved March 22, 2009, from www.kidney.org/atoz/content/warning.cfm

Patel, P. (2008). *End-stage kidney disease.* Retrieved May 31, 2009, from www.nlm.nih.gov/medlineplus/ency/article/000500.htm

Paz, J. C. (2009). Genitourinary system. In J. C. Paz & M. P. West (Eds.), *Acute care handbook for physical therapists* (pp. 327–351). St. Louis, MO: W. B. Saunders.

Prostrate Cancer Foundation. (2010). *Frequently asked questions about prostrate cancer.* Retrieved October 29, 2010, from www.pcf.org/site/c.leJRIROrEpH/b.5800851/k.645A/Prostate_Cancer_FAQs.htm

Ramakrishnan, K., & Mold, J. W. (2005). Urinary catheters: A review. *Internet Journal of Family Practice, 3*(2). Retrieved May 31, 2009, from http://www.ispub.com/ostia/index.php?xmlFilePath=journals/ijfp/vol3n2/urinary.xml

Recent evidence suggests. (2004). Benign prostatic hyperplasia. In *Handbook of diseases* (3rd ed., pp. 91–94). Philadelphia: Lippincott Williams & Wilkins.

Stoller, M. L., Kane, C. J., & Carroll, P. R. (2007). Urology. In S. J. McPhee, M. A. Papadakis, & L. M. Tierney, Jr. (Eds.), *Current medical diagnosis and treatment* (pp. 954–997). New York: McGraw-Hill.

Watnick, S., & Morrison, G. (2007). Kidney. In S. J. McPhee, M. A. Papadakis, & L. M. Tierney, Jr. (Eds.), *Current medical diagnosis and treatment* (pp. 918–953). New York: McGraw-Hill.

11

Oncology

Helene Smith-Gabai, OTD, OTR/L, BCPR

Hearing a diagnosis of cancer is emotionally distressing because it is usually associated with severe disease and death. Cancer is the second leading cause of death in the United States after heart disease ("Cancer," 2007; Shelton, Lipoma, & Oertli, 2008). Cancer occurs in more than 100 forms. It is a disease in which cells are characterized by abnormal growth and division, often traveling to distant organs or tissues through the circulatory or lymphatic systems (Mailoo & Williams, 2004; Oertli, 2007). If untreated, cancer cells continue to grow into a benign or malignant tumor (Cooper, 2006). *Oncology* is the branch of medicine that deals with the diagnosis, treatment, and prevention of cancer.

Cancer death rates have declined steadily over the past 30 years as a result of earlier detection, constantly improving treatment options, and heightened public awareness about prevention and screening (American Cancer Society [ACS], 2010a). Despite a half-million cancer deaths per year, this decreased mortality rate indicates an overall increase in cancer survivors ("Cancer," 2006). *Cancer survivors* are people with any type of cancer, past or present, who are still living. American cancer survivors number more than 11 million, with more than 1.5 million new cases estimated for 2010 (ACS, 2010a). However, cancer remains a life-threatening disease with profound implications for patients and their families (Lyons, 2006). Generally, the earlier cancer is detected and treated, the better the prognosis is.

Because patients are surviving longer, they continue to deal with the prolonged side effects of cancer treatments (Cooper, 2006; Purcell, Fleming, Haines, & Bennett, 2009). Cancer is increasingly being viewed as a chronic condition requiring a chronic disease management approach, including new physical and emotional support strategies (Taylor & Currow, 2003).

A variety of approaches are used in treating cancer, which include, but are not limited to, radiation, chemotherapy, surgery, hormone therapy, and targeted therapy (ACS, 2010a). Any approach to cancer treatment has to be holistic, addressing the patient's physical, mental, emotional, and spiritual needs, and requires sensitivity and compassion on the part of health care providers (Shelton et al., 2008). Cancer can interfere with occupational performance, disrupting roles and routines and affecting self-identity, self-esteem, and quality of life. One of the challenges of working with cancer patients is that patients face occupational challenges not only from the disease, but also from the cancer treatments themselves (Cooper & Littlechild, 2004; Taylor & Currow, 2003).

Risk Factors

Intrinsic and extrinsic risk factors predispose a person to develop cancer. *Intrinsic factors* are those risk factors over which the person has no control, whereas *extrinsic factors* may be modifiable and preventable.

Intrinsic Factors

Intrinsic factors can include age, heredity, hormones, immune system competence, and metabolic abnormalities (ACS, 2010a). These factors, individually or sequentially, can increase the risk of developing a cancerous condition.

Age
The incidence of cancer increases with age. More than 77% of cancers are detected in adults older than age 55 (ACS, 2010a). It is generally believed that cumulative insults or repeated exposures may be a factor in increased cancer incidence in the aging population ("Cancer," 2006).

Heredity

Only a small percentage of cancers are the result of heredity (approximately 5%); most are a result of gene mutation or damage that occurs during a person's lifetime (ACS, 2010a).

Hormones

Levels of sex hormones (e.g., estrogen, progesterone, testosterone) are linked to the development of breast, ovarian, endometrial, and prostate cancers ("Cancer," 2006). Prostate cancer is the most common form of cancer in men, and breast cancer is the most common form of cancer in women (Shelton et al., 2008).

Immune System Competence

A compromised immune system (e.g., HIV, transplant organ recipient) has been linked to increased risk of cancer. When the immune system does not recognize cancer cells as foreign bodies, it does not respond to them, which allows cancer cells to continue proliferating until the immune system can no longer destroy them ("Cancer," 2007).

Metabolic Abnormalities

Obesity and diabetes have been linked to increased risk of colorectal cancer (Stürmer, Buring, Lee, Gaziano, & Glynn, 2006).

Extrinsic Factors

Extrinsic factors are those that can be controlled for or are preventable. These risk factors fall into three general categories: the environment, occupation, and lifestyle. Most cancers result from extrinsic causes.

Environment

The environment is a large source of carcinogens, for example,

- *Ionizing radiation:* X-rays, radon, uranium. Exposure to X-rays is associated with cancers of the breast, lung, thyroid, stomach, colon, and urinary tract; leukemia; and multiple myeloma ("Cancer," 2006).
- *Solar radiation:* Ultraviolet B radiation damages the DNA of skin cells ("Cancer," 2007).

- *Air pollution:* Has links to lung cancer. Indoor air pollutants (e.g., cigarette smoke, radon) are considered more harmful than outdoor air pollution ("Cancer," 2006, 2007).
- *Chemicals:* Exposure to pesticides, diesel exhaust, nicotine, benzene, nitrates, asbestos, wood dust, and polyvinyl chloride.
- *Irritants:* Can include tobacco tar, asbestos, wood, coal, and leather dust.
- *Viruses and infections:* May include Epstein–Barr virus, HIV, hepatitis B virus, human papillomavirus, and *Helicobacter pylori* (*H. pylori*).

Occupation

Various occupations can significantly increase a person's exposure to environmental carcinogens. For example, shipyard workers and firefighters are more likely to be exposed to asbestos (mesothelioma). Leather- and woodworkers are more likely to be exposed to leather and wood dust, miners to coal dust, tire plant workers to carbon black, and farm workers and exterminators to pesticides ("Cancer," 2006). Bladder cancer is linked to people who manufacture rubber paint and dyes.

Lifestyle

Lifestyle factors are the most preventable risk factors for cancer. Lifestyle choices such as alcohol intake, sunbathing and tanning booth use, use of tobacco products, sexual practices, and dietary choices can contribute to a person's risk of developing cancer. For example, alcohol consumption has been associated with liver (developed from cirrhosis), breast, and colorectal cancer ("Cancer," 2006). Environmental exposure to ultraviolet rays has been directly linked to skin cancers (basal cell and squamous cell carcinomas). The number of severe sunburns also compromises the system because the greater the number of sunburns, the greater the risk for developing skin cancer.

Smokers have a 10 times greater risk of developing lung cancer than nonsmokers. This risk is directly related to duration and frequency: How long the person has been smoking, and how many cigarettes he or she smokes a day. Even chewing tobacco has been associated with oral cancers. Tobacco has been linked to 30% of all cancer deaths and 87% of lung cancer deaths (ACS, 2010a). However, that risk is reduced if the smoker quits. The number of sexual partners or being in a relationship with someone who has had multiple sexual partners increases a woman's risk of developing cervical cancer. Hormonal drugs, such as birth control pills, estrogen replacement, and anabolic steroids, are additional risk factors. Obesity and physical inactivity have also been linked to increased cancer risk (ACS, 2010a; Shelton et al., 2008).

Many cancers are preventable by changing one's lifestyle, including wearing sunscreen or limiting exposure to ultraviolet sunlight, avoiding tanning beds, not smoking, avoiding foods containing nitrates, eating a healthy diet, and early cancer screenings. One of the challenges in addressing the causal links between carcinogenic substances and cancer is that cancer can take many years to manifest between exposure and development (ACS, 2010a). Table 11.1 lists

Table 11.1. **American Cancer Society Screening Guide**

Site	Recommendation
Breast	• Annual mammogram, beginning at age 40 • Breast self-examination, beginning at age 20 • Screening MRI for women with a 20%–25% lifetime risk of breast cancer; family history of breast or ovarian cancer; women treated for Hodgkin's disease • Clinical breast exam every 3 years for women < age 40; annually for women > age 40
Colon and rectum	Beginning at age 50, one of these methods should be chosen: • FSIG every 5 years • Annual fecal occult blood test or fecal immunochemical test • A combination of a FSIG with either a FOBT or a FIT is preferable over either test by itself • Double contrast barium enema every 5 years • Colonoscopy every 10 years
Prostate	• Beginning at age 50, annual rectal exam and PSA test • Beginning at age 45, people at high risk
Uterus (cervix)	• 3 years after beginning intercourse or after age 21, pap smear every year • At or after age 30, with 3 normal tests in a row, can be screened every 2–3 years • After age 70, with 3 normal pap smears within 10 years, no longer have to be screened for cervical cancer • High-risk patients (HIV or weak immune system) may need to be screened more frequently • After hysterectomy, screening no longer necessary unless hysterectomy was because of cervical cancer

Note. FIT = fecal immunochemical test; FOBT = fecal occult blood test; FSIG = flexible sigmoidoscopy; PSA = protein-specific antigen.

Source. American Cancer Society. (2010). *Cancer facts and figures 2010* (p. 62). Retrieved September 14, 2010, from http://www.cancer.org/acs/groups/content/@nho/documents/document/acspc-024113.pdf. Copyright © 2010 by American Cancer Society. Adapted with permission.

the American Cancer Society's recommended guidelines for cancer screening.

Cell Growth

Normal cell division is orderly and controlled. It is also programmed so that the cells that die off balance new cell formation (Packel, 2006). As normal cells develop, they differentiate or become specialized for a specific function and with a specific structure ("Cancer," 2007). The immune system usually protects the body from cancerous cells. However, if the body's immune system is compromised or loses its ability to stop the growth of mutated cells, then cancer develops (Shelton et al., 2008).

Many mechanisms may cause an abnormality in cell reproduction, growth, and differentiation. Hormones, growth factor, infection, and inflammation are factors that can affect cell growth. When a mutation occurs, normal cells can change to cancer cells. These new cells differ from the original cell, in that they lose the ability to differentiate and function differently than their cell of origination.

The approximately 100 cancer genes are called *oncogenes*. These genes are either *proto-oncogenes* (cancer-causing genes) or *anti-oncogenes* (genes that suppress tumor development). Proto-oncogenes and impaired anti-oncogenes transform normal cells into malignant cells ("Cancer," 2006). Tumor cells may also release

substances (e.g., enzymes, antigens, hormones) that are biologic markers indicative of cancer presence (Gould, 2006). Tumor markers are used to screen those at high risk for cancer, to diagnose certain cancers, to monitor response to treatments, or to detect recurrence ("Cancer," 2007). These tumor markers may be found on the cells of tumors, in the bloodstream, in cerebrospinal fluid, or in urine ("Cancer," 2007).

Cancer cells share various characteristics: (1) They undergo abnormal mitosis, (2) their function is abnormal and does not resemble the cells of origin, (3) they are not encapsulated, and (4) they can travel to other sites ("Cancer," 2007). The growth of cancer cells is disorderly and rapid and tends to be aggressive. Tumors grow like normal cells and require a blood supply, oxygen, and nutrients but grow at a much faster rate, replacing and destroying normal cells ("Cancer," 2006, 2007).

Not all abnormal cells are malignant. *Dyplasia* is a reversible condition in which cells change in response to various conditions and agents. If untreated, dysplasia can progress to malignancy (Goodman, 2009). Table 11.2 compares the characteristics of both benign and malignant cancer cells. Tumors may also cause tissue death by growing large enough to impair or block the blood supply of neighboring tissue ("Cancer," 2006). Unlike normal cells, cancer cells lack "contact inhibition" and do not stop dividing when they touch other cells (Packel, 2006).

Table 11.2.   Characteristics of Benign and Malignant Tumors

Characteristic	Benign Tumors	Malignant Tumors
Potential to metastasize	No	Yes; may invade surrounding tissues or spread to distant sites via blood circulation, the lymph system, or both
Encapsulated	Yes	No
Morphologically typical of tissue of origin	Yes	No
Rate of growth	Slow	Unpredictable
Recurrence after surgical removal	Rare	Common

Metastasis

When cancerous cells are malignant, they no longer divide normally. Cancer cells that travel to different locations in the body are known as *metastases*. As cancer cells continue to grow and develop at the primary site, they can become invasive, infiltrating neighboring tissue. Cancerous cells can also spread by penetrating nearby blood vessels and the lymphatic system, breaking off and traveling to a distant secondary site and invading other tissues and organs ("Cancer," 2007). In addition, cancerous cells can be transported externally from one site to another within the same person via surgical tools or gloves ("Cancer," 2006, 2007). Table 11.3 lists primary organs and common metastasis sites.

Table 11.3. **Metastasis, by Primary Site**

Primary Site	Metastasis
Bladder	• Lungs • Liver • Other pelvic organs • Bone
Breast	• Bone • Lung • Liver • Axillary lymph nodes • Brain
Colon/rectum	• Liver • Lung • Bone • Brain • Peritoneum
Esophagus	• Bone • Lung • Liver • Nodes
Head and neck	• Lung
Kidney	• Lung • Bone
Lung	• Bone • Adrenal glands • Liver • Brain • Spinal cord

(continued)

Table 11.3.   (continued)

Primary Site	Metastasis
Melanoma	• Bone • Lung • Liver • Lymph nodes • Brain
Ovaries	• Lung • Liver • Peritoneum • Diaphragm
Pancreas	• Liver • Lung • Bone • Brain
Prostate	• Bone • Lung • Brain
Stomach	• Liver • Lung
Testicles	• Liver • Lung
Uterus	• Lung • Other pelvic organs

Note. The most common metastasis sites are bone, lungs, liver, and lymph nodes.
Sources. ACS (2010c), "Cancer" (2007).

Staging and Classification

Staging is important in determining the extent and spread of cancer to other parts of the body of the individual patient. It is used in determining prognosis and treatment and based on tumor size and location and whether the cancer has metastasized from one organ to another. The Union Internationale Contre le Cancer and the American Joint Committee on Cancer developed the TNM system in staging cancer ("TNM Staging System," 2010). The TNM system is outlined in Box 11.1. Once the T, N, and M are determined, an overall stage number of 0, I, II, III, or IV is given. The higher the stage number is, the more severe the disease and the higher the degree of differentiation from normal cells.

For example, *Stage I* indicates early disease in which cancer is present and cells are well differentiated but have not spread. *Stage IV* indicates advanced disease in which tumors are

---

Box 11.1. The TNM System

T Is for Tumor

- The *T* category describes the primary tumor.
- *TX:* Tumor cannot be evaluated (cannot be measured or found).
- *T0:* No evidence of primary tumor.
- *Tis:* Cancer in situ (i.e., tumor has not started growing into surrounding tissue or structures).
- *T1–T4:* Describes the size, level of invasion, or both. The higher the *T* number, the larger and more invasive the tumor is considered.

N Is for Node

- The *N* category describes lymph node involvement.
- *NX:* Nearby lymph nodes cannot be evaluated.
- *N0:* Nearby lymph node does not contain cancer.
- *N1–N3:* Describes size, location, number of lymph node involvement, or all of these. The greater the *N* is, the greater the lymph node involvement.

M Is for Metastasis

- The *M* category indicates the presence of metastases.
- *MX:* Metastasis cannot be evaluated.
- *M0:* No known distant metastases.
- *M1:* Distant metastases are present.

Source. TNM staging system (2010).

poorly differentiated with infiltration to other tissues and lymph nodes. Stage IV is associated with aggressive fatal tumors (Polich & Paz, 2009). Tumors can also be classified as in situ (in their original location), local, regional, or distant (ACS, 2010a; National Cancer Institute [NCI], 2009).

Although the TNM designation is used with many forms of cancer, it is not used for all. For instance, cell type is used to grade the severity of brain and spinal cord tumors. The Ann Arbor staging classification (presented later in Table 11.7) is used for staging lymphoma; at present, no staging system exists for leukemia (NCI, 2008). Staging and classification are referred to as *stage grouping,* and they assist in providing information on prognosis and tumor aggressiveness. This information can help guide the direction of intervention provided by occupational therapists.

Signs and Symptoms of Cancer

According to the American Cancer Society, the 7 cancer warning signs that should prompt people to seek medical attention are

- Change in bowel or bladder habits
- *A* sore throat that does not heal
- *Unusual* bleeding or discharge
- *Thickening* or lump in breast or elsewhere
- *Indigestion* or difficulty swallowing
- *Obvious* change in a wart or mole
- *Nagging* cough or hoarseness ("Cancer," 2006, 2007).

Patients may be asymptomatic initially, but as the cancer progresses certain symptoms become more apparent. These symptoms generally include cachexia, infection, pain, fatigue, and blood count abnormalities (e.g., anemia, thrombocytopenia, leukopenia; "Cancer," 2006, 2007):

- *Cachexia:* A physical wasting syndrome in which the patient appears emaciated. Malignant cells confiscate nutrients, blood, and oxygen from normal cells, leading to normal tissue starvation and wasting. Patients may also experience anorexia (loss of appetite), altered taste sensation, mucositis, nausea, and vomiting as a side effect of cancer treatments (e.g., chemotherapy). *Mucositis* is the inflammation of the mucous membranes of the gastrointestinal (GI) tract, which makes eating difficult, painful, or both. Cooper (2006) recommended addressing anorexia and mucositis by eating smaller, more frequent meals, determining which food textures are easiest for patients to chew and swallow, adapting feeding utensils, and maintaining good oral hygiene.

- *Infection:* Malnutrition, anemia, and immunosuppression resulting from cancer treatments increase the risk of infection. For example, pneumonia may develop because of physical inactivity, a weak cough reflex, and impaired ability to clear secretions (Gould, 2006).

- *Pain:* Refer to "Cancer Pain" section.

- *Fatigue:* Refer to "Cancer-Related Fatigue" section.

- *Blood count disorders:* Anemia may be caused by hematological cancers or chronic bleeding, or it may be a side effect of cancer treatments (e.g., chemotherapy, radiation therapy). Leukopenia and thrombocytopenia may also be secondary to cancer treatments or cancer with bone marrow involvement. Therapists should verify patient blood counts before treating because leukopenia indicates increased risk of infection, and thrombocytopenia indicates increased risk of bleeding.

Cancer Pain

Chronic pain is present in 50%–70% of patients with early disease and 60%–90% of patients with advanced disease (Cohen, 2005; Goodman, 2009). Pain may be a consequence of bone or tissue destruction, visceral surface stretching, cord compression, collapse of vertebra, nerve inflammation, or immobility ("Cancer," 2007; Goodman, 2009; Packel, 2006).

Pain management strategies may include massage, acupuncture, guided imagery, relaxation training, cryotherapy, thermotherapy, electrical stimulation, biofeedback, or use of pain medications (Goodman, 2009). For those patients using physical agent modalities, always check with the physician to be sure that thermal or electrical modalities are not contraindicated for the type of cancer being treated. Refer to Table 11.4 for the etiology and symptoms of cancer-related pain. According to Barsevick, Newhall, and Brown (2008), pain can also contribute to cancer-related fatigue (CRF).

Cancer-Related Fatigue

CRF is one of the most commonly experienced symptoms of cancer (Oertli, 2007; Purcell et al., 2009; Wang, 2008). CRF affects 70%–100% of cancer patients and may manifest as exhaustion, drowsiness, difficulty with concentration, or feelings of depression and weakness (Packel, 2006). CRF differs from regular fatigue in that it does not correspond to levels of exertion and is not relieved by rest (Purcell et al., 2009). Approximately 30% of cancer survivors report continued problems with fatigue even years after undergoing cancer treatment (Goodman, 2009). Radiation-related fatigue peaks 4 weeks after treatment, and chemotherapy-related fatigue peaks 4–5 days after infusion but may return with each new cycle of chemotherapy (Packel, 2006).

The exact mechanism of CRF is unknown. However, it has been linked to the disease process itself, medical treatments (e.g., chemotherapy, radiation therapy, biologic response modifiers, hormone therapy), infection, other comorbidities, or other cancer-related symptoms (e.g., pain, emotional distress, sleeping disorders, anemia, deconditioning, malnutrition; Barsevick et al., 2008; Packel, 2006;

Table 11.4. **Cancer-Related Pain**

Type	Descriptors	Possible Etiology	Exam
Neuropathic pain	• Tingling • Burning • Numbness • Shocklike • Intermittent • Constant	• Tumor adjacent to or adhered to peripheral nerves • Vertebral collapse causing nerve compression • Radiation fibrosis, causing tissue adherence to nerve	• Motor weakness • Altered sensation • (+) neural tension tests • Pain along a myotome or dermatome • Numbness/tingling in distal fingertips and toes
Skeletal pain	• Sharp • Intermittent or constant • Escalating back pain • Pain in supine • Pain with ambulation • Pain in groin with standing	• Altered bone stability • Cord compression • Avascular necrosis	• Pain with weightbearing • Pain with joint compression • Pain that radiates to groin/anterior thigh with weightbearing • Pain in a band across chest • Pain with coughing
Joint pain	• Pain with functional activity • Ache	• Tumor encroaching joint space • Neupogen pain • Arthralgia syndrome associated with Taxanes	• Possible palpation of tumor • Pain with passive and active ROM
Postsurgical pain	• Pain with coughing • Pain with mobility • Sharp • Constant ache • Intermittent or chronic	• Positioning during surgery • Manipulation of nerves during surgery • Altered biomechanics from nerve palsy • Muscle spasm from positioning	• Pain along surgical site • Tingling along nerve distribution • Pain with deep inspiration

(*continued*)

Type	Descriptors	Possible Etiology	Exam
Soft tissue pain	• Ache • Stiffness with movement	• Radiation fibrosis • Soft tissue changes from graft-vs.-host disease • Contracture from immobility • Protective muscle spasm	• Reproduction of symptoms with passive stretching • Decreased skin elasticity • (+) trigger points • Decreased passive or active ROM

Source. Reprinted with permission from SLACK Incorporated: Malone D. J., & Lindsay, K. L. B, 2006, *Physical Therapy in Acute Care: A Clinician's Guide.* Thorofare, NJ: SLACK Incorporated.

Wang, 2008). The National Comprehensive Cancer Network and the Oncology Nursing Society have both established guidelines for managing CRF. However, these guidelines differ on the basis of where the patient is in the course of his or her disease (i.e., receiving active treatment, long-term follow-up, or nearing end of life; Barsevick et al., 2008).

Deconditioning as a result of the disease or the treatment of cancer is a common issue in cancer therapy (Crannell & Stone, 2008). Bedside treatments may be appropriate to maximize patient endurance and engagement in occupations and activities. According to Barsevick et al. (2008), evidence has shown that exercise (e.g., aerobic, interval, strengthening) is an effective approach to CRF. However, they urge caution for patients who are neutropenic or have bone metastases, anemia, or low platelet counts.

CRF can have a profound effect on the ability to engage in occupations and on quality of life. Therapy focuses on energy conservation, aerobic activity, stress reduction, and relaxation techniques (Barsevick et al., 2008; Packel, 2006). Education, counseling, and addressing the underlying causes of fatigue (e.g., pain, insomnia, emotional distress) can help alleviate symptoms and help patients cope with CRF (Barsevick et al., 2008). In planning interventions, adapting activities, and modifying tasks and the environment, therapists need to consider the contexts in which CRF occurs and the patient's response and recovery.

Types of Cancer

This section provides a brief review of the most common cancers, including the breast, lung, skin, the gastrointestinal and genitourinary systems, and hematological cancers, head and neck cancer, soft tissue and bone cancer, and cancerous tumors of the brain and spinal cord are also discussed.

Breast Cancer

Breast cancer is more prevalent in women (99%) than in men and is one of the most common cancers among American women (Cohen, 2005; Packel, 2006). It is estimated that in 2010 more than 207,000 women and almost 2,000 men will develop breast cancer (ACS, 2010a).

Breast cancer is initially asymptomatic and usually detected with a mammogram; however, breast abnormalities or lumps may be identified through thorough self-examination. As the disease progresses, the patient may experience changes in the breast tissue (e.g., thickening, swelling, redness) or discharge (ACS, 2010a). Risk factors for breast cancer include age, heredity, obesity, use of oral contraceptives, never having children or first child after age 30, hormone replacement therapy, sedentary lifestyle, and alcohol consumption (ACS, 2010a). However, maintaining a healthy body weight, remaining physically active, and breastfeeding are all associated with lowered risk (ACS, 2010a).

In addition to the general symptoms of cancer and cancer-related treatments, breast cancer has many psychological and physical issues. Self-esteem and body image may be altered because of the emotional distress, disfigurement, losing a breast, or disability. Symptoms of breast cancer can include fatigue; pain; chemotherapy-induced peripheral neuropathy; radiation-induced brachial plexopathy; lymphedema; hot flashes; depression; anxiety; shortness of breath (from secondary lung tumors); pathological fractures (from secondary bone tumors); and the neurological, cognitive, sensory, and perceptual deficits associated with central nervous system involvement (Vockins, 2004). Breast cancer may form in the ducts or lobules. The five types of breast cancer are defined in Table 11.5.

Medical management of breast cancer can include chemotherapy, radiation, hormone therapy, and surgical intervention, depending on the type and location of the tumor. Chemotherapy and radiation may be used first to decrease tumor size or determine the most effective type of follow-up radiation or chemotherapy. However, radiation carries the risk of brachial plexopathy, a rare side effect of radiation treatment that can result in nerve and tissue injury secondary to lymphedema constriction of the brachial plexus (Cooper, 2006). Symptoms of brachial plexopathy may present even years after radiation therapy has been completed (Cooper, 2006).

Common types of surgical intervention for breast cancer include lumpectomy, partial mastectomy or segmental mastectomy, subcutaneous mastectomy, simple or total mastectomy, modified radical mastectomy, and radical mastectomy (see Table 11.6). After surgical removal of the tumor, people may choose to have reconstructive surgery, which is used to correct an acquired defect from surgical removal of the tumor or breast and to improve quality of life. In preparation for breast reconstruction, a patient may have tissue expanders placed to stretch the remaining tissue and underlying muscle for future breast reconstruction. Tissue

Table 11.5. **Types of Breast Cancer**

Type	Definition
Ductal carcinoma in situ	Early form of noninvasive breast cancer. Abnormal cells grow within the milk ducts of the breast.
Lobular carcinoma in situ	Abnormal growth of cells within the milk-producing glands of the breast.
Invasive ductal carcinoma	Most common form of breast cancer in which cancer cells form within the lining of the milk duct, break through the ductal wall, and invade nearby breast tissue. Can spread to the lymph nodes, and other parts of the body.
Invasive lobular carcinoma	Cancer begins in the lobules but breaks through and invades surrounding breast tissue. Can spread to the lymph nodes, and other parts of the body.
Inflammatory breast cancer	Aggressive but rare form of cancer in which cancer cells block the lymph vessels of the breast. Breast often appears inflamed (red and swollen).

Table 11.6.   Types of Surgical Intervention for Breast Cancer

Type	Body Tissue Removed
Radical mastectomy	Breast tissue, skin, pectoralis major and minor, rib, and lymph nodes (Levels 1, II, and III)
Modified radical mastectomy	Breast, skin, and axillary lymph nodes (Levels I and II)
Simple or total mastectomy	The whole breast with the possibility of a sentinel node biopsy in a later procedure
Subcutaneous mastectomy	Entire breast, but the nipple and areola are spared
Prophylactic mastectomy	The entire breast without the presence of cancer
Partial mastectomy or segmental mastectomy	Tumor and surrounding wedge of tissue to clear margins. Complete axillary node dissection is performed when a sentinel node biopsy is positive
Lumpectomy	Tumor, margin of healthy surrounding tissue, sentinel lymph node biopsy (complete axillary node dissection is performed after a positive sentinel lymph node biopsy)

Sources. Feledy, Hanasono, and Robb (2006); Hunt, Newman, Copelan, and Bland (2009).

expanders consist of a silicone balloon filled with saline. The expander is placed below the pectoralis major muscle. Saline is then added during routine visits to the plastic surgeon until the desired size has been achieved in preparation for the permanent breast implants. The most commonly used types of reconstruction are *transverse rectus abdominus myocutaneous (TRAM) flap, deep inferior epigastric perforator (DIEP) flap,* and *latissimus dorsi myocutaneous (LDMF) flap.* Reconstructive surgery may be immediate or delayed.

Lymph node involvement is an important issue after surgery because of complications that may arise from the removal of lymph nodes. This involvement will also affect how occupational therapists educate patients on postsurgical precautions for lifelong lymphedema management. Patients can experience impaired hand function, brachial plexopathy, and chronic pain with lymph node resection that can result in immobility and limited range of motion (ROM; Cooper & Littlechild, 2004; Nesbit, 2004). Surgeons will often complete a

sentinel lymph node biopsy for the involved side, and sometimes the uninvolved side, to check for any positive lymph node involvement. The type of postsurgical intervention will be dependent on the type, size, and location of the tumor.

When the lymphatic system is compromised by the removal of lymph nodes, it can lead to *lymphedema,* which is a buildup of lymph fluid in tissue, resulting in swelling of the arm, chest, or breast. Lymphedema management requires special training. Lymphedema treatment may consist of manual lymphatic drainage therapy, fitting patients for special compression garments, educating patients on how to bandage with lymphedema bandages, self-massage, instruction in a home exercise program, and general precautions (e.g., avoiding infection; Cohen, 2005). Refer to Appendix 6.A for a list of general precautions for patients at risk for lymphedema.

After reconstructive surgery that involves a DIEP or TRAM flap reconstruction, the person is instructed to walk flexed forward at the waist to a 45° angle to protect the incision site, anastomosis, and muscles. A rolling walker may be necessary for initial support. Generally, patients are restricted from lifting more than 10 pounds on the ipsilateral side to prevent lymphedema and to protect the integrity of blood vessels, muscles, and tissue involved in the surgical procedure.

Postsurgical interventions for patients with postoperative drains include active range of motion to 90° shoulder flexion and abduction of the ipsilateral side to protect surgical incisions. People may reach overhead, but high repetitious movements at that level are not encouraged because it increases the output in the postsurgical drains. However, normal functional movement is encouraged.

Precautions for Breast Surgery and Reconstruction

- DIEP and TRAM flap.
- Walk in a flexed-forward position.
- Use "beach chair" positioning while sitting; back may be reclined, but hips (flexed 90° or greater) and knees should be flexed.
- Log roll when getting out of bed to avoid straining abdominal muscles.
- Limit abdominal muscle movement with out-of-bed and daily activities.
- Avoid scapular retraction.
- Avoid high repetitious bilateral movement of the upper extremities until cleared by the physician. Consult with physician regarding any other ROM limitations or precautions.
- Observe weight-lifting restrictions of 5–10 pounds on the ipsilateral side.

Precautions for Bilateral Mastectomy With Spacers

- Avoid scapular retraction.
- Avoid high repetitious bilateral movements of the upper extremity until drains are removed.

In addition, therapists can assist patients with positioning, adaptive equipment, sensory stimulation, compression garments, relaxation and stress management techniques, and therapeutic touch (Cohen, 2005).

Lung Cancer

The National Cancer Institute (2009) estimates that approximately 222,000 new cases and 157,000 deaths from *lung cancer* will occur in the United States in 2010. Lung cancer, which is often undiagnosed until advanced, is the leading cause of cancer death, even exceeding breast cancer in women (ACS, 2010a). *Small-cell lung cancer* and *non–small-cell lung cancer* are the two major types of lung cancer. Of the two, small-cell lung cancer grows rapidly and has a poorer prognosis (Packel, 2006). Non–small-cell lung cancer accounts for 85% of lung cancers and consists of three types: *squamous cell carcinoma, adenocarcinoma,* and *large-cell undifferentiated carcinoma* (Politch & Paz 2009).

By far the greatest risk factor for lung cancer is tobacco, which increases with frequency and duration. Additional risk factors include exposure to toxic heavy metals (e.g., cadmium, arsenic, chromium), asbestos (a mineral fiber), radon (a radioactive gas), radiation, organic chemicals, air pollution, and secondhand smoke and a history of tuberculosis (ACS, 2010a; NCI, 2009). Symptoms of lung cancer include cough, dyspnea, recurrent pneumonia or bronchitis, chest pain, hemoptysis, fever, and weight loss (ACS, 2010a; "Cancer," 2007; Polich & Paz, 2009).

Lung cancer is diagnosed on the basis of the appearance of abnormal cells, using a microscope. These cells may be retrieved from a sputum sample, bronchoscopy, fine-needle aspiration, or thoracentesis (NCI, 2009). X-ray, positron emission tomography, and computed tomography scans are also used diagnostically. Treatment for lung cancer may include chemotherapy, radiation, surgery, or biotherapies. Surgery is the predominant treatment approach and may include pneumonectomy, lobectomy, lung wedge resection, or pleurectomy (Polich & Paz, 2009). Laser therapy and photodynamic therapy have been identified by the NCI (2009) as additional forms of treatment.

In addition, the University of Texas M. D. Anderson Cancer Center (UTMDACC), a preeminent cancer center, uses proton therapy for the treatment of lung cancer (UTMDACC, 2010a). The benefit of photodynamic and proton therapy is that they cause minimal damage to healthy tissue. According to Morris et al. (2009), evidence has also shown that participation in a pulmonary rehabilitation program is beneficial to patients with primary lung cancer or pulmonary symptoms (e.g., dyspnea, fatigue, limited activity tolerance) associated with other forms of cancer or cancer treatments. Refer to Chapter 5 for more information on pulmonary rehabilitation.

Regardless of treatment options, lung cancer has no known cure. The 5-year survival rate for most lung cancers is only 16% (ACS, 2010a; Shelton et al., 2008).

Skin Cancer

Skin cancer is the most commonly diagnosed form of cancer in the United States. However, nearly all skin cancer can be successfully treated with early detection (UTMDACC, 2009). The ACS (2010a) estimates more than 68,000 new cases of melanoma and more than 8,700 deaths will occur in 2010. Risk factors for all skin cancers include (ACS, 2010a; UTMDACC, 2009):

- Easily sunburned;
- Blonde or red hair;
- Excessive exposure to the sun;
- Use of tanning booths;
- History of basal cell or squamous cell carcinoma;
- Immune system disorders; and
- Occupational exposure to coal tar, pitch, arsenic, creosote, or radiation

Skin cancer occurs in multiple forms:

- *Melanoma:* Forms in the melanocytes (skin cells that make pigment).
- *Basal cell carcinoma:* Derives from epithelial cells and is the most common form of skin cancer. This carcinoma usually develops in areas exposed to sunlight. People with fair skin and light eyes are at increased risk. This carcinoma is highly curable.

- *Squamous cell carcinoma:* Arises from the squamous cells. Prolonged sun exposure is also a risk factor for this carcinoma, which is known to metastasize to the lungs, bone, lymph nodes, and brain (Polich & Paz, 2006).
- *Neuroendocrine carcinoma:* Originates from the neuroendocrine cells (cells that release hormones in response to signals from the nervous system NCI, 2008).

However, considering all types of skin cancer, melanoma has the highest rate of mortality and is the most likely to spread to other organs (UTMDACC, 2009). Signs and symptoms of melanoma include changes in the size, color, and shape of skin lesions. Risk factors for melanoma include family history, many moles (>50), and atypical moles. Children with a history of blistering sunburns are also at greater risk of developing melanoma as adults (ACS, 2010a).

The ABC warning signals of melanoma include (ACS, 2010a; UTMDACC, 2009):

- *A:* asymmetry in the mole
- *B:* border irregularity (ragged or blurred edges)
- *C:* color (uneven pigmentation)
- *D:* diameter (>6 millimeters)
- *E:* evolution (lesion that grows larger in size: height and width)
- *F:* feeling (changes in sensation at mole site).

Treatments for most skin cancers include surgical excision and, in some cases, radiation. Malignant melanoma may warrant a lymph node dissection, radiation, immunotherapy, chemotherapy, palliative surgery, or all of these, depending on the stage and progression of the disease (ACS, 2010a).

Gastrointestinal Cancer

Cancers of the GI tract include those of the esophagus, stomach, liver, pancreas, colon, and rectum (refer to Chapter 9 for more information on these organs). Cancers of the GI tract can result in malabsorption and nutritional deficiencies. Many of these cancers are initially asymptomatic and as a result are not diagnosed until at an advanced stage. Treatment may include chemotherapy, radiation, surgery, or a combination.

Esophagus

Risk factors for esophageal cancer include smoking, alcohol, obesity, gastroesophageal reflux disease, Barrett's esophagus, achalasia, age, race, and gender. Symptoms include pain with swallowing, difficulty swallowing, hoarse voice, persistent cough, heartburn, and weight loss.

An *esophagectomy* (removal of esophageal tissue) may be performed for advanced dysplasia of the esophagus. Therapists should note that patients with esophageal cancer often have swallowing precautions or restrictions.

Stomach

Risk factors for stomach cancer include *H. pylori* infection, diet, tobacco, obesity, type A blood type, pernicious anemia, Epstein–Barr virus, heredity, age, gender, previous stomach surgery, and certain occupations (ACS, 2010b).

Surgical procedures for stomach cancer may include removal of a portion of (*sub-total* or *near-total gastrectomy*) or the entire stomach (*total gastrectomy*). Sections of the intestines may also be removed, along with portions of the stomach (e.g., *gastroduodenostomy* or *gastrojejunostomy*). After these frequently extensive surgeries, pain may limit engagement in activities of daily living (ADLs) and functional mobility.

Liver

Liver cancer may refer to *metastatic liver disease* or *hepatocellular carcinoma* (e.g., primary site). Risk factors include hepatitis, alcohol-related cirrhosis, drugs, exposure to certain chemicals, or heredity disorders. Symptoms can include abdominal pain, jaundice, ascites, and weakness.

Surgical intervention may include liver resection, tumor ablation, or transplantation. Refer to Chapter 14 for more information on liver transplantation. The survival rate is only 2% for advanced metastasized liver cancer (ACS, 2010a).

Pancreas

The ACS (2010a) estimates more than 43,000 new cases and over 36,000 deaths from *pancreatic cancer* will occur in 2010. Risk factors include tobacco use, obesity, heredity, chronic pancreatitis, and diabetes. Symptoms can include weight loss, anorexia, hyperglycemia, abdominal pain, nausea, vomiting, malaise, bloody stools, and jaundice (ACS, 2010a; "Cancer," 2006).

Surgical treatment may include a Whipple procedure (*pancreatoduodenectomy*), *distal pancreatectomy*, or *total pancreatectomy*. The prognosis for pancreatic cancer is poor. One-year survival rates are 25%, and 5-year survival rates are only 6% (ACS, 2010a).

Colon and Rectum

The ACS (2010a) estimates approximately 142,000 new cases of colon and rectal cancers and 51,000 deaths for 2010. *Colorectal cancer* is the third most common type of cancer and the most common type of GI cancer (Packel, 2006; Polich & Paz, 2009). Risk factors include age, heredity, and history of inflammatory bowel disease. Lifestyle factors include sedentary lifestyle, tobacco use, obesity, alcohol consumption, and diets rich in red and processed meats but low in fruits and vegetables (ACS, 2010a). Symptoms can include rectal bleeding, blood in stools, cramping, and changes in bowel habits (ACS, 2010a).

As with other cancers, colorectal cancer is treated by chemotherapy, radiation, and surgery. Surgical intervention for colorectal cancer may include a *colectomy, hemicolectomy,* or *perineal resection.*

Genitourinary Cancers

Genitourinary (GU) cancers include cancers of the prostate, testicles, cervix, uterus, ovaries, fallopian tubes, bladder, and kidneys. However, only the most common GU cancers (eg., prostate, cervical, bladder, kidney) are reviewed in this section. Patients with GU cancers may experience side effects from the cancer, as well as cancer treatments. These side effects can result in peripheral neuropathy, pelvic pain, lymphedema, incontinence, and sexual dysfunction (Packel, 2006).

Prostate

Prostate cancer is the second leading cause of death from cancer for men. The ACS (2010a) estimates over 217,000 new cases of prostate cancer and 32,000 deaths for 2010. The best chance for prostate cancer survival is through early detection, usually performed through a prostate-specific antigen test (PSA) and through digital rectal exam. Prostate cancer may not be diagnosed until advanced, when metastatic disease to the bone is present. Prostate cancer is usually graded using the Gleason score (i.e., 1–5 range), which microscopically compares the appearance of cancer cells to normal prostate cells. The lower the Gleason grade, the more closely cells resemble normal prostate tissue.

There are only a few identified risk factors associated with prostate cancer. These include age (>age 50), diet, heredity, race, and high testosterone levels or testosterone therapy (Mayo Clinic, 2010). Symptoms of prostate cancer include urinary problems, hematuria, blood in sperm, and lower-extremity edema.

Prostate cancer is often treated with external beam radiation therapy, radioactive seed implants (brachytherapy), hormone therapy (to reduce the production of testosterone), or radical prostatectomy (surgical removal of the prostate gland).

Cervix

For women, *cervical cancer* is one of the most common cancers of the reproductive system. Human papillomavirus, a sexually transmitted virus, is one of the known causes of cervical cancer. However, other risk factors include heredity, tobacco, a weak immune system, and certain lifestyle choices (e.g., early sexual relations, many sexual partners, history of other sexually transmitted diseases, tobacco use; ACS, 2010a; Mayo Clinic, 2010). Pap smears (or pap test) are used as a screening tool in detecting cervical cancer.

The two types of cervical cancer are *squamous cell carcinoma* and *adenocarcinoma.* Squamous cell carcinoma (the predominant type of cervical cancer) develops from the lining of the cervix, and adenocarcinoma develops from the gland cells of the cervix. Symptoms can include vaginal pain with intercourse or bleeding between periods, after intercourse, or with menopause. Most cases of cervical cancer are now prevented by a vaccine against human papillomavirus.

Cervical cancer may be treated with chemotherapy, radiation, or surgically by removing the uterus and cervix through a *total abdominal hysterectomy.* A removal of the uterus but not the cervix is called a *subtotal abdominal hysterectomy.* In a *radical hysterectomy* the cervix, uterus, and part of the vagina are removed. However, the surrounding tissue, ligaments and organs (e.g., ovaries, fallopian tubes) may also be removed. Cervical cancer has also been treated by electrocoagulation, cryotherapy, and ablation (ACS, 2010a).

Bladder

The ACS (2010a) estimates approximately 70,000 new cases of *bladder cancer* and 14,000 deaths for 2010. Risk factors for urinary cancer include smoking and working in industries such as leather, dye, or rubber manufacturing (ACS, 2010a). Symptoms include urinary tract infections, painful urination, increased frequency of urination, and hematuria.

Surgical treatment includes transurethral resection of the bladder tumor or segmental or radical cystectomy (partial or total removal of the bladder). In a *radical cystectomy,* a urinary conduit may be constructed from a piece of intestine to divert urine from the kidneys to a pouch outside the body (urostomy bag) or an internal reservoir that can be drained by a catheter through a hole in the abdomen (Mayo Clinic, 2010). The intestine may also be used to fashion an internal bladder reservoir or neobladder that allows normal urination. The 5-year survival rate for bladder cancer is 80% (ACS, 2010a).

Kidney

The most common form of *kidney cancer* is *renal cell carcinoma.* Risk factors include tobacco, obesity, hypertension, age (>age 60), gender (male), workplace chemicals, and treatment for kidney failure (e.g., long-term dialysis, immunosuppression medication for kidney transplantation; ACS, 2010a; Mayo Clinic, 2010). Symptoms include lower back pain, fatigue, weight loss, hematuria, hypertension, polycythemia, hypercalcemia, urinary retention, and pulmonary embolism resulting from obstruction of renal veins ("Cancer," 2007; Mayo Clinic, 2010). Surgical treatment for renal cancer can include partial or complete *nephrectomy* (surgical removal of the kidney).

Hematological Cancers

Cancers of the blood and stem cells include leukemia, lymphoma, and multiple myeloma. Combined, this group is responsible for 60,000 deaths annually and is the second leading cause of cancer deaths in the United States (Shelton et al., 2008).

Leukemia

Leukemia is cancer of the white blood cells or bone marrow that results in abnormal blood cell counts leading to anemia or thrombocytopenia. In the United States, approximately 43,000 new cases of leukemia and almost 22,000 deaths are estimated for 2010 (ACS, 2010a). Leukemia occurs 10 times more frequently in adults than in children (ACS, 2010a). The most common types of adult leukemia are *acute myeloid leukemia* and *chronic lymphocytic leukemia;* however, two other forms of leukemia exist, *acute lymphocytic leukemia* and *chronic myeloid leukemia.* Chronic leukemias grow and mature more slowly than acute leukemias.

Risk factors for leukemia include exposure to benzene, tobacco, radiation, or genetic disorders such as Down syndrome (Leukemia and Lymphoma Society [LLS], 2010). Symptoms of leukemia include fatigue, fever, dyspnea on exertion, paleness, bone and joint pain, edema, excessive bleeding, slow healing of cuts, low white cell counts, and increased risk of pathologic fracture and infection (LLS; Shelton et al., 2008).

Leukemia is primarily treated with chemotherapy; however, it may also be treated with bone marrow or stem cell transplantation. Refer to Chapter 14 for detail on hematopoietic transplantation.

Five-year survival rates for acute myeloid leukemia are approximately 23%; for chronic lymphocytic leukemia, 79% (ACS, 2010a). Before working with patients with leukemia, therapists are advised to verify patient blood counts and modify or defer therapy as appropriate (refer to Appendix P for blood counts and their implications).

Lymphoma

Lymphoma is cancer that begins in the cells of the immune and lymphatic systems (lymph nodes and spleen; LLS, 2010; NCI, 2008; Polich & Paz, 2009). *Hodgkin lymphoma* and *non-Hodgkin lymphoma* are two basic categories of lymphoma. The ACS (2010a) estimates approximately 74,000 new cases of lymphoma including Hodgkin and non-Hodgkin lymphoma and 21,000 deaths will occur in 2010. In lymphoma, malignant lymphocytes "crowd out" normal cells, resulting in enlarged lymph nodes (LLS, 2010).

Symptoms may include swollen lymph nodes, night sweats, itching, fatigue, weight loss, and fever (ACS, 2010a). The etiology of lymphoma is not known; however, it has been associated with increased risk from exposure to organic compounds, hepatitis C, HIV, Epstein–Barr virus, *H. pylori* (e.g., gastric lymphoma), and human T-cell lymphocytotrophic virus and in patients who with immunosuppression (e.g., organ transplant recipients; ACS, 2010a).

Lymphomas are categorized using the Ann Arbor classification system rather than the TNM staging system (see Table 11.7). Treatment includes chemotherapy, radiation, or bone marrow transplantation. One-year survival rates for Hodgkin lymphoma are 92% and non-Hodgkin lymphoma are 80%. If untreated, lymphomas are fatal because malignant cells invade organs and blood vessels, leading to infarction (Polich & Paz, 2009).

Multiple Myeloma

Multiple myeloma is cancer of the *plasma cells* (B-lymphocyte white blood cells found in bone marrow), which are responsible for producing antibodies for the immune system. It is estimated there will be more than 20,000 new cases of multiple myeloma diagnosed in 2010 (LLS, 2010).

Multiple myeloma is initially asymptomatic and progresses over a long period. Malignant cells invade bone, which may result in symptoms

Table 11.7. Ann Arbor Classification System for Lymphoma

Stage	Disease Distribution and Involvement
I	Cancer present in a single lymph node region or single extralymphatic organ or structure (e.g., spleen, Waldeyer's ring [a ring of lymphoid tissue near the tonsils], or thymus).
II	Cancer is present in two or more lymph node regions on the same side of the diaphragm, or one or more lymph node regions and one extralymphatic organ are involved on the same side of the diaphragm.
III	Cancer is present in lymph node regions, organs, or structures on both sides of diaphragm.
IV	Involvement of multiple extranodal lymphoma sites (e.g., gastrointestinal tract or skin) outside the primary site (lymph nodes or lymphatic system may or may not be involved).

Sources. Armitage (2005), Polich and Paz (2009).

of bone pain, pathologic fracture, spinal cord compression, anemia, and decreased immunity to fight infection (Mayo Clinic, 2010; Packel, 2006; Polich & Paz, 2009). Released calcium and phosphorous from destroyed bone can also result in kidney stones and renal failure (Polich & Paz, 2009).

The International Staging System is used rather than the TNM system for staging this cancer. Multiple myeloma has no cure. Treatment consists of chemotherapy, radiation, biotherapy, or bone marrow transplantation. If untreated, the prognosis is 7 months; however, with treatment this may be expanded to 2–3 years (Packel, 2006).

Occupational therapists are advised to consult with physicians before mobilizing patients at risk for pathologic fracture. If the patient has skeletal stability, weight-bearing exercises are encouraged to prevent osteopenia (Packel, 2006).

Head and Neck Cancers

Head and neck cancers may include cancers of the oral cavity (e.g., lip, tongue, mouth, salivary glands), nasal cavities, thyroid gland, and pharynx. Risk factors include smoking, using smokeless or chewing tobacco, and excessive alcohol consumption (ACS, 2010a). One-year survival rates are 83%; 5-year survival rates are 61% (ACS, 2010a).

All cancers are more successfully treated when identified early; however, symptoms of oropharyngeal cancer may not initially appear dangerous. Symptoms may include small plaquelike areas that are white or red; bleeding sores; neck mass; headaches; ear pain; coughing up blood; and difficulty swallowing, breathing, or clearing secretions (ACS, 2010a; NCI, 2005; Polich & Paz, 2009).

Treatment predominantly includes surgery and radiation. Surgical procedures may include radical neck dissection or laryngectomy. A *radial neck dissection* usually involves the lymph nodes, the internal jugular vein, sternocleidomastoid muscle, submandibular gland, and the spinal accessory nerve on one side of the neck, unless both sides are involved. If the spinal accessory nerve is not spared, the patient will experience shoulder dysfunction and weakness resulting in loss of scapular stability. Sternocleidomastoid muscle weakness can also result in decreased ability to rotate to the contralateral side.

Reconstruction surgery is important to correct disfigurement, and patients frequently need emotional support before reconstruction (Packel, 2006). Reconstructive therapy can include skin or muscle flaps or grafts. Therapy after a neck dissection may initially be deferred to allow time for wound healing (Packel, 2006).

When therapy is initiated, the focus is generally on conservative cervical ROM. However, always verify parameters and precautions with medical staff, especially plastic surgeons, before beginning therapy (see Table 11.8 for postsurgical precautions).

Sarcoma

Sarcomas are rare malignant tumors of soft tissue and bone that can be found in any part of the body (including the trunk, head, and neck areas) but are predominantly found in the lower extremities (UTMDACC, 2010c). The two main types of sarcomas are osteosarcoma (primary bone sarcoma) and soft tissue sarcoma. Primary bone tumors account for less than 1% of all cancers and can develop at any age, but they most frequently develop in those age 20 or younger. Soft tissue sarcomas are approximately 4 times more common and may come from nerve, muscle, fat, fibrous tissue, joint tissue, blood vessels, or deep skin tissues (ACS, 2009a; Shelton et al., 2008). The 5-year survival rate for soft tissue sarcomas is more than 90% if treated early (Shelton et al., 2008).

The most common types of sarcoma in adults are *malignant fibrous histiocytoma* and *liposarcoma* (tumors that arise from fat tissue) and *leiomyosarcoma* (tumors that arise from the smooth muscle tissue usually found in the abdominal cavity). Malignant fibrous histiocytomas and liposarcomas are most commonly found in the legs; leiomyosarcoma, in the abdomen (ACS, 2009b).

Some sarcomas, especially those located close to the surface of the skin, may be detected early. They can appear as a lump, which may or may not change in size or cause pain. However, tumors that are deeper in the tissue are not easily detected and may not be noticed until they become larger or present with symptoms of pain, discomfort, unexplained anemia, and blood in vomit or feces. Approximately 50% of sarcomas are detected only after they have spread. Symptoms of sarcoma include weakness, impaired circulation, edema, nerve compression, pain, limited ROM, and increased risk for pathologic fracture (Shelton et al., 2008).

The treatment of sarcoma varies by type and location. Treatment may include surgery, chemotherapy, radiation therapy, or a combination. Surgery is the most common treatment approach and may include amputation or limb preservation, both of which have high levels of patients who return to engagement in routine activities including driving, work, and sexual relations (Shelton et al., 2008). However, almost 25% of patients with sarcoma who undergo surgery have trouble with adjustment (Oertli, 2007). People treated for sarcoma can develop impairments in mobility, dependence in ADLs, and varying levels of fatigue.

Table 11.8. **Head and Neck Postsurgical Precautions**

Without Reconstruction	**With Reconstruction**
• Keep head of bed 30° or higher • Gentle neck exercises as tolerated (generally to the point of pain only)	• Keep head of bed 30° or higher • No extensive neck exercises for approximately 3 weeks • Try to keep head in a neutral position • Check weight-bearing status depending on flap site of origin (e.g., trapezius, pectoralis, forearm, fibula)

Brain and Spinal Cord Tumors

The ACS (2010a) estimates 22,000 new cases of *cancer of the brain and nervous system* and 13,000 deaths for 2010. Brain tumors may occur as a primary source or secondary to metastases. Primary brain tumors may occur in astrocytes, meninges, or nerve cells (Polich & Paz, 2009). Brain tumors are more common in adults after age 45 (Cooper, 2006). Common types of cancer that may metastasize to the brain are breast cancer, lung cancer, and melanoma. Symptoms of central nervous system cancers can include headaches, seizures, lethargy, hemiparesis, dysphasia, dysphagia, weakness, nausea, dizziness, vertigo, cranial nerve dysfunction, cognitive deficits, personality changes, and impaired sensation, coordination, or balance ("Cancer," 2007; Cooper, 2006).

Treatment usually consists of chemotherapy, radiation or surgery. The four major types of brain tumors are classified according to the cells of origination and are discussed in the following section (Polich & Paz, 2009; UTMDACC, 2010b).

Glioma

Glioma is a general term for a group of tumors that start in glial cells. The three types of glial cells are astrocytes, oligodendrocytes, and ependymal cells. Many tumors can be considered gliomas, including glioblastoma multiforme, astrocytomas, oligodendrogliomas, and ependymomas.

Most *astrocytomas* can spread widely throughout the brain and blend with the normal brain tissue, which can make them very hard to remove surgically. A *glioblastoma multiforme* is the most rapid growing, aggressive, and lethal brain tumor in adults. It accounts for 67% of all astrocytomas.

Oligodendrogliomas are formed out of the myelin sheath around nerve cells. These tumors usually occur in adults older than age 45. The most aggressive of this type of tumor is called *anaplastic oligodendroglioma*. Like astrocytomas, they usually infiltrate nearby brain tissue and cannot fully be removed with surgery.

Ependymomas arise out of the cells that line the ventricles (ependymal cells) and can sometimes block the movement of cerebrospinal fluid through the ventricles, causing an enlargement of the ventricles called *hydrocephalus*. Ependymomas do not typically infiltrate other brain tissue.

Meningioma

Meninges are the layer of tissues that make up the outer covering or lining of the brain and spinal cord. Tumors that grow from meningeal tissue account for approximately one-quarter to one-third of all spinal cord and brain tumors. The risk of developing meningiomas increases with age, and it occurs more frequently in women and in some cases runs in families. However, meningiomas are frequently benign.

Acoustic Neuromas and Schwannomas

Acoustic neuromas and schwannomas are tumors that develop from the Schwann cells that line the cranial and peripheral nerves. When they develop on the VIIIth cranial nerve that manages hearing and balance, they are called *acoustic neuroma* or *vestibular schwannoma*. These tumors can cause buzzing and ringing of the ears, balance impairments, facial numbness, and one-sided hearing loss (Mayo Clinic, 2010; UTMDACC, 2009).

Medulloblastoma

Medulloblastomas are most often found in children younger than age 10. They arise from the fetal cells in the cerebellum. These fast-growing tumors can be spread easily through cerebrospinal fluid pathways and can invade other nearby brain tissue or spread outside of the central nervous system.

As with all cancers, the location of the brain tumor is important in understanding and identifying related functional deficits. Both benign and malignant tumors can cause cognitive and neurological deficits as a result of compressed tissue or cerebral edema. Symptoms may include cognitive deficits, bowel and bladder disorders, sexual dysfunction, or skin changes (Polich & Paz, 2009). In addition, tumor resections can also result in hemiplegia or ataxia (Polich & Paz, 2009). Tumors located in the spinal cord can cause cord compression and can even result in permanent paralysis if treatment is unsuccessful.

Medical Management of Cancer

Cancer can be treated medically in several ways, including radiation, chemotherapy, biotherapy, surgery, or a combination. Generally, the four goals of cancer treatment are

1. *Cure (eradication):* No reoccurrence within 5 years of time of diagnosis and treatment.
2. *Control:* Slowing or stopping cancer growth.
3. *Palliation:* Alleviation of symptoms with advanced disease and with a focus on quality of life.
4. *Prophylaxis:* For patients at high risk of cancer or recurrence ("Cancer," 2006; Gould, 2006).

One of the challenges of cancer treatment is that treatments often have adverse effects that affect occupational performance and daily functioning. For example, treatments may cause peripheral neuropathy, tremors, fibrosis, edema, arthritis, fatigue, and pain, which can limit movement and the ability to engage in meaningful and purposeful activities (Shelton et al., 2008). Common side effects of cancer treatments are listed in Table 11.9.

Radiation

Radiation (radiotherapy) produces cell death by damaging DNA. An increased dose of radiation equals an increase in the number of cells destroyed. Unfortunately, it destroys normal cell tissue as well. An X-ray beam may be used to destroy cancer cells on the surface or deeper in the body. The higher the energy of the X-ray beam is, the deeper in the body it can target. Curative radiation therapy is mostly limited to localized tumors. This form of treatment may be used as palliative treatment to relieve or prevent symptoms and minimize complications. External beam radiation therapy is the most common type of radiation therapy (Polich & Paz, 2009).

Because radiation is delivered directly to the tumor site, the patient is tattooed at various points on the body to indicate where the radiation is to be delivered. If the patient has any scarring (e.g., scar tissue from a mastectomy), that region may become tight from the radiation. This area would benefit from massage, and passive ROM (PROM) is generally applied to the extremity on the ipsilateral side.

Brachytherapy, another form of radiation treatment, is the placement of radioactive implants directly into a tumor or body cavity. When a patient is receiving brachytherapy, an occupational therapist is unlikely to work with him or her because the patient is considered radioactive and is generally in an isolation room with lead doors. This type of treatment approach is most commonly used for cancers of the tongue, uterus, or cervix and some sarcomas, but it may also be used for brain, prostate, head, neck, and esophageal tumors (Polich & Paz, 2009).

Another type of radiation therapy is proton therapy, a more recent form of radiotherapy. Benefits include little to no damage to surrounding healthy tissues, patients are not radioactive, and side effects are fewer than with other forms of radiotherapy. Image-guided therapy targets treatment directly to the tumor site (UTMDACC, 2010a).

Chemotherapy

Chemotherapy, or *anticancer drugs,* is used frequently to reduce tumor size, prevent metastasis, and treat disseminated cancers. Many advanced cancers will respond to this type of treatment approach. Chemotherapy can be delivered intravenously or orally, and it may be given once or in multiple rounds or cycles.

Occupational therapists can work with patients while they are actively receiving chemotherapy. However, some precautions need to be maintained when handling the bodily fluids of patients actively receiving treatment. Because of the toxic nature of bodily fluids after the administration of chemotherapy, protective gloves should be used. Major side effects of chemotherapy include nausea, vomiting, *mucositis* (inflammation of mucous membranes), and infection. Mucositis can lead to difficulty with

(*Text continues on p. 433*)

Table 11.9. Side Effects of Common Cancer Treatments and Suggested Management Strategies

Treatment	Side Effect	Lifestyle Management Strategies
Chemotherapy, radiation therapy, biotherapy, and surgery	Fatigue	• Prioritize • Adopt energy conservation strategies • Incorporate rest breaks into daily routines • "Listen to your body"; when feeling tired, rest • Use adaptive equipment and modify environment when warranted • Exercise regularly • When possible, delegate responsibilities; "allow" people to help • Engage in a balanced lifestyle • Modify and grade activities
Chemotherapy, radiation therapy, and biotherapy	Gastrointestinal problems (e.g., nausea, vomiting, anorexia, diarrhea, constipation)	• Avoid greasy, fried, and spicy foods • Avoid strong odors • Drink small sips of water throughout the day, and stay well hydrated • Eat 5–6 smaller more frequent meals than 3 large meals • Eat and drink slowly • Use adapted feeding utensils if needed • For nausea, take antiemetic medication • For anorexia, try changing the context in which meals are eaten (e.g., eat out with friends); try new foods to stir interest; prepare foods that are easy to eat and swallow (e.g., milkshakes, soups, gelatin); increase activity level to increase appetite; avoid filling up on drinks before meals • For diarrhea, adopt the BRAT diet (i.e., *b*ananas, *r*ice, *a*pplesauce, *t*oast); stay well hydrated; avoid foods high in fiber, dairy products, greasy foods, gaseous vegetables (e.g., cabbage), raw fruits and vegetables, alcoholic drinks, and caffeinated beverages • For constipation, eat fresh fruits and vegetables, whole grains, nuts, seeds; drink plenty of liquids

Table 11.9. (continued)

Treatment	Side Effect	Lifestyle Management Strategies
Chemotherapy and biotherapy	Fluid retention	• Avoid foods with high salt content • Elevate feet when sitting • Avoid constricting clothing • Regularly weigh self • Avoid standing for long periods of time • Wear compression stockings if warranted
Chemotherapy and radiation therapy	Sore mouth or throat	• Perform good oral care (e.g., use soft toothbrush, rinse mouth with salt water and baking soda, brush teeth after meals and before bed) • Avoid alcohol-based mouthwash (e.g., Listerine) replace with Biotene-type mouthwash or oral products • Keep mouth and lips moist (e.g., suck ice chips, take frequent sips of water, use lip balm) • Eat foods that are easy to swallow (e.g., cooked cereal, milkshakes); cut food into small manageable pieces; mash food or add broth or gravy to soften foods • Avoid foods that are very cold or very hot (e.g., extreme temperatures) • Avoid salty, hard, or spicy foods; citrus drinks (e.g., orange, lemon, or grapefruit juices); or foods or drinks high in sugar • Sit up for at least 30 minutes after meals • Avoid tobacco products and alcohol
Chemotherapy and radiation therapy	Alopecia (hair loss)	• Use a mild shampoo • Pat, do not vigorously towel dry hair • Adopt a short hairstyle or wear a wig, hat, or other head covering • Shave head • Apply sunscreen, or wear a hat, when out in the sun • Wear a hat or scarf in cold weather to protect head • Wear a soft cap with no seams to bed to keep head warm if needed • Wear glasses to protect eyes if eyelashes fall out (also helps keep dust and particles from getting in eyes)

(continued)

Table 11.9.   (continued)

Treatment	Side Effect	Lifestyle Management Strategies
Chemotherapy, radiation therapy, and biotherapy	Increased risk of infection (e.g., leukopenia, neutropenia, bone marrow suppression, immunosuppresion)	• Practice good hand hygiene • Maintain good oral hygiene • Wash raw fruits and vegetables before eating them • Avoid crowds or people who are sick or contagious; avoid people recently vaccinated (e.g., mumps, measles, chickenpox) • Wear a mask if outside in crowded areas (e.g., grocery store or shopping mall) • Avoid swimming in lakes or pools • Avoid getting cuts (e.g., use an electric shaver instead of a razor)
Chemotherapy	Bleeding problems (e.g., thrombocytopenia, hemorrhage)	• Use electric shaver, not sharp razor • Avoid blowing nose; instead wipe nose gently • Use soft toothbrush when brushing teeth • Avoid using dental floss • Use sanitary pads, not tampons • Avoid contact sports
Chemotherapy and biotherapy	Anemia	• Incorporate energy conservation strategies • Schedule rest breaks into daily routines • Eat a high-protein diet, and foods high in iron • Drink at least 8 glasses of liquid daily
Chemotherapy, radiation therapy, biotherapy, and hormonal therapy	Sexual and fertility changes (e.g., pain with intercourse, irregular menstruation, menopausal symptoms, decreased libido, erectile dysfunction)	• Maintain good communication with your partner • Talk to a health care professional • Join a support group • Use birth control (e.g., use condoms, as chemotherapy may damage sperm resulting in birth defects) • Use creams and lubricants for vaginal dryness
Chemotherapy and radiation therapy	Changes in urination (e.g., frequency; trouble with urination; urine that is a different color, is cloudy, or has a strong odor)	• Increase fluid intake but avoid drinks with caffeine and alcohol • Wear clothing that is easy to get on and off for easier toileting • Use of bedside commode or raised toilet seat to increase independence in toilet transfers and speed of accessing toilet

Table 11.9.   (continued)

Treatment	Side Effect	Lifestyle Management Strategies
Chemotherapy	Sensory changes (e.g., peripheral neuropathy)	• Increase safety awareness during routine activities • Incorporate home and bathroom safety strategies • Employ fall prevention strategies • Use compensatory strategies for impaired sensation • If experiencing nerve pain (e.g., bottom of feet) that keeps you awake at night, consult MD about medication (e.g., Neurotin)
Biotherapy	Memory changes	• Plan ahead • Be organized (e.g., use pill box to keep track of medicines) • Write things down or record them (e.g., use a calendar to keep track of appointments) • Get adequate rest • Involve all stakeholders • Ask for help when needed
Chemotherapy	Psychological issues (e.g., anxiety, depression)	• Engagement in stress management and relaxation techniques (e.g., controlled breathing, mindfulness meditation, progressive muscle relaxation, guided imagery) • Pharmacology (e.g., anti-depressants) • Address issues of loss, grief, and anger • Join a support group • Engage in occupations that are purposeful and meaningful • Exercise • Consult a health care professional
Chemotherapy and radiation therapy	Skin changes (e.g., dry itching skin, rash)	• Keep skin clean and dry • Avoid perfume or alcohol-based products; use mild soaps, lotions, and creams • If receiving radiation therapy, moisturize area but wash off thoroughly before treatment • Use intense cream (e.g., Cere Ve, Eucerin) on bottoms of feet and palms of hands to prevent cracking if skin is peeling or very dry • Shower with warm, not hot, water

(*continued*)

Table 11.9. (continued)		
Treatment	**Side Effect**	**Lifestyle Management Strategies**
		• Pat self dry after showering (instead of rubbing skin) • Wear loose-fitting clothes (e.g., wear loose bra or camisole if receiving radiation therapy in breast area). • Wear sunscreen (e.g., SPF 30+), long sleeves, long pants, and hat when outdoors • Avoid tanning booths • Keep nails clean and short • Wear gloves when washing dishes, using cleansers, or working in garden • Avoid heating pads and ice packs over areas that received radiation therapy • For dry eyes (dried mucous membranes), consider wearing eye glasses instead of contact lenses, and use rewetting drops or artificial tears
Surgery	Disfigurement, deformity, scar tissue, fibrosis, incisional pain, bleeding, infection	• Emotional support • Reconstructive surgery • Splinting and positioning to prevent contracture and maintain function • Pharmacological and non-pharmacological approaches to address issues of pain • Adherence to standard precautions to minimize risk of infection • Anticoagulation and early mobilization to prevent clots
Hormonal therapy	Steroid-induced myopathy	• Range of motion and flexibility exercise program • Functional mobility retraining and activities • Engagement in basic activities of daily living • Modify and grade activities • Use of adaptive equipment and durable medical equipment to maximize independence

Sources. Cooper (2006), Goodman (2009), Lim & Foye (2009), NCI (2010).

eating and speaking, mouth sores, pain, and bleeding (Redman, 2004). Chemotherapy treatment may include

- *Gliadel®,* a biopolymer wafer about the size of a dime, designed to deliver *carmustine* (a type of slow-release chemotherapy) directly into the surgical cavity created when a brain tumor is resected. Gliadel dissolves slowly, which allows chemotherapy to take place immediately after surgery. Gliadel wafers are used in the treatment of newly diagnosed high-grade malignant gliomas, as an adjunct to surgery and radiation, and for recurrent glioblastoma multiforme (Uddin & Jarmi, 2010).

- *Omaya Reservoir,* a device surgically inserted under the scalp for direct injection of chemotherapy into the spinal fluid. Drugs can be administered through this reservoir rather than through the back during a spinal tap.

- *CHOP,* a regimen used in treating non-Hodgkin lymphoma. It combines four different chemotherapy agents: cyclophoshamide, doxorubicin hydrochloride, oncovin, and prednisolone. CHOP is administered in 3-week cycles. Side effects include fatigue and increased risk of infection, bruising, or anemia.

Chemotherapy and radiation can be used in conjunction to more effectively reduce the tumor size. The type and amount of chemotherapy and radiation delivered is determined by the site and stage of the tumor.

Biotherapy

Biotherapy, also referred to as *immunotherapy* or *biological response modifiers,* works with the body's own natural defenses to fight cancer. Also included in this group are hormone therapies. Hormonal therapy focuses on eliminating the hormonal source of cancer through surgery or medication and is commonly used in treating breast and prostate cancers (Polich & Paz, 2009). Immunotherapy involves improving the immune system's response to cancer or boosting the patient's immune system (Goodman, 2009; Polich & Paz, 2009). Stem cell and bone marrow transplantation are also considered biotherapies.

Surgery

Surgery is primarily performed to remove tumors and is guided by several factors including the patient's age and functional status, tumor size and location, and type of cancer (Polich & Paz, 2009). In addition to tumor resection, lymph node dissection may be performed to control the spread of cancer by removing malignant lymph nodes (Polich & Paz, 2009). A radical excision involves removing the primary tumor, surrounding tissue, and lymph nodes ("Cancer," 2007). *Debulking* is a procedure in which the cancer is not completely excised, but tumor size is reduced to alleviate symptoms or to increase the success of radiation or chemotherapy. Surgery may also be exploratory to stage the cancer or reconstructive to repair the area of resection using skin flaps, muscle, or fascia.

Surgery has also been performed as a palliative or prophylactic measure. Palliative surgery may be performed to alleviate symptoms and complications of cancer, and prophylactic surgery may be performed if the patient has a high risk for a specific type of cancer but does not have active disease (e.g., mastectomy for breast cancer risk).

Transplantation

Transplantation may be indicated when other forms of treatment are unsuccessful and cancerous organs are removed. Refer to Chapter 14 for more information on solid organ transplantation.

Hematopoietic cell transplantation generally refers to bone marrow transplantation and peripheral stem cell transplantation. This approach is used in treating blood disorder cancers such as leukemia, lymphoma, and multiple myeloma. Hematopoietic cell transplantation is performed by ridding the body of cancerous cells and replacing them with stem cells that engraft, producing normal blood cells. The transplanted marrow may be from the patient *(autologous)* or from a donor *(allogeneic)*. Autologous stem cells are collected from the patient's own marrow or bloodstream through apheresis. In this procedure, blood is drawn from the patient, the stem cells are removed, and the blood is returned to the patient. Patients undergo high-dose chemotherapy before the transplant and are therefore at a high risk of infection with immunosuppression. In allogeneic transplants, patients may receive human leukocyte antigens from matched siblings or from a matched, unrelated donor. A high histocompatability between donor and recipient results in a lowered risk of developing graft-versus-host disease (GVHD; Packel, 2006).

Side effects of stem cell transplantation may include nausea, vomiting, GVHD, delayed wound healing, cataracts, thyroid dysfunction, osteoporosis, and veno-occlusive disease (Goodman, 2009). GVHD occurs when the graft perceives the host body as foreign, proceeding to attack the patient's organs. GVHD is often treated with steroids, which have their own side effects with chronic use, including myopathy, weakness, and osteopenia. Refer to Chapter 14 for information on hematopoietic cell transplantation and the signs and symptoms of chronic GVHD.

Oncological Emergencies

Oncological emergencies can arise as a complication of therapy or because of metabolic or obstructive changes of the disease itself. If the patient, family, and medical team are aware of and alert to these potential complications, they can be recognized early and treated effectively. Complications may include

- *Superior vena cava syndrome,* which is associated with small-cell lung cancer, breast cancer, and lymphoma. The vena cava is occluded, impairing venous return, which may result in dilated neck veins and face and upper-extremity lymphedema.
- *Electrolyte disorders,* which are associated with breast, lung, renal cancers, and multiple myeloma resulting in hypercalcemia.

- *Tumor lysis syndrome,* which is caused by chemotherapy and rapid tumor growth. It is associated with myeloproliferative disorders (e.g., leukemia, lymphoma) and may cause acute renal failure, tachycardia, decreased blood pressure, and arrhythmias.
- *Spinal cord compression,* which is invasive metastasis of the spine associated with lung, breast, cervical, prostate, kidney, and colon cancers and multiple myeloma. It can be the result of vertebral collapse or displacement resulting in back pain, muscle weakness, and gait abnormalities.
- *Hypercoagulable states,* which are associated with hematological cancers in which widespread clotting and simultaneous bleeding of small blood vessels occur.
- *Severe thrombocytosis ($<10,000$ cells/ millimeter^3),* which is associated with increased risk of spontaneous bleeding.
- *Increased pressure or fluid accumulation,* which may result in cardiac tamponade, malignant peritoneal infusion, or malignant pleural effusion. It may be due to hematological, breast, lung, testicular, ovarian, or GI tract cancers. ("Cancer," 2007; Goodman, 2009; Shelton et al., 2008)

Palliative Care

The focus of cancer is on curative measures, but when that is not possible, it may shift to palliation. *Palliative care* focuses on pain control, symptom management, and emotional support. The focus is on patients, families, and quality of life rather than the disease. According to Schleinich, Warren, Nekolaichuk, Kaasa, and Watanabe (2008), unmet occupational needs and unmet symptom control are the two major issues identified by terminally ill patients.

Occupational therapists can help patients near the end of life find meaning, despite waning physical abilities or the state of their disease (Cohen, 2005). Occupational therapy continues to focus on autonomy, maintenance of independence, and emotional support. Pizzi and Briggs (2004) advocated a positive approach by focusing on client-centered care and family-centered care with a focus on activity, mobility, and pain management. Occupational therapy interventions can also focus on environmental modifications, equipment needs, and instruction in stress management and energy conservation strategies.

The most important role for occupational therapists is validating activities that are meaningful to the patient. According to Pearson, Todd, and Futcher (2007), therapists can assist patients with developing coping strategies, help patients with their daily tasks, facilitate engagement in social and leisure activities, and help patients increase their control over their environment.

Impact of Cancer

Cancer affects a variety of the body systems both physically and cognitively, and it also raises issues that affect self-esteem, relationships, work, finances, and end-of-life issues. Cancer can cause psychosocial distress for both patients and their families or caregivers. Many adverse side effects also result from the very treatments used to eliminate the cancer. Anemia, nausea, pain, alopecia, weight gain, weight loss, physical disfigurement, sleep disturbances, and fatigue are just a few of the side effects of cancer and cancer treatments. Radiation, chemotherapy, surgery, and biologic response modifiers can also cause cognitive changes, including problems with memory, problem solving, and concentration, which may be more pronounced with central nervous system involvement (Redman, 2004).

Psychosocial Implications

A diagnosis of cancer is a life-altering experience with physical and psychosocial implications (Cohen, 2005; Massie, 2004; Watterson, Lowrie, Vockins, Ewer-Smith, & Cooper, 2004). Patients with cancer often experience uncertainty about the future; emotional distress surrounding issues of loss of control; and loss of ability to engage in normal, valued, and meaningful occupations. Patients find it distressing to, in many cases, no longer engage in valued occupations that help define them (Lyons, 2006).

A diagnosis of cancer can prompt patients to reflect on their mortality and their understanding and personal meaning of illness, life, and death (Lyons, 2006). In addition, cancer may also be associated with stigma, loss, and impending death. The patient may experience loss of control, body function, self-esteem, and hope and a sense of grief and altered self-image. Loss may also be experienced not only by the patient but also by his or her caregivers, family, and friends, who may also feel helpless and inadequate in coping with the patient's disease (Massie, 2004; Redman, 2004).

A diagnosis of cancer may also mean prolonged hospitalization for patients who are immunosuppressed.

According to Mailoo and Williams (2004), lack of social support and grief are linked to shorter survival and increased incidence and recurrence of certain cancers. They also suggested a link between the mind and an anti-cancer immune system response that would complement occupational therapy's holistic approach to patient care.

Psychosocial and emotional stress can manifest as physical symptoms of headache, dizziness, rapid breathing, palpitations, dry mouth, and cognitive symptoms of negative thinking, jumping to conclusions, catastrophizing, or all-or-nothing thinking (Cooper, 2006), which is why it is important for therapists to be empathetic, sensitive, client centered, and holistic in their approach. Cooper (2006) recommended taking the time to hear patients' stories and acknowledging that you "hear" what they are saying to you. When emotional and psychosocial issues are acknowledged and addressed, including coping strategies, the result is greater patient satisfaction (Massie, 2004). Occupational therapists can be instrumental in helping patients with coping strategies and stress management techniques.

Occupational Therapy Approach

Cancer is a disease that is disruptive to occupational balance, productivity, life roles, self-identity, and self-esteem (Watterson et al., 2004). Therapists need to recognize that a diagnosis of cancer has physical, cognitive, emotional, and spiritual implications that affect function and occupational performance. The focus of occupational therapy should be on "promoting health in the face of disease, restoring performance skills and patterns; preventing disability; modifying contexts, activity demand, or performance patterns; and providing support that help patients maintain function" (Shelton et al., 2008, p. 1371).

According to Oertli (2007), the role of occupational therapy is to collaboratively identify roles that are meaningful to patients and their ability to engage in these roles. Loss of control is a difficult issue that cancer patients face, and occupational therapists can help their patients adapt to cancer-related loss though occupation (Oertli, 2007). Engagement in occupation helps cancer patients cope with the physical and psychosocial challenges of having cancer by imbuing normalcy, routine, and control over their lives and health care–related decisions (Lyons, 2006; Vockins, 2004).

Symptom management can be addressed through education, structuring and modifying activities and environments, and implementing interventions that support independence and engagement in meaningful occupations. Education may focus on an understanding of the disease process, instruction in energy conservation principles, safety strategies, stress management, relaxation techniques, pain management, and coping strategies. Relaxation techniques have been shown to relieve certain symptoms of cancer and cancer treatments, such as pain, nausea, and vomiting (Mailoo & Williams, 2004). Occupational tasks can also be analyzed and modified to ensure successful completion, building on patients' perceived self-efficacy.

In addressing the performance skills and performance patterns of occupational therapy interventions, the focus may be on increasing activity tolerance, ROM, strength, flexibility, sensory reeducation, desensitization or compensation, scar management, and opportunities provided for engagement in routine occupations (e.g., ADLs).

The literature provides support for exercise being beneficial in improving activity tolerance and quality of life for patients with cancer; however, it may be contraindicated for patients with bony metastases (Monga et al., 2007; Morris et al., 2009). Prolonged physical inactivity and a sedentary lifestyle are also detrimental to patients with cancer, whereas physical activity assists with flexibility, endurance, and improved sleep, as well as helping to reduce fatigue, anxiety, and depression (Monga et al., 2007). However, attention should be paid to the meanings of selected activities and not just the outcome. According to Mailoo and Williams (2004), working on donning a hospital gown for the sake of working on the task of dressing may not be meaningful to the patient.

Occupational therapy is unique in that it has a holistic approach to patient care that recognizes that engagement in occupation can influence health and well-being. Occupational therapists can help patients with cancer engage in or reclaim valued occupations and meaningful roles or explore new occupations or ways to engage in meaningful occupations but alter the form (Lyons, 2006). Therapy should be client centered and occupation based and take into consideration not just physical abilities but also coping mechanisms and psychosocial issues (self-identity, locus of control, emotional distress) that affect not just the patients but also their families and caregivers. Whatever approach is taken, the following guidelines are offered to assist the therapist working with this population:

- Verify blood counts and coagulation profiles before treating patients; observe precautions for abnormal levels (refer to Appendix P for blood counts and their implications).
- Always monitor vital signs, because chemotherapy and other cancer treatments may affect cardiopulmonary and nervous system function.
- Be aware of bulbs, drains, tubes, and lines that may interfere with therapy or pose a safety hazard.

- Observe standard precautions, including good hand hygiene, because patients may be at increased risk for infection.
- Consult with the physician before mobilizing patients with bone cancer.
- Manual muscle testing may be contraindicated for patients with multiple myeloma or metastatic disease to bones because of bone fragility and risk of pathologic fracture.
- Verify weight-bearing status of patients with bone cancer or bone grafts.
- Verify any contraindications to using resistive exercises or activities for patients with bone lesions or with thrombocytopenia (low platelet count).
- Do not actively stretch patients with 20,000 platelets per microliter or less because they are at increased risk for uncontrolled bleeding and bruising.
- Observe neutropenic precautions if white blood cell count is less than 4,000 per millimeter cubed (refer to Appendix P for more information on precautions).
- Monitor patients for signs of fatigue or activity intolerance, and modify interventions accordingly.
- Be aware of signs of oncological emergency.
- Reinforce any weight-lifting restrictions when patients engage in ADLs.
- Instruct patients in fall prevention and safety. Patients may be at risk for falls because of steroid myopathies or peripheral neuropathies.
- Assess the patient's need for adaptive equipment, positioning (to prevent skin breakdown), splinting (to prevent contracture), balance, and cognitive retraining, as warranted.
- Keep the head of the bed at least 30° for patients with head, neck, or facial tumors to minimize risk of aspiration.
- Instruct postsurgical breast cancer patients in bed mobility and log-roll techniques to minimize use of surgically affected abdominal muscles when going from supine to sitting.

- Refer lymphedema patients to a specialist for instruction in lymphedema management.
- Avoid exercising muscles under new muscle flaps; consult the physician for specific precautions.
- Avoid exercising areas of recent skin graft; consult the physician for specific precautions.
- Be cautious when exercising areas with blue or black markings from radiation because the area underneath may be fragile.
- Defer therapy for patients with implanted radioactive seeds.
- Encourage ROM exercises to maintain flexibility and prevent contractures.
- Use early mobilization to help prevent postoperative complications (e.g., ileus, deep vein thrombosis, pneumonia). Simply sitting at the bedside participating in simple hygiene activities will assist in improving endurance and preventing complications.
- Instruct patients in deep-breathing exercises to prevent postoperative pulmonary complications, especially for patients on bedrest precautions.
- Instruct patient and family in energy conservation strategies, use of proper body mechanics, and use of recommended equipment.

Conclusion

Occupational therapy can play a key role in addressing ADLs; work; leisure; discharge planning; equipment recommendations; and instruction in pain, stress, fatigue, and dyspnea management (Cooper & Littlechild, 2004). Lifestyle management can be addressed by helping patients assess their priorities and facilitate achievement of balance in life. Patients with cancer can be enabled and empowered to engage in activities that support their self-worth, self-identity, and acknowledged values. Working with cancer patients requires a holistic approach that deals with both physical and psychosocial issues. The occupational therapist's role is to enable patients and to maximize their ability to engage in everyday tasks, reaching their functional goals regardless of life expectancy (Strzelecki, 2006; Vockins, 2004).

References

American Cancer Society. (2009a). *Lymphedema: What every woman with breast cancer should know.* Retrieved September 2010, from http://www.cancer.org/acs/groups/cid/documents/webcontent/002876-pdf.pdf

American Cancer Society. (2009b). *Sarcoma—Adult soft tissue cancer.* Retrieved August 2009, from www.cancer.org/docroot/CRI/content/CRI_2_4_1X_What_is_sarcoma_38.asp

American Cancer Society. (2010a). *Cancer facts and figures 2010.* Retrieved September 2010, from http://www.cancer.org/acs/groups/content/@epidemiologysurveilance/documents/document/acspc-026238.pdf

American Cancer Society. (2010b). *Stomach cancer.* Retrieved September 2010, from http://www.cancer.org/Cancer/StomachCancer/DetailedGuide/stomach-cancer-risk-factors

American Cancer Society. (2010c). *Which cancers spread where. Learn about cancer.* Retrieved September 2010, from http://www.cancer.org/Cancer/AdvancedCancer/DetailedGuide/advanced-cancer-where-cancers-spread

Armitage, J. O. (2005). Staging non-Hodgkin lymphoma. *CA: A Cancer Journal for Clinicians, 55*(6), 368–376.

Barsevick, A. M., Newhall, T., & Brown, S. (2008). Management of cancer-related fatigue. *Clinical Journal of Oncology Nursing, 12*(5, Suppl.), 21–25. doi: 10.1188/08.cjon.S2.21-25

Cancer. (2006). In *Atlas of pathophysiology* (pp. 6–12). Philadelphia: Lippincott Williams & Wilkins.

Cancer. (2007). In J. Munden (Ed.), *Professional guide to pathophysiology* (2nd ed., pp. 12–50). Philadelphia: Lippincott Williams & Wilkins.

Cohen, S. (2005). Breast cancer: The OT role. *OT Practice, 10*(9), 16–20.

Cooper, J. (2006). *Occupational therapy in oncology and palliative care* (2nd ed.). West Sussex, England: Wiley.

Cooper, J., & Littlechild, B. (2004). A study of occupational therapy interventions in oncology and palliative care. *International Journal of Therapy and Rehabilitation, 11,* 329–333.

Crannell, C. E., & Stone, E. (2008). Bedside physical therapy project to prevent deconditioning in hospitalized patients with cancer. *Oncology Nursing Forum, 35,* 343–345.

Feledy, J. A., Hanasono, M. M., & Robb, J. L. (2006). Reconstruction surgery in the cancer patient. In B. W. Feig, D. H. Berger, & G. M. Fuhrman (Ed.), *The M. D. Anderson surgical oncology handbook* (4th ed., pp. 635–649). Philadelphia: Lippincott Williams & Wilkins.

Goodman, C. C. (2009). Oncology. In C. C. Goodman & K. S. Fuller (Eds.), *Pathology: Implications for the physical therapist* (pp. 348–391). St. Louis, MO: W. B. Saunders.

Gould, B. E. (2006). Neoplasms. In *Pathophysiology for the health professions* (3rd ed., pp. 104–126). Philadelphia: W. B. Saunders.

Hunt, K. K., Newman, A. L., Copelan, E. M., & Bland, K. T. (2009). Breast. In F. C. Brunicardi, D. R. Anderson, T. R. Billar, D. L. Dunn, J. G. Hunter, J. B. Matthews, et al. (Ed.), *Schwartz's principles of surgery* (9th ed., pp. 423–474). New York: McGraw-Hill.

Leukemia and Lymphoma Society. (2010). *Disease information.* Retrieved September 2010, from http://www.leukemia-lymphoma.org/all_toplevel.adp?item_id=4187

Lim, S. S., & Foye, P. M. (2009). Corticosteroid-induced myopathy: Treatment and medication. *eMedicine.* Retrieved September 2010, from http://emedicine.medscape.com/article/313842-treatment

Lyons, K. D. (2006). Occupation as a vehicle to surmount the psychosocial challenges of cancer. *Occupational Therapy in Health Care, 20*(2), 1–16.

Mailoo, V., & Williams, C. J. (2004). Psychoneuroimmunology: A theoretical basis for occupational therapy in oncology. *International Journal of Therapy and Rehabilitation, 11,* 7–12.

Massie, D. K. (2004). Psychosocial issues for the elderly with cancer: The role of social work. *Topics in Geriatric Rehabilitation, 20,* 114–119.

Mayo Clinic. 2010. *Diseases and conditions.* Retrieved September 2010, from www.mayoclinic.com/health/DiseasesIndex/DiseasesIndex

Monga, U., Garber, S. L., Thornby, J., Vallbona, C., Kerrigan, A. J., Monga, T. N., et al. (2007). Exercise prevents fatigue and improves quality of life in prostate cancer patients undergoing radiotherapy. *Archives of Physical Medicine and Rehabilitation, 88,* 1416–1422. doi: 10.1016/j.apmr.2007.08.110

Morris, G. S., Gallagher, G. H., Baxter, M. F., Brueilly, K. E., Scheetz, J. S., Ahmed, M. M., et al. (2009). Pulmonary rehabilitation improves functional status in oncology patients. *Archives of Physical Medicine and Rehabilitation, 90,* 837–841.

National Cancer Institute. (2005). *Head and neck cancer: Questions and answers* (National Cancer Institute Fact Sheet). Retrieved September 2010, from http://www.cancer.gov/cancertopics/factsheet/Sites-Types/head-and-neck

National Cancer Institute. (2008). *Staging: Questions and answers* (National Cancer Institute Fact Sheet). Retrieved November 16, 2008, from www.cancer.gov/cancertopics/factsheet/detection/staging

National Cancer Institute. (2009). *Cancer topics: Small cell lung cancer treatment.* Retrieved September 2010, from http://www.cancer.gov/cancertopics/pdq/treatment/non-small-cell-lung/healthprofessional

National Cancer Institute. (2010). Types of treatment. *Cancer Topics.* Retrieved September 2010, from http://www.cancer.gov/cancertopics/treatment/types-of-treatment

Nesbit, S. G. (2004). My breast cancer: An occupational therapist's perspective. *Occupational Therapy in Mental Health, 20*(2), 51–67.

Oertli, S. (2007). Cancer: Many diagnoses, one occupation-based approach. *OT Practice, 12*(11), 16–19.

Packel, L. (2006). Oncological diseases and disorders. In D. J. Malone & K. L. B. Lindsay (Eds.), *Physical therapy in acute care: A clinician's guide* (pp. 503–544). Thorofare, NJ: Slack.

Pearson, E. J. M., Todd, J. G., & Futcher, J. M. (2007). How can occupational therapists measure outcomes in palliative care? *Palliative Medicine, 21,* 477–485.

Pizzi, M., & Briggs, R. (2004). Occupational and physical therapy in hospice: The facilitation of

meaning, quality of life, and well-being. *Topics in Geriatric Rehabilitation, 20*(2), 120–130.

Polich, S., & Paz, J. C. (2009). Oncology. In J. C. Paz & M. P. West (Eds.), *Acute care handbook for physical therapists* (3rd ed., pp. 199–217). St. Louis, MO: W. B. Saunders.

Purcell, A., Fleming, J., Haines, T., & Bennett, S. (2009). Cancer-related fatigue: A review and a conceptual framework to guide therapists' understanding. *British Journal of Occupational Therapy, 72,* 79–86.

Redman, B. K. (2004). Cancer self-management preparation. In *Patient self-management of chronic disease: The health care provider's challenge* (pp. 33–52). Boston: Jones & Bartlett.

Schleinich, M. A., Warren, S., Nekolaichuk, C., Kaasa, T., & Watanabe, S. (2008). Palliative care rehabilitation survey: A pilot study of patients' priorities for rehabilitation goals. *Palliative Medicine, 22,* 822–830.

Shelton, M. L., Lipoma, J. B., & Oertli, E. S. (2008). Oncology. In M. V. Radomski & C. A. T. Latham (Eds.), *Occupational therapy for physical dysfunction* (6th ed., pp. 1358–1375). Philadelphia: Wolters Kluwer.

Strzelecki, M. V. (2006). Careers: An OT approach to clients with cancer. *OT Practice, 11*(15), 7–8.

Stürmer, T., Buring, J. E., Lee, I.-M., Gaziano, J. M., & Glynn, R. J., (2006). Metabolic abnormalities and risk for colorectal cancer in the Physicians' Health Study. *Cancer Epidemiology Biomarkers and Prevention, 15,* 2391–2397.

Taylor, K., & Currow, D. (2003). A prospective study of patient identified unmet activity of daily living needs amongst cancer patients at a comprehensive cancer care centre. *Australian Occupational Therapy Journal, 50*(2), 79–85.

TNM staging system. (2010). In *Encyclopædia Britannica.* Retrieved September 13, 2010, from Encyclopædia Britannica Online: http://www.britannica.com/EBchecked/topic/765936/TNM-staging-system

Uddin, A. S., & Jarmi, T. (2010). Glioblastoma multiforme: Treatment and medication. *eMedicine.* Retrieved September 20, 2010, from http://emedicine.medscape.com/article/1156220-treatment

University of Texas M. D. Anderson Cancer Center. (2009). *Just the facts... Skin cancer.* Retrieved

September 2010, from http://www.mdanderson. org/patient-and-cancer-information/cancer-information/community-services/brochures/ pdfs/mda42044-skin.pdf

University of Texas M. D. Anderson Cancer Center. (2010a). *Benefits of proton therapy.* Retrieved September 20, 2010, from http://www. mdanderson.org/patient-and-cancer-information/ proton-therapy-center/what-is-proton-therapy/ benefits-of-proton-therapy/index.html

University of Texas M. D. Anderson Cancer Center. (2010b). *Brain cancer.* Retrieved September 2010, from http://www.mdanderson.org/patient-and-cancer-information/cancer-information/cancer-types/brain-cancer/index.html

University of Texas M. D. Anderson Cancer Center. (2010c). *Soft tissue sarcoma.* Retrieved September 2010, from http://www.mdanderson.org/patient-and-cancer-information/cancer-information/ cancer-types/soft-tissue-sarcoma/index.html

Vockins, H. (2004). Occupational therapy intervention with patients with breast cancer: A survey. *European Journal of Cancer Care, 13,* 45–52.

Wang, X. S. (2008). Pathophysiology of cancer-related fatigue. *Clinical Journal of Oncology Nursing,* 12(5, Suppl.), 11–20. doi: 10.1188/08.cjon. S2.11-20

Watterson, J., Lowrie, D., Vockins, H., Ewer-Smith, C., & Cooper, J. (2004). Rehabilitation goals identified by inpatients with cancer using the COPM. *International Journal of Therapy and Rehabilitation, 11,* 219–224.

Appendix 11.A.

Guidelines for Lymphedema

The lymph system assists the body in fighting against infection. With breast cancer, the chest or arm on the involved side may swell and be more prone to infection because of the removal of lymph vessels and nodes. The following guidelines are from the American Cancer Society (2009a) to help prevent infection and swelling in the involved arm. The emphasis is on maintaining good hygiene and skin protection.

General Precautions

- Use the affected arm normally as you would for all activities of daily living.
- Do simple stretching exercises each day to keep full movement in your chest, arm, and shoulder.
- Avoid muscle strain when engaging in activities.
- Avoid burns.
- Avoid constricting clothing.
- Do not have a blood pressure cuff applied to the affected arm.
- Try to avoid infection.
- Maintain good hand hygiene.
- Clean any cuts, scratches, insect bites, or hangnails by first washing with soap and water, applying an antiseptic ointment, and then covering with a clean bandage.
- Have your blood drawn from, IVs inserted in, and any injections given in the unaffected arm, including vaccinations and flu shots.
- Avoid gaining weight, which can increase the burden on the remaining lymph nodes.

Basic Activities of Daily Living

- Regularly moisturize hands and cuticles with lotion or cream to prevent chapping and cracking skin.
- Do not use a scissor to cut cuticles; push them back with a cuticle stick.
- Do not shave with sharp razor. Use an electric razor.
- Avoid tight clothing, tight sleeves, or elastic bands.
- Do not wear tight jewelry.
- Wear watch on the uninvolved arm.
- Wear comfortable fitting shoes.
- Wear loose-fitting bra and pad straps to prevent them from digging into your shoulders.
- After a mastectomy, avoid wearing a heavy prosthesis (breast form).
- If wearing a back pack, use one that is equally weighted on both shoulders. Avoid using a pocketbook or briefcase with shoulder straps.

Instrumental Activities of Daily Living

- Wear gloves when using chemical cleansers or washing dishes.
- Use long oven mitts when cooking or baking. Avoid oil burns from frying foods and steam burns from boiling liquids or microwaved foods.
- Wear gloves when gardening or doing yard work.

- If your arm becomes sore during activity, rest and raise it above the level of your heart.
- Avoid heavy lifting, pulling, or vigorous repetitive activities.
- Use the unaffected arm or both arms for carrying children, groceries, or other heavy objects.
- Use insect repellant and sunscreen when outdoors.
- Avoid sunburns. Use at least SPF 15, or wear long sleeves, and avoid the sun during the hottest part of the day.
- Avoid extreme cold that can chap skin or cause rebound swelling.
- Avoid high heat from saunas, hot tubs, or even heating pads.
- Avoid hot pads or cold packs.
- When flying, wear a prescribed compression sleeve and exercise the arm.

General Guidelines Regarding Activities for People With Upper-Extremity Lymphedema

High Risk

- Gardening
- Tennis or racquet sports
- Golfing
- Shoveling snow
- Moving furniture
- Carrying luggage or grocery bags
- Scrubbing
- Weight lifting with affected arm
- Intense horse riding (gripping reins)
- Bowling
- Traveling on airplanes.

Medium Risk

- Jogging or running
- Biking (minimize gripping)
- StairMaster
- NordicTrack
- General weight lifting of rest of body
- Easy horseback riding.

Beneficial

- Swimming
- Walking
- StairMaster (no grip and elevate arm occasionally)
- Yoga
- Water aerobics.

Note. Compiled by Stephanie Hood, MPT, CDT. Reprinted with permission.

12

Infectious Diseases and Autoimmune Disorders

Debra A. Kerrigan, MS, OTR/L

The *immune system* is the body's mechanism for fighting infectious microbes. *Infectious microbes* include bacteria, viruses, parasites, and fungi. Nonliving toxins such as foreign particles, drugs, and chemicals may also trigger an immune response. Protective barriers (e.g., the skin, mucous membranes, cilia, stomach acids) provide the first line of defense in preventing infections by preventing microbes from entering the body. When microbes do enter the bloodstream or the skin, the immune system works to combat the infection.

Immune System Structure and Function

Unlike other body systems, the immune system is a functional system rather than an organ system. The immune system consists of many individual immune cells that use the lymphatic and circulatory pathways for transportation throughout the body. The two types of immune system responses to infection are innate (nonspecific) immunity and adaptive (specific or acquired) immunity (see Appendix 12.A for additional resources on the immune system).

The *innate immune system* responds immediately to protect the body from all foreign substances. It is not specific to any particular pathogen. *Innate immunity* is also referred to as *natural* or *native immunity* because all people are born with it. It uses nonspecific cellular and chemical defenses to kill and destroy pathogens and to promote tissue healing. Components of innate immunity include

- *Phagocytes:* Macrophages and neutrophils that kill pathogens by ingesting them;
- *Natural killer cells:* Large granular lymphocytes that kill virus and tumor cells via the release of cytolytic chemicals;
- *Antimicrobial proteins:*
  - *Interferons:* Small proteins secreted by virus-infected cells that limit the spread of viral infections by protecting uninfected tissue cells, and
  - *Complement:* A group of approximately 20 plasma proteins that (1) kill bacteria and certain other cell types by cell lysis; (2) enhance phagocytosis by coating the bacterial surface (osponization), allowing phagocytes to recognize and engulf the bacteria; and (3) enhance the inflammatory and immune responses;
- *Fever:* A systemic response to harmful microorganisms. Mild to moderate fevers are beneficial in fighting infections by increasing metabolism and boosting the production of white blood cells and antibodies; and
- *Inflammation:* Nonspecific response to bodily injury such as physical trauma, extreme temperatures, chemicals, foreign bodies, ischemia, and infection. The cardinal signs of inflammation are heat, redness, swelling, and pain.

The *adaptive immune system* is specific to particular foreign substances and enhances the protective mechanisms of the innate immune system. It develops with exposure to various antigens and provides protection from subsequent infections from the same microbes. The characteristics of the acquired immune system are that it is antigen specific and systemic, and it has memory. The two types of adaptive immunity are

1. *Humoral immunity:* Mediated by the antibodies in bodily fluids (e.g., blood, lymph, saliva, secretions). Antibodies are produced and secreted by B lymphocytes (B cells) or plasma cells that recognize specific antigens.

   - *Active humoral immunity* results from the production of antibodies in response to encountering antigens during bacterial or viral infections (naturally acquired) or through vaccinations (artificially acquired).

   - *Passive humoral immunity* results when antibodies are obtained from a human or animal donor. This immunity occurs naturally in a fetus when the mother's antibodies cross the placenta and artificially through the injection of immune serum (e.g., gamma globulin) to treat diseases such as hepatitis, poisonous snake bites, and rabies. Passive humoral immunity is fast acting and short lived.

2. *Cell-mediated immunity:* Mediated by T cells to destroy microbes that are inside a cell and cannot be reached by antibodies. Types of T cells include

   - *Killer T cells (cytotoxic)*, which kill virus-invaded body cells and cancer cells;

   - *Helper T cells*, which stimulate production of other cells (killer T cells and B cells); and

   - *Suppressor T cells*, which slow or stop activity of B and T cells when infection has cleared.

Infectious Disease

The immune system is active during periods of health and illness. In times of health, the immune system actively fights pathogens that enter the body. Infectious disease occurs when the pathogens cause signs and symptoms of illness. *Colonization* refers to the state in which microbes are present in the skin or mucous membrane, without signs and symptoms of an active infection. The following factors can lead to a weakened immune system, placing a person at a higher risk for acquiring an infectious disease:

- Compromised skin or mucous membranes (e.g., IV sites, urinary catheters, chest tubes);
- Malnutrition;
- Chronic illnesses such as diabetes or cancer;
- Circulatory problems;
- Old age;
- Stress;
- Surgery; and
- Immune system defects.

Neutropenia is a condition characterized by a low number of neutrophils in the blood, causing the patient to be at an increased risk for acquiring an infection. Patients who have a compromised immune system, including patients who have blood cancers; receive chemotherapy or radiation treatment; receive hemodialysis; have aplastic anemia; have Vitamin B12 deficiency; or have a disease that affects the immune system, such as HIV or autoimmune diseases, may have neutropenia. Patients with neutropenia are generally placed on neutropenic precautions. All people entering the patient's room must perform hand hygiene and wear personal protective equipment (see Appendix 12.B). Restrictions may also specify that no fresh flowers or uncooked foods be allowed in the room. Always refer to the posted precautions or check with the patient's nurse regarding specific restrictions for patients on neutropenic precautions.

Health Care–Associated Infections

Infectious diseases are one of the leading causes of death in the United States and worldwide. In United States hospitals, health care–associated infections (HAIs) account for approximately 1.7–2 million infections per year and are associated with as many as 103,000 deaths per year, making HAIs one of the top 10 leading causes of death (Carrico & Ramirez, 2007; Klevens, Edwards, et al., 2007; Marinella, Pierson, &

Chenoweth, 1997). Although patients may be admitted to the hospital with a known infectious disease, such as pneumonia, other patients may be admitted with an unidentified or unknown infectious disease, like methicillin-resistant *Staphylococcus aureus* (MRSA) or HIV. In addition, patients who were not infectious at the time of admission may acquire an infectious disease (e.g., *Clostridium difficile*) during their hospitalization.

The term *nosocomial infection* refers specifically to an infection acquired in the hospital. The Centers for Disease Control and Prevention (CDC; 2008) has defined HAIs more broadly as infections that patients acquire during the course of receiving treatment for other conditions within a health care setting.

Any patient in the hospital is at risk for acquiring a HAI. At the hospital level, administrators and physicians work to create and implement policies and procedures to detect, treat, and prevent the spread of infectious diseases. Policies and procedures cover all aspects of hospital care from triage and admission through discharge, including infectious disease testing, operating room procedures, patient transport, house cleaning, equipment sterilization, use of antibiotics, patient and visitor education, and employee education about the importance of following standard precautions and hand hygiene guidelines.

One of the most pressing issues is the prevalence of antimicrobial-resistant (also known as *multidrug-resistant*) organisms, such as MRSA and vancomycin-resistant enterococci (VRE). *Multidrug-resistant organisms (MDROs)* are microorganisms, predominantly bacteria, that are resistant to one or more classes of antimicrobial agents. The CDC Campaign to Reduce Antimicrobial Resistance in Healthcare Settings (CDC, 2001) has reported that more than 70% of the bacteria that cause HAIs are MDROs that are resistant to at least one of the drugs commonly used to treat them. Treatment options for patients with these infections are extremely limited.

Hospitalized patients, especially patients in the intensive care unit (ICU), tend to be at higher risk than nonhospitalized patients for acquiring MDRO infections (Siegel, Rhinehart, Jackson,

Chiarello, & Healthcare Infection Control Practices Advisory Committee, 2006). Hospitalized patients infected with MDROs are more likely to have longer hospital stays and to require treatment with second- or third-choice drugs that may be less effective, more expensive, more toxic, or all of these (CDC, 2001).

Evidence has shown that MDROs are carried from one person to another via the hands of health care workers, which are easily contaminated through direct contact with an infected patient or with surfaces in close proximity to the infected patient. Poor adherence to published recommendations for hand hygiene and glove use among health care workers increases the risk of transmitting MDROs to patients (Siegel et al., 2006). Preventing the emergence and spread of antimicrobial-resistant organisms in hospitals requires (1) diagnosing and treating the infection effectively, (2) prescribing the appropriate antimicrobial agent, and (3) consistent application of infection control practices by all health care workers (CDC, 2001; Goldman et al., 1996; Siegel et al., 2006). Poor hand hygiene increases the risk of patient-to-patient transmission of health care-associated infections. Siegel et al. (2006) found that health care workers are more receptive to and compliant with recommended control measures when organizational leaders participate in efforts to reduce the transmission of MDROs.

In addition to poor hand hygiene, the body of evidence implicating long and artificial nails to HAIs is growing. Winslow and Jacobson (2000) reviewed several research studies that linked artificial nails and long natural nails to the transmission of infectious organisms. Colony counts of bacteria were higher both before and after hand washing or surgical scrubbing in artificial and long natural nails compared with shorter natural nails. The CDC (2002) recommended that health care workers having direct contact with patients at high risk (e.g., patients in ICUs or operating rooms) not wear artificial nails or nail extenders and that natural nail tips be less than 0.25 inches long.

Some facilities have made the decision to extend the CDC guidelines to all health care workers having direct patient care. Evidence linking nail polish to increased transmission of HAIs is conflicting, except in the case of chipped nail polish, for which the evidence has supported higher colonization of bacteria compared with fresh polish and natural nails (Winslow & Jacobson, 2000). This evidence has suggested that health care workers with direct patient care who choose to wear nail polish should remove chipped and worn polish and reapply a fresh coat.

Although patient-to-patient transmission of infectious organisms via the hands of health care workers is the prevalent vehicle for dissemination of HAIs, contaminated equipment such as stethoscopes, blood pressure cuffs, thermometers, gloves, and gowns can also increase the risk of transmission of HAIs. Marinella, Pierson, and Chenoweth (1997) found that most stethoscopes are contaminated with bacteria and that the bacteria can be transmitted to human skin. They also found that isopropyl alcohol was the most effective agent for cleaning stethoscopes. Zachary et al. (2001) found a high rate of contamination in health care workers' gowns, gloves, and stethoscopes during routine medical examination of patients with known VRE. They also found that patients not known to be colonized with VRE could serve as sources for dissemination.

The CDC and other government and professional groups continue to work to define best practices with respect to prevention of HAIs in acute care hospitals and other health care settings. Occupational therapists working in acute care hospitals can do their part in helping to prevent transmission of HAIs by consistently adhering to hand hygiene practices and other infection control practices required by their facility.

Infectious Diseases in Health Care Settings

Table 12.1 contains a list of the infectious diseases that American occupational therapists working in acute care hospitals are most likely to encounter. The CDC has published an updated comprehensive guideline for preventing the transmission of infectious agents in health care settings (Siegel, et al., 2007). Portions of this document that are applicable to occupational therapists working in an acute care setting are summarized in Appendixes 12.B and 12.C.

Sepsis

Sepsis is also known as *systemic inflammatory response syndrome* (*SIRS*). It is the leading cause of death in critically ill patients in the United States (Hotchkiss & Karl, 2003). Sepsis results from the spread of infection from its initial site to the bloodstream, leading to widespread inflammation and decreased blood flow to vital organs. Sepsis is most commonly caused by bacterial infections but can be caused by fungal, parasitic, and viral infections. People with sepsis are generally critically ill and are treated in the hospital's intensive care unit.

According to the Cleveland Clinic Center for Consumer Health Information (2008), the following types of infections can commonly lead to sepsis:

- Appendicitis, peritonitis, gallbladder infections, liver infections;
- Infections of the brain or spinal cord;
- Pneumonia;
- Cellulitis; and
- Urinary tract infections, especially when the patient has a urinary catheter.

At an increased risk for sepsis are

- People with a weakened or compromised immune system;
- People who are very young or very old;
- People with severe injuries; and
- People who are in the hospital.

Occupational Therapy Approach for Working With Patients With Infectious Diseases

Occupational therapists working in acute care hospitals are likely to encounter patients with

(*Text continues on p. 461*)

Table 12.1. **Common Infectious Diseases Seen by Occupational Therapists in Acute Care Hospitals in the United States**

Disease	Characteristics and Incidence	Method of Transmission	Precautions	Special Considerations
Burkholderia cepacia (*B. cepacia*)	A group of bacteria, often resistant to common antibiotics, that are a known source of infection in hospitalized patients. Symptoms vary and can lead to serious respiratory infections. *B. cepacia* infections have been linked to contaminated mouthwash and nasal spray and exposure to sublingual probes. *At-Risk Population* • Patients with weakened immune systems • Patients with chronic lung disease, especially cystic fibrosis	• Person-to-person contact • Contact with contaminated surfaces • Exposure to *B. cepacia* in the environment	Contact	Highly contagious; strict adherence to hand hygiene and infection control practices is a must.
Chickenpox (*varicella zoster*) or shingles (*herpes zoster*)	A highly contagious disease caused by VZV. Characterized by a rash that generally appears first on the head and is most concentrated on the trunk. The rash progresses rapidly from macules to papules to vesicles before crusting. Crops of lesions can be present in different stages of development. There may be a slight elevation of temperature and general malaise at the onset. Generally, mild and self-limiting. Primary infection with VZV results in chickenpox. Shingles is the result of recurrent infection. *Complications* • Bacterial infection of skin lesions • Pneumonia (viral or bacterial) • Central nervous system manifestations • Reye syndrome • Postherpetic neuralgia	Person to person, through the air or contact with fluid from chickenpox blisters	• Contact • Airborne	Do not treat this patient if • Pregnant • Have never had chickenpox or the vaccine • Immunocompromised

(*continued*)

Table 12.1. (continued)

Disease	Characteristics and Incidence	Method of Transmission	Precautions	Special Considerations
	At-Risk Populations • Age >15 years • Infants <1 year • Immunocompromised people • Newborns of women with rash within 5 days before to 2 days after delivery *Incidence* Before the vaccine, about 11,000 people were hospitalized for chickenpox, and about 100 people died each year in the United States. Numbers have decreased by 90% since 1996.			
Clostridium difficile (C. difficile)	A bacterium that causes diarrhea and more serious intestinal conditions such as colitis. The bacteria are found in the feces. A common cause of AAD, it accounts for 15%–25% of all episodes of AAD. *Characterized by* • Watery diarrhea (at least 3 bowel movements/day for ≥2 days) • Fever • Loss of appetite • Nausea • Abdominal pain or tenderness *At-Risk Population* • Older adults • People with other illnesses requiring prolonged antibiotic use	• Person to person via contact with the feces of an infected person • Touching contaminated surfaces	Contact	• Wash hands with soap and water, which is the only way this bacterium can be killed. Alcohol-based hand rubs are not effective against *C. difficile* spores. • If a patient has diarrhea even if he or she is not being tested for *C. difficile*, use the precautions anyway.

Disease	Description	Transmission	Precautions
	• Person undergoing gastrointestinal surgery • Long length of stay in health care settings • Serious underlying illness • Immunocompromised people *C. difficile* infections can result in *C. difficile* diseases such as colitis; more serious intestinal conditions; sepsis; and, rarely, death.		• Wear a gown if the treatment plan involves sitting the patient where the diarrhea may leak out of the diaper or if toileting is the treatment plan. • Make sure the diaper is fastened tightly.
CMV	Herpes virus found in body fluids, including urine, saliva, breast milk, blood, tears, semen, and vaginal fluids. Once in a person's body, CMV stays there for life. CMV infections in healthy adults and children are usually silent, with no signs or symptoms. Some children and adults infected with CMV may experience mild symptoms such as fever, sore throat, fatigue, and swollen glands. CMV may cause disease in unborn babies and in people with weakened immune systems. *At-Risk Populations* • Unborn children • People who work with young children • Immunocompromised people (e.g., transplant recipients, HIV) Babies with congenital CMV may develop temporary symptoms such as liver problems, spleen problems, jaundice, purple skin splotches, lung problems, small size at birth, and seizures. They may also develop permanent symptoms or disabilities such as hearing loss, vision loss, mental disability, small head, lack of coordination, seizures, and death.	• Person to person, through close contact with body fluids • Pregnant woman to unborn baby • Blood transfusions and organ transplants	Standard • Good hand hygiene is essential, especially for pregnant women. • Avoid contact with saliva of young children (e.g., through kissing; sharing food, drinks, and utensils).

(continued)

Table 12.1. (continued)

Disease	Characteristics and Incidence	Method of Transmission	Precautions	Special Considerations
	Symptoms may appear at birth or months or years after birth. Babies born with CMV who have symptoms at birth are more likely to have permanent disabilities or symptoms that get worse over time. *Incidence* CMV is the most common virus transmitted to a pregnant woman's unborn child, with approximately 1 in 150 children born with congenital CMV. Approximately 1%–4% of uninfected mothers in the United States have primary (or first) CMV infection during a pregnancy. Between 50% and 80% of adults in the United States are infected with CMV by age 40. Very small risk of getting CMV infection from casual contact.			
Gastroenteritis norovirus	Noroviruses are a group of highly contagious, related viruses that cause acute gastroenteritis in humans. Norovirus was recently approved as the official genus name for the group of viruses provisionally described as "Norwalk-like viruses." Characterized by acute-onset vomiting, watery, nonbloody diarrhea with abdominal cramps, and nausea. In addition, myalgia, malaise, and headache are commonly reported. Low-grade fever is present in about half of cases. Dehydration is the most common complication and may require intravenous replacement fluids.	• Primarily through the fecal–oral route, either by direct person-to-person spread or fecally contaminated food or water	• Standard (when virus is suspected)	Wear a gown, if the treatment plan involves sitting the patient where the diarrhea may leak out of the diaper; if toileting is the treatment plan, or if the patient is vomiting.

	• Through hand transfer via contact with materials and surfaces that have been contaminated with either feces or vomitus	• Contact (when caring for diapered or incontinent patients or when risk of splashing is present)	Make sure the diaper is fastened tightly.
Hepatitis A	Liver disease caused by the hepatitis A virus. The virus is found in the stool of people infected with hepatitis A. Health care–associated hepatitis A occurs infrequently, and transmission to personnel usually occurs when the source patient has unrecognized hepatitis and is incontinent of bowel or has diarrhea. Once a person has been infected with hepatitis A, they cannot get it again. Symptoms include jaundice, fatigue, abdominal pain, loss of appetite, nausea, diarrhea, and fever. *Risk Factors* • Eating or drinking in patient care areas • Not washing hands after contact with an infected person • Sharing food, beverages, or cigarettes with patients, their families, or other staff members. *Incidence* 35,000 reported cases/year before the hepatitis A vaccine. Vaccine has been more widely used since the late 1990s, with a significant decrease in number of reported cases.	Person to person, by putting something in the mouth that has been contaminated with the stool of a person with hepatitis A	Standard contact (for diapered or incontinent patients)	• Do not eat or drink in patient care areas. • Do not share food, beverages, or cigarettes with patients, their families, or other staff members.

(*continued*)

Table 12.1. (continued)

Disease	Characteristics and Incidence	Method of Transmission	Precautions	Special Considerations
Hepatitis B	Liver disease caused by HBV. Can cause lifelong infection, cirrhosis (scarring) of the liver, liver cancer, liver failure, and death. Spread when blood from an infected person enters the body of a person who is not infected. *At-Risk Population* Affects people of all ages. Causes approximately 5,000 deaths/year. *Incidence* Occupational infections have decreased by 95% per year since hepatitis B vaccine became available: >10,000 infections in 1983, <400 infections in 2001. All HCWs who might be exposed to blood in an occupational setting should receive the hepatitis B vaccine. Risk for infection in HCWs who have been immunized is virtually nonexistent. Infected HCWs who adhere to standard precautions and who do not perform invasive procedures pose no risk for transmitting HBV to patients.	Percutaneous (i.e, puncture through the skin) or mucosal contact with infectious blood or body fluids	Standard	• All health care workers should be vaccinated against HBV. • Wear appropriate PPE when contact with blood or body fluids is anticipated. • Be familiar with facility's postexposure guidelines. If exposure occurs, do the following immediately: 1. Wash cuts with soap and water. 2. Flush splashes to the nose, mouth, or skin with water. 3. Irrigate eyes with clean water, saline, or sterile irrigates.

4. Report the exposure to the department responsible for managing exposures (e.g., employee health, infection control).

Disease	Description	Transmission	Precautions
Hepatitis C	Liver disease caused by HCV, which is found in the blood of people who have this disease. Can lead to chronic infection (75%–85% of infected people) and cirrhosis (20% of chronically infected people). Leading indication for liver transplant. 1%–5% of infected people may die. Symptoms include jaundice, fatigue, dark urine, abdominal pain, loss of appetite, and nausea. *At-Risk Populations* • Injecting drug users • Recipients of clotting factors made before 1987 • Patients on hemodialysis • Recipients of blood, solid organs, or both before 1992 • People with undiagnosed liver problems • Infants born to infected mothers • Health care workers through needlesticks or sharps Average risk for infection after a needlestick or cut exposure to HCV-infected blood is approximately 1.8%. Low risk of transmission from infected HCWs to patients. Infected HCWs should follow strict hand hygiene and standard precautions, use protective barriers as indicated, and cover cuts and skin sores to keep from spreading HCV.	Contact with the blood of an infected person	Standard Infected health care workers should cover cuts and skin sores and strictly follow hand hygiene and standard precautions.

(continued)

Table 12.1.   (continued)

Disease	Characteristics and Incidence	Method of Transmission	Precautions	Special Considerations
HIV/AIDS	HIV is the virus that causes AIDS. HIV attacks the immune system by destroying white blood cells (T cells or CD4 cells) that the immune system must have to fight disease. AIDS is the final stage of HIV infection. Having AIDS means that the virus has weakened the immune system to the point at which the body has difficulty fighting infections. Neurological, cognitive, and musculoskeletal impairments may also occur. Symptoms vary with progression of disease. The Centers for Disease Control and Prevention classifies HIV in 4 stages: • *Group I:* Primary HIV infection syndrome • *Group II:* Asymptomatic HIV infection • *Group III:* HIV infection with symptoms of lymphadenopathy • *Group IV:* AIDS *At-Risk Populations* • IV drug users • People having unprotected vaginal, anal, or oral sex with homosexual or bisexual men, multiple partners, or anonymous partners • People diagnosed with or being treated for hepatitis, tuberculosis, or a sexually transmitted disease • Having received a blood transfusion or clotting factor between 1978 and 1985 • Having unprotected sex with someone who has any of the risk factors listed earlier	Percutaneous (i.e., puncture through the skin) or mucosal contact with infectious blood or body fluids	Standard	• Wear appropriate PPE when contact with blood or body fluids is anticipated. • Be familiar with postexposure guidelines. If exposure occurs, do the following immediately: 1. Wash cuts with soap and water. 2. Flush splashes to the nose, mouth, or skin with water. 3. Irrigate eyes with clean water, saline, or sterile irrigates.

	Incidence HIV is primarily found in the blood, semen, or vaginal fluid of an infected person. In 2003, 1 million people in the United States were infected with HIV, with approximately 47% Black, 34% White, and 17% Hispanic. Approximately 74% of people living with HIV are males. Low risk of acquiring HIV in the United States through receiving a blood transfusion or blood products. Since 1985, all donated blood in the United States has been tested for HIV. Low risk of HCWs being exposed to HIV on the job if precautions are carefully followed. *Additional reference:* Fauci, Touchette, and Folkers (2005)			4. Report the exposure to the department responsible for managing exposures (e.g., employee health, infection control).
Influenza	Contagious respiratory disease caused by influenza viruses. The two main types of influenza (flu) virus, Types A and B, are responsible for seasonal flu epidemics each year. Can cause mild to severe illness and can lead to death. Outbreaks of health care–associated influenza affect both patients and personnel in hospitals. *At-Risk Populations* • Older adults • Young children • People with certain health conditions or weakened immune systems. *Incidence* Affects up to 20% of Americans/year, with >200,000 people hospitalized because of complications and approximately 36,000 deaths. *Worldwide:* Affects 3 to 5 million people/year with 250,000–500,000 deaths/year.	• Person to person via large virus-laden droplets that are generated when infected people cough or sneeze and settle on the mucosal surfaces of the upper respiratory tracts of susceptible people who are near (e.g., within about 6 feet)	• Droplet • Contact	• Get annual flu shot. • Do not go to work with the flu.

(continued)

Table 12.1.   (continued)

Disease	Characteristics and Incidence	Method of Transmission	Precautions	Special Considerations
	Influenza vaccination of both health care personnel and patients combined with basic infection control practices can help prevent outbreaks. *Additional references:* Fauci et al. (2005)	• Direct or indirect contact with surfaces/items contaminated with the virus and then touching the eyes, nose, or mouth.		
MRSA	Type of bacteria that causes staph infections and is resistant to certain antibiotics, such as methicillin, oxacillin, penicillin, and amoxicillin. 85% of MRSA infections are health care related, with one-third occurring during hospitalization. Commonly causes serious and potentially life-threatening infections, such as bloodstream infections, surgical site infections, or pneumonia. *At-Risk Populations* • People who have undergone invasive medical procedures • People with a weakened immune system • Treatment in hospital or health care facility • Age >65 • Male • Black Patients who already have a MRSA infection or who are colonized are the most common sources of transmission.	Person to person via human hands, especially HCWs' hands, that become contaminated with MRSA bacteria by contact with infected or colonized patients or devices and surfaces contaminated with body fluids containing MRSA.	Contact	Locate source of MRSA. • MRSA in a covered wound is easier to manage than MRSA in the sputum. • If a patient is coughing, wear a mask.

(continued)

Incidence

Becoming more prevalent in health care settings. MRSA accounted for 2% of total staph infections in 1974, 22% in 1995, and 63% in 2004. 20% death rate in U.S. hospitals in 2005.

MRSA can infect healthy people in the community. Community-associated MRSA infections may result in skin infections that look like pimples or boils and can be swollen and painful and have draining pus.

Additional reference: Klevens, Morrison, et al. (2007)

			Standard

PNA (hospital associated) — Cross-colonization via HCWs' hands

Second most common hospital-associated infection. Accounts for

- 15% of all hospital-associated infections
- 27% of all infections acquired in the medical ICU
- 24% of all infections acquired in the coronary care unit
- 20%–33% deaths from health care–associated infections.

Primary risk factor is mechanical ventilation with endotracheal intubation.

At-Risk Populations

- People with depressed level of consciousness
- People with dysphagia resulting from neurological or esophageal disorders
- People with endotracheal (naso- or orotracheal) tubes
- People with a tracheostomy
- People with enteral (naso- or orogastric) tubes
- People postsurgery

Incentive spirometer and deep breathing recommended to decrease the risk of postsurgical PNA.

Elevating head of the bed (30°–45°) recommended to prevent aspiration in patients with decreased consciousnesses, dysphagia, or endotracheal or enteral tubes.

Table 12.1.   (continued)

Disease	Characteristics and Incidence	Method of Transmission	Precautions	Special Considerations
TB	Lung disease caused by *Mycobacterium tuberculosis* bacteria. Can move to any part of the body such as the kidney, spine, and brain. Can be fatal. *Symptoms of Active TB Disease:* • Bad cough that lasts ≥3 weeks • Pain in the chest • Coughing up blood or sputum (phlegm from deep inside the lungs) • Weakness or fatigue • Weight loss • No appetite • Chills • Fever • Sweating at night Latent TB infections occur in people who breathe in TB bacteria and whose bodies are able to fight the bacteria to stop them from growing. The bacteria become inactive, but they remain alive in the body and can become active later. People with latent TB infections have no symptoms, cannot spread it to others, and usually have a positive skin test. They may develop active TB disease if the latent infection is not treated.	Person to person through the air. Spread by airborne particles when people with active TB disease sneeze, cough, speak, or sing and the particles are inhaled by people who share the same airspace. Transmission in health care settings most likely to occur when patients who have unrecognized TB are not on anti-TB therapy and are not in isolation.	Airborne	Must have an N-95 mask that is properly fitted.

	At-Risk Populations • People with HIV • People in high-risk environments such as correctional facilities, homeless shelters, hospitals, and nursing homes • Racial and ethnic minorities • People born outside the United States in areas with high prevalence of TB • People with weakened or compromised immune systems *Incidence* • Declining number of cases over 11 years, with 14,517 cases in 2004 • Estimated 9–14 million with latent infection; 10% will develop active TB disease *Worldwide:* • Affects one-third of the world's population • 9 million new TB cases/year • 2 million TB-related deaths/year *Additional reference:* Fauci et al. (2005)	Multidrug-resistant cases of TB are on the rise and are more difficult to treat.		
VRE	Infection of the urinary tract, blood, or wounds caused by enterococci bacteria that are resistant to vancomycin. Enterococci are often colonized in human intestines and the female genital tract and are often in the environment. In 2006–2007, enterococci caused 1 out of 8 hospital infections. Of these, approximately 30% were VRE.	Person to person via human hands, especially HCWs' hands that become contaminated with VRE bacteria by contact with infected or colonized	Contact	Be particularly diligent if toileting is part of the treatment plan.

(continued)

Table 12.1. (continued)

Disease	Characteristics and Incidence	Method of Transmission	Precautions	Special Considerations
	At-Risk Populations • People who have been treated with antibiotics, including vancomycin, for long periods of time • People who are hospitalized • People with weakened or compromised immune systems • People who have undergone surgical procedures • People with medical devices that stay in for some time such as urinary catheters or central IV catheters • People who are colonized with VRE	patients or devices and surfaces contaminated with body fluids containing VRE		

Note. Most of the information in this table has been summarized from information provided by the Centers for Disease Control and Prevention's Diseases and Conditions A–Z Index Web site (www.cdc.gov/DiseasesConditions/) or the CDC Division of Healthcare Quality Promotion Infection Control A–Z Index Web site (www.cdc.gov/ncidod/dhqp/a_z.html). When information has come from another source, this source is indicated in the table. AAD = antibiotic-associated diarrhea; CMV = cytomegalovirus; HCV = hepatitis C virus; HCWs = health care workers; HPV = hepatitis B virus; ICU = intensive care unit; MRSA = methicillin-resistant *Staphylococcus aureus*; PNA = pneumonia; PPE = personal protective equipment; TB = tuberculosis; VRE = vancomycin-resistant enterococci; VZV = *varicella zoster* virus.

HAIs. Many of the activities that occupational therapists use in treating their patients (e.g., toileting, bathing, dressing) have the potential to transfer infectious organisms. Therefore, it is imperative that occupational therapists be knowledgeable about and diligent in following infection control practices. Snaith and Rugg (2006) found that most studies investigating infection control knowledge and practice among health care workers have focused primarily on nursing. They also found that occupational therapists do not always apply infection control guidelines, even when the therapists acknowledged that such precautions were necessary.

Occupational therapists should follow standard precautions when working with all patients. Standard precautions assume all patients are potentially infectious; therefore, occupational therapists should perform hand hygiene and wear personal protective equipment as described in Appendix 12.B. In addition, occupational therapists must be knowledgeable about transmission-based precautions and alter their treatment as needed to comply with the recommended precautions. The following guidelines should be followed.

Adaptive Equipment

All *adaptive equipment* (e.g., reachers, sock aids, shoehorns, dressing sticks) must be cleaned after each use following the facility's infection control guidelines. Facility policies and procedures should delineate responsibilities for cleaning the equipment and how the equipment should be cleaned (e.g., using germicidal wipes, alcohol).

When patients are on transmission-based precautions, the equipment should be dedicated for use with this patient and left in the patient's room. Before removing the equipment from the patient's room, it must be cleaned using the facility's approved disinfectant. Only equipment that is absolutely necessary and can be easily cleaned should be brought into the patient's room. For example, use of a terry cloth–covered sock aid or a cloth-covered leg lifter is not advisable, unless that sock aid or leg lifter is issued to that patient or the facil-

ity has the means to disinfect cloth-covered equipment.

Monitoring Equipment

Monitoring equipment such as stethoscopes and pulse oximeters must be cleaned after being used with any patient. Alcohol wipes are effective and appropriate for use when following standard precautions. Most facilities have dedicated monitoring equipment kept in the room of patients who are on transmission-based precautions. Before removing monitoring equipment from a patient's room, it must be cleaned using the facility's approved disinfectant.

Transfer Equipment

Transfer equipment (e.g., sliding boards, lifts, standing aids, gait belts) must be cleaned after each use, following facility guidelines. When patients are on transmission-based precautions, only equipment that is absolutely necessary, and can be easily cleaned, should be brought into the patient's room. This equipment should be left in the patient's room for the duration that it is needed. Before removing transfer equipment from the patient's room, it must be cleaned using the facility's approved disinfectant. Cloth gait belts should always be applied over clothing (e.g., hospital gown) and avoid contact with patient's skin. Noncloth (plastic) gait belts that can be easily disinfected are recommended when patients are on transmission-based precautions.

Toileting

Perform hand hygiene after helping patients with any toileting-related activities such as placing or removing bed pans, handling Foley catheters, transferring on or off a toilet or a commode, emptying commodes, adjusting commode heights, and performing toilet hygiene. Wear gloves during these activities when contact with urine or feces is possible. Wear gloves and gown when patients are on contact precautions. Extra care should be taken when working with patients who have

Foley catheters. Be sure that the tubing has enough slack while transferring or moving a patient to help prevent the catheter from accidentally being pulled out. The drainage bag should be kept below the level of the patient's bladder to prevent backflow from the tube toward the bladder, which can increase the patient's risk for acquiring a urinary tract infection.

Bathing and Dressing

Perform hand hygiene after helping patients with bathing and dressing activities. Wear gloves during these activities when contact with urine or feces is possible. Wear gloves and gown when patients are on contact precautions.

Activity Modification

When patients have an active infectious disease, they may experience several symptoms, including fatigue, pain, loss of appetite, nausea, diarrhea, and fever, that may interfere with their ability to participate in daily activities, and goals may need to be modified. For example, a patient with acute *C. difficile* who normally toilets independently may need to use a bedside commode until the frequent diarrhea resolves. Infections can cause increased heart rate, respiration rate, and blood pressure. Similarly, vasodilation from an inflammatory response can cause orthostatic hypotension. Therefore, vital signs should be monitored closely and activities may need to be modified according to the patient's activity tolerance.

Mental Status Changes

Older patients may experience mental status changes such as confusion and memory loss when they have an acute infection, which is often the reason elderly patients are admitted to the hospital. Occupational therapists may be the first to notice mental status changes in a hospitalized patient and should report these changes to the patient's nurse or doctor.

Autoimmune Diseases

The immune system predominantly works to prevent and fight infectious diseases. However, in a patient with an autoimmune disorder, the immune system is unable to distinguish between healthy body tissue and antigens. The immune system reacts to normal body tissues, resulting in a response that destroys them. Although the causes of autoimmune diseases are not completely known, epidemiological and animal studies have suggested that infections can induce autoimmune diseases (Barzilai, Ram, & Shoenfeld, 2007; Fairweather & Rose, 2004). For example, the Epstein–Barr virus has been classically linked to systemic lupus erythematosus (Barzilai et al., 2007).

Autoimmune diseases can affect one or more body systems, tissues, or cells such as connective tissues, muscles, joints, skin, endocrine glands, heart, kidneys, blood vessels, and blood cells. Although the prevalence of autoimmune diseases is low (approximately 8% of the population), significantly more women (78%) than men are affected (Davidson & Keiser, 1997; Fairweather & Rose, 2004). Table 12.2 lists common autoimmune diseases that occupational therapists may encounter.

Occupational Therapy Approach for Working With Patients With Autoimmune Diseases

Most likely, patients with autoimmune diseases will have the disease as a comorbidity rather than as the reason for admission to the hospital. However, in the acute care setting, the autoimmune disease may be interfering with occupational performance and may be the primary reason for an occupational therapy consult. For example, a patient with rheumatoid arthritis may be admitted with an acute illness, but the nurses then notice the patient is having difficulty with self-feeding or other activities of daily living (ADLs) and requests an occupational therapy consult.

Acute care therapists need to be aware of the impact of autoimmune diseases on occupational performance. For example, therapists may need to modify activities and teach energy conservation and pacing techniques for patients

Table 12.2. Common Autoimmune Diseases

Disease	Characteristics and Description	Cross-Reference
Rheumatoid arthritis	Systemic disease that is generally characterized by inflammation and pain in joints on both sides of the body. May affect fingers, wrists, elbows, toes, ankles, knees, and the neck. Can cause joint destruction, deformity, and loss of mobility.	Chapter 7. Orthopedic and Musculoskeletal Disorders
Lupus erythematosus	Chronic autoimmune disorder that may affect the skin, joints, kidneys, and other organs. Systemic lupus erythematosus is the most common form of the disease.	Chapter 7. Orthopedic and Musculoskeletal Disorders
Scleroderma	Chronic connective tissue disease, with hardening of the skin being the most visible manifestation of the disease.	Chapter 7. Orthopedic and Musculoskeletal Disorders
Guillain–Barré syndrome	Disorder that affects the peripheral nervous system. Causes muscle weakness and abnormal sensations. Can lead to total paralysis.	Chapter 6. The Nervous System
Multiple sclerosis	Progressive disease affecting the central nervous system. Can cause problems with movement, coordination, strength, cognition, vision, tone, sensation, and urinary function.	Chapter 6. The Nervous System
Myasthenia gravis	Neuromuscular disorder that affects voluntary muscles. May cause muscle weakness and vision problems.	Chapter 6. The Nervous System

with decreased activity tolerance. For patients with joint pain and deformity, occupational therapists can use positioning and splinting to promote functional positions, decrease pain, and minimize deformities. Table 12.2 lists other chapters in this book in which more information about common autoimmune diseases and occupational therapy guidelines can be found. Many times, the acute hospitalization is the first contact a patient with an autoimmune disease has with an occupational therapist. It is appropriate to educate the patient about long-term management of the disease and resources available, including outpatient occupational therapy, community resources (e.g., disease-specific organizations, local classes, local senior centers), and support groups.

References

Barzilai, O., Ram, M., & Shoenfeld, Y. (2007). Viral infection can induce the production of autoantibodies. *Current Opinion in Rheumatology, 19,* 636–643.

Carrico, R., & Ramirez, J. (2007). A process for analysis of sentinel events due to health care–associated infection. *American Journal of Infection Control, 35,* 501–507.

Centers for Disease Control and Prevention. (2001). *Campaign to prevent antimicrobial resistance in healthcare settings.* Retrieved November 12, 2008, from www.cdc.gov/drugresistance/healthcare/problem.htm

Centers for Disease Control and Prevention. (2002). Guideline for hand hygiene in healthcare settings: Recommendations of the healthcare Infection Control Practices Advisory Committee and the HICPAC/SHEA/APIC/IDSA Hand Hygiene Task Force. *MMWR, 51*(RR-16), 1–48.

Centers for Disease Control and Prevention. (2008). *Infection control in healthcare settings.* Retrieved September 28, 2008, from www.cdc.gov/ncidod/dhqp/index.html

Cleveland Clinic Center for Consumer Health Information. (2008). *Sepsis overview.* Retrieved September 28, 2008, from www.clevelandclinic.org/health/health-info/docs/3800/3887.asp?index=12361

Davidson, A., & Keiser, H. D. (1997). Diagnosing and treating the predominantly female problems of systemic autoimmune diseases. *Medscape General Medicine.* Retrieved September 28, 2008, from www.medscape.com/viewarticle/719238_2

Fairweather, D., & Rose, N. R. (2004). Women and autoimmune diseases. *Emerging Infectious Diseases, 10,* 2005–2011. Retrieved September 28, 2008, from www.cdc.gov/ncidod/eid/vol10no11/04-0367.htm

Fauci, A. S., Touchette, N. A., & Folkers, G. K. (2005). Emerging infectious diseases: A 10-year perspective from the National Institute of Allergy and Infectious Diseases. *Emerging Infectious Diseases, 11,* 519–525.

Goldman, D. A., Weinstein, R. A., Wenzel, R., Tablan, O., Duma, R. J., Gaynes, R. P., et al. (1996). Strategies to prevent and control the emergence and spread of antimicrobial-resistant microorganisms in hospitals: A challenge to hospital leadership. *JAMA, 275,* 234–240.

Hotchkiss, R., & Karl, I. E. (2003). Medical progress: The pathophysiology and treatment of sepsis. *New England Journal of Medicine, 348,* 138–150.

Klevens, R. M., Edwards, J. R., Richards, C. L., Horan, T. C., Gaynes, R. P., Pollock, D. A., et al. (2007). Estimating health care-associated infections and deaths in U.S. hospitals, 2002. *Public Health Reports, 122,* 160–166.

Klevens, R. M., Morrison, M. A., Nadle, J., Petit, S., Gershman, K., Ray, S., et al. (2007). Invasive methicillin-resistant *staphylococcus aureus* infections in the United States. *JAMA, 298,* 1763–1771.

Marinella, M. A., Pierson, C., & Chenoweth, C. (1997). The stethoscope: A potential source of nosocomial infection? *Archives of Internal Medicine, 157,* 786–790.

Siegel, J. D., Rhinehart, E., Jackson, M., Chiarello, L., & Healthcare Infection Control Practices Advisory Committee. (2006). *Management of multidrug-resistant organisms in healthcare settings, 2006.* Retrieved September 28, 2008, from www.cdc.gov/ncidod/dhqp/pdf/ar/mdroGuideline2006.pdf

Siegel, J. D., Rhinehart, E., Jackson, M., Chiarello, L., & Healthcare Infection Control Practices Advisory Committee. (2007). *2007 guideline for isolation precautions: Preventing transmission of infectious agents in healthcare settings.* Retrieved September 28, 2008, from www.cdc.gov/ncidod/dhqp/pdf/guidelines/Isolation2007.pdf

Snaith, L., & Rugg, S. (2006). Occupational therapists' knowledge and practice of infection control procedures: A preliminary study. *British Journal of Occupational Therapy, 69,* 124–129.

Winslow, E. H., & Jacobson, A. F. (2000). Can a fashion statement harm the patient? Long and artificial nails may cause nosocomial infections. *American Journal of Nursing, 100,* 63–65.

Zachary, K. C., Bayne, P. S., Morrison, V. J., Ford, D. S., Silver, L. C., & Hooper, D. C. (2001). Contamination of gowns, gloves, and stethoscopes with Vancomycin-resistant enterococci. *Infection Control and Hospital Epidemiology, 22,* 560–564.

Appendix 12.A.

Further Reading

Kapasi, Z. F. (2006). The immune system and infectious diseases and disorders. In D. J. Malone & K. L. Bishop Lindsay (Eds.), *Physical therapy in acute care: A clinician's guide* (pp. 111–138). Thorofare, NJ: Slack.

Parry, M. F., Grant, B., Yukna, M., Adler-Klein, D., McLeod, G. X., Taddonio, R., et al. (2001). *Candida osteomyelitis* and diskitis after spinal surgery: An outbreak that implicates artificial nail use. *Clinical Infectious Diseases, 32,* 352–357.

Passaro, D. J., Waring, L., Armstrong, R., Bolding, F., Bouvier, B., Rosenberg, J., et al. (1997).

Post-serratiamarcescens wound infections traced to an out-of-hospital source. *Journal of Infectious Diseases, 175,* 992–995.

Tablan, O. C., Anderson, L. J., Besser, R., Bridges, C., & Hajjeh, R. (2003). *Guidelines for preventing health-care–associated pneumonia, 2003: Recommendations of CDC and the Healthcare Infection Control Practices Advisory Committee.* Retrieved September 28, 2008, from www.cdc.gov/ncidod/dhqp/pdf/guidelines/CDCpneumo_guidelines.pdf

Appendix 12.B.

Standard Precautions

The Centers for Disease Control and Prevention (CDC) have combined the major features of universal precautions and body substance isolation into a single guideline called *standard precautions* (Siegel, Rhinehart, Jackson, Chiarello, & Healthcare Infection Control Practices Advisory Committee, 2007). These guidelines are based on the principle that all blood, body fluids, secretions, excretions, nonintact skin, and mucous membranes may be contaminated with an infectious agent that could be transmitted within the health care setting. Standard precautions assume that all patients are potentially infected or colonized with an infectious organism, regardless of suspected or confirmed infection status. Standard precautions are intended not only to protect health care workers but also to protect patients by ensuring that health care workers do not carry infectious agents to patients via their hands or equipment used during patient care (Siegel, et al., 2007). Standard precautions include the following practices.

Hand Hygiene

Health care workers can contaminate their hands by touching intact areas of a patient's skin (e.g., while taking vitals or assisting with a transfer) or by touching surfaces contaminated by the patient (e.g., bed rails, bedside tables, commodes, walkers). Hand hygiene reduces the incidences of health care–associated infections (HAIs) and should be performed before and after any patient contact. The following hand hygiene guidelines are excerpted from the *Guideline for Hand Hygiene in Healthcare Settings* (CDC, 2002).

1. Avoid unnecessary touching of surfaces in close proximity to the patient.

2. Decontaminate hands by washing with soap and water when they are visibly soiled with blood or other body fluids. Use an alcohol-based hand rub for routinely decontaminating hands when they are not visibly soiled.

3. In each of the following clinical situations, decontaminate hands with an alcohol-based

hand rub. If an alcohol-based hand rub is not available, hands may be decontaminated by washing with soap and water.

a) Before direct contact with patients;

b) After contact with a patient's intact skin;

c) After contact with body fluids or excretions, mucous membranes, nonintact skin, and wound dressings if hands are not visibly soiled;

d) After contact with inanimate objects, including medical equipment, in the patient's vicinity; and

e) After removing gloves.

4. Wash hands with soap and water in the following situations:

a) Before eating;

b) After using the restroom; and

c) When exposure to spores (e.g., *Clostridium difficile* [*C. difficile*] or *Bacillus anthracis*) is suspected or proven. The physical action of washing and rinsing hands is recommended because alcohols and other antiseptic agents have poor activity against spores.

5. When decontaminating hands with an alcohol-based rub, apply the product to one hand and rub hands together, covering all surfaces of hands and fingers, until hands are dry. It is not necessary or desirable to routinely wash hands after each application of alcohol-based hand rubs.

6. When decontaminating hands by washing with soap and water, use the following procedure:

a) Prepare to have access to a paper towel;

b) Wet hands with water;

c) Apply soap product to hands;

d) Rub hands together vigorously for at least 15 seconds, covering all surfaces of hands and fingers;

e) Rinse hands with warm running water;

f) Dry hands thoroughly with a disposable towel;

g) Use the towel to turn off the faucet; and

h) Avoid using hot water because repeated exposure to hot water may increase the risk of dermatitis.

7. Hand lotions or creams can minimize the occurrence of dermatitis associated with frequent hand washing or frequent use of alcohol-based hand rubs.

8. Do not wear artificial nails or extenders when having direct contact with patients at high risk for infection (e.g., those in intensive care units). Keep natural nail tips less than 0.25 inches long. Facilities may have their own policies regarding artificial nails and fingernail length that are more stringent than these guidelines.

9. The CDC considers wearing rings in health care settings an unresolved issue and has not made any recommendations with regard to wearing rings. Facilities may have their own policies regarding wearing rings.

Personal Protective Equipment

The following personal protective equipment (PPE) guidelines are excerpted from the *Guideline for Isolation Precautions: Preventing Transmission of Infectious Agents in Healthcare Settings 2007* (Siegel et al., 2007).

1. General principles

a) Wear PPE when the nature of the anticipated patient interaction indicates that contact with blood or body fluids is likely to occur.

b) Prevent contamination of clothing and skin during the removal of PPE.

c) Remove and discard PPE before leaving the patient's room.

2. Gloves

a) Wear gloves when you can reasonably anticipate contact with blood, body fluids, mucous membranes, nonintact skin, or intact skin that is potentially contaminated (e.g., the skin of a patient who is incontinent of stool or urine).

b) Remove gloves after contact with a patient, the surrounding environment, or both, including medical equipment.

c) Do not wear the same pair of gloves for the care of more than one patient.

d) Do not wash gloves for the purpose of reuse.

e) Change gloves during patient care if hands will move from a contaminated body site to a clean body site.

3. Gowns

a) Wear a gown to protect skin and prevent soiling of clothing during patient care activities when contact with blood, body fluids, secretions, or excretions is anticipated.

b) Wear a gown for direct patient contact if the patient has uncontained secretions or excretions.

c) Remove gown and perform hand hygiene before leaving the patient's environment.

d) Do not reuse gowns, even for repeated contact with the same patient.

4. Mouth, nose, and eye protection

a) Use PPE to protect the mucous membranes of eyes, nose, and mouth during patient care activities that are likely to generate splashes or sprays of body fluids, blood, secretions, and excretions.

b) Select masks, goggles, face shields, and combinations on the basis of the anticipated need of the task to be performed.

5. Donning PPE. When donning PPE, put it on in the following order:

a) *Gown:* Make sure the gown fully covers the torso from the neck to knees and that the arms of the gown reach the wrist. Fasten the gown at both the neck and the waist.

b) *Mask or respirator:* Secure ties or elastic band at middle of the head and neck. Fit flexible band to the bridge of

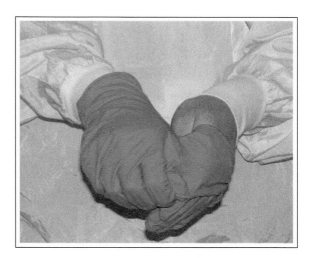

Figure 12.B1. Removing glove from one hand.
Source. Debra A. Kerrigan.

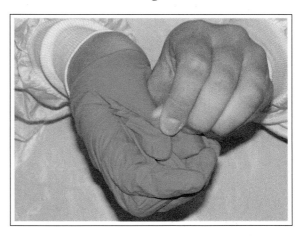

Figure 12.B2. Removing glove from second hand.
Source. Debra A. Kerrigan.

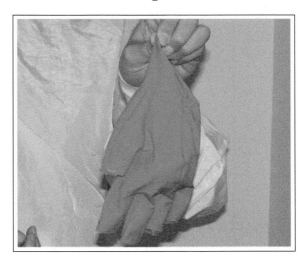

Figure 12.B3. Discarding gloves.
Source. Debra A. Kerrigan.

the nose. Make sure it fits snugly to the face and below the chin. Respirators must be fit tested, which is usually done by employee health when health care workers are hired. Health care workers must be fit tested again whenever their faces change as a result of weight loss, weight gain, or surgery.

c) *Gloves:* Select gloves according to hand size. Make sure the glove covers the wrist of the gown.

6. Doffing PPE. Always remove PPE before leaving the patient's room. Remove PPE in the following order to prevent contamination:

a) *Gloves:* Note that the outside of gloves are contaminated. Grasp outside of one glove with the opposite gloved hand; peel off. Hold removed glove in gloved hand. Slide fingers of ungloved hand under remaining glove at wrist to remove and discard in trash can (see Figures 12.B1, 12.B2, and 12.B3).

b) *Gown:* Note that the front of the gown and the sleeves are contaminated. Unfasten neck ties, then waist ties. Remove gown using a peeling motion; pull gown from each shoulder toward the same hand. The gown will turn inside out. Hold removed gown away from the body, roll into a bundle, and discard into waste or linen receptacle (see Figure 12.B4).

c) *Mask or respirator:* Note that the front of the mask or respirator is contaminated. Grasp only bottom ties, then top ties or elastics, and remove. Discard in waste container (see Figure 12.B5).

d) *Hand hygiene:* Perform immediately after removing all PPE.

Respiratory Hygiene and Cough Etiquette

Respiratory hygiene and cough etiquette is a new component of standard precautions. The

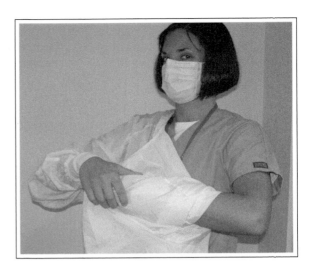

Figure 12.B4. Removing gown using peeling motion.
Source. Debra A. Kerrigan.

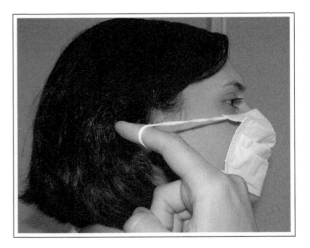

Figure 12.B5. Removing mask by grasping elastic or ties.
Source. Debra A. Kerrigan.

2007 guideline for preventing the transmission of infectious agents in health care settings (Siegel et al., 2007) includes measures that health care facilities should implement to contain respiratory secretions in patients and accompanying people who have signs and symptoms of a respiratory infection. These measures begin at the point of initial encounter in the health care setting (e.g., triage, reception, waiting areas in emergency departments). Occupational therapists working in the acute care setting should be aware of their facility's policies and guidelines for respiratory hygiene and cough etiquette. Occupational therapists with a known respiratory infection should adhere to respiratory hygiene and cough etiquette by doing the following (Siegel et al., 2007):

1. Cover mouth and nose (preferably with an arm rather than a hand, if possible) when sneezing or coughing;

2. Dispose of used tissues promptly;

3. Wear a mask when coughing; and

4. Perform hand hygiene after hands have been in contact with respiratory secretions.

Patient Care Equipment

All adaptive equipment (e.g., sock aid, reacher), mobility devices (e.g., wheelchairs, walkers), and patient monitoring equipment (e.g., stethoscope, pulse oximeter) should be properly disinfected after being used in treating a patient and before being used with another patient. Facility guidelines for cleaning agents should be followed. Care should be used when selecting adaptive equipment to ensure that it can be easily cleaned and disinfected. Equipment that cannot be easily cleaned and disinfected should be dedicated for single-patient use. PPE (gloves or gown) should be used when handling equipment that is visibly soiled or has come in contact with blood or body fluids. Commodes should be sanitized between patient use, following facility guidelines.

Appendix 12.C.

Transmission-Based Precautions

Transmission-based precautions are used in addition to standard precautions when the route of transmission is not completely interrupted using standard precautions alone. The three categories of transmission-based precautions are contact precautions, droplet precautions, and airborne precautions. The following guidelines for transmission-based precautions are based on the *Guideline for Isolation Precautions: Preventing Transmission of Infectious Agents in Healthcare Settings 2007* (Siegel et al., 2007).

Contact Precautions

Contact precautions are intended to prevent transmission of infectious agents, which are spread by direct or indirect contact with the patient or the patient's environment. Contact precautions are also indicated when the presence of excessive wound drainage, fecal incontinence, or other bodily discharges pose an increased potential for environmental contamination and an increased risk for transmission. In acute care

hospitals, patients requiring contact precautions are usually in single-patient rooms or in rooms with other patients who are infected or colonized with the same pathogen. In addition to *Standard Precautions*, occupational therapists should adhere to the following guidelines when working with patients who require contact precautions:

1. Wear personal protective equipment (PPE), as described in the Personal Protective Equipment section of Appendix 12.B.

2. Handle patient care equipment in accordance with standard precautions. In acute care hospitals, use disposable noncritical patient care equipment (e.g., blood pressure cuffs, stethoscopes, pulse oximeters). When disposable equipment is not available (e.g., reacher, sock aid), equipment should be dedicated for use with a single patient. If use of the equipment for multiple patients cannot be avoided, clean and disinfect the equipment before using it with another patient.

3. The Centers for Disease Control and Prevention (CDC) has recommended that in acute care hospitals, transport or movement of patients outside the room should be limited to medically necessary purposes. Occupational therapy treatment for patients on contact precautions should be confined to the patient's room. However, some facilities may allow patients on contact precautions to leave their room for therapy. If the patient's source of infection is not easily containable by dressings or diapers, do not take the patient from the room. If the source of infection is containable by dressings, diapers, or Foley catheters (in the case of patients with vancomycin-resistant enterococci in the urine), do the following before leaving the patient's room:

- Decontaminate the patient's hands and place a gown on the patient;
- Remove your PPE and decontaminate your hands; and
- Do not touch anything in the room, including bed rails and tables, after decontaminating your hands.

Outside the room, stay with the patient and do not allow the patient to touch things in common areas (e.g., hallways, bathrooms, kitchens). Facility-specific policies vary in whether they recommend that patients on contact precautions wear gloves when outside their rooms. Occupational therapists should be aware of and adhere to their facility's specific policies.

Droplet Precautions

Droplet precautions are intended to prevent transmission of pathogens spread through close respiratory or mucous membrane contact with respiratory secretions. Examples of infectious agents for which droplet precautions are indicated include *B. pertussis* and influenza virus. In acute care hospitals, patients on droplet precautions are usually in single-patient rooms or in rooms with other patients who are infected or colonized with the same pathogen.

Because transport or movement of patients on droplet precautions should be limited to medically necessary purposes, occupational therapists should plan to treat these patients in their rooms. Occupational therapists should only bring into the patient's room adaptive equipment or stationary items (e.g., clipboards, pens) that can be easily cleaned and disinfected or that can be dedicated to the use of that single patient. In addition to following standard precautions, occupational therapists should don a mask on entry into the patient's room.

Airborne Precautions

Airborne precautions are intended to prevent transmission of infectious agents that remain infectious over long distances when suspended in the air. Examples of infectious agents for which airborne precautions are indicated include rubeola virus (measles), varicella virus (chickenpox), and tuberculosis. In acute care hospitals, occupational therapists will likely find patients who require airborne precautions in an airborne *infection isolation room (AIIR)*. AIIRs are also known as *monitored negative-pressure rooms*. Occupational therapists who are susceptible or nonimmune should not care for patients with vaccine-preventable airborne diseases such as measles, chickenpox, and smallpox.

In addition to following standard precautions, occupational therapists should don a mask or respirator (fit-tested National Institute for Occupational Safety and Health–approved N95 or higher) on entry into the patient's room. The recommendation for using a mask or respirator when caring for patients on airborne precautions is disease specific, so occupational therapists should check the precautions sign posted on the patient's door or check with the patient's nurse before entering the room. For example, a respirator is required when entering the room of a patient when tuberculosis or smallpox are suspected or confirmed.

13

Dysphagia

Wendy Avery, MS, OTR/L

Difficulty in swallowing is referred to as *dysphagia. Swallowing* is the act in which food and fluids are manipulated and transported from the mouth to the stomach. Other terms associated with swallowing are *feeding* and *eating. Feeding* is "the process of setting up, arranging, and bringing food [or fluid] from the plate or cup to the mouth" (O'Sullivan, 1995, p. 19; American Occupational Therapy Association [AOTA], 2007). *Eating* is "the ability to keep and manipulate food [or] fluid in the mouth and swallow it" (O'Sullivan, 1995, p. 19; AOTA, 2007).

Occupational therapists are well qualified as primary dysphagia therapists in the acute care setting. AOTA endorses the role of occupational therapists as primary dysphagia therapists (AOTA, 2007) and offers Specialty Certification in Feeding, Eating, and Swallowing for occupational therapists and occupational therapy assistants. AOTA (2007) also delineated entry- and advanced-level dysphagia skills for occupational therapists and occupational therapy assistants. The occupational therapist's skills in addressing all elements of a client's function encompass basic activities of daily living (BADLs), which include and have an impact on swallowing. Occupational therapists can address a variety of the client's feeding and swallowing needs in the challenging unhomelike hospital context. In this environment, nutritional needs compete with pressing medical and surgical procedures but are very important to both medical and rehabilitative interventions.

This chapter provides an introduction to dysphagia care for occupational therapists practicing in the acute care setting. Dysphagia is an advanced practice skill (AOTA, 2007), and although this chapter does not provide a sufficient knowledge base for the occupational therapist

to begin practice in this area, it does provide an introduction. Readers are strongly encouraged to explore a wide range of learning opportunities and mentorship to develop skills in this practice area. Suggestions for further learning are listed in Appendix 13.A.

Prevalence of Dysphagia in the Acute Care Setting

Patients in the acute care setting often have dysphagia, and its prevalence may be 28% (Young & Durant-Jones, 1990). Dysphagia's prevalence is likely higher in specific disease populations; Warnecke et al. (2008) noted that as many as 81% of acute stroke patients demonstrate a risk for aspiration.

Dysphagia occurs in acute care settings as a result of one or more of three etiologies: (1) acute dysphagia that is a symptom of a current diagnosis; (2) chronic dysphagia; or (3) dysphagia as a consequence of hospitalization because of immobility, illness, or hospital interventions. Often, two or three of these circumstances occur in a single patient. Dysphagia in the acute care setting can be more severe than in other settings because medical acuity worsens its presentation. Dysphagia may be associated with dehydration (Leibovitz et al., 2007), malnutrition (Patel & Martin, 2008), pneumonia, and death (Masiero, Pierobon, Previateo, & Gomiero, 2008).

Swallowing Physiology and Pathophysiology

Swallowing is a complex process that involves numerous muscles and nerves and consists of both voluntary and reflexive components. Figure 13.1 illustrates the primary anatomical

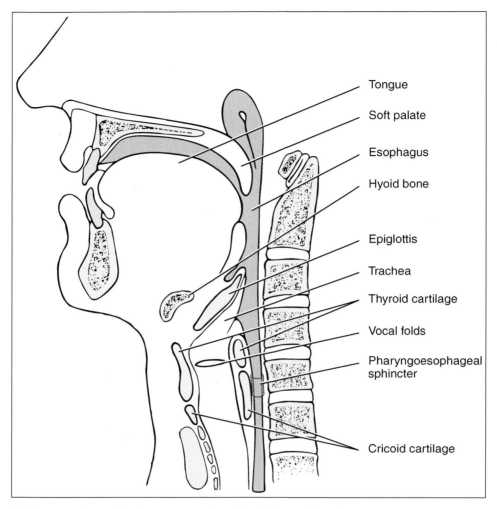

Figure 13.1. Primary anatomical structures involved in swallowing.
Source. Richard Fritzler, Medical Illustrator, Roswell, GA.

structures involved in swallowing. Eating is an integral part of swallowing, and so is included in the following description of the stages of swallowing. The motor functions involved in the phases of swallowing are listed in Table 13.1.

Phases of Swallowing

- *Preoral phase:* Cognitive and physical orientation to the eating activity occurs. Feeding takes place during the preoral phase, during which the client moves food or liquid to the mouth. This phase is primarily voluntary.

- *Oral preparatory phase:* A solid or liquid bolus is prepared by the structures of the

oral cavity to be swallowed, which involves tasting, chewing, manipulation, and containment of the bolus in the mouth. This phase is also primarily voluntary.

- *Oral phase:* The bolus is propelled toward the pharynx by motion of the tongue against the hard and soft palates. Both voluntary and involuntary controls occur during the oral phase.

- *Pharyngeal phase:* The soft palate elevates to close off the nasopharynx. The larynx lifts and protracts, and the epiglottis moves posteriorly to cover the opening to the larynx, protecting it from the entry of the food or liquid bolus. The swallow response is initiated as the bolus is propelled through

Table 13.1. Phases of Swallowing

Action	Purpose	Muscles	Cranial Nerve Innervation
Oral preparatory phase functions			
Lip closure	Retain bolus in mouth	Orbicularis oris	VII
Cheek	Retain bolus on teeth surfaces and centrally in mouth	Buccinator	VII
Jaw closure	Elevation, closure of mandible and mouth, chewing	Temporalis	V
		Masseter	V
		Lateral pterygoid	V
Jaw opening	Open mouth and jaw, chewing	Lateral pterygoid	V
Bolus reception and manipulation	Pull tongue forward, backward, up, down	Extrinsic tongue muscles: genioglossus, hyoglossus, chondroglossus, styloglossus	XII
Bolus manipulation	Change the shape of the tongue during bolus manipulation	Intrinsic tongue muscles: vertical transverse, superior longitudinal, inferior longitudinal	XII
Oral phase functions			
Tongue holds bolus against the hard palate	Hold bolus in place before initiating swallow	Intrinsic and extrinsic tongue muscles	XII
Bolus is propelled posteriorly	Moves bolus into pharynx	Extrinsic tongue muscles:	
		Digastric	V
		Mylohyoid	V
		Geniohyoid	XII
Pharyngeal phase functions			
Hyoid bone elevates and moves anteriorly	Elevates larynx, opens upper esophageal sphincter	Digastric	V
		Mylohyoid	V
		Geniohyoid	XII
		Hyoglossus	XII

(*continued*)

Table 13.1.   (continued)

Action	Purpose	Muscles	Cranial Nerve Innervation
Posterior tongue elevates	Closes opening between oral cavity and pharynx	Palatoglossus	X
Velum (soft palate) elevates	Prevents food material from entering nasopharynx	Palatopharyngeus Levator velum palatinum	X and XI X, XI
Vocal folds close	Keeps food from entering trachea and airway	True vocal folds False vocal folds	X, recurrent branch
Pharynx elevates and shortens	Bolus propulsion through pharynx	Palatopharyngeus Stylopharyngeus	X, XI IX
Upper esophageal sphincter relaxes as bolus passes through	Allows food to pass into body of esophagus	Superior constrictor Middle constrictor Inferior constrictor (These muscles relax, signaled by pull from hyoid motion, above)	X, XI X X, XI
Esophageal phase functions			
Sequential contraction of esophageal muscle	Bolus propulsion through esophagus	Upper third of esophagus: Striated muscle Lower two-thirds of esophagus: Smooth muscle	Nucleus ambiguus, X Dorsal motor nucleus of X
Lower esophageal sphincter relaxes	Allows food to pass into stomach	Lower esophageal sphincter	Spinal afferents: X Efferents: X

the pharynx during closure of the larynx and the opening of the upper esophageal sphincter (UES). This phase is primarily involuntary, although voluntary controls may alter its motions.

- *Esophageal phase:* The UES returns to its closed position to keep food from reentering the pharynx. The bolus travels through the esophagus, and the lower esophageal sphincter opens, allowing the bolus to pass into the stomach. This phase

is involuntary, although body position changes may alter the movement of the bolus through the esophagus.

Cranial Nerves

Cranial nerve functions in swallowing with respect to motor and sensory functions are provided in Table 13.2. Sensory inputs are critical to many aspects of swallowing, including motor response to the bolus, awareness of

Table 13.2. **Cranial Nerves Involved in Normal Swallowing**

Cranial Nerve	Central Nervous System	Autonomic Nervous System
V; trigeminal	*Sensory:* Touch, pressure in oral cavity *Motor:* Muscles of mastication, tensor velum palatini, mylohyoid, digastric	None
VII; facial	*Sensory:* Taste, anterior tongue *Motor:* Lips	*Visceral motor:* Sublingual, submandibular glands
IX; glossopharyngeal	*Sensory:* Taste, posterior tongue *Motor:* Stylopharyngeus, parasympathetic fibers	*Visceral motor:* Parotid gland
X; vagus	*Sensory:* Sensations from larynx, pharynx, trachea, esophagus	*Visceral motor:* Smooth muscle of abdominal viscera
XI; spinal accessory	Same as cranial nerve X, except for palatoglossus	None
XII; hypoglossal	*Motor:* Intrinsic tongue muscles, extrinsic tongue muscles except mylohyoid and anterior digastric	None

the swallowing process, and protection of the airway.

Pumps and Valves

The swallow may be conceived as a series of valves and pumps that sequentially contain and propel the bolus (Crary & Groher, 2003). This series of valves and pumps is listed in Table 13.3.

Characteristics of Dysphagia

Dysphagia may be noticed by the client, who describes *symptoms* (feelings or observations that the client notices). Gathering information from the client about dysphagia symptoms is part of the evaluation process and helps the occupational therapist to understand the client's perspective. In the acute care setting, clients may not have observed their symptoms and may have difficulty communicating them.

A client's swallowing function is also observed by the caregiver, occupational therapist, physician, and other skilled health care providers, who observe *signs,* or observations noted by others. Signs are noted during structured observation in a clinical bedside evaluation. Because much of the swallow is not directly visible, instrumental (imaging) procedures like the *modified barium swallow (MBS)* and *fiberoptic endoscopic evaluation of swallowing (FEES)* are necessary to obtain objective information about unseen aspects of the swallow. Instrumental procedures provide essential information with regard to aspiration (entry of

Table 13.3. Pumps and Valves in the Swallow Mechanism

Valve	Purpose	Associated Pump	Disruption Caused by Valve Failure
Lips	Containment of bolus within the oral cavity. Creation of pressure around the bolus.	Intraoral motion of bolus: manipulation Posterior bolus propulsion toward pharynx	Leakage of bolus out of lips Bolus falls apart in the oral cavity
Velum	Closes off the naso-pharynx to maintain oral pressure. Protects the nasopharynx from entry of bolus.	Intraoral motion Posterior bolus propulsion toward pharynx	Nasal regurgitation Bolus falls apart because of lack of pressure
True and false vocal cords	Seal the airway as the bolus passes through the pharynx.	Swallow response: bolus passes through pharynx	Airway penetration by bolus Aspiration of the bolus
Upper esophageal sphincter	The tonic "resting" state keeps the bolus from passing into the esophagus prematurely. Prevents regurgitation of the bolus back into the pharynx.	Pharyngeal Swallow response propels the bolus through this valve	Reflux of the bolus from the esophagus back into the pharynx
Lower esophageal sphincter	Opens to allow passage of the bolus into the stomach. The tonic "resting" state of the lower esophageal sphincter prevents bolus material from refluxing back into the esophagus.	Esophageal contractions propel bolus through this valve	Reflux of the bolus from the stomach back into the esophagus

food or fluid into the larynx from which it may easily be aspirated).

Symptoms and signs vary greatly with the individual patient and with the diagnosis. They may include cough while eating, wet vocal quality, complaints of pain with swallowing, throat clearing, effortful swallowing, drooling, residual food in the oral cavity, and weight loss. Typical signs of dysphagia through the phases of the swallow are presented in Table 13.4. Comparison of these signs with the physiology

of the swallow described earlier can assist the therapist in determining which aspect of the swallow is impaired. Although some of these signs can be observed while the patient is eating or during a bedside swallow, other signs can only be observed during an MBS or FEES.

Dysphagia is associated with a number of diagnoses commonly seen in acute care. The signs and symptoms of dysphagia in major disease categories are summarized in Table 13.5. The occupational therapist is cautioned not to

Table 13.4. Dysphagia in the Phases of Swallowing

Clinical or Instrumental Observation	Cause
Oral preparatory phase dysphagia	
Bolus is not formed; residual food on tongue, sulci of mouth, hard palate	Reduced tongue motion or incoordination, sensory loss, inattention
Bolus falls anteriorly in front of teeth, drooling	Weak lip musculature, sensory loss, inattention
Bolus "pockets" laterally between teeth and cheek or on one side of the tongue	Weak cheek musculature, sensory loss, inattention
Difficulty chewing	Reduced or weak jaw motion
Food residue on tongue, difficulty controlling bolus, bolus spilling into pharynx	Weak or reduced tongue motions
Limited or absent oral manipulation of the bolus	Oral apraxia (in the absence of weakness or sensory loss)
Oral phase dysphagia	
Reduced opposition of tongue to soft palate (velum) and hard palate	Weak tongue elevation
Bolus residue on hard palate	Weak tongue motions limiting posterior bolus movement
Reduced sequential opposition of tongue to hard palate, then soft palate	Weak or uncoordinated tongue motions
Soft or liquid bolus "spills" into pharynx prematurely, residue in valleculae	Reduced tongue control; reduced seal between posterior tongue base and velum
Reduced epiglottic closure	Weak base of tongue
"Piecemeal deglutition": small amounts of bolus left on tongue	Weak tongue or oral manipulation: Bolus cannot be gathered in one mass for swallowing
Slowed "transit" of bolus to posterior oral cavity	Weak or uncoordinated tongue motions
Aspiration (material entering the airway) before the swallow	Bolus not controlled and falls into airway (especially liquids)
Pharyngeal phase dysphagia	
Reduced propulsion of bolus through pharynx	Base of tongue weakness; decreased strength of pressure wave through pharynx
Residue in valleculae	Weakness of base of tongue and laryngeal elevation; reduced posterior movement of base of tongue

(continued)

Table 13.4. (continued)

Clinical or Instrumental Observation	Cause
Incomplete closure of epiglottis	Weakness of base of tongue and laryngeal elevation
Coating of food or barium on pharyngeal walls	Reduced bilateral pharyngeal contractions
Nasal penetration of food during swallow	Inefficient closure of nasopharynx by the velum, especially with liquids
Penetration or aspiration of bolus	Reduced closure of epiglottis over airway (laryngeal closure); weak laryngeal elevation
Stasis of bolus in pyriform sinuses	Reduced anterior laryngeal pressure
Residue in pyriforms, valleculae (aspiration of residue overflow)	Delayed swallow response
Aspiration during the swallow	Incomplete airway (vocal fold) closure
Aspiration after the swallow	Absent or weak swallow (pharyngeal residue in valleculae, pyriform sinuses overflow drops into airway)
Esophageal phase dysphagia	
Movement of bolus from esophagus to pharynx	Esophageal motility disorder; incompetence of upper esophageal sphincter
Reflux	Incompetence of lower esophageal sphincter
Aspiration after swallow	Bolus refluxes from esophagus up through lower esophageal sphincter into pharynx and into airway

assume a specific presentation for an individual patient's diagnosis.

Dysphagia Screening, Clinical Evaluation, and Assessment

Dysphagia screening determines the need for evaluation and assessment. Evaluation should include use of an assessment, or a standardized test of swallowing dysfunction.

Screening

Screening is the process of determining whether a patient requires a full formal dysphagia evaluation. Screening does not require a physician's

referral because no intervention is completed. Screening may be done through a combination of oral report from caregivers and observation of the patient. If any doubt whether dysphagia is present remains once the screening is completed, a full dysphagia evaluation is recommended. Screening rather than completing a full evaluation can save time, efficiently meeting client and staffing needs. In some facilities, nursing staff may complete the dysphagia screening.

Several standardized screening tools are listed in Appendix 13.B. In the dysphagia literature, some standardized screenings involve giving the patient food or water, and some do not. Physicians often use those that provide food and water. Once an occupational therapist

(Text continues on p. 482)

Table 13.5.   Signs and Symptoms of Dysphagia in Commonly Seen Diagnoses

Diagnosis	Signs and Symptoms
Aging	Age-related muscle loss (*sarcopenia*) in oral–motor structures. Pharyngeal constriction is reduced during swallow in older patients with dysphagia (Kendall & Leonard, 2001b). Common medical conditions in elders may be associated with slowed pharyngeal bolus transit (Kendall, Leonard, & McKenzie, 2004). Delayed airway closure and resulting aspiration may be accompanied by the weaker pharynx in this population (Kendall & Leonard, 2001a). Upper esop hageal sphincter pressure at rest is reduced, and higher pressure during the swallow is also slower to relax than in younger people (van HerWaarden et al., 2003).
Amyotrophic lateral sclerosis	Oral and pharyngeal weakness, as well as laryngeal weakness, is seen in amyotrophic lateral sclerosis. Both upper and lower motor neurons may be affected. Airway protection and pharyngeal motions that propel the bolus may be lost (Ertekin et al., 2000).
Alzheimer's disease	Slowed oral and pharyngeal responses accompany difficulty with self-feeding and reduced attention span. Texture intolerance may be present with preference for purees and sweets. Eating and swallowing apraxia are often seen.
Brain injury	Different injuries may vary in presentation. Oral phase challenges may include reduced lip closure and tongue control and bolus pocketing in the cheek (Mackay, Morgan, & Bernstein, 1999). Slowed trigger of pharyngeal swallow, reduced base of tongue motions, and reduced laryngeal elevation may be present (Logemann, Pepe, & Mackay, 1994). Behavioral and cognitive issues frequently interfere with eating (Avery-Smith & Dellarosa, 1994).
Brain tumors	Nature of the swallowing deficit varies with tumor location and size. Interventions are similar to those used for clients with stroke. Swallowing may be affected by interventions for tumor (radiation, chemotherapy).
Chronic obstructive pulmonary disease	Shortness of breath may make swallowing difficult and create a risk for aspiration. Challenges with airway closure and aspiration may be seen (Martin-Harris, 2008).

(continued)

Table 13.5.   (*continued*)

Diagnosis	Signs and Symptoms
Developmental disorders: Cerebral palsy and mental retardation	Cerebral palsy or mental retardation may affect the ability to form and manipulate a bolus, move it through the pharynx, and swallow it without aspirating (Rogers et al., 1994). Abnormal postural reflexes and abnormal and fluctuating muscle tone may affect swallowing structures as well as mobility and stability of the trunk and limbs, affecting feeding and swallowing.
Guillain–Barré syndrome	Guillain–Barré syndrome attacks the peripheral nervous system. It can affect respiratory muscles; as a result, reduced breath support for swallowing and airway protection challenges may be seen. Pharyngeal deficits may be more serious than oral deficits (Chen, Donofrio, Frederick, Ott, & Pikna, 1996). Patients may require dysphagia intervention after the need for ventilator support for breathing.
Head and neck tumors	Clients who are receiving treatment for head and neck cancers require intensive swallowing intervention (Pauloski, 2008). Modified barium swallow is a critical part of assessment because surgeries remove tissue in oral cavities, pharyngeal cavities, or both. Surgical removal of oral tumors and tumors at the juncture of the oral cavity and the pharynx necessitate compensatory techniques for oral manipulation of the bolus because oral structures and muscular tissues are removed along with the tumor. Individual presentations vary depending on tumor size and location and how fast it grows.
	Pharyngeal cancers may be treated with partial or total laryngectomy. *Partial laryngectomy* includes *hemilaryngectomy* (vertical removal of half of the larynx) and *supraglottic laryngectomy* (removal of structures above the *glottis*, defined as the vocal cords and the space between them). Airway protection resulting from reduced airway closure can be a side effect of both procedures (Crary & Groher, 2003). Patients with *total laryngectomy* cannot aspirate because the esophagus and the airway have been surgically separated, but they may have difficulty with bolus propulsion.
	Chemotherapy reduces appetite, resulting in weakened musculature for eating. Radiation therapy causes *xerostomia* (dry mouth because of reduced salivary flow), reduced sense of taste, and reduced blood flow to affected musculature, causing weakness and often eventual muscle fibrosis. *Trismus* or inability to move the jaw may result. Surgery often includes tracheostomy for airway protection, which may further complicate rehabilitation efforts.
Multiple sclerosis	Oral and pharyngeal weakness may be seen, especially during flare-up events. Delayed pharyngeal swallow, difficulty with airway protection, and aspiration may be observed (Abraham & Yun, 2002).

Table 13.5. **(continued)**

Diagnosis	Signs and Symptoms
Parkinson's disease	Slow motions of arm and oral motions for preoral and oral phases of swallow. Impulsivity and poor safety judgment, poor bolus manipulation, oral residue, delayed laryngeal elevation, and delayed oral and pharyngeal transit times (Nagaya, Kachi, Yamada, & Igata, 1998).
Pneumonia	Aspiration caused by the presence of reduced laryngeal protection during swallowing may cause aspiration pneumonia, particularly in older adults (Marik & Kaplan, 2003). For that reason, many hospital patients have pneumonia. Pneumonia can be concurrent with any diagnosis; therefore, its presentation cannot be typified. Pneumonia may also cause aspiration because the cough reflex may be depressed in older adults (Sekizawa et al., 1990).
Spinal cord injury	Patients with spinal cord injury can demonstrate dysphagia at the C5 level of injury and above, although concerns with pulmonary health may be an issue at lower levels because of immobility (risk of pneumonia), presence of tracheostomy, and ventilator dependence (Kirshblum, Johnston, Brown, O'Connor, & Jarosz, 1999). Aspiration may be a concern. Anterior cervical decompression may be a complicating factor (Riley, Skolasky, Alber, Vaccaro, & Heller, 2005).
Stroke, left hemisphere	Patients demonstrate slow oral stage initiation; slow trigger of the pharyngeal phase; apraxia for feeding and swallowing; pharyngeal and laryngeal sensory deficits (Aviv et al., 1997); and possibly unilateral weakness (right side) of oral and pharyngeal structures.
Stroke, right hemisphere	Clients may demonstrate oral phase delays and delays in pharyngeal trigger and laryngeal elevation; slowed pharyngeal phase, penetration, and aspiration (Robbins et al., 1993); pharyngeal and laryngeal sensory deficits (Aviv et al., 1997); oral sensory deficits (left side); unilateral weakness (left side) of oral and pharyngeal structures; neglect or denial of dysphagia; impulsive behavior at mealtime.
Stroke, brainstem or subcortical	Clients may demonstrate pharyngeal and laryngeal sensory deficits (Aviv et al., 1997), oral phase delays, delay in trigger of the swallow, weakness in oral and pharyngeal motions.
Tracheostomy	Tracheostomy reduces vocal cord closure, reducing coughing ability (Shaker et al., 1995). Subglottic pressure is reduced, which may "pull" food into the larynx during the swallow (Fornataro-Clerici & Roop, 1997). Tracheostomy with cuff inflation may decrease elevation of the larynx during swallow and increase aspiration (Ding & Logemann, 2005), although some recent studies have indicated otherwise. Terk, Leder, and Burrell (2007) did not find that a tracheostomy tube restricted hyoid bone and laryngeal motion during the swallow.

(continued)

Diagnosis	Signs and Symptoms
Table 13.5.	*(continued)*
Mechanical ventilation	Clients on positive pressure mechanical ventilation are at risk for both dysphagia and aspiration pneumonia. The ventilator provides an artificial inhale and exhale, making normal timing of the swallow relative to breathing difficult and increasing potential for aspiration. The inflated tracheostomy tube cuff, necessary to maintain the airway while on mechanical ventilation, may create a barrier, as discussed earlier, although case studies have shown that for some patients, ventilation is adequate when the cuff is deflated for swallowing (Tippett & Siebens, 1991). The occupational therapist and the team must decide whether it is better to wait until a client is off the ventilator to begin eating. Some clients on long-term ventilation may have no major challenges with swallowing.

provides food or water, an intervention or evaluation is taking place, which necessitates physician referral. Screening tools may serve occupational therapists as brief evaluation tools in some acute care settings, and relevant screening tools are listed in Appendix 13.B.

Clinical Evaluation

In the acute care setting, dysphagia evaluation can serve different purposes. Physicians may refer clients for dysphagia evaluation to determine the diet that will minimize the risk of aspiration. Clients may be referred to determine whether eating, drinking, and taking medications by mouth provides a risk of aspiration or whether an alternative nutritional route such as a nasogastric tube or a feeding tube (a surgically or endoscopically placed tube that places food directly into the stomach) is needed. A third reason for dysphagia evaluation in this setting is to determine whether a patient is eating sufficiently for recovery from his or her illness; this determination may be made in conjunction with the dietitian.

Dysphagia evaluation usually uses a feeding trial. Providing oral hygiene activities before eating allows the occupational therapist to observe elements of oral motor function and sensation, as well as a BADL skill. Oral hygiene

tasks also clear the oral cavity of bacteria that may contribute to pneumonia if aspirated (Scannapieco, 2006). Some patients in the acute care setting may not yet be candidates for eating by mouth. Criteria for patients who are not yet ready to attempt eating by mouth are listed in Table 13.6.

Assessment

Many standardized dysphagia assessments are available, some of which are provided in Appendix 13.C. Some assessments are comprehensive and collect much of the information that is required to initiate intervention, and they may be considered evaluations. A key feature of an assessment is its protocol, which dictates how each test item is assessed and scored.

Dysphagia assessments commonly include information on cognitive status, including alertness and orientation; motor control, including posture and positioning and the ability to self-feed; oral and pharyngeal control without test foods; and oral and pharyngeal control during swallowing. Individual occupational therapy departments may develop their own dysphagia evaluations. Standardizing a department evaluation with a protocol transforms it into an assessment and allows uniformity of patient care and, ultimately, data collection if desired.

Table 13.6. **When to Defer a Dysphagia Evaluation**

1. The client has newly suspected aspiration since the physician initiated the referral.

2. The client is transferred to an intensive care unit with a change in medical status after the referral was initiated.

3. The client has unstable or decompensated cardiac status or new complaints of shortness of breath since the referral was initiated.

4. The client has had acute neurologic changes since the referral was initiated.

5. The client requires additional pulmonary support to breathe or has unsatisfactory blood gas values (or pulse oximetry values).

6. The client has had a new tracheostomy placed since the referral was initiated.

7. The client is being weaned from a ventilator and is being assessed for tolerance of the current ventilatory mode. Evaluation during such trials may affect the success of the ventilatory trials or the client's ability to swallow.

Source. From Avery-Smith, W., Brod Rosen, A., & Dellarosa, D. (1997). *Dysphagia Evaluation Protocol* (p. 23). San Antonio, TX: Harcourt Assessment. Copyright © by Harcourt. Reprinted with permission.

Instrumental Evaluation

Instrumental evaluations, which provide moving images of the swallow, complement the clinical evaluation and help to assess the unseen parts of the swallow. The therapist's clinical evaluation along with physician input determines whether an instrumental evaluation is recommended. Instrumental evaluations for dysphagia used in acute care (as well as postacute care) are the MBS and the FEES. The rationale for these procedures is that much of the swallow is unseen, and the presence of silent aspiration cannot be reliably assessed in a clinical evaluation (Smith Hammond & Goldstein, 2006). Many occupational therapists are trained to assist with or perform these two procedures. Although pulse oximetry might appear to be a convenient way to assess for aspiration, research has not borne this out (Ramsey, Smithard, & Kalra, 2006), but it can help to assess whether a client's respiratory status is adequate for attempting eating by mouth.

The *MBS* is sometimes known as *videofluoroscopy*. It is called a *modified* barium swallow to differentiate it from the barium swallow procedure, which assesses esophageal function. During this procedure, which usually occurs in the hospital imaging department, the patient eats therapist-selected textures of food and fluid that have been combined with barium. In some settings, the patient may eat barium that has been manufactured in different textures. Swallowing images are captured on videotape or DVD. The study can then be viewed later, including frame-by-frame analysis if necessary, to note elements of the swallow. This evaluation can assess efficacy of rehabilitative swallowing strategies. Some hospitals have technology available that allows MBS to be accomplished at the client's bedside, which is useful for clients who are too ill to be transported to the imaging department.

FEES is an endoscopic swallowing evaluation. During this evaluation, a small flexible fiberoptic endoscope is passed through one of the patient's nares through the nasopharynx to the level of the valleculae. Pharyngeal and vocal cord function may be observed during phonation and while the patient eats selected textures. This evaluation is easily done at the patient's bedside and may be particularly useful in the intensive care unit setting (Hafner, Neuhaber, Hirtendelder, Schmedler, & Eckel, 2008). Controversy over reliability, validity, and necessity

Table 13.7.   Comparison of Modified Barium Swallow and Fiberoptic Endoscopic Evaluation of Swallowing

Modified Barium Swallow	Fiberoptic Endoscopic Evaluation of Swallowing
Quick	Quick
Noninvasive	Minimally invasive
Some radiation exposure	No radiation exposure
Image is X-ray shadows	Image is actual anatomy
Images all phases of swallow	Visualizes primarily the pharynx and larynx
Food mixed with barium or barium of different consistencies must be given to assess function	Barium not needed; administration of food is optional

of both MBS and FEES exists (Kelly, Drinnan, & Leslie, 2007). See Table 13.7 for a comparison of MBS and FEES.

Blue Dye Testing

The *Modified Evans Blue Dye Test* (Belafsky, Blumenfeld, LePage, & Nahrstedt, 2003) is used to assess for aspiration in clients with tracheostomy or during FEES. During this test, FD&C Blue Dye No. 1 is given to the patient, either mixed with food or by itself. If the patient has a tracheostomy, tracheal secretions are observed for blue food color; during FEES, a blue tinge is observed below the level of the vocal cords.

Blue dye use raises several important concerns. Blue dye has in the past been used to color enteral tube feeding and to assess for reflux by coloring secretions. Its use has caused two deaths when the blue dye entered the bloodstream in clients with medical conditions that caused increased gut permeability (Maloney et al., 2002). Some medical centers have ceased using blue dye for any studies or for use in enteral feedings. Additionally, this test's reliability may be variable because the procedure has been found to be inaccurate in detecting trace amounts of aspiration in both clients with

tracheostomy (Brady, Hildner, & Hutchins, 1999) and clients undergoing FEES (Donzelli, Brady, Wesling, & Craney, 2001). Indeed, Leder, Acton, Lisitano, and Murray (2005) found a high level of inter- and intrarater reliability for FEES testing without blue dye.

Interventions for Dysphagia

Different occupational therapy interventions may be considered preparatory for a feeding session or meal. These interventions include positioning and mobility, oral care, and self-feeding, and they may have great impact on the patient's ability to manage safe oral intake over the course of an initial intervention session.

Positioning and Mobility

Stable trunk position with core and extremity symmetry can optimize the client's swallowing skills. Naturally, eating in a chair is best, and it encourages arousal when the patient is drowsy. The client should be seated in an upright chair or wheelchair with legs supported on the floor and arms on the table. Props and supports should be provided to optimize symmetrical and upright position. If assisting the client out of bed is not possible, the client should be assisted into a stable, symmetric upright position in bed with some knee flexion to encourage some anterior pelvic tilt, with the arms up on an overbed table.

Oral Care

Meticulous regular oral care is a critical part of any dysphagia program. Good oral care has been shown to reduce pneumonia rates because the same organisms that colonize the oral cavity can enter the airway and cause pneumonia in the lungs (Yoneyama et al., 2002). Oral care also provides important sensory and motor stimulation for the client in preparation for a meal or the feeding-trial portion of the dysphagia assessment.

The client should be assisted to remove and clean dentures and partial plates. Use of mouthwash and toothbrush should be incorporated into the occupational therapy care plan, with these ADL items adapted as needed. Emphasis should be placed on oral care before and after meals as needed for the client and caregivers. Use of toothbrushes is best, even for gums; however, soft, sponge-tipped swabs may be dipped in mouthwash if the toothbrush is not tolerated. If the client cannot spit out secretions, the toothbrush or swab must be only moistened and surfaces of the oral cavity gently cleaned. Alternately, a suctioning toothbrush can be used.

Self-Feeding

Although no firm research has been done on this subject, assisting the patient to self-feed likely improves the quality of the swallow and, of course, reinforces independent self-care goals. Barriers to self-feeding and strategies to encourage it are suggested in Table 13.8.

Dysphagia Interventions

Rehabilitation dysphagia interventions are continually being refined with research findings. Dysphagia interventions are commonly grouped into *restorative* (rehabilitative) or *modified* (compensatory) interventions. Restorative interventions seek to help the client regain lost function. Modified interventions seek to provide ways to compensate for lost function and anatomic structures lost to injury or surgery.

Restorative approaches are often used with patients with diagnoses in which recovery is expected within a short time frame, such as stroke, although more recently, the literature has demonstrated that even clients with long-term swallowing deficits can make gains in eating and swallowing with intensive therapy programs (Huckabee & Cannito, 1999; Leelamanit, Limsakul, & Geater, 2002). In clients with central nervous system deficits, new concepts of neuroplasticity encourage occupational therapists to help patients learn to reuse motor and sensory functions required for safe swallowing (Robbins, 2006). For those with peripheral nervous system deficits, exercise approaches are used for development of muscle strength in oral motor structures (Robbins, 2006).

Modified approaches are used when potential for recovery of function may be limited or once recovery has plateaued. A modified approach may be used concurrently with a rehabilitative approach, for example, in the use of a particular swallow maneuver to temporarily reduce potential for aspiration after a stroke. An example of a permanently needed modified approach would be the permanent use of a head rotation maneuver after hemilaryngectomy (which removes muscle and other tissues in one side of the pharynx), permitting food to bypass the permanently affected side of the pharynx.

In acute care, these two approaches are often combined, in the interest of providing maximal independence with eating and swallowing in a very short period of time, to permit discharge to a least restrictive environment. Clients who are expected to recover quickly participate in restorative therapy. Clients who enter the acute care setting with a preexisting chronic dysphagia compounded by acute dysphagia require a combination of approaches.

Indirect Intervention

Indirect dysphagia interventions are those that do not involve swallowing of food or fluids. A wide variety of indirect interventions may

Table 13.8. Strategies to Encourage Self-Feeding

Challenge	Strategy
Disorientation or distractibility to activity	• Remove distractions (visual and auditory) from environment; turn off TV. • Present one food container at a time. • Provide verbal cues to orient the client as needed during eating.
Unilateral neglect or visual field cut	• Present one food container at a time, and cue the client to observe it as needed. • Provide an anchor (a colorful piece of paper at the side of the plate).
Low vision	• Use clock method to describe location of food on the plate. • Present a limited number of food containers at one time. • Use a dark tray or placemat and a light-colored plate. (Refer to Appendix F for other low-vision strategies.)
Lack of appetite	• Present favorite or preferred foods. • Discontinue pump feedings 1–2 hours before meals or snacks. • Limit portion size so as not to overwhelm patients with large amounts of food on the tray.
Difficulty bringing food to mouth	• Provide adapted eating tools: utensils, plate guards, lidded cups, universal cuffs. • Provide finger foods to start.
Difficulty using dominant arm to eat	• Use hand-over-hand guiding techniques. • Provide splints, overhead slings, or mobile arm supports as needed. • If motion is absent, retrain self-feeding with nondominant arm.

enhance swallowing, including positioning, oral care, and eating strategies, as discussed earlier. Other indirect interventions include exercise programs and sensory stimulation programs.

Exercise programs involve strengthening of or neuromuscular facilitation programs for oral and pharyngeal structures, depending on whether the patient's diagnosis is the result of weakness or central nervous system pathology. Programs for weakness involve gentle passive exercises progressing to active and resistive exercises to oral structures. Neuromuscular facilitation programs may be based on proprioceptive neuromuscular facilitation or neurodevelopmental therapy approaches. Readers are referred to other resources for more information on these topics; suggestions are located in Appendix 13.A.

Sensory stimulation programs involve providing graded sensory input to enhance sensation. Again, the reader is referred to additional resources in Appendix 13.A for further information.

Direct Intervention

Direct dysphagia interventions include dietary modifications, modified swallowing techniques, and sometimes use of free water protocols.

Dietary Modifications

Dietary modifications are a cornerstone of dysphagia rehabilitation, and dysphagia diets are a diet option in most hospital nutrition departments. These diets are based on the concept that softer foods require less oral manipulation and are more cohesive; thus, they are more easily swallowed. Thickened fluids are also theorized to move more slowly through the oral and pharyngeal cavities and to be less likely to enter the airway (Groher et al., 2007). In 2002, the American Dietetic Association published the National Dysphagia Diet (see Table 13.9) in an effort to standardize dysphagia diets throughout the United States.

Note, however, that no one set of diet textures or diet progression is appropriate for all diagnoses, and indeed not even for one single diagnosis. Some generalizations may be made; research has suggested that, for example, many people with left hemiplegia demonstrate slowness in oral manipulations and a delayed trigger of the swallow and therefore benefit from thickened fluids to reduce the risk of food material entering the larynx. However, individual clients must be evaluated on the basis of foods and fluids that they appear to tolerate either on clinical assessment or on imaging tests.

Modified Swallowing Techniques

Different ways of swallowing help to direct the bolus in different ways to ensure airway protection. These techniques are described in Table 13.10. Lazarus, Logemann, Song, Rademaker, and Kahrilas (2002) suggested that supersupraglottic swallow, effortful swallow, Mendelsohn maneuver, and tongue-hold (Masako) maneuver all serve to pull the base of the tongue back to the posterior pharyngeal wall and improve contact between the two structures.

Table 13.9. National Dysphagia Diet: Food and Fluid Levels From Easiest to Most Difficult

National Dysphagia Diet Level	Description
Solid foods	
1: Dysphagia pureed	Homogeneous, cohesive, and puddinglike; little chewing required
2: Dysphagia mechanical–altered	Cohesive, moist, semisolid foods requiring some chewing
3: Dysphagia–advanced	Soft foods requiring more chewing
Regular	All foods allowed
Fluids	
Spoon-thick	1–50 cP
Honeylike	351–1.750 cP
Nectarlike	51–350 cP
Thin	1–50 cP

Note. cP = centipoise, a unit of measurement used to assess viscosity. Water has a viscosity of 0.0089 poise at 25° C and of 1 centipoise at 20° C.
Source. American Diabetic Association (2002).

Table 13.10. Modified Swallowing Techniques

Technique	Movement Required	Effect
Chin tuck	Capital flexion.	Chin tuck narrows the entrance to the larynx, reducing the chance of food or fluid falling into the airway; chin tuck has been shown to reduce aspiration of thin liquids (Logemann et al., 2008).
Supraglottic swallow	Breath hold, swallow while maintaining swallow, cough, then reswallow.	Supraglottic swallow causes a prompt upper esophageal sphincter opening, prolongs the pharyngeal swallow, and helps to close off the larynx (Ohmae, Logemann, Kaiser, Hanson, & Kahrilas, 1996). Any bolus that drips into the airway is coughed up above the vocal cords and can be reswallowed.
Mendelsohn maneuver	Push the tongue up into the hard palate and maintain laryngeal elevation during the swallow.	Increases extent and duration of laryngeal elevation, which increases duration and width of cricopharyngeus opening, allowing easier bolus passage (Boden, Hallgren, & Witt Hedstrom, 2006).
Effortful swallow	Contract the throat muscles hard while swallowing.	Moves the base of the tongue posteriorly, thus helping to clear food material from the valleculae during swallow (Pouderoux & Kahrilas, 1995). Also, it further elevates the hyoid bone and reduces oral residue during the swallow (Hind, Nicosia, Roecker, Carnes, & Robbins, 2001) and increases pressure in the pharynx during the swallow (Steele & Huckabee, 2007; Witte, Huckabee, Doeltgen, Gumbly, & Robb, 2008).
Neck rotation	Turning the head to the weaker or hemiparetic side during the swallow as far as range of motion and comfort will allow.	Rotation closes off the side of the pharynx to which the head is turned (Ohmae, Ogura, Kitahara, Karaho, & Inouye, 1998).

Free Water Protocols

Recent years have seen a trend to presenting unthickened water to dysphagia clients, on the assumption that even in the worst-case scenario, aspiration of a small amount of water will not cause aspiration pneumonia and that provision of a small amount may help to counteract dehydration. A small study by Garon, Engle, and Ormiston (1997) demonstrated that pneumonia and dehydration did not occur in a study group of stroke patients who received free water. Because organisms that colonize in the oral cavity cause pneumonia, meticulous oral hygiene is a prerequisite for providing water to patients with dysphagia.

Caregiver Training

Caregiver training is critical in follow-through on all swallowing instructions, particularly if the client is unable to correctly follow through on his or her own. "Return demonstration" during client and caregiver instruction assures the occupational therapist that recommendations are understood. Written information that the patient and caregiver can take home ensures carryover, and discussions about food textures should be completed depending on the client's intervention program.

Discharge Recommendations

Many acute care clients with dysphagia are at the beginning of the health care continuum. The occupational therapist must be sure that dysphagia programs and recommendations are communicated to professionals in the discharge setting, whether inpatient rehabilitation, skilled nursing, home, or outpatient care.

Occupational Therapy Approach

Dysphagia interventions in acute care differ from dysphagia interventions in other settings. Although clients with chronic dysphagia may be seen, all clients referred have acute diagnoses that may precipitate or worsen dysphagia. An understanding of the typical course of an acute illness and its medical and surgical interventions is helpful in developing goals and prioritizing dysphagia interventions. The occupational therapist must have ready access to current, relevant informational resources to deal with diagnoses and treatment regimes that have not been previously encountered. Other considerations in the acute care setting include

- Rapid changes in an individual's medical acuity and the presence of concomitant diagnoses that influence client and therapist goals and interventions.

- Variations in medication routines often experienced by patients in acute care; they may be receiving medications given only in the hospital setting. Many types of medications can affect the ability to swallow (Spieker, 2000).

- Alterations to intervention plans, which occur by necessity with changes in medical status, both positive and negative.

- Short hospital stays, which necessitate rapid and sometimes frequent therapist interventions. Repeated brief visits, particularly at mealtime, may be needed.

- Staffing levels influence the nature of assessment or intervention. For instance, in some departments, occupational therapists may complete a dysphagia evaluation and then turn functional interventions over to nursing staff; they may even direct volunteers to supervise individual mealtime sessions.

- Consideration of dysphagia intervention by a trained occupational therapist as conservative treatment because it does not involve medical or surgical interventions.

- Therapeutic interventions by occupational therapists occurring simultaneously with more invasive medical or imaging procedures. For example, a patient with aspiration pneumonia referred for dysphagia intervention may have a barium swallow test to assess for gastroesophageal reflux that may have caused the pneumonia. These assessments and their results must be reviewed by the treating occupational therapist and discussed with the managing physician if they affect intervention planning.

- Dysphagia patients in the hospital often being seen in intensive care, neurology, and neurosurgery units. In these hospital settings, rehabilitation efforts of occupational therapy, physical therapy, and speech–language pathology are intensive. If a speech–language pathologist is the primary dysphagia therapist, it is advantageous for the occupational therapist to understand the patient's dysphagia goals, just as it is important that the speech–language pathologist understand occupational therapy goals for eating and positioning. As such, mutual client outcome goals are achieved. Thus, team communication is critical, and goal setting is ideally done collaboratively.

- Occupational therapists addressing not only the client's immediate, acute care management but also helping to plan for the client's future needs and progress. Given the severity of the illnesses that often precipitate dysphagia, swallowing intervention in the hospital is only the beginning of long-term dysphagia care for more involved clients. The hospital occupational therapist must set the stage for continued interventions, bearing in mind the discharge plan for an individual. Planning in the acute care setting precipitates a continuum of care for many patients. Short-term goals must be reasonable, attainable, and ideally consistent with longer-term goals that will be addressed in subsequent settings. Communication with swallowing therapists through the next location of rehabilitation is critical in providing progressive and logical interventions and in ensuring that rehabilitation is reimbursed.

Efficacy of Acute Care Dysphagia Interventions

Although numerous studies have demonstrated the efficacy of dysphagia therapy, few have been based on large randomized controlled trials. Likewise, studies that focus on acute care dysphagia interventions are limited, and few have been published within the past 10 years. A summary of some studies found in the literature is provided in Table 13.11. Dysphagia management has been shown to reduce hospital lengths of stay in acute stroke patients (Odderson, Keaton, & McKenna, 1995).

Table 13.11. **Dysphagia Intervention Effects**

Intervention Effect	Patient Population	Study Citation
Reduction of aspiration pneumonia incidence	Acute care population	Kaprisin, Clumeck, & Nino-Murcia (1989)
Reduction of aspiration pneumonia incidence	Patients with stroke	Agency for Healthcare Research and Quality (1999)
Weight gain, increased oral intake, reduction in aspiration pneumonia	Neurology and neurosurgery patients	Martens, Cameron, & Simonson (1990)
Reduction in pneumonia rates	Patients with stroke	Foley et al. (2008)
Improvement in ability to safely eat by mouth	Various diagnoses, primarily neurologic disease	Schindler et al. (2008)

References

Abraham, S. S., & Yun, P. T. (2002). Laryngopharyngeal dysmotility in multiple sclerosis. *Dysphagia, 17*, 69–74.

Agency for Healthcare Research and Quality. (1999). *Diagnosis and treatment of swallowing disorders (dysphagia) in acute-care stroke patients.* Retrieved June 29, 2008, from http://www.ncbi.nlm.nih.gov/bookshelf/br.fcgi?book=erta8

American Dietetic Association. (2002). *National Dysphagia Diet: Standardization for optimal care.* Chicago: Author.

American Occupational Therapy Association. (2007). Specialized knowledge and skills in feeding, eating, and swallowing for occupational therapy practice. *American Journal of Occupational Therapy, 61*, 686–700.

Avery-Smith, W., & Dellarosa, D. M. (1994). Approaches to treating dysphagia in patients with brain injury. *American Journal of Occupational Therapy, 48*, 235–259.

Avery-Smith, W., Brod Rosen, A., & Dellarosa, D. (1997). *Dysphagia Evaluation Protocol.* San Antonio, TX: Harcourt Assessment.

Aviv, J. E., Martin, J. H., Sacco, R. L., Diamond, B., Tandon, R., Thompson, J., et al. (1997). Silent laryngopharyngeal sensory deficits after stroke. *Annals of Otology, Rhinology, and Laryngology, 106*, 87–93.

Belafsky, P. C., Blumenfeld, L., LePage, A., & Nahrstedt, K. (2003). The accuracy of the modified Evan's blue dye test in predicting aspiration. *Laryngoscope, 113*, 1969–1972.

Boden, K., Hallgren, A., & Witt Gedstrom, J. (2006). Effects of three different swallow maneuvers analyzed by videomanometry. *Acta Radiologica, 47*, 628–633.

Brady, S. L., Hildner, C. D., & Hutchins, B. F. (1999). Simultaneous videofluoroscopic swallow study and modified Evans blue dye procedure: An evaluation of blue dye visualization in cases of known aspiration. *Dysphagia, 14*, 146–149.

Chen, M. Y. M., Donofrio, P. D., Frederick, M. G., Ott, D. J., & Pikna, L. A. (1996). Videofluoroscopic evaluation of patients with Guillain–Barré syndrome. *Dysphagia, 11*, 11–13.

Crary, M. A., & Groher, M. E. (2003). *Introduction to adult swallowing disorders.* St. Louis, MO: Butterworth-Heinemann.

DePippo, K. L., Holas, M. A., & Reding, M. J. (1994). The Burke Dysphagia Screening Test: Validation of its use in patients with stroke. *Archives of Physical Medicine and Rehabilitation, 75*, 1284–1286.

Ding, R., & Logemann, J. A. (2005). Swallow physiology in patients with trach cuff inflated or deflated: A retrospective study. *Head and Neck, 27*, 809–813.

Donzelli, J., Brady, S., Wesling, M., & Craney, M. (2001). Simultaneous modified Evans blue dye procedure and video-nasal endoscopic evaluation of the swallow. *Laryngoscope, 111*, 1746–1750.

Ertekin, C., Aydogdu, I., Yuceyar, N., Kiylioglu, N., Tarlace, S., & Ulagaf, B. (2000). Pathophysiological mechanisms of oropharyngeal dysphagia in amyotrophic lateral sclerosis. *Brain, 123*, 125–140.

Foley, N., Teasell, R., Salter, K., Kruger, E., & Martino, R. (2008). Dysphagia treatment post stroke: A systematic review of randomized controlled trials. *Age and Aging, 37*, 258–264.

Fornataro-Clerici, L., & Roop, T. A. (1997). *Clinical management of adults requiring tracheostomy tubes and ventilators.* Gaylord, MI: Northern Speech Services.

Garon, B. R., Engle, M., & Ormiston, C. (1997). A randomized control study to determine the effects of unlimited oral intake of water in patients with identified aspiration. *Journal of Neurological Rehabilitation, 11*, 139–148.

Groher, M. E., Crary, M. A., Carnaby Mann, G., Vickers, Z., & Aguilar, C. (2007). The impact of rheologically controlled materials on the identification of airway compromise on the clinical and videofluoroscopic swallowing examinations. *Dysphagia, 21*, 218–225.

Hafner, G., Neuhaber, A., Hirtenfelder, S., Schmedler, B., & Eckel, H. E. (2008). Fiberoptic endoscopic evaluation of swallowing in intensive care unit patients. *European Archives of Otorhinololaryngology, 265*, 441–446.

Hind, J. A., Nicosia, M. A., Roecker, E. B., Carnes, M. L., & Robbins, J. (2001). Comparison of effortful and noneffortful swallows in healthy middle-aged and older adults. *Archives of Physical Medicine and Rehabilitation, 82*, 1661–1665.

Huckabee, M. L., & Cannito, M. P. (1999). Outcomes of swallowing rehabilitation in chronic brainstem dysphagia: A retrospective evaluation. *Dysphagia, 14,* 93–109.

Kaprisin, A. T., Clumeck, H., & Nino-Murcia, M. (1989). The efficacy of rehabilitative management of dysphagia. *Dysphagia, 4,* 48–52.

Kelly, A. M., Drinnan, M. J., & Leslie, P. (2007). Assessing penetration and aspiration: How do videofluoroscopy and fiberoptic endoscopic evaluation of swallowing compare? *Laryngoscope, 117,* 1723–1727.

Kendall, K. A., & Leonard, R. J. (2001a). Bolus transit and airway protection coordination in older dysphagic patients. *Laryngoscope, 111,* 2017–2021.

Kendall, K. A., & Leonard, R. J. (2001b). Pharyngeal constriction in elderly dysphagia patients compared with young and elderly nondysphagic controls. *Dysphagia, 16,* 272–278.

Kendall, K. A., Leonard, R. J., & McKenzie, S. (2004). Common medical conditions in the elderly: Impact on pharyngeal bolus transit. *Dysphagia, 19,* 71–77.

Kirshblum, S., Johnston, M. V., Brown, J., O'Connor, K. C., & Jarosz, P. (1999). Predictors of dysphagia after spinal cord injury. *Archives of Physical Medicine and Rehabilitation, 80,* 1101–1109.

Lazarus, C., Logemann, J. A., Song, C. W., Rademanker, A. W., & Kahrilas, P. J. (2002). Effects of voluntary maneuvers on tongue base function for swallowing. *Folia Phoniatrica et Logopaedica, 54,* 171–176.

Leder, S. B., Acton, L. M., Lisitano, H. L., & Murray, J. T. (2005). *Fiberoptic endoscopic evaluation of swallowing (FEES) with* and without blue-dyed food. *Dysphagia, 20,* 17–162.

Leelamanit, V., Limsakul, C., & Geater, A. (2002). Synchronized electrical stimulation in treating pharyngeal dysphagia. *Laryngoscope, 112,* 2204–2210.

Leibovitz, A., Baumoehl, Y., Lubart, E., Yaina, A., Platinovitz, N., & Segal, R. (2007). Dehydration among long-term care elderly patients with oropharyngeal dysphagia, *Gerontology, 53,* 179–183.

Logemann, J. A., Gensler, G., Robbins, J., Lindblad, A. S., Brandt, D., Hind, J. A, et al. (2008). A randomized study of three interventions for aspiration of thin liquids in patients with dementia or Parkinson's disease. *Journal of Speech, Language, and Hearing Research, 51,* 173–183.

Logemann, J. A., Pepe, J., & Mackay, L. E. (1994). Disorders of nutrition and swallowing: Intervention strategies in the trauma center. *Journal of Head Trauma Rehabilitation, 9,* 43–56.

Logemann, J. A., Veis, S., & Colangelo, L. (1999). A screening procedure for oropharyngeal dysphagia. *Dysphagia, 14,* 44–51.

Mackay, L. E., Morgan, A. S., & Bernstein, B. A. (1999). Swallowing disorders in severe brain injury: Risk factors affecting return to oral intake. *Archives of Physical Medicine and Rehabilitation, 80,* 365–371.

Maloney, J. P., Ryan, T. A., Brasel, K. J., Binion, D. G., Johnson, D. R., Halbower, A.C., et al. (2002). Food dye use in enteral feedings: A review and a call for a moratorium. *Nutrition in Clinical Practice, 17,* 169–181.

Marik, P. E., & Kaplan, D. (2003). Aspiration pneumonia and dysphagia in the elderly. *Chest, 124,* 328–336.

Martens, L., Cameron, T., & Simonsen, M. (1990). Effects of a multidisciplinary management program on neurologically impaired patients with dysphagia. *Dysphagia, 5,* 147–151.

Martin-Harris, B. (2008). Clinical implications of respiratory–swallowing interactions. *Current Opinions in Otolaryngology and Head and Neck Surgery, 16,* 194–199.

Masiero, S., Pierobon, R., Previateo, C., & Gomiero, E. (2008). Pneumonia in stroke patients with oropharyngeal dysphagia: A six month follow-up study. *Neurological Science, 29,* 139–145.

Massey, R., & Jedlicka, D. (2002). The Massey Bedside Swallowing Screen. *Journal of Neuroscience Nursing, 34,* 252–253, 257–269.

Nagaya, M., Kachi, T., Yamada, T., & Igata, A. (1998). Videofluorographic study of swallowing in Parkinson's disease. *Dysphagia, 13,* 95–100.

Odderson, I., Keaton, J., & McKenna, B. (1995). Swallow management in patients on an acute stroke pathway: Quality is cost effective. *Archives of Physical Medicine and Rehabilitation, 76,* 1130–1133.

Ohmae, Y., Logemann, J. A., Kaiser, P., Hanson, D. G., & Kahrilas, P. J. (1996). Effects of two breath-holding maneuvers on oropharyngeal swallow. *Annals of Otology, Rhinology, and Laryngology, 105,* 123–131.

Ohmae, Y., Ogura, M., Kitahara, S., Karaho, T., & Inouye, T. (1998). Effects of head rotation on pharyngeal function during normal swallow. *Annals of Otology, Rhinology, and Laryngology, 107*, 344–348.

O'Sullivan, N. (1995). *Dysphagia care: Team approach.* Fairfield, CA: Cottage Square Press.

Patel, M. D., & Martin, F. C. (2008). Why don't elderly hospital inpatients eat adequately? *Journal of Nutrition, Health, and Aging, 12*, 227–231.

Pauloski, B. R. (2008). Rehabilitation of dysphagia following head and neck cancer. *Physical Medicine Rehabilitation Clinics of North America, 19*, 889–928.

Pouderoux, P., & Kahrilas, P. J. (1995). Deglutitive tongue force modulation by volition, volume, and viscosity in humans. *Gastroenterology, 108*, 1418–1426.

Ramsey, D. J., Smithard, D. G., & Kaira, L. (2006). Can pulse oximetry or a bedside swallowing assessment be used to detect aspiration after stroke? *Stroke, 37*, 2984–2988.

Riley, L. M., Skolasky, R. L., Alber, T. J., Vaccaro, A. R., & Heller, J. G. (2005). Dysphagia after anterior cervical decompression and fusion: Prevalence and risk factors from a longitudinal cohort study. *Spine, 30*, 2564–2569.

Robbins, J. (2006). Preface: New frontiers in dysphagia rehabilitation. *Seminars in Speech and Language Pathology, 27*, 217–218.

Robbins, J., Levine, R. L., Maser, A., Rosenbek, J. C., & Kempster, G. B. (1993). Swallowing after unilateral stroke of the cerebral cortex. *Archives of Physical Medicine and Rehabilitation, 74*, 1295–1300.

Rogers, B., Stratton, P., Msall, M., Andres, M., Champlain, M. K., Koerner, P., et al. (1994). Long-term morbidity and management strategies of tracheal aspiration in adults with severe developmental disabilities. *American Journal of Mental Retardation, 98*, 490–498.

Scannapieco, F. A. (2006). Pneumonia in nonambulatory patients: The role of oral bacteria and oral hygiene. *Journal of the American Dental Association, 137*(Suppl.), 21S–25S.

Schindler, A., Vincon, E., Grosso, E., Miletto, A. M., DiRosa, R., & Schindler, O. (2008). Rehabilitative management of oropharyngeal dysphagia in acute care settings: Data from a large Italian teaching hospital. *Dysphagia, 23*, 230–236.

Sekizawa, K., Ujiie, Y., Itgabashi, S., Sasaki, H., & Takishma, T. (1990). Lack of cough reflex in aspiration pneumonia. *Lancet, 335*, 1228–1229.

Shaker, R., Milbrath, M., Ren, J., Campbell, B., Toohill, R., & Hogan, W. (1995). Deglutitive aspiration in patients with tracheostomy: Effect of tracheostomy on the duration of vocal cord closure. *Gastroenterology, 108*, 1357–1360.

Smith Hammond, C. A., & Goldstein, L. B. (2006). Cough and aspiration of food and liquids due to oral–pharyngeal dysphagia: ACCP Evidence-Based Clinical Practice Guidelines. *Chest, 129* (1, Suppl.), 154S–168S.

Spieker, M. R. (2000). Evaluating dysphagia. *American Family Physician, 61*, 3639–3648.

Steele, C. M., & Huckabee, M. L. (2007). The influence of orolingual pressure on the timing of pharyngeal pressure events. *Dysphagia, 22*, 30–36.

Terk, A. R., Leder, S. B., & Burrell, M. I. (2007). Hyoid bone and laryngeal movement dependent upon presence of a tracheotomy tube. *Dysphagia, 22*, 89–93.

Tippett, D. C., & Siebens, A. A. (1991). Using ventilators for speaking and swallowing. *Dysphagia, 6*, 94–99.

Trapi, M., Enderle, P., Nowotsy, M., Teuschi, Y., Matz, K., Dachenhausen, A., et al. (2007). Dysphagia bedside screening for acute-stroke patients: The Gugging Swallowing Screen. *Stroke, 38*, 2948–2952.

van Herwaarden, M. A., Katz, P. O., Gideon, R. M., Barrett, J., Castell, J. A., Achem, S., et al. (2003). Are manometric parameters of the upper esophageal sphincter and pharynx affected by age and gender? *Dysphagia, 18*, 211–217.

Warnecke, T., Teismann, I., Maimann, W., Olenber, S., Zimmersman, J., Kramer, C., et al. (2008). Assessment of aspiration risk in acute ischaemic stroke—Evaluation of the simple swallowing provocation test. *Journal of Neurology, Neurosurgery, and Psychiatry, 79*, 312–314.

Witte, U., Huckabee, M. L., Doeltgen, S. H., Gumbly, F., & Robb, M. (2008). The effect of effortful swallow on pharyngeal manometric measurements during saliva and water swallowing in healthy participants. *Archives of Physical Medicine and Rehabilitation, 89*, 822–828.

Wood, P., & Errich-Herring, B. (1997). Dysphagia: A screening tool for stroke patients. *Journal of Neuroscience Nursing, 29*, 325–330.

Yoneyama, T., Yoshida, M., Ohrui, T., Mukaiyama, H., Okamoto, H., Hoshiba, K., et al. (2002). Oral care reduces pneumonia in older clients in nursing homes. *Journal of the American Geriatrics Society, 50,* 430–433.

Young, E. C., & Durant-Jones, L. (1990). Developing a dysphagia program in an acute care hospital: A needs assessment. *Dysphagia, 5,* 159–165.

Appendix 13.A.

Resources and Continuing Education Opportunities in Dysphagia

Print Materials and Recommended Reading

Avery, W. (Ed.). (2010). *Dysphagia care and related feeding concerns for adults* (AOTA Self-Paced Clinical Course, 2nd ed.). Bethesda, MD: American Occupational Therapy Association.

Clark, H. (2003). Neuromuscular treatments for speech and swallowing: A tutorial. *American Journal of Speech–Language Pathology, 12*, 400–415.

Fornataro-Clerici, L., & Roop, T. A. (1997). *Clinical management of adults requiring tracheostomy tubes and ventilators.* Gaylord, MI: Northern Speech Services.

Groher, M. E. (1997). *Dysphagia: Diagnosis and management.* Boston: Butterworth-Heinemann.

Assessments

Avery-Smith, W., Brod Rosen, A., & Dellarosa, D. M. (1997). *Dysphagia Evaluation Protocol.* San Antonio, TX: Harcourt Assessment.

Mann, G. (2002). *MASA: The Mann Assessment of Swallowing Ability.* Clifton Park, NY: Singular.

Murray, J. (1999). *Manual of dysphagia assessment in adults.* San Diego, CA: Singular.

Web-Based Materials and Courses

- *American Dietetic Association:* www.eatright. org provides information on nutrition and the National Dysphagia Diet.

- *Ciao Seminars:* http://ciaoseminars.com. Offers a variety of live and Web-based courses on anatomy and physiology of swallowing, dysphagia intervention, and VitalStim® certification.

- Daniels, S. (2006). Neurological disorders affecting oral, pharyngeal swallowing. *GI Motility Online.* Retrieved December 24, 2008, from http://www.nature.com/gimo/contents/pt1/full/gimo34.html

- *Dysphagia.com:* http://dysphagia.com offers many resources on dysphagia care and a link to the dysphagia electronic mailing list.

- The *American Occupational Therapy Association (AOTA)* offers a forum for feeding, eating, and swallowing disorders for AOTA members at http://otconnections.com

- *Winkings Skull:* www.winkingskull.com offers interactive images of oral, pharyngeal, and esophageal structures.

CD-ROM and DVD

- Berkovitz, B., Kirsch, C., Moxham, B. J., Alusi, G., & Cheeseman, T. *Interactive head and neck* [CD-ROM]. London: Primal Pictures. Available from Primalpictures.com. Demonstrates anatomy of head and neck structures including anatomy involved in swallowing.

- *3D Swallow:* http://3dswallow.com offers a DVD of animations of the anatomic structures of swallowing, normal swallow, and samples of abnormal swallows.

Other Resources

AOTA offers advanced practice certification in feeding, eating, and swallowing. Visit AOTA at http://aota.org/Practitioners/ProfDev/Certification.aspx for more information on this program. Feeding, eating, and swallowing competencies and indicators are listed in the certification manual.

Appendix 13.B.

Standardized Dysphagia Screening Tools

Screening Tool	Format	Standardization and Comments	Availability
Observational screenings			
Nutrition and Swallowing Screen	Observational checklist		Wood & Errich-Herring (1997)
Screenings that include administration of food or liquid			
Burke Dysphagia Screening Test	Checklist	Uses 3 oz. of water to screen Stroke patients Standardized protocol	DePippo, Holas, & Reding (1994)
Northern Dysphagia Patient Check	Checklist	Uses thin liquid of pudding texture and cookie Standardized protocol	Logemann, Veis, & Colangelo (1999)
Gugging Swallowing Screen	Checklist	Standardized protocol; reliability and predictive and concurrent validity tested	Trapi et al. (2007)
Massey Bedside Swallowing Screen	Checklist	Content validity, predictive validity, and interrater reliability tested	Massey & Jedlicka (2002)

Appendix 13.C.

Standardized Dysphagia Assessments

Assessment	Description	Patient Population	Reliability and Validity Testing	Comprehensive?	Publisher and Availability
Dysphagia Evaluation Protocol	• Standardized • Developed by occupational therapists in an acute care setting	All dysphagia diagnoses	Yes	Yes	Harcourt Assessment, 1997, www. Harcourt Assessment. com
MASA: Mann Assessment of Swallowing Ability	• 24-point scale • Quickly administered	Neurogenic dysphagia	Yes	No	Singular Publishing, 2002
Clinical Swallowing Examination	• Uses a scoresheet form • Developed by a speech–language pathologist	All dysphagia diagnoses	No	Yes, although does not include dysphagia history and demographic information collection	www.Delmar Learning.com, 1999
Occupational Therapy Clinical Dysphagia Assessment	• Scoresheet form • Developed by occupational therapists	All dysphagia diagnoses	No	Yes	American Occupational Therapy Association, 2003, http:// AOTA.org

14

Transplantation

Helene Smith-Gabai, OTD, OTR/L, BCPR

The concept of *transplantation* has been of interest to physicians for centuries as a potential cure for disease, but not until the late 20th century did it become a viable treatment option for end-stage organ disease. Advancements in surgical technique, organ preservation, immunosuppression therapies, and closer candidate selection have increasingly improved survival rates and quality of life for transplant recipients (Lee & Moinzadeh, 2009; Malone & Lindsay, 2006; Petechuk, 2006; Wells & Goodman, 2009). According to data from the United Network of Organ Sharing (UNOS, 2009), more than 23,000 transplantations occurred in the United States from January to October 2008, with 77 people receiving an organ transplant every day (UNOS, 2009). Transplantation as a "highly technical and demanding specialty is now considered the standard of care for end-stage organ disease" (Malone & Lindsay, 2006, p. 545).

Background

Human organ transplantation has been performed since the 1950s with varying degrees of success. In 1954, Dr. Joseph Murray of Boston performed the first successful living donor kidney transplant between 24-year-old identical twins. The recipient survived for 8 years. The first successful heart transplant was performed in 1968 in South Africa by Dr. Christiaan Barnard. However, the patient survived less than 2 weeks. The advent of cyclosporine (an immunosuppressant) in the 1980s, which works by blocking T-helper cell production, revolutionized the viability of and survival rate for transplantation (Barter, 2006; Kanter, Vega, & Smith, 1998; McClellan, 2003). With increased knowledge about immunosuppression, several immunosuppression regimens have since been developed in

addition to cyclosporine. Refer to Appendix B for more information on transplant medications. Transplantation as a treatment option has become so successful that recently a heart transplant recipient was reported to have survived 31 years. Public awareness and education about organ donation is also increasing. April is not only Occupational Therapy Month but also National Donate Life Month.

Before the 1980s, a person's chance of obtaining an organ was determined by his or her length of time on a waiting list and not by medical urgency. That system has now changed to make it more equitable by considering other factors for placement on the transplant list. For example, the prospects of success and benefits of transplantation are weighed against the risk of undergoing major surgery and long-term survival (Freundenberger, Hoffman, Gottlieb, Robinson, & Fisher, 2000). The Scientific Registry of Transplant Recipients is a national organization responsible for analysis and reporting on transplant allocation equitability (McClellan, 2003; Petechuk, 2006; Scientific Registry of Transplant Recipients, 2009).

However, the biggest challenge to organ transplantation remains the shortage of donor organs (McClellan, 2003; Petechuk, 2006; Steinman et al., 2001; Wells & Goodman, 2009). Many more candidates are on waiting lists than there are available organs. In 2004, a new name was added to a transplant waiting list every 13 minutes, while each day 17 people on the list died waiting for a donor (Petechuk, 2006). As of January 2009, more than 100,000 candidates were on waiting lists for organs but fewer than 12,000 donors were available (UNOS, 2009). Many candidates do not survive the wait because a donor is not located in time. Fortunately, in the case of liver disease, using living donors providing partial (or split) liver organs has become a viable option. However, this procedure is not without risk to both the donor and the recipient. The number of candidates

Table 14.1. Number of Candidates in 2008 on Transplant Waiting Lists

Organ	Number
All	100,457
Kidney	78,170
Pancreas	1,578
Kidney–pancreas	2,238
Liver	15,848
Intestine	216
Heart	2,715
Lung	2,010
Heart–lung	89

Source. United Network for Organ Sharing (2009).

in 2008 on organ waiting lists by organ type are listed in Table 14.1.

Another challenge that posttransplant patients face is the lifelong balance between organ rejection and infection. The body's natural defense system recognizes the donor organ as foreign tissue. Immunosuppression therapy increases the chances that the recipient's body will not reject the donor organ. However, immunosuppression therapy also makes the recipient's body more vulnerable to infection. In rare cases, *chimerism* may occur, in which the donor's leukocytes take root in the recipient's body (McClellan, 2003). White blood cells from both the donor and the recipient's immune system intermingle and coexist (Petechuk, 2006). The recipient's body does not recognize the donor organ as foreign and successfully accepts the donor organ, requiring smaller amounts of immunosuppression therapy (McClellan, 2003). This rare phenomenon is being studied as a possible future direction in transplantation.

Occupational therapists may work with patients before or after transplantation. Goals are similar for both stages, namely to increase function, strength, and participation in desired occupations. Before transplant, patients are often deconditioned and require assistance with performing functional activities, owing to limitations secondary to their end-stage organ disease. The goals of pretransplant rehabilitation are improvement or maintenance of functional abilities and endurance while the candidate awaits transplantation. In contrast, posttransplant patients now have a healthy organ and no longer have an end-stage organ disease. They must recuperate from major surgery and build their endurance back up to engage in former roles and desired occupations. Posttransplant patients also benefit from education on lifestyle changes to protect their new organ (refer to the "Implications for Occupational Therapy" section; see also Appendix 14.A).

Organ Procurement and Allocation

Transplantation is a process, not just a surgical procedure. Many factors determine its success. Transplant candidates must first undergo an extensive evaluation by a transplant center team before being placed on a waiting list. All pertinent candidate information is then entered into the UNOS national database. *UNOS* is a nonprofit organization under contract with the U.S. Department of Health and Human Services that assists with matching donor organs with potential candidates. Once a candidate is accepted on the waiting list, information about the candidate's disease, blood and tissue type, body size, age, gender, number of previous transplants, and time on the waiting list is entered into the UNOS databank (Barter, 2006; McClellan, 2003). Waiting time on the transplant list can last several weeks to years.

UNOS is made up of all U.S. transplant centers, tissue-matching laboratories, and organ procurement centers (Wells & Goodman, 2009). UNOS is also involved in the collection and management of data and outcomes relating to donations and transplantation in the United States. In addition, it is responsible for the *Organ Procurement and Transplantation Network (OPTN)*, a national registry of organ matching, established through the National Organ Transplant

Act of 1984 (P. L. 98–507; OPTN, n.d.). OPTN brings together all members of the transplant community and is available 24 hours a day, 7 days a week. Approximately 59 organ procurement organizations (OPOs) are included in the OPTN, which are distributed between 11 national UNOS regions across the United States. Refer to Appendix 14.B for a list of the 11 UNOS membership regions.

All OPOs and hospital transplant centers must be OPTN members to receive Medicare funds (UNOS, 2009). Hospitals that receive Medicare funds are also required to notify their OPO of all patients who have died or are near death, so the OPO can identify potential donors (McClellan, 2003; Petechuk, 2006). Historically, patients were considered dead when their hearts stopped beating, which limited organ viability and recovery because of tissue ischemia. The previous definition has now largely been replaced by cessation of brain activity. Potential donors are people who are brain dead, even though their hearts and lungs may still be functioning with mechanical ventilation, cardiopulmonary bypass, or both (Lee & Moinzadeh, 2009). According to the Uniform Determination of Death Act of 1980, an individual who has sustained either (1) irreversible cessation of circulatory and respiratory functions or (2) irreversible cessation of all functions of the entire brain, including the brainstem, is dead. A determination of death must be made in accordance with accepted medical standards. (Uniform Determination of Death Act, 1980). Most transplant donors have sustained brain death because of injury from a motor vehicle accident, intracerebral bleed, or gunshot wound (Kanter et al., 1998).

Once a donor has been identified, organs cannot be recovered without the donor's presumed consent (e.g., identified on a driver's license or organ donation card). In addition, the family or legal guardian must also give informed consent. Physicians who care for the dying patient are never the same physicians who approach the family about donation or who harvest the organs. Once the donation process is set in motion, the local OPO conducts organ recovery, evaluates the suitability of the organs, and identifies compatible candidates through the UNOS computer databank. Donor organs are stored in a cold organ preservation solution for transportation to the transplant centers in which the recipients are located. The OPO handles all costs associated with organ donation, recovery, and transportation. In the United States, selling or receiving payment for organs is illegal.

When a donor organ becomes available, the UNOS computer database generates a list of matching candidates that is based on objective criteria, including histocompatibility, size of the donor organ, medical urgency of the candidate (e.g., status code), time on the waiting list, and geographic distance between the donor and the recipient (UNOS, 2009). The distance between the donor hospital to the potential transplant center must be considered because some organs have a very limited preservation time (e.g., heart, lungs). Donor organs are offered first to matched recipients within the OPO's UNOS region, which helps minimize organ preservation time with improved organ quality and outcomes (UNOS, 2009). If a suitable candidate cannot be found in their area, then the organ is offered to other regions.

According to UNOS guidelines, transplant centers have 1 hour to decide whether they will accept the donor organ for their patient before it is offered to another center (Petechuk, 2006). Even if a donor organ is accepted by a transplant center, the transplant surgeon may decide that the organ is not acceptable or the candidate is not healthy enough at the time to undergo the surgery. Organ transplantation procedures performed in the United States in 2008 are listed in Table 14.2.

Transplant Team

Many disciplines are involved in transplant care. Each plays an important function in ensuring a successful transplant. The different members of the transplant team and their functions are listed Table 14.3. It is up to the individual transplant center to decide whether to submit a patient's name as a candidate for the waiting list (Steinman et al., 2001). Different transplant centers may specialize in different transplant procedures, and their criteria for listing may also differ. Therefore, candidates

Table 14.2. Organ Transplants Performed in the United States, January–October 2008

Organ	Number
Kidney	13,743
Deceased donor	8,815
Living donor	4,928
Pancreas	370
Deceased donor	370
Kidney and pancreas	705
Deceased donor	705
Liver	5,273
Deceased donor	5,053
Living donor	220
Intestines	155
Deceased donor	155
Heart	1,802
Deceased donor	1,802
Lung	1,221
Deceased donor	1,221
Heart and lung	19
Deceased donor	19

Source. Organ Procurement and Transplantation Network data (United Network for Organ Sharing, 2009).

An additional transplantation procedure reviewed in this chapter is hematopoietic transplantation, which includes bone marrow and peripheral blood stem cells. Corneas, heart valves, skin, veins, bone, ligaments, and tendons can also be donated and transplanted (Wells & Goodman, 2009) but are beyond the scope of this chapter.

Solid organ transplantations are classified as *single organ* or *multiple organ* (e.g., heart–lung, kidney–pancreas), but multiple-organ procedures are not as common as single-organ procedures. Donor organs may be procured from cadavers (*deceased donor*) or from a living person (*living donor*). More than 6,300 live donor transplant surgeries were performed in 2007 (UNOS, 2009). Living donors have been used for kidney, liver, lung, and stem cell transplantation. Living donor kidney transplantation is possible because humans can function with only one kidney. Living donor liver or split-liver transplantation is feasible because the liver is the only organ that can regenerate itself. This procedure is often performed between a parent and child.

In addition, transplants can be classified as *allograft* (*homograft*), meaning within the same species but from a nonidentical member, or *isograft* (*syngeneic*), meaning from an identical twin. In *autograft transplantation*, tissue is transplanted from one site to another within the same person, as in a skin graft (Wells & Goodman, 2009). A *xenograft* (*heterograft*) is a transplant between two different species (e.g., use of porcine heart valves or a baboon heart).

Criteria for Organ Donation and Candidacy for Transplantation

There are specific criteria for both living and deceased donor organs to be acceptable for transplantation. There are also specific criteria for a candidate to be placed on a transplant waiting list. Select factors from both donors and candidates must match in order to increase the odds of a successful transplantation.

may choose to register at multiple transplantation centers, and doing so will not affect their status on the UNOS waiting list.

Types of Transplantations

Solid organ transplantation includes the heart, lungs, kidneys, pancreas, liver, and intestines.

Table 14.3. Interdisciplinary Transplant Team

Team Member	Function
Transplant coordinator	• Coordinates the pretransplant evaluation. • Liaison between the transplant team and the candidate; guides the candidate and family through the transplant process. • Verifies candidate's name on the waiting list. • Notifies candidate when a donor has been located. • May suggest candidate obtain a beeper for quick notification. • Follows patient's progress before and after transplant. • Needs to be notified if patient is sick or out of town. • Available 24 hours a day, in case of urgent patient problem.
Transplant surgeon	• Performs the transplant surgery and is responsible for immediate postsurgery care. • Performs routine biopsies. • May be involved in follow-up care.
Transplant physician	• Manages medical care (not surgery), including tests and medications before and after transplant (e.g., cardiologist, nephrologist, pulmonologist). • Works closely with the transplant coordinator. • May be involved in follow-up care.
Social worker	• Addresses financial issues; provides information on insurance coverage and fund raising. • Provides emotional support and counseling, including coping strategies. • Educates candidate about transplant resources.
Psychiatrist	• Assesses candidate's mental health and psychological stability; may address issues of family and community support, stress, anxiety, substance abuse (e.g., drug, alcohol, tobacco use), and coping strategies. • Assesses cognitive functioning; determines whether patient has the capacity to give informed consent and his or her level of comprehension. • Assesses whether patient will be able to comply with posttransplant regimen (e.g., lifelong medications; keeping scheduled lab and office visits; diet, exercise, and self-monitoring of vital signs; signs of infection, rejection, or both).
Clinical nutritionist	• Addresses patient nutritional status before and after transplant. • May address issues of malnutrition or posttransplant obesity.

(continued)

Table 14.3. *(continued)*

Team Member	Function
Pharmacist	• Instructs patient in medication schedule, purpose, dosages, and side effects.
Rehabilitation professionals (e.g., occupational, physical, speech therapists)	• Assesses rehabilitation potential. • Evaluates functional limitations. • Assists candidates in improving strength, endurance, and ability to engage in occupations before and after transplantation. • Assists with discharge recommendations to next level of care (e.g., home vs. rehabilitation stay). • Assesses equipment needs.
Financial coordinator	• Explains cost of transplantation and insurance issues. • Works with insurers, administration, and transplant team to coordinate finances related to all aspects and phases of the transplantation process. • Although the donor organ is donated, many charges are associated with transplantation, including hospital charges, physician charges, and posttransplant medication charges. • Charges may be higher if patient stays in an intensive care unit before a donor is located or has posttransplant complications that necessitate a longer intensive care unit stay.
Clergy	• Assists with spiritual and emotional issues related to transplant; offers support.
Staff nurses	• Address daily care and progress. • Instruct recipients in monitoring vital signs, signs and symptoms of infection and rejection, and care of incision site.

Living Donors

The criteria for living donors include age (< age 50, but possibly ≤ age 60) and no history of drug abuse, alcohol abuse, cancer, syphilis, tuberculosis, HIV, or hepatitis B. In addition, it is ideal if the donor's body size approximates the candidate's. Donors must match through ABO blood typing (A, B, AB, or O blood type) and tissue typing. *Histocompatibility* (tissue typing) refers to the person's immune system antigens, which release antibodies that attack foreign tissue. If a positive cross-match between the donor and recipient is found, then they are incompatible because the recipient has antibodies that will react against the donor organ (McClellan, 2003).

Organ preservation time is not an issue with living donors as it is with deceased donors because living organ donation is a scheduled procedure. In addition, associated risk to the live donor is generally little. However, cases of living donor morbidity have been reported, resulting from perioperative complications, poor postprocedure care, or unknown medical conditions that should have disqualified the donor from being selected (Petechuk, 2006).

Deceased Donors

Criteria for deceased donors include no evidence of sepsis, cancer, infectious disease, hepatitis B, HIV, or trauma to the organ. Donors must match through ABO blood typing and tissue typing. Additional factors include the donor organ's size and condition and geographic distance from a matched recipient (McClellan, 2003). As previously mentioned, distance is an issue because different organs have different preservation or ischemic times, which can limit donor organ allocation.

With deceased donor transplantation, information about the donor is kept confidential. However, recipients may send a letter to the donor family via the transplant coordinator or, if both the donor family and the recipient wish it, contact between both parties may be established.

Transplant Candidate

To be placed on a transplant waiting list, the candidate must have an end-stage organ disease that no longer responds to traditional medical or surgical treatments. Candidates should present with psychological and emotional stability, good family support, and stable financial support for the procedure and posttransplant care. In addition, cancer or any diseases or infections that would attack the new organ cannot be present, nor can a recent history of tobacco, drug, or alcohol abuse (Lee & Moinzadeh, 2009). As with donors, candidates also have an age limit, typically up to age 60; however, this age limit may differ on the basis of the type of transplantation. Each transplant procedure also has absolute and relative contraindications (refer to the sections for each individual organ for detail).

Contraindications are associated with increased risk of mortality, poorer outcomes, or poor quality of life. Recent cancer is usually a contraindication because posttransplant immunosuppression medications can accelerate the spread of cancer (Petechuk, 2006). Patients with HIV are generally not transplant candidates because their compromised immune systems would not tolerate posttransplant immunosuppression medications. Transplantation may also be contraindicated if the patient lacks adequate psychosocial support, financial resources, or even adequate transportation to keep medical appointments. Most important, the candidate must be willing to adhere to a lifelong medication regimen and constant vigilance to minimize the risk of and exposure to infection and injury.

Pretransplant Tests and Screening

Candidates, as part of their transplant evaluation, must undergo a series of tests before being placed on the transplant list. Patients are screened not just to determine blood and tissue type for matching but also to determine whether they are healthy enough to survive the transplantation surgery. Most candidates have an end-stage disease that can significantly weaken them before the transplantation surgery is performed. On the basis of the type of transplantation, the pretransplant evaluation may include

- *Blood and tissue typing:* Matching of donor organs to candidates by blood type (e.g., A, B, O) and human leukocyte antigen (HLA) compatibility (*HLAs* are proteins found on the surface of cells that help the immune system differentiate between native tissue and foreign substances);
- Complete blood count, basic metabolic panel, and coagulation values (complete blood count, basic metabolic panel, prothrombin time, partial thromboplastin time; refer to Appendix P for more information on laboratory values);
- Arterial blood gas analysis;
- Liver function testing;
- Sputum culture;
- Glomerular filtration rate;
- Urinalysis (to assess kidney function and presence of protein, blood, drugs, or nicotine);
- Stool guaiac (to test for presence of occult blood);

- Screening for presence of virus, infection, or cancer (e.g., HIV, cytomegalovirus [CMV], Epstein–Barr virus, toxoplasma, purified protein derivative [test for tuberculosis], hepatitis B, hepatitis C, prostate-specific antigen, pap smear, mammogram);
- Pulmonary function test;
- Ventilation–perfusion scan;
- Six-minute walk test, exercise stress test, or both;
- Echocardiogram or transesophageal echocardiogram;
- Electrocardiogram;
- Cardiac catheterization;
- *Imaging studies:* Computed tomography scan, MRI, Doppler ultrasound, or X-ray;
- Psychosocial evaluation, including support system, coping mechanisms, and ability to comply with posttransplant regimen; and
- Financial resources (including insurance coverage) to pay for the procedure, pre- and posttransplant care, and the required lifelong medication regimen.

Posttransplant care includes many of the same tests, including biopsy for early signs of rejection.

Rejection and Infection

Posttransplant care involves a constant balance between preventing organ rejection, preventing risk of infection, and minimizing the side effects of immunosuppressant medications. The immune system produces white blood cells, which originate in bone marrow. B-cells mature in bone marrow, and T-cells mature in the thymus gland. B-cells (*humoral immunity*) release antibodies to attack pathogens or foreign substances, and T-cells (*cell-mediated immunity*) destroy them. Antigens are substances that stimulate the body to produce antibodies in response to it. "Foreign antigens from transplanted organs [will] trigger an immune response. That stimulates the production of antibodies to launch an attack when an organ is transplanted into a new body" (McClellan, 2003, p. 57). The immune system has a memory, so repeated exposure to the same foreign substance, virus, or infection results in an increasingly rapid and stronger immune system response. Refer to Chapter 11 for more information on the immune system.

When the immune system is suppressed with medication, the risk of organ rejection is minimized. Unfortunately, as essential as immunosuppressant medications are, they increase susceptibility to infection and are associated with a host of negative long-term effects, including osteoporosis, avascular necrosis, atherosclerosis, prolonged wound healing, and skin and lip cancers, particularly squamous cell (Wells & Goodman, 2009). However, without immunosuppression medication, most transplanted organs would be rejected within 2 weeks (McClellan, 2003). To stay on top of rejection, patients often undergo routine tissue biopsies. Traditionally, a cocktail of three medications (e.g., calcineurin inhibitors, antiproliferative agents, and steroids) is used to prevent rejection and minimize the side effects of using a high dose of any one medication (Wells & Goodman, 2009).

The three types of rejection experienced after transplantation are hyperacute, acute, and chronic (Lee & Moinzadeh, 2009; Malone & Lindsay, 2006; Wells & Goodman, 2009).

Hyperacute Rejection

- *Time frame:* Occurs within the first 48 hours after transplant; rejection is quick and immediate. The recipient's antibodies immediately attack donor tissue. Destruction of the graft's vascular endothelium results in organ failure and death.
- *Cause:* May be caused by ABO (blood type) incompatibility or reaction of recipient antibodies to donor organ antigens; risk is minimized by pretransplant antibody screening and tissue typing.
- *Signs and symptoms:* Generalized malaise and high fever.
- *Treatment:* Generally does not respond to treatment, requiring immediate retransplantation. Plasmapheresis and immunoglobulin therapy may be used in an attempt

to remove antibodies from the recipient's blood.

Acute Rejection

- *Time frame:* Occurs within the first year of transplantation; can be detected as early as 4–10 days after transplantation. Acute rejection can also occur years after transplantation, and patients may experience multiple episodes of acute rejection over the course of their life.
- *Cause:* Immune system response to a foreign organ. Most patients experience some level of acute rejection.
- *Signs and symptoms:* Patient may initially be asymptomatic. Sudden weight gain, fever, malaise, electrolyte imbalances, graft tenderness, hypertension, decreased exercise capacity, decreased urine output, increased blood urea nitrogen, increased creatinine, dyspnea, fatigue, nausea, vomiting, sweating, or chills. If untreated, will result in graft failure.
- *Treatment:* Change in immunosuppressant medications, course of Orthoclone OKT3 and steroids (refer to Appendix B for more information on these medications).

Chronic Rejection

- *Time frame:* Occurs after the first year posttransplantation, resulting in a gradual and progressive deterioration of the organ graft.
- *Cause:* Immune response formed in organ blood vessels.
- *Signs and symptoms:* Varies depending on the organ. May be asymptomatic initially. Refer to individual organ sections for detail.
- *Treatment:* Immunosuppressant medication is not effective in preventing chronic rejection but can slow progression. Chronic rejection leads to organ loss. The only definitive treatment is retransplantation.

Solid organ transplantation rejection is typically a phenomenon of *host versus graft disease.* However, a fourth type of rejection is known as *graft versus host disease (GVHD).* In this type of rejection, the donor organ perceives the recipient's tissue as foreign and rejects it. GVHD is more common with hematopoietic transplantation than with solid organ transplantation. Symptoms include skin rash, vomiting, diarrhea, weight loss, abdominal pain, ileus, and hepatitis, whereas chronic GVHD can lead to bronchiolitis; generalized polyneuropathy; muscle wasting; joint contractures; or eventual hemorrhage, infection, and death (Wells & Goodman, 2009). Treatment includes corticosteroids and immunosuppression medication. "The overall fatality rate is about 20%; in the severe form, this rate exceeds 80%. Most people with grade 4 disease do not survive" (Wells & Goodman, 2009, p. 1054).

After transplant, the patient faces a lifelong delicate balance between preventing rejection and infection. Sources of infection may be bacterial, viral, or fungal and can manifest in the lungs, colon, liver, urinary tract, mouth, or site of indwelling devices (e.g., ventilators, catheters; Lee & Moinzadeh, 2009). Signs and symptoms of infection may include fever (>100.4 °F or >38 °C); cough; shortness of breath; sore throat; chills; sweating; fatigue; and gastrointestinal symptoms of nausea, vomiting, or diarrhea. Treatment consists of adjusting immunosuppressant medications and a course of antibiotics.

In addition to rejection and infection, transplant medications increase the patient's risk of developing hypertension, diabetes, and CMV. An additional complication of transplantation includes *reperfusion injuries,* an inflammatory response that occurs when blood is returned to the donor organ during transplantation surgery. This injury predominantly occurs in heart and lung transplant patients with pulmonary hypertension (Wells & Goodman, 2009). Reperfusion injuries can be mild or lead to organ failure.

Solid Organ Transplantation

This section highlights the criteria, contraindications, surgical procedure, and post transplant care, for solid organ transplantation. There is also a brief description of multi-organ transplantation and retransplantation.

Kidney

Although patients with end-stage renal disease can live through dialysis (peritoneal or hemodialysis), kidney transplantation offers better quality of life and increased survival (Steinman et al., 2001). However, dialysis may provide time for candidates to delay transplantation until a suitable organ is donated. Of the two types of dialysis, peritoneal dialysis is associated with a lower rate of delayed graft function than is hemodialysis (Wells & Goodman, 2009). Refer to Chapter 10 for more information on dialysis. Box 14.1 lists information related to kidney transplantation.

Renal transplantation is the most common type of transplant surgery performed. It can be deceased or living donor, because only one functioning kidney is necessary for survival. Of kidney donations in the 21st century, 50% are from living donors (Petechuk, 2006). On rare occasions, both kidneys may be transplanted if both deceased donor kidneys are less than optimal (UNOS, 2009). Recipients of living donor organs have a higher survival rate ($\leq$15 years) than recipients of deceased donor organs (7–8 years; Lee & Moinzadeh, 2009).

According to UNOS (2009), common diagnoses appropriate for kidney transplantation include

- *Glomerular diseases:* Chronic glomerulonephritis, chronic glomerulosclerosis, chronic pyelonephritis, hemolytic uremic syndrome, systemic lupus erythematosus, amyloidosis, Goodpasture's syndrome, sickle cell anemia, and Wegener's granulomatosis;

- *Diabetes:* Type 1 and Type 2, diabetic nephropathy;

- *Vascular diseases:* Primary uncontrolled hypertension, polycystic kidney disease, neoplasms; and

- *Tubular and interstitial diseases:* Gout, nephritis, nephrolithiasis, radiation nephritis, sarcoidosis, acute tubular necrosis, urolithiasis.

Procedure

In a kidney transplant procedure, an incision is made in the lower abdomen and the donor kidney is placed below the native kidney. The renal artery and veins of the donor organ are attached to the recipient's iliac artery and vein, and the donor ureter is connected to the recipient's bladder (see Figure 14.1.). The native kidney is generally not removed and remains in its normal anatomical position.

Box 14.1. Kidney Transplantation

Criteria	Contraindication	Preservation Time	Survival Rate
Type 1 diabetes and end-stage renal disease that does not respond to conventional treatment. Diabetes is the most common cause of end-stage renal disease.	Reversible kidney disease, advanced cardiopulmonary disease, metastatic cancer or recent malignancy, active substance abuse, obesity, active or recurring infection, or HIV with a CD4 count of <200 cells/mm.^{3}	Kidneys can be maintained $\leq$72 hr before transplant and are usually the last organs to be harvested.	*One year:* >95% (living, related donor), >91% (deceased donor).

Sources. Lee & Moinzadeh (2009), Malone & Lindsay (2006), Steinman et al. (2001), Wells & Goodman (2009).

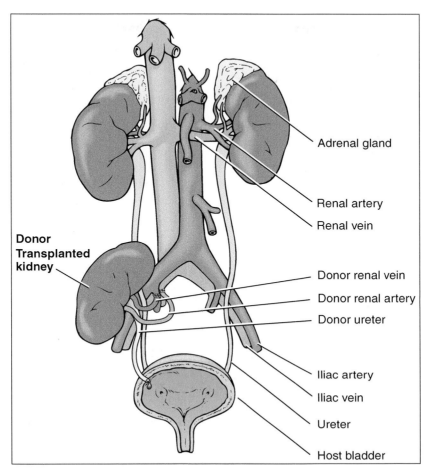

Adrenal gland

Renal artery

Renal vein

Donor Transplanted kidney

Donor renal vein

Donor renal artery

Donor ureter

Iliac artery

Iliac vein

Ureter

Host bladder

Figure 14.1. Kidney transplantation.
Source. Richard Fritzler, Medical Illustrator, Roswell, GA.

Posttransplant Care

Care includes daily weight measurement and strict intake and output monitoring. Therapists should note that kidney transplant patients' blood pressures tend to be higher than normal with exercise (Lee & Moinzadeh, 2009).

Complications

- Dialysis, which may still be required for the first few weeks after transplantation because of delayed graft function, which occurs when renal failure persists after transplantation but is rare with living donor transplantation (Malone & Lindsay, 2006). Return of renal function is judged by urine output and normalization of serum blood urea nitrogen and creatinine levels (Lee & Moinzadeh, 2009).

- Acute tubular necrosis, which may result in delayed kidney function and causes delayed graft function.

- Nephrotoxicity.

- Urethral obstruction, requiring placement of nephrostomy tube or surgical correction.

- Urine leakage (initially).

- Diabetes.

- Renal artery thrombosis or stenosis.

- Hypertension, which occurs in as many as 80% of recipients (Wells & Goodman, 2009).

- Hyperkalemia.

- Urinary tract infection.
- Hepatitis.
- Cancer.
- Lymphoproliferative disease.

Symptoms of Rejection

Symptoms include a gradual increase in creatinine and blood urea nitrogen, electrolyte imbalances, weight gain, new-onset hypertension, presence of sediment in urine, decreased urine output, and peripheral edema (Lee & Moinzadeh, 2009; Malone & Lindsay, 2006).

Symptoms of Chronic Rejection

Symptoms include nephropathy and worsening hypertension.

Liver

Liver transplants are the second most commonly performed transplant procedure. Box 14.2 lists information on the criteria, contraindications, preservation time, and survival rates for liver transplantation. Liver transplant procedures may be *orthotopic* (whole deceased donor liver), *living donor*, or *split liver* (e.g., liver segment). With a living donor, a single donor lobe is transplanted into the recipient. Donor and recipient liver regeneration can take several months. The donor experiences no loss of function; however, people receiving living liver donations have a higher risk of morbidity and mortality than people receiving living kidney donation (Johnson, Jha, & Lu, 2004).

In a split-liver transplant, a deceased donor liver is divided into two and transplanted into two different recipients. A reduced liver transplant may also be performed when the donor liver is too large for the recipient (UNOS, 2009). The most famous liver transplant recipient is Chris Klug, who won a 2002 Olympic bronze medal for snowboarding just 18 months after his liver transplant surgery (Barter, 2006; McClellan, 2003).

Candidates are prioritized by their Model for End-Stage Liver Disease (MELD) score, which is based on mortality risk, ensuring that deceased donor organs are allocated according to medical urgency (Ahmad, Bryce, Cacciarelli, & Roberts, 2007). MELD is based on serum creatinine levels, bilirubin levels, and international normalization ratio values. Creatinine levels measure kidney function, often associated with liver disease, whereas bilirubin levels reflect the liver's ability to excrete bile, and the international normalization ratio reflects the liver's ability to produce blood-clotting factors (UNOS, 2009). MELD scores range from 6 (*less ill*) to 40 (*gravely ill;* Ahmad et al., 2007; UNOS, 2009). A UNOS modification calculator for computing MELD scores is available at http://www.mayoclinic.org/meld/mayomodel6.html.

Box 14.2. Liver Transplantation			
Criteria	**Contraindication**	**Preservation Time**	**Survival Rate**
End-stage liver disease refractory to conventional treatment. Wait time on the transplant list is determined by the patient's Model for End-Stage Liver Disease score.	Continued alcohol or drug abuse, active infection, age (>65), advanced heart or lung disease, recent myocardial infarction (within past 6 months), HIV, or cancer.	*Deceased donor liver:* ≤24 hr.	*1 year:* 83%. *5 years:* 74%. *9 years:* 55%.

Sources. Lee & Moinzadeh (2009), Malone & Lindsay (2006).

The Child–Turcotte–Pugh is an additional scoring method and prognostic measure for cirrhotic liver failure that looks at the five features of end-stage liver disease: prothrombin time, serum bilirubin, albumin levels and the presence or absence of ascites, and encephalopathy (Ebell, 2006; Steinman et al., 2001).

Common diagnoses appropriate for liver transplantation may include

- Hepatitis C, the most common condition requiring an orthotopic liver transplant (Steinman et al., 2001);
- Alcoholic cirrhosis;
- Primary biliary cirrhosis;
- Sclerosing cholangitis;
- Chronic viral hepatitis B or D;
- Cancer of the bile ducts or liver (e.g., cholangiocarcinoma, cholangioma, hepatocellular carcinoma);
- Metabolic diseases, including hemochromatosis, Wilson's disease, or alpha-1 antitrypsin deficiency;
- Cystic fibrosis;
- Budd–Chiari syndome;
- Total parenteral nutrition (hyperalimentation) liver disease; and
- Portal hypertension with variceal bleeding.

Procedure

With *orthotopic liver transplantation*, the native organ is removed, and the donor liver is put in its anatomical position. A transverse incision is made in the abdomen below the ribs (subcostal) with an extension toward the xiphoid. The donor liver is subsequently connected to the recipient's blood vessels (e.g., inferior vena cave, portal vein, hepatic artery) and bile ducts. In *living donor transplantation*, only a section of the donor's left lobe is removed (Wells & Goodman, 2009).

Posttransplant Care

Occupational therapists should be aware that because of the nature of end-stage liver disease, ascites, anasarca, malnutrition, deconditioning, and muscle wasting may still persist even after the procedure. The patient's balance will likely be compromised secondary to ascites, which also restricts reaching the feet for lower-body activities of daily living (ADLs).

After transplant, deep breathing and increased activity should be encouraged to prevent pulmonary complications (Lee & Moinzadeh, 2009). However, resistive exercise should be avoided until the abdominal incision is healed. Consult with the patient's physician for any restrictions before treating. Engagement in ADLs may also be hindered by T tubes for collecting bile and Jackson–Pratt tubes and bulbs, which collect drainage from around the liver (see Figure 14.2). Liver transplant patients routinely undergo liver biopsies, liver function tests, and coagulation panels to monitor for signs of rejection and liver function. Prolonged coagulation time is a sign of decreased liver function, and production of bile, hyperglycemia, and hypokalemia are signs of returning liver function (Lee & Moinzadeh, 2009). Defer treatment if the patient's international normalization ratio is elevated (consult with physician for parameters).

Complications

Complications are not limited to graft dysfunction, rejection, and infection. Additional complications with liver transplants may include (Wells & Goodman, 2009) the following:

- *Extrahepatic complications:* Renal failure, neurological disorders, pulmonary disorders (atelectasis, pneumonia, pleural effusion, respiratory distress syndrome), hepatocellular carcinoma, hepatitis B, and Budd–Chiari syndrome; and
- *Central nervous system complications:* Encephalopathy; intracranial, intracerebral, or subarachnoid hemorrhage or infarct; confusion, coma, cortical blindness, quadriplegia, tremors, CMV, psychosis, focal seizures, and locked-in syndrome.

Additional complications can include hepatic blood vessel stenosis or thrombosis, biliary leaks, diabetes, decreased urine output, or jaundice.

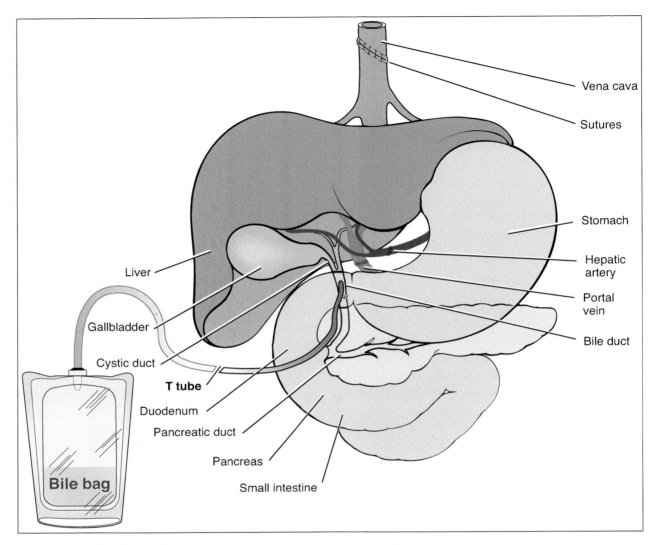

Figure 14.2. T tube for bile drainage after liver transplantation.
Source. Richard Fritzler, Medical Illustrator, Roswell, GA.

In addition, issues of hypervolemia; impaired cardiopulmonary functioning; weakness; fatigue; pneumonia; and wound, line, or urinary tract infections may arise (Malone & Lindsay, 2006). Liver transplant patients may also be at increased risk for colorectal cancer.

Symptoms of Acute Rejection

Patients may be asymptomatic or may present histologically with portal inflammation and bile duct injury.

Symptoms of Chronic Rejection

Symptoms may include ductopenic rejection or vanishing bile duct syndrome marked by liver tissue fibrosis and necrosis, a rise in bilirubin and aspartate aminotransferase levels, thickening of hepatic arteries, narrowing of bile ducts, and progressive liver failure (Lee & Moinzadeh, 2009; Malone & Lindsay, 2006). Split-liver transplants have the additional risk of leaking bile, which can destroy surrounding tissue (Barter, 2006).

Pancreas

Unlike other transplant procedures, pancreas transplantation is not considered life saving but instead aims to improve quality of life, stabilizing the complications associated with

Type 1 diabetes, and free the patient from exogenous insulin therapy (Lee & Moinzadeh, 2009; Malone & Lindsay, 2006; Wells & Goodman, 2009). Living donor transplantation is a rare procedure in which a segment of the body or tail of the pancreas is used; however, a whole deceased donor organ is preferable (Lee & Moinzadeh, 2009). Pancreas transplantation is often combined with kidney transplantation because patients with pancreas failure frequently have renal failure as well (UNOS, 2009). Refer to Box 14.3 for information on the criteria, contraindications, preservation time, and survival rates for pancreas transplantation.

The goal of pancreas transplantation is to return the patient to normoglycemia and prevent progression of diabetic complications (Lee & Moinzadeh, 2009). This type of procedure may reverse neuropathy but not other long-term complications of diabetes (e.g., retinopathy or vascular stenosis; Robertson, Davis, Larsen, Stratta, & Sutherland, 2000; Wells & Goodman, 2009).

Procedure

Pancreas transplantation requires a lower abdominal incision. The donor pancreas, and often part of the donor duodenum (for draining exocrine secretions), is placed near the native pancreas, which remains in place to aid digestion. The donor pancreas is also connected to blood vessels that supply blood to the lower extremities.

Posttransplant Care

The two types of drainage systems for pancreatic exocrine secretions are enteric or bladder. In *enteric drainage*, the donor duodenum is attached to the small bowel; in *bladder drainage* (the more common procedure), the duodenum is attached to the urinary bladder (Lee & Moinzadeh, 2009; Robertson et al., 2000). The advantage with bladder drainage is that urine amylase can be used as a marker of rejection. Signs of a functioning graft include insulin production. Blood sugar levels are routinely monitored and should be between 80 milligrams/deciliter and 150 milligrams/deciliter within several hours of the transplant with normalization between 2 and 3 days after transplant (Lee & Moinzadeh, 2009).

Occupational therapists should ensure that patients have adequate hydration when working in therapy because patients with pancreas transplantation need 3–4 liters of fluid daily (Lee & Moinzadeh, 2009). Electrolyte values must be monitored until metabolic and fluid levels are stabilized because the pancreas transplant with bladder attachment secretes large volumes of water and bicarbonate (Malone & Lindsay, 2006).

Box 14.3. Pancreas Transplantation

Criteria	Contraindication	Preservation Time	Survival Rate
Insulin dependent with Type 1 or Type 2 diabetes mellitus (that is poorly controlled with standard treatment), pancreatic cancer, bile duct cancer, diabetes secondary to cystic fibrosis, or diabetes secondary to chronic pancreatitis.	Severe cardiovascular disease, complete blindness, morbid obesity, active tobacco use, major amputation, > age 45, or hepatitis C.	Approximately 12–24 hr.	*One year:* >90%, with 60%–85% of patients no longer requiring insulin. *Five years;* 52%.

Sources. Lee & Moinzadeh (2009), Malone & Lindsay (2006), Wells & Goodman (2009), UNOS (2009).

Complications

Complications may include metabolic acidosis with urinary bladder drainage, dehydration, and hypovolemia if the patient is not adequately hydrated; reflux of urine into the donor organ, causing pancreatitis; urinary tract infections; urethral stricture; dysuria; chronic hematuria; hyperkalemia; duodenal leaks; graft pancreatitis; peritonitis; and abscess or graft thrombosis (Lee & Moinzadeh, 2009; Malone & Lindsay, 2006). Enteric drainage increases the risk of infection and development of small bowel complications. Further complications from pancreatic transplant may include ileus, leukocytosis, decrease in bicarbonate, or decrease in urine pH (Lee & Moinzadeh, 2009).

Symptoms of Chronic Rejection

Chronic rejection is indicated by hyperglycemia. Retransplantation is indicated with graft failure.

Islet Cells

A less invasive alternative to pancreas transplantation is islet cell transplantation, an emerging option for improving glycemic control in treating brittle or labile Type 1 diabetes mellitus (Shapiro & Ricordi, 2004; Shapiro et al., 2006; see also Box 14.4). In diabetes mellitus Type 1, the body's immune system destroys pancreatic islet of Langerhans beta cells that produce insulin. Type 1 diabetes is a serious disorder that predisposes the patient to a host of potentially devastating conditions, including blindness, stroke, renal failure, nerve damage, heart attack, and premature death. Most islet cell transplantations are based on the Edmonton Protocol, in which islet cells from two or more deceased donors are infused into a patient along with glucocorticoid-free immunosuppression therapy (Shapiro et al., 2000). Combined islet cell and kidney transplantations have also been performed for patients with end-stage diabetic nephropathy (Robertson et al., 2000; Shapiro et al., 2000).

In islet cell transplantation, extracted pancreatic islet cells are injected by needle into the portal vein, where they lodge in the small blood vessels of the liver (National Diabetes Information Clearinghouse [NDIC], 2007). If successful, this procedure negates the use of daily insulin medication by the patient because the transplanted cells begin producing insulin. However, it does not reverse the preexisting diabetic damage to other organs.

A disadvantage of islet cell transplantation is that insulin independence is not sustainable, often requiring subsequent transplantation or resumption of some exogenous insulin therapy (Ryan et al., 2005; Shapiro et al., 2000, 2006). In addition, islet cell transplantation is not a common procedure and is still considered experimental. In many ways, islet cell transplantation is preferable to pancreas transplantation because it is less invasive. However, pancreas transplantation is associated with better long-term glycemic control (Shapiro et al., 2000).

Procedure

Islet cells are extracted from at least two cadaver donors to obtain the 800,000 cells required for one transplant. However, the normal

Box 14.4. **Islet Cell Transplantation**	
Criteria for Islet Cell Transplantation	**Prognosis**
Poorly controlled severe Type 1 diabetes or complications of Type 1 diabetes.	As of 2006, 40% of patients no longer required insulin medication; by 3 years that number decreased to 17%. However, hypoglycemia and glycemic lability were better controlled after transplantation.

Sources. NDIC (2007), Ryan et al. (2005).

pancreas has approximately 1–1.5 million islet cells. The procedure itself lasts approximately 1 hour; however, isolation of islet cells may take up to 10 hours (see Figure 14.3).

Complications

Islet cell transplantation is considered a relatively minor procedure but has associated risks of bleeding at the catheter site, blood clots in the portal vein or liver, infection, or hypoglycemia. Islet cell immunosuppression medication has been associated with mouth ulcers, diarrhea, anemia, leukopenia, and ovarian cysts (Ryan et al., 2005; Shapiro et al., 2006).

Posttransplant Care

In addition to immunosuppression medication, the patient may initially require insulin, which

gradually decreases as the new islet cells begin working. Patients remain in the hospital approximately 2 days.

Symptoms of Rejection

A rise in blood glucose levels may be indicative of rejection.

Heart

Heart transplantation has a certain aura, different from that of the other organs, because of its symbolism in most cultures as being sacred and the center of being (Barter, 2006; McClellan, 2003). Unlike other transplantation procedures, it can be performed only with a deceased donor organ. Because of the shortage of donor hearts, transplant centers are increasingly using

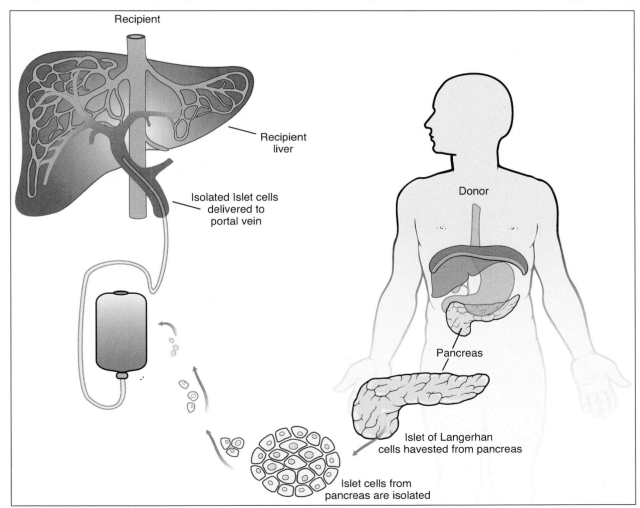

Figure 14.3. Islet cell transplantation.
Source. Richard Fritzler, Medical Illustrator, Roswell, GA.

	Box 14.5.	**Orthotopic Heart Transplantation**	
Criteria	**Contraindication**	**Preservation Time**	**Survival Rate**
End-stage heart disease refractory to conventional medical and surgical treatment, with <1-year life expectancy. The age limit is commonly ≤60; in some cases, however, it may be ≤65 or 70.	Type 1 diabetes with diabetic complications, chronic obstructive pulmonary disease, fixed pulmonary hypertension, unresolved pulmonary infarction, irreversible liver disease, or active peptic ulcer disease.	Heart valves can be preserved for years; however, preservation time for a donor heart is approximately 4 hrs.	*1 year:* 87%. *5 years:* 71%.
Sources. D'Amico (2005), Lee & Moinzadeh (2009).			

ventricular assist devices (VADs) as a bridge to transplantation; however, patients with a VAD are at increased risk for acute rejection (Lee & Moinzadeh, 2009). (Refer to Chapter 3 for information on VADs.) Heart transplantation is predominantly orthotopic. Refer to Box 14.5 for information on the criteria, contraindications, preservation time, and survival rates for orthotopic heart transplantation.

The patient is placed on a cardiopulmonary bypass machine, the native heart is removed, and the donor heart is put in its anatomical place (see Figure 14.4). However a small percentage (<1%) of heart transplant procedures

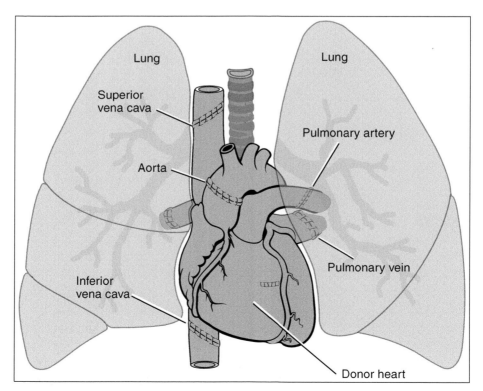

Figure 14.4. Orthotopic heart transplantation.
Source. Richard Fritzler, Medical Illustrator, Roswell, GA.

are heterotopic or piggyback, in which the native heart is left in its place and the donor heart is attached to it.

In a heterotopic transplant, the donor heart assists the remaining native heart (see Figure 14.5). This procedure may be indicated for patients with fixed pulmonary hypertension (Lee & Moinzadeh, 2009; Wells & Goodman, 2009). Heterotopic heart transplants may also be performed for patients who are considered poor candidates for orthotopic heart transplantation (e.g., donor–recipient size mismatch or a suboptimal donor organ; Kanter, 1990; Malone & Lindsay, 2006). Pulmonary hypertension is also a contraindication for orthotopic heart transplantation because it may lead to right ventricular dysfunction of the donor heart, graft failure, and eventual death (D'Amico, 2005; Kanter et al., 1998).

Heterotopic transplantation is the preferred procedure because the right ventricle of the native heart is typically hypertrophied from pulmonary hypertension and can better handle this condition, whereas the donor heart handles left ventricular function and cardiac output (Kanter, 1990). However, heterotopic heart transplantation also carries a greater risk of emboli, dysrhythmia, and angina from the native heart (Kanter, 1990; Malone & Lindsay, 2006).

Common diagnoses treated by heart transplantation include

- Ischemic heart disease or coronary artery disease,
- Cardiomyopathy (dilated, hypertrophic, or restrictive),
- Valvular heart disease,
- Congestive heart failure,
- Congenital heart diseases,
- Primary cardiac tumors that have not metastasized, and
- Malignant ventricular dysrhythmias.

Patients with left ventricular ejection fraction of less than 20% and New York Heart Association Class III and Class IV are also candidates for transplantation (Steinman et al., 2001; Wells & Goodman, 2009). Refer to Chapter 3 for more information on New York Heart Association categories. Candidates are classified on the transplant lists on the basis of urgency as Status 1A, 1B, or 2 (D'Amico, 2005):

- *Status 1A:* Patients are critically ill and remain in the intensive care unit while

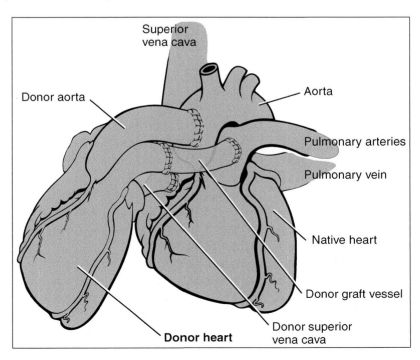

Figure 14.5. Heterotrophic (piggyback) heart transplant.
Source. Richard Fritzler, Medical Illustrator, Roswell, GA.

awaiting a donor organ. They require one of the following:

— VAD (implanted <30 days)

— Intra-aortic balloon pump

— Extracorporeal membrane oxygenator

— Continuous mechanical ventilation

— High dosage or multiple IV inotropes.

- *Status 1B:* Patients may also be in the intensive care unit or on a regular floor. They require at least one of the following:

— VAD (implanted >30 days)

— Inotrope support.

- *Status 2:* Patients do not require special medications to support cardiac function, do not require VAD support, and have a 1-year mortality risk of more than 15% (Wells & Goodman, 2009). Status 2 patients may wait at home until a donor is located.

- *Status 7:* Inactive.

Status 1A patients have first priority on the basis of urgency. If a donor organ becomes available and is not compatible with the Status 1A candidate, the donor organ may then go to a Status 1B candidate. If a donor organ does not match a Status 1B candidate, then a Status 2 patient is considered.

Contraindications

As mentioned in Box 14.5, heart transplantation has numerous contraindications. Poorly controlled diabetes is a relative contraindication because diabetes is associated with poor wound healing, retinopathy, neuropathy, and nephropathy (D'Amico, 2005; Steinman et al., 2001). Chronic obstructive pulmonary disease may result in difficulty weaning from ventilator support and predisposes the heart transplant patient to pulmonary infection (D'Amico, 2005). Pulmonary infarction increases the risk of recurrent emboli, and because many transplant medications are hepatotoxic, irreversible liver disease is also a contraindication (D'Amico, 2005). Peptic ulcer disease increases the risk of hemorrhage during the surgery.

Additional contraindications include patients with cardiac amyloid, systemic illness (e.g., systemic lupus erythematosis, sarcoidosis), HIV/AIDS, age older than 65, peripheral vascular disease, intrinsic renal disease, dementia, or history of poor medical compliance. In addition, heart transplantation is contraindicated in patients with active seizure disorder, stroke with poor rehabilitation, morbid obesity (ideal body weight >135% or body mass index >30), recent pulmonary infarction, severe osteoporosis, or substance abuse (D'Amico, 2005; Freundenberger et al., 2000; Malone & Lindsay, 2006; Steinman et al., 2001). Obesity is a contraindication because it increases the patient's risk for morbidity and mortality, including poor wound healing, pulmonary complications, and lower extremity thrombosis (Mehra et al., 2006). Posttransplant tobacco use is associated with coronary allograft vasculopathy and malignancy (Mehra et al., 2006). Adults with congenital heart disease, patients requiring short-term extracorporeal mechanical circulatory support, pretransplant patients requiring dialysis or ventilation, or patients with diabetes requiring insulin have the highest risk of mortality with heart transplantation (Taylor et al., 2007).

Procedure

A cardiac bypass machine is used to maintain blood circulation throughout the body during the surgery. The incision is combined with a median sternotomy in which the native heart is removed, but the posterior right atrium with the sinus node, left atrium, aorta, and pulmonary artery remain. The donor heart is then placed in the heart's normal anatomical position. The surgical procedure may last 4–6 hours.

After surgery, patients will have an arterial line for measuring blood pressure, a pulmonary artery catheter for measuring left ventricle function, and chest tubes to drain blood and fluids (Lee & Moinzadeh, 2009). Temporary pacing wires and medications (e.g., inotrope support) are also used to regulate heart rhythm until the donor heart begins to function properly on its own.

Posttransplant Care

Cardiac biopsies are performed on a prescribed schedule to monitor for rejection. Biopsies are initially performed frequently, then with progressively longer intervals between them. Biopsies are rated on a scale ranging from 0 (*no rejection*) to 4 (*severe rejection*). The International Society of

Table 14.4. **International Society of Heart and Lung Transplantation Grading System for Acute Rejection**

Grade	Acute Rejection
0	No rejection
1R	Mild
2R	Moderate
3R	Severe

Source. From the ISHLT Standardized Cardiac Biopsy Grading: Acute Cellular Rejection (Stewart, et al., 2005). *Note.* "R" denotes revised grade from 1990 model.

Heart and Lung Transplantation Grading System for Acute Rejection is provided in Table 14.4.

Occupational therapists working with heart transplant recipients must adhere to strict hand washing, because transplant patients are at increased risk of infection. Therapists must also incorporate sternal precautions, which include lifting no more than 5–10 pounds, no heavy pulling or pushing with upper extremities, and avoidance of activities that result in shoulder retraction with chest expansion. Refer to Chapter 3 for details on sternal precautions.

In monitoring response to therapy, the donor heart is denervated so anginal pain is not felt, and complaints of pain are usually attributed to incisional pain. Rate of perceived exertion scales (e.g., Borg scale) are good indicators of a patient's activity tolerance. Monitor for dyspnea, arrhythmias, or dizziness. The patient's electrocardiogram will now have two P waves (one from the native sinoatrial node and the other from the donor heart). The P wave from the native sinoatrial node cannot cross the incision and therefore cannot stimulate ventricular contraction; Lee & Moinzadeh, 2009).

Because the donor heart is denervated, no autonomic nervous system input controls the patient's heart rate, so resting heart rates are elevated (usually 90–110 beats per minute). Patients require warm-up and cool-down periods of 5–10 minutes with any exercise or activity because the heart now relies on circulating catecholamines (e.g., epinephrine, norepinephrine: fight-or-flight hormones) to increase heart rate, resulting in a slower-than-normal increase in heart rate and return to resting rate (Lee & Moinzadeh, 2009; Wells & Goodman, 2009). "If the recipient does not warm up sufficiently, the feeling of fatigue and stress (similar to an athlete 'hitting the wall') is experienced due to the inability to increase cardiac output to meet demands. The recipient is functioning in anaerobic metabolism" (Wells & Goodman, 2009, p. 1081).

Patients can usually begin therapy 2–3 days after surgery, and exercises are progressed to the patient's tolerance. The sternum is held together with wire, which should not be compromised until healed, in approximately 4–6 weeks. Therefore, upper-body resistive exercise is contraindicated for the first 4–6 weeks (depending on the surgeon). However, active range of motion exercises and ADLs that do not retract the shoulders while expanding the chest are appropriate. Isometric exercises should also be avoided because of the volume of stress they put on the heart (Wells & Goodman, 2009). Therapists are also advised to change positions slowly because patients frequently have orthostatic hypotension the first few days (Lee & Moinzadeh, 2009).

At discharge, patients are instructed not to drive, lift, push, or pull for approximately 6–8 weeks. They are instructed on their medication schedule and on infection prevention. Heart transplant patients can also benefit from a referral to an outpatient cardiac rehabilitation program.

Complications

Complications include postoperative bleeding; cardiac tamponade; cyclosporine-induced hypertension; diabetes mellitus; thrombosis; right or biventricular heart failure; reduced cardiac output; elevated central venous pressure; new cardiac arrhythmias; hypotension; pulmonary hypertension; low urine output; pericardial effusion; or patient complaints of fatigue, lethargy, depression, dyspnea, or renal dysfunction (Lee & Moinzadeh, 2009; Wells & Goodman, 2009). Approximately 25% of heart transplant recipients develop kidney disease within the first year. Skin cancer, particularly squamous cell, is also commonly associated with long-term immunosuppression after cardiac transplantation. In addition, long-term corticosteroid use is also associated with a host of adverse side effects.

Symptoms of Acute Rejection

The patient may be asymptomatic or present with low-grade fever, lethargy, fatigue, palpitations, arrhythmias, increased shortness of breath, dyspnea on exertion, hypotension with activity, or increased resting blood pressure (Malone & Lindsay, 2006).

Symptoms of Chronic Rejection

Coronary allograft vasculopathy is a condition of accelerated atherosclerosis with obstruction of coronary arteries leading to cardiac ischemia or infarct. It is associated with a history of CMV, tobacco use, and diabetes (Wells & Goodman, 2009). Coronary allograft vasculopathy is the leading cause of death 1 year after transplant, and retransplantation is the only treatment recourse (Bishay, 2006; Kanter et al., 1998).

Lung

The three different types of lung transplantation are single lung, double lung, or living donor lobe. *Single-lung transplant* is the most common procedure; however, *double-lung transplant* is commonly used for patients with cystic fibrosis. *Living donor transplant* is a rare procedure in which an adult donates a segment or lobe to be transplanted into a child (National Heart, Lung, and Blood Institute, 2008). Box 14.6 lists information on the criteria, contraindications, preservation time, and survival rates for lung transplantation.

The Lung Allocation System helps determine placement on the waiting list and is based on length of survival without a transplant and length of survival during the first year with transplant (UNOS, 2005). Forced vital capacity, oxygen requirements at rest, New York Heart Association functional class, continuous mechanical ventilation, body mass index, age, and diagnosis are some of the variables used in calculating the Lung Allocation System category (Wells & Goodman, 2009). Lung Allocation System diagnostic categories (UNOS, 2005) include

- *Group A:* Chronic obstructive pulmonary disease, emphysema, alpha-1 antitrypsin deficiency, bronchiectasis, lymphangioleiomyomatosis, sarcoidosis, or primary ciliary dyskinesia;

Box 14.6. Lung Transplantation

Criteria	Contraindication	Preservation Time	Survival Rate
End-stage lung disease with a life expectancy of <18–24 mos.	Poor left ventricular function; severe coronary artery disease; severe lung, kidney, or central nervous system disease; or active tobacco use. Poorer outcomes are also associated with prolonged ventilator use, infectious disease, and immobility.	Approximately 4–6 hr for deceased donor lungs.	For both single- and double-lung transplants: *1 year:* 83%. *5 years:* 46%.

Sources. Lee & Moinzadeh (2009), Malone & Lindsay (2006).

- *Group B:* Primary pulmonary hypertension, Eisenmenger's syndrome, scleroderma;
- *Group C:* Cystic fibrosis or hypogamma-globulinemia; and
- *Group D:* Interstitial pulmonary fibrosis, sarcoidosis, lung retransplant, obliterative bronchiolitis, pulmonary fibrosis (not interstitial pulmonary fibrosis), eosinophilic granuloma, amyloidosis, mixed connective tissue disease, or restrictive scleroderma.

Diseases appropriate for transplantation (UNOS, 2009) include

- Congenital Eisenmenger's syndrome,
- Emphysema,
- Chronic obstructive pulmonary disease,
- Cystic fibrosis,
- Idiopathic pulmonary fibrosis,
- Primary pulmonary hypertension,
- Alpha-1 antitrypsin deficiency,
- Sarcoidosis,
- Bronchiectasis,
- Scleroderma,
- Occupational lung disease,
- Pulmonary vascular disease,
- Rheumatoid disease, and
- Inhalation burns or trauma.

Procedure

An anterolateral or posterolateral thoracotomy is used for single-lung transplantation. When both lungs are transplanted as in cystic fibrosis, bronchiectasis, or pulmonary hypertension, the procedure is a bilateral anterior thoracotomy or a transverse sternotomy ("clamshell") in which the more damaged lung is replaced first, followed by the second lung (Lee & Moinzadeh, 2009; Malone & Lindsay, 2006; see Figure 14.6). In a living donor lobe transplant, two lower lobes are donated from two different donors.

Posttransplant Care

Posttransplant care includes short-term mechanical ventilation and supplemental

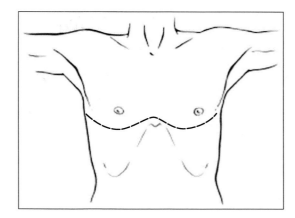

Figure 14.6. Lung transplant using a clamshell incision.
Source. Richard Fritzler, Medical Illustrator, Roswell, GA.

oxygen, which is usually weaned before the patient is discharged from the hospital. "Lung volumes and flow rates improve to two-thirds of normal in single-lung transplantation" (Lee & Moinzadeh, 2009, p. 417). Bronchopulmonary hygiene including postural drainage, airway suctioning, incentive spirometry, diaphragmatic breathing, and coughing exercises are strongly encouraged to prevent atelectasis and pneumonia (Malone & Lindsay, 2006).

Occupational therapy focuses on functional mobility, increasing endurance and strength, incorporating proper breathing techniques (e.g., diaphragmatic and pursed lip breathing), and facilitating engagement in normal occupations. Early mobilization should be encouraged. Check physician or facility policy regarding thoracotomy precautions. Patients are generally instructed to avoid lifting more than 10 pounds and only partial weight bearing of upper extremities (Lee & Moinzadeh, 2009). The patient with a median sternotomy or anterolateral thoracotomy is cautioned to avoid any strenuous or resistive upper-extremity exercises for approximately 4–6 weeks (American Association of Cardiovascular and Pulmonary Rehabilitation, 1998). However, an active range of motion exercise program should be incorporated for flexibility and conditioning. Oxygen saturation levels should be monitored throughout the treatment session. Modify interventions according to the patient's tolerance.

Standard precautions should be observed, including strict hand washing, because lung transplant patients are at increased risk of infection. The patient's cough reflex is impaired because of denervation of the new lung or lungs; therefore, the risk of atelectasis, mucous plugs, pulmonary edema, pulmonary effusion, acute respiratory distress syndrome, wound dehiscence, and bronchial anastomoses is increased (Lee & Moinzadeh, 2009). Lung transplant patients are also more susceptible to and have a higher rate of infections than other transplant patients because the transplanted organ is constantly exposed to air, bacteria, and germs that are breathed in (McClellan, 2003). Because of the heightened risk of pneumonia and respiratory infections, patients need to wear a mask if leaving their room and ambulating in the hallways. Lung transplant recipients are also at increased risk for osteopenia, osteoporosis, renal disease, and diverticulitis requiring a colectomy (Wells & Goodman, 2009).

Lung transplant patients may benefit from an outpatient pulmonary rehabilitation program after discharge to increase strength and endurance for functional activities. Program modifications for patients before and after lung transplantation are given in Table 14.5.

Symptoms of Acute Rejection

Symptoms may include dyspnea on exertion, nonproductive cough, leukocytosis, hypoxemia, decreased pulmonary function tests, increased white blood cell counts, fever, chills, fatigue, desaturation with activity, and increased oxygen requirements or need for mechanical ventilation (Lee & Moinzadeh, 2009; Malone & Lindsay, 2006; Wells & Goodman, 2009). Patients undergo routine bronchoscopy and biopsy to monitor for signs of acute rejection. Bronchoscopy is also used to clear secretions and examine the airway for patency.

Symptoms of Chronic Rejection

Bronchiolitis obliterans leads to scarring and fibrosis of lung tissue and is the leading cause of death with lung transplantation (Malone & Lindsay, 2006). Bronchiolitis obliterans is responsible for 30% of deaths during the first year (Wells & Goodman, 2009).

Intestines

Most intestinal transplants are whole-organ transplantation; however, segments can also be transplanted. Intestinal transplant is usually combined with a liver transplant (UNOS, 2009).

Criteria

Criteria for implantation include

- Irreversible intestinal failure or liver failure secondary to hyperalimentation (total parenteral nutrition; Wells & Goodman, 2009),
- Short gut syndrome (volvulus secondary to adhesions or malrotation, inflammatory bowel disease, tumors, or mesenteric vascular thrombosis), and
- Functional bowel problems (pseudoobstruction, Hirschsprung's disease).

Complications

Infections are responsible for 60% of graft loss; rejection, for 14%.

Survival Rate

The 1-year survival rate is more than 78%; the 5-year survival rate is 40%.

Multiple Organ Transplantation

Pancreas–kidney transplant is performed for those patients with both Type 1 diabetes and renal failure. This surgery is more involved and has more potential complications than a single-organ procedure. Pancreas–kidney transplantation can result in normal blood sugar levels without the need for dialysis. "Graft and recipient survival rates in diabetic recipients are higher when the recipient receives simultaneous pancreas–kidney transplantation" (Wells & Goodman, 2009, p. 1095). The 1-year survival rate is 92%; the 5-year rate is 76%. Survival rates with a living related kidney donor are even higher.

- Patients younger than age 45 with no history of congestive heart failure or minimal atherosclerotic disease are the most appropriate candidates for pancreas–kidney transplantation (Steinman et al., 2001).

Table 14.5.   Program Modification for Patients Before and After Lung Transplantation

Pretransplant

- Age-specific patient/family training
- Intensity of exercise training reduced
- Exercise as tolerated by dyspnea
- Stable patient may exercise at home
- Waiting time to transplant unknown, so disease can progress, requiring reassessment and modification of exercise and medical program
- Periodic review of home exercise program and maintenance exercise attendance

Immediate Posttransplant

- Optimize airway clearance and lung expansion
- Decreasing requirement for supplemental oxygen
- Improving stability in erect posture
- Directed cough
- Encourage proper breathing techniques for all activities
- Modify activities to accommodate chest tubes and other lines
- Facilitate upper- and lower-extremity range of motion, strengthening, and functional mobility

Postdischarge

- Oxygen saturation monitored
- Postural awareness
- Back protection and instruction in proper body mechanics (patients on long-term immunosuppressants are at risk for osteoporosis)
- Increased tolerance for engagement in activities of daily living
- Emotional support and reassurance
- Monitor for signs of infection or rejection (decrease in functional endurance and exercise tolerance)

Source. Adapted with permission, American Association of Cardiovascular and Pulmonary Rehabilitation, 1998, *Guidelines for Pulmonary Rehabilitation Programs*, 2nd ed. (Champaign, IL: Human Kinetics), p. 106.

- Serum creatinine levels are used to detect and monitor graft rejection of both the pancreas and the kidney (Robertson et al., 2000).

Heart–lung transplant is performed for patients with both end-stage heart and lung disease, which includes cystic fibrosis, congenital heart disease, primary pulmonary hypertension, idiopathic pulmonary fibrosis, Eisenmenger's syndrome, or retransplantion resulting from graft failure (Malone & Lindsay, 2006; UNOS, 2009). The heart and lungs are removed together as a whole and attached to the recipient's trachea, right atrium, and aorta (Lee & Moinzadeh, 2009). Heart–lung transplant typically involves transplantation of both lungs, not the heart with a single lung (UNOS, 2009). The autonomic nervous system provides no input because both the heart and lungs are denervated, so treatment needs to be modified accordingly. Survival rate at 1 year is 66%; at 5 years, it is 38%.

Retransplantation

When a primary graft fails, retransplantation may be the only recourse to ensure patient survival. However, retransplantation patients are at a higher risk of morbidity and mortality. In addition, retransplantation is controversial because of the scarcity of donor organs and the many people waiting for a primary transplantation. Table 14.6 lists survival rates for primary transplant and retransplantation procedures. Retransplantation is often contraindicated for patients with a history of noncompliance.

Hematopoietic Cell Transplantation

Hematopoietic cell transplantation refers to bone marrow and peripheral blood stem cell transplantation. The purpose of hematopoietic cell transplantation is to return the patient's hematologic and immune function to normal (Lee & Moinzadeh, 2009). Stem cells located in marrow develop into the three types of blood cells (red blood cells, white blood cells, and platelets) through differentiation. When blood cells are fully developed and functional, they are released into the bloodstream. Although stem cells reside in bone marrow, a small percentage circulate in the bloodstream.

In *bone marrow transplantation*, stem cells are aspirated from donor marrow; in *peripheral blood stem cell transplantation*, patients are given growth factor to stimulate the release of large amounts of stem cells from the marrow into the bloodstream, where they are then collected through a process called *hemapheresis*. Before donated stem cells are transplanted, the recipient's diseased bone marrow is destroyed through high-dose chemotherapy, radiation, or both (Stewart, 2000). The donor stem cells are then infused into the recipient, where they eventually engraft, producing normal healthy cells.

The four types of hematopoietic cell transplantation procedures (Leukemia & Lymphoma Society [LLS], 2005; Wells & Goodman, 2009) are

- *Allogeneic,* in which the donor has a closely matched HLA, as in a sibling;
- *Syngeneic,* in which the donor is an identical twin;
- *Autologous,* in which the patient's own stem cells are harvested and then reinfused; and
- *Cord blood stem cells,* in which placental or umbilical cord blood—a rich source of blood-forming stem cells—is drained from the afterbirth and frozen for later use (LLS, 2009).

Seventy percent of patients need to look outside their families for a match (National Marrow Donor Program, 2008), because the probability of a sibling being a match is only 1 in 4 (LLS, 2005). The National Marrow Donor Program has a registry of HLA typing information to match patients with unrelated donors. According to the National Marrow Donor Program (2008) listing, more than 7 million potential donors have been listed, 90,000 cord blood units have been donated by parents after their baby's birth, and more than 33,000 transplants have occurred since inception of the registry.

Criteria

Patients generally are younger than age 50, with cancer, a bone marrow failure syndrome, or genetic disease (Wells & Goodman, 2009). Age is a factor because older adults are at greater risk for developing GVHD, have less tolerance for pretreatment conditioning (e.g., chemotherapy, radiation therapy), and are more likely to have comorbidities than younger patients (LLS, 2005).

Bone marrow injury may be a result of primary marrow failure, destruction of marrow from disease, or exposure to chemicals or radiation (LLS, 2005). Stem cell transplantation is indicated for patients with immune-deficiency

Table 14.6. **Survival Rate Percentages for Primary Transplant and Retransplantation Surgeries, 1997–2004**

Organ	1 Year	3 Year	5 Year
Heart			
Primary	87.1	78.5	71.5
Retransplantation	81.6	66.4	57.5
Lung			
Primary	83.1	62.2	46.3
Retransplantation	65.1	38.3	27.6
Heart–lung			
Primary	66	48	38.6
Retransplantation		1 person	
Kidney			
Primary	91.9	82.4	71.9
Retransplantation	89.2	78.0	66.7
Pancreas			
Primary	78.4	65.5	53.4
Retransplantation	70.6	60.4	45.2
Kidney–pancreas			
Primary	91.8	84.2	76.2
Retransplantation	85.2	64.1	59.4
Liver			
Primary	83.4	73.7	67.4
Retransplantation	67	55.5	46.2
Intestines			
Primary	77.9	53.7	39.7
Retransplantation	64.1	31	39.7

Source. United Network for Organ Sharing (2009). Reprinted with permission.

diseases, inherited severe blood cell diseases (e.g., thalassemia, sickle cell disease), and aplastic anemia (LLS, 2005). However, the most common diseases treated with stem cell transplantation are non-Hodgkin lymphoma, multiple myeloma, and acute and chronic myelogenous leukemia (Wells & Goodman, 2009).

Procedure

Before transplantation, the patient undergoes conditioning or pretreatment with high-dose chemotherapy, radiation therapy, or both to destroy all cancerous cells, achieving a state of immunosuppression (LLS, 2005; Wells & Goodman, 2009).

Chemotherapy or radiation prior to transplant helps in these ways: it decreases the risk that the recipient's immune cells will reject the transplanted stem cells and it rids the recipient of the disordered lymphocytes that are often the cause of the condition (e.g., an attack by the patient's own lymphocytes on developing blood cells). (LLS, 2005, p. 9)

Some patients with leukemia, lymphoma, and myeloma may be treated with total body irradiation (Stewart, 2000).

In allogeneic bone marrow transplantation, bone marrow is aspirated from the donor's iliac crest or sternum. It takes 4–6 weeks for donor marrow to be completely replaced (LLS, 2005). With peripheral blood stem cell transplantation, growth factor stimulates the release of large amounts of stem cells into the bloodstream, where they are collected. With hemapheresis, blood is separated into its various components. White blood cells and platelets are harvested because they contain the stem cells, and the red blood cells and plasma are returned to the donor. It may take more than one session to collect enough stem cells for transplantation (LLS, 2005).

Once stem cells are collected from either marrow or the peripheral blood system, they are infused through an IV line in the recipient's chest. This process can take several hours. However, it takes several weeks for engraftment (production of new blood cells) to occur and 1–2 years for the immune system to normalize. Patients are not discharged from the hospital until their bodies can produce a sufficient amount of blood cells (Stewart, 2000; see Figure 14.7).

In autologous transplantation, stem cells are removed from blood rather than marrow and undergo a process of *leukapheresis,* in which the white blood cells are removed (Stewart, 2000; Wells & Goodman, 2009). The harvested stem cells are cryopreserved (frozen) until needed for reinfusion (Stewart, 2000). After the patient has undergone high-dose chemotherapy or radiation to destroy his or her diseased cells, the collected stem cells are injected back into the patient. The patient must have an adequate number of healthy stem cells for this procedure

to be successful. It can be more than 6 months before the transplant recipient is well enough to resume normal routines, roles, and occupations (Stewart, 2000).

Complications

GVHD occurs when the donor organ forms antibodies that attack the recipient's tissues because it recognizes the host as a foreign body. Host versus graft disease may also occur if the recipient's body rejects the donor stem cells as foreign. However, GVHD does not occur with autologous or syngeneic donors because HLA matching is not an issue. GVHD may be minimized through stem cell T lymphocyte depletion (LLS, 2005), and it is often treated with steroids, which have their own side effects with chronic use including myopathy, weakness, and osteopenia.

Effects of chronic GVHD may include other organ systems (Packel, 2006):

- *Skin:* Rash (in acute GVHD) and fibrosis;
- *Liver:* Right upper-quadrant pain, hepatic dysfunction, elevated liver function tests, encephalopathy, and jaundice; and
- *Gastrointestinal system:* Malabsorption, nutritional deficiency, vomiting, diarrhea, and loss of lean body mass.

Additional complications may occur from the chemotherapy and radiation therapies used to prepare the patient for hematopoietic cell transplantation. These conditioning pretreatment complications (LLS, 2005; Stewart, 2000) can include

- *Skin:* Rashes and hyperpigmentation;
- *Hair:* Alopecia (hair loss);
- *Mouth:* Oral mucositis (mouth sores), which interfere with eating and maintaining proper nutrition;
- *Eyes:* Cataracts;
- *Gastrointestinal system:* Nausea, vomiting, diarrhea, and abdominal cramps;
- *Bladder:* Hemorrhagic cystitis (bloody or painful urination);
- *Lungs:* Interstitial pneumonitis (noninfectious pneumonia), congestion, and shortness of breath;

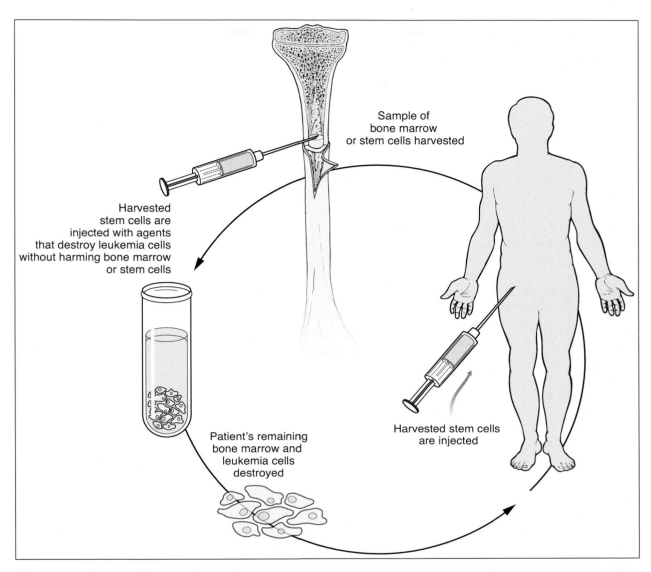

Figure 14.7. Stem cell transplantation.
Source. Richard Fritzler, Medical Illustrator, Roswell, GA.

- *Liver:* Jaundice, ascites, mental status changes, lethargy, abnormal liver enzymes, and veno–occlusive disease (blood vessels of the liver become obstructed);

- *Heart:* Congestive heart failure and temporary arrhythmia;

- *Muscle cramping and spasms:* Associated with electrolyte imbalances;

- *Thyroid:* Decreased thyroid function necessitating oral thyroid hormones; and

- *Reproductive organs:* Premature menopause or male sterility.

For the first few weeks after hematopoietic cell transplantation, patients are at a severe risk of infection until engraftment occurs. Patients may remain immunocompromised for 6 months to 1 year after the transplant (Stewart, 2000). When working with hematopoietic transplantation patients, occupational therapists are advised to monitor vitals, check blood counts, minimize risk of infection, note any GVHD symptoms, and consult with the physician about exercise and activity parameters. Good hand hygiene is essential in preventing infection. In addition to gloves, therapists may need to wear a mask when working with patients and ensure that patients wear a face mask when leaving their room.

Psychological Impact of Transplantation

It is important that transplant candidates undergo psychological screening before transplantation because it can have a profound effect on transplant success. The evaluation focuses on coping strategies, social and family support, and pretransplant psychiatric history (Dew et al., 1996). Transplant recipients need good coping skills and a good support system. It may seem obvious that family support is important for successful transplantation; however, the whole transplantation process can be stressful not just for the patient but also for family members. In addition, transplantation involves changing roles from sickness to wellness and changes in life expectancy that can affect patient and family dynamics (Malone & Lindsay, 2006).

Graft success is also dependent on patients' compliance with their posttransplant regimen. Noncompliance is a major risk factor for organ rejection, quality of life, and ultimately survival (Bunzel & Laederach-Hofmann, 2000; Butler, Roderick, Muller, Mason, & Peveler, 2004; Mehra et al., 2006). "The odds of graft loss are increased seven-fold in nonadherent patients compared with adherent patients" (Butler et al., 2004, p. 775). The posttransplant regimen includes taking prescribed medications; lifestyle changes, including diet and exercise; avoiding substance abuse; and keeping all follow-up appointments, including labs and biopsies to monitor for rejection. People with substance abuse, mental retardation, dementia, severe personality disorder, and emotional instability have an increased risk of noncompliance (Bunzel & Laederach-Hofmann, 2000; Mehra et al., 2006). Conversely, patients may stop taking their posttransplant medication over time because they feel so good after the transplant. Unfortunately, nonadherence to medication protocols increases the risk of rejection.

In addition, the transplant process can be emotionally laden. Transplant recipients may feel guilty knowing they benefited from someone else's death. Transplant recipients may even undergo a type of posttraumatic stress disorder related to their transplant experience and confront issues of their mortality because they suffered from an end-stage organ disease (Dew et al., 1996). Those on the waiting list also experience a great deal of anxiety and uncertainty, not knowing whether they will survive until a matched donor is located. Anxiety disorders are the most commonly reported psychiatric disorder associated with long-term transplantation (Dew et al., 1996). Some immunosuppression medications are also associated with psychiatric disturbances and mental status changes. In addition, stem cell transplant patients must cope with a prolonged hospital stay, uncomfortable side effects, and social isolation until engraftment occurs (LLS, 2005).

The ongoing financial commitment is another stress factor. Insurance coverage does not cover the total expense, and patients and their families often have to fund raise to secure enough money for transplantation. In addition to the surgery, the patient's posttransplant care, including lifelong medication, is very costly. Associated transplantation costs include hospital charges, physician fees, medical supplies, medications, and outpatient visits, including biopsies and other tests. Table 14.7 lists the National Foundation of Transplant's estimated cost of transplant procedures by organ.

Future Trends

Advancements in areas of research and in transplantation are continuous. Some of these areas include xenotransplantation (cross-species transplantation), artificial organ technology, embryonic stem cell transplantation (because stem cells can develop into any type of cell, replacing damaged tissue anywhere in the body), cloning, and domino transplants. Additional areas include new immunosuppression approaches, including long-term tolerance, and induced chimerism through infusion of donor marrow during transplantation. Hand and face transplantation have also shown recent success.

Table 14.7. National Foundation of Transplant Estimated Cost of Transplant Procedures, by Organ or Organs

Procedure	Cost ($)
Bone marrow	250,000
Heart	300,000
Heart–lung	300,000–350,000
Isolated small bowel	350,000
Kidney	75,000–100,000
Kidney–pancreas	150,000
Liver	250,000
Lung	200,000–250,000
Pancreas	100,000

Note. Costs may vary by transplantation center and with development of complications.
Source. Petechuk (2006).

However, these topics and ethical issues related to transplantation procurement, allocation, use of embryonic stem cells, and retransplantation are beyond the scope of this chapter.

Implications for Occupational Therapy

Goals for occupational therapy both before and after transplantation are similar. Therapy focuses on strength training, increasing endurance, and return to engagement in valued occupations. Pretransplant patients may be deconditioned and have poor activity tolerance, muscle wasting, dyspnea, or poor nutritional status because of their end-stage organ disease. Because any individual patient's time on the waiting list is unknown, every effort should be made to keep patients as strong and as healthy as possible for their upcoming surgery. Patients should be encouraged to continue with regular occupations within their tolerance with an emphasis on both physical and mental health and wellness.

Posttransplant interventions may also need to be modified because patients remain deconditioned as a result of their end-stage organ disease before transplantation. Patients often have incisional pain in the acute phase, which may further restrict ability to participate in desired occupations. In addition, transplant patients commonly develop hypertension, diabetes, and osteoporosis, and interventions need to be modified accordingly. Patients may also continue to experience stress and uncertainty and require encouragement and emotional support. During periods of rejection or active infection, treatment should be modified secondary to increased metabolic demands; adaptations include decreasing intensity, frequency, and duration of exercise.

Therapists should be aware of several precautions when working with transplant patients, which may include awareness of patient lines, tubes, and drains and observance of standard precautions for infection control. Therapists are advised to observe good hand hygiene, clean all equipment before bringing it into patients' rooms, and wearing a face mask if sick. Patient vital signs should also be routinely monitored as a barometer of patient tolerance for therapy.

Education for patients returning to home (and work) should focus on

- Minimizing risk of infection;
  - Avoiding crowds (e.g., shopping centers and malls, religious services, parties, entertainment venues);
  - Avoiding people with colds, flu, or other respiratory infections;
  - Avoiding children who have recently been immunized with live vaccine;
  - Keeping up to date on immunizations but with inactive organisms;
  - Performing good hand hygiene;
  - Performing good oral hygiene;
  - Bathing or showering frequently to remove bacteria from skin;
  - Cleaning cuts and scrapes with antibacterial soap;
  - Properly washing all fruits and vegetables;
  - Avoiding foods with raw meat and raw eggs;
  - Avoiding exposure to mold;
  - Washing hands after handling pets; and
  - Possibly taking antibiotics before any dental procedures; and
  - Avoiding gardening and wearing a face mask when outside in areas of high air pollution (lung transplant patients).
- Using energy conservation strategies (refer to Appendix D);
- Managing stress;
- Understanding the importance of exercise, diet, nutrition, weight control, and other lifestyle issues;
- Stretching, warming up, and cooling down for any activity;
- Avoiding contact sports, driving a car, or lifting until cleared by physician;
- Protecting skin from sunburn; transplant patients may burn more easily; and
- Self-monitoring.
  - Rate of perceived exertion (refer to Chapter 3);

- Blood pressure (many transplant recipients develop high blood pressure from the medications they must take); and
- Blood glucose levels and signs of diabetes (transplant medications may cause development of diabetes; LLS, 2005; Stewart, 2000).

Transplantation is not a cure but a treatment option for end-stage organ disease. However, the scarcity of donor organs continues to limit the number of transplant procedures performed annually. Occupational therapists working in acute care settings (especially hospitals designated as transplant centers) will increasingly work with patients with transplantation as their primary or secondary condition. With an increased understanding of body structures and their functions and the transplant process and its sequelae, therapists will have a more holistic understanding of and approach to working with this population.

References

Ahmad, J., Bryce, C. L., Cacciarelli, T., & Roberts, M. S. (2007). Differences in access to liver transplantation: Disease severity, waiting time, and transplantation center volume. *Annals of Internal Medicine, 146,* 707–713.

American Association of Cardiovascular and Pulmonary Rehabilitation. (1998). Pulmonary rehabilitation for patients with special conditions. In *Guidelines for pulmonary rehabilitation programs* (2nd ed., pp. 105–107).Champaign, IL: Human Kinetics.

Barter, J. (2006). *Organ transplants.* Detroit: Thomson Gale.

Bishay, R. (2006). Cardiac allograft vasculopathy: The silent, long-suffering enemy. *Hypothesis, 4*(1), 19–27.

Bunzel, B., & Laederach-Hofmann, K. (2000). Solid organ transplantation: Are there predictors for posttransplant noncompliance? A literature review. *Transplantation, 70,* 711–716.

Butler, J. A., Roderick, P., Muller, M., Mason, J. C., & Peveler, R. C. (2004). Frequency and impact of nonadherence to immunosuppressants after renal transplantation: A systematic review. *Transplantation, 77,* 769–789.

D'Amico, C. L. (2005). Cardiac transplantation: Patient selection in the current era. *Journal of Cardiovascular Nursing, 55,* S4–S13.

Dew, M. A., Roth, L., Schulberg, H. C., Simmons, R. G., Kormos, R. L., Trzepacz, P. T., et al. (1996). Prevalence and predictors of depression and anxiety-related disorders during the year after heart transplantation. *General Hospital Psychiatry, 18,* 48S–61S.

Ebell, M. H. (2006). Point of care guides: Predicting prognosis in patients with end-stage liver disease. *American Family Physician, 74,* 1762–1763.

Freundenberger, R., Hoffman, J., Gottlieb, S., Robinson, S., & Fisher, M. (2000). Characteristics of patients referred for cardiac transplantation: Implications for the donor organ shortage. *American Heart Journal, 140,* 857–860.

Johnson, L. B., Jha, R. C., & Lu, A. D. (2004). Adult living-donor liver transplantation. In P. C. Kuo, R. D. Davis, D. C. Dafoe, & R. R. Bollinger (Eds.), *Comprehensive atlas of transplantation* (p. 115). Baltimore: Lippincott Williams & Wilkins.

Kanter, K. R. (1990). Heterotopic heart transplantation. *Emory University Journal of Medicine, 4,* 77–85.

Kanter, K. R., Vega, J. D., & Smith, A. L. (1998). Heart transplantation—Current perspectives. *Journal of the Medical Association of Georgia, 87,* 141–144.

Lee, J., & Moinzadeh, L. (2009). Organ transplantation. In J. C. Paz & M. P. West (Eds.), *Acute care handbook for physical therapists* (3rd ed., pp. 401–425). St. Louis, MO: W. B. Saunders.

Leukemia & Lymphoma Society. (2005). *Blood and marrow stem cell transplantation.* Retrieved March 22, 2009, from www.leukemialymphoma.org/attachments/National/br_1203086953.pdf

Malone, D. J., & Lindsay, K. L. B. (2006). Transplantation. In D. J. Malone & K. L. B. Lindsay (Eds.), *Physical therapy in acute care: A clinician's guide* (pp. 545–575). Thorofare, NJ: Slack.

McClellan, M. (2003). *Organ and tissue transplants: Medical miracles and challenges.* Berkeley Heights, NJ: Enslow.

Mehra, M. R., Kobashigawa, J., Starling, R., Russell, S., Uber, P. A., Parameshwar, J., et al. (2006). Listing criteria for heart transplantation: International Society for Heart and Lung Transplantation guidelines for the care of cardiac transplant candidates—2006. *Journal of Heart Lung Transplantation, 25,* 1024–1042.

National Diabetes Information Clearinghouse. (2007). *Pancreatic islet transplantation.* Retrieved September, 2010 from http://diabetes.niddk.nih.gov/dm/pubs/pancreatic islet/

National Heart, Lung, and Blood Institute. (2008). *What is a lung transplant?* Retrieved January 14, 2009, from www.nhlbi.nih.gov/health/dci/Diseases/lungtxp/lungtxp_whatis.html

National Marrow Donor Program. (2008). *National Marrow Donor Program: Connecting patients with donors.* Retrieved March 3, 2009, from www.marrow.org/index.html

National Organ Transplant Act of 1984, Pub. L. 98–507, 98 Stat. 2339.

Organ Procurement and Transplantation Network. (n.d.). *Policy management: National Organ Transplant Act.* Retrieved September 13, 2010, from http://optn.transplant.hrsa.gov/policiesAndBylaws/nota.asp

Packel, L. (2006). Oncological diseases and disorders. In D. J. Malone & K. L. B. Lindsay (Eds.), *Physical therapy in acute care: A clinician's guide* (pp. 503–544). Thorofare, NJ: Slack.

Petechuk, D. (2006). *Organ transplantation.* Westport, CT: Greenwood Press.

Robertson, R. P., Davis, C., Larsen, J., Stratta, R., & Sutherland, D. E. R. (2000). Pancreas and islet transplantation for patients with diabetes. *Diabetes Care, 23,* 112–116.

Ryan, E. A., Paty, B. W., Senior, P. A., Bigam, D., Alfadhli, E., Kneteman, N. M., et al. (2005). Five-year follow-up after clinical islet transplantation. *Diabetes, 54,* 2060–2069.

Scientific Registry of Transplant Recipients. (2009). *Scientific registry of transplant recipients.* Retrieved February 14, 2009, from www.ustransplant.org/

Shapiro, A. M. J., Lakey, J. R. T., Ryan, E. A., Korbutt, G. S., Toth, E., Warnock, G. L., et al. (2000). Islet transplantation in seven patients with Type 1 diabetes mellitus using a glucocorticoid-free immunosuppressive regimen. *New England Journal of Medicine, 343,* 230–238.

Shapiro, A. M. J., & Ricordi, C. (2004). Unraveling the secrets of single donor success in islet transplantation. *American Journal of Transplantation, 4,* 295–298.

Shapiro, A. M. J., Ricordi, C., Hering, B. J., Auchincloss, H., Lindblad, R., Robertson, R. P., et al. (2006). International trial of the Edmonton Protocol for islet transplantation. *New England Journal of Medicine, 355,* 1318–1330.

Steinman, T., Becker, B. N., Frost, A. E., Olthoff, K. M., Smart, F. W., Suki, W. N., et al. (2001). Guidelines for the referral and management of patients eligible for solid organ transplantation. *Transplantation, 71,* 1189–1204.

Stewart, S., Winters, G. L., Fishbein, M. C., Tazelaar, H. D., Kobashigawa, J., Abrams, J., et al. (2005). Revision of the 1990 Working Formulation for the Standardized of Nomenclature in the Diagnosis of Heart Rejection. *Journal of Heart and Lung Transplantation, 24,* 1710–1720.

Stewart, S. K. (2000). *Autologous stem cell transplants: A handbook for patients.* Highland Park, IL: Blood and Marrow Transplant Information Network.

Taylor, D. O., Edwards, L. B., Boucek, M. M., Trulock, E. P., Aurora, P., Christie, J., et al. (2007). Registry of the International Society for Heart and Lung Transplantation: Twenty-Fourth Official Adult Heart Transplant Report—2007. *Journal of Heart Lung Transplantation, 26,* 769–781.

Uniform Determination of Death Act. (1980). Retrieved April 30, 2009, from www.law.upenn.edu/bll/archives/ule/fnact99/1980s/udda80.htm

United Network for Organ Sharing. (2005). *Lung allocation score system update.* Retrieved September 13, 2010, from http://www.unos.org/docs/DataSlides _Fall_2005.pdf

United Network for Organ Sharing. (2009). *United Network for Organ Sharing.* Retrieved January 15, 2009, from www.unos.org/

Wells, C. L., & Goodman, C. C. (2009). Transplantation. In C. C. Goodman & K. S. Fuller (Eds.), *Pathology: Implications for the physical therapist* (3rd ed., pp. 1037–1097). St. Louis, MO: W. B. Saunders.

Appendix 14.A.

Transplant Organizations and Additional Resources

- **American Society of Multicultural Health and Transplant Professions:** www.asmhtp.org/
- **American Society of Transplant Surgeons:** www.asts.org
- **Association of Organ Procurement Organizations:** www.aopo.org
- **Donate Life America:** www.shareyourlife.org
- **International Islet Transplantation Registry:** www.med.uni-giessen.de/itr/
- **International Society for Heart and Lung Transplantation:** www.ishlt.org/
- **National Donor Family Council:** www.kidney.org/transplantation/ donorfamilies/ index.cfm

- **National Marrow Donor Program:** www.marrow.org/
- **National Transplant Assistance Fund and Catastrophic Injury Program:** www.ntafund.org
- **Organ Procurement and Transplantation Network:** www.optn.org
- **Scientific Registry of Transplant Recipients:** www.ustransplant.org
- **Transplant Olympics:** http://www.kidney.org/transplantation/athletics/index.cfm
- **Transplant Week:** www.transplantweek.org
- **United Network for Organ Sharing:** www.unos.org

Appendix 14.B.

U.S. UNOS Membership Regions

Region	States
1	Connecticut, Maine, Massachusetts, New Hampshire, Rhode Island, eastern Vermont
2	Delaware, District of Columbia, Maryland, New Jersey, Pennsylvania, West Virginia, Northern Virginia
3	Alabama, Arkansas, Florida, Georgia, Louisiana, Mississippi, Puerto Rico
4	Oklahoma, Texas
5	Arizona, California, Nevada, New Mexico, Utah
6	Alaska, Hawaii, Idaho, Montana, Oregon, Washington
7	Illinois, Minnesota, North Dakota, South Dakota, Wisconsin
8	Colorado, Iowa, Kansas, Missouri, Nebraska, Wyoming
9	New York, western Vermont
10	Indiana, Michigan, Ohio
11	Kentucky, North Carolina, South Carolina, Tennessee, Virginia

Source. United Network for Organ Sharing (2009).

15

Burns

Marcy D. Bearden, MS, OTR

Each year, the 125 specialized burn units in the United States report more burn injuries. According to the National Burn Repository, 181,836 burns were treated in medical facilities between 1998 and 2007 (Miller et al., 2008). A burn injury can have a devastating effect on a person's daily functioning, lifestyle preferences, and psychological health. Burns, along with other injuries to the skin, can lead to severe scarring and contractures, which can result in decreased range of motion (ROM) and strength of affected joints. The earlier a burn injury is treated and the proper protocols initiated, the better the outcomes and the lower the risk of functional deficits.

Many factors affect the survival, healing, and outcomes of a burn injury; these factors may include age, depth of burn, mechanism of burn, treatment options, comorbidities, infection, and medical complications. As reported in the 2007 National Burn Repository, mortality rates range from 0.7% in burns that cover less than 10% of the body to 81.2% in burns that cover 90% or more of the body. The average mortality rate reported among burn centers is 4.4% (Miller et al., 2008).

Because of the skin's complexity, the healing process, and the multitude of factors affecting recovery, it is imperative that burn victims be evaluated by occupational and physical therapists within the first 24 hours after injury. Early positioning and splinting of affected body areas can minimize or prevent edema, provide a functional position, and reduce the risk of contracture. In many burn centers, physical and occupational therapists have merged their roles to encompass more comprehensive treatment and are referred to nonspecifically as *burn therapists*. This chapter focuses mainly on the contributions of occupational therapists as members of the burn team.

Burn Centers and Burn Teams

Hospitals with designated burn centers are the best places for burns to be treated. The American Burn Association criteria for a burn center referral include burns of the hands, feet, face, genitalia, perineum, or major joints. The criteria also include partial-thickness burns covering more than 10% of total body surface area, preexisting conditions that may complicate recovery, and traumatic injury in which burn injury poses a greater risk than the trauma injury (Holmes, 2008).

Many people in a burn center are involved in the patient's successful recovery from a burn injury. These people make up the burn team, and each has an important function. A burn team may consist of a burn or plastic surgeon; nurses; burn therapists (physical therapist, occupational therapist, or both); a nutritionist; a pharmacist; a case manager; and, in some cases, an aesthetician. All members work together to provide the patient with the most comprehensive care and strive to obtain the best aesthetic and functional results as possible.

Skin Composition and Burn Characteristics

Skin is the largest organ in the body and part of the integumentary system, which encompasses skin, hair, nails, and glands. Three distinct layers make up the skin: the epidermis, dermis, and subcutaneous tissue, or hypodermis (see Figure 15.1). The *epidermis* is the outermost layer of skin and is made up of five sublayers that work together to continually rebuild the skin's surface. The epidermis contains *melanocytes* (cells that produce the melanin that gives skin its pigmentation), the *Langerhans cells* (cells involved in the immune system), *Merkel cells* (tactile cells), and *sensory nerves*. In adults, the epidermis is shed and replaced by new cells every 4–6 weeks (Reddy, 2008).

535

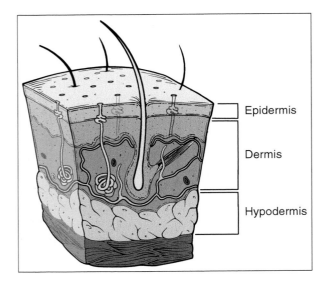

Figure 15.1. Layers of the skin.
Source. Richard Fritzler, Medical Illustrator, Roswell, GA.

The *dermis* consists of living cells and houses blood capillaries, hair follicles, glands, nerve endings, and receptors. The three types of tissue found throughout the dermal layer are *collagen, elastic tissue,* and *reticular fibers.*

The *subcutaneous tissue* or *hypodermis* is a layer of fat that contains larger blood vessels and nerve endings. The primary functions of the hypodermis are to help regulate body temperature and protect the internal organs from external impact (Kita, 2009). The function of the skin disrupted when a burn injury occurs depends on the depth of the burn (Kao & Garner, 1999).

Burns are characterized by their thickness or depth: *superficial, partial,* or *full thickness.* Table 15.1 describes the general characteristics and healing times for the different depths of burn injuries. Depending on the mechanism of injury, a burn wound typically varies in depth. These depths are identified as three zones:

- *Zone of coagulation:* Generally found at the center of the burn and characterized as the portion of the burn with maximum damage. Tissue in this zone has incurred permanent damage.

- *Zone of stasis:* Surrounds the zone of coagulation and is defined by tissue with decreased profusion. The zone of stasis can convert to the zone of coagulation, but the tissue can potentially be salvaged depending on treatment. Occlusive dressings, splints, edema, and inadequate fluid resuscitation can lead to the conversion of the zone of stasis and further tissue loss.

- *Zone of hyperemia:* The outermost area of the burn injury, characterized by increased tissue profusion and viable tissue.

Table 15.1. **Types of Burn Injuries**

Thickness	Layer of Skin Affected	Characteristics	Healing Time and Method
Superficial	Epidermis	Red, painful, intact skin	Heals spontaneously in 1–3 days
Partial thickness	Epidermis, parts of the dermis	Red, wet, edematous, painful, blisters	Reepithelialize in 7–21 days
Full thickness	Epidermis; dermis; hypodermis; and, in very severe cases, the muscle and bone	White or gray, leathery, insensate, contracted	5–14 days via skin grafting

Source. Kao and Garner (1999).

The tissue in this zone will recover unless complications such as sepsis occur (Hettiarachy & Dziewulski, 2004).

Types of Burns

Burns can result from a variety of different sources or exposures. This section discusses thermal, electrical, and chemical burns as well as frostbite, along with the associated treatment options.

Thermal Burns

Thermal burns are burns caused by flame, scald, or contact with a hot surface. Thermal burns can vary in depth on the basis of the length of exposure to the heat source and the heat source itself. The mechanism of injury and the depth of burn will determine treatment options. Scald wounds account for 30% of burns reported in the 2007 American Burn Repository (Miller et al., 2008) and are most common in children and older adults. The most common mechanisms of a scald are spilling a hot drink and hot bath water. A scald burn typically results in superficial and partial-thickness burns. Flame burns account for 40% of burns (Miller et al., 2008) and are usually partial and full thickness in nature. Contact burns (4%) result from coming in contact with a hot surface for a prolonged period of time or brief exposure to an extremely hot liquid. These burns are partial to full thickness in nature (Hettiarachy & Dziewulski, 2004).

Typically, flame and scald burns are thought to be "dirty wounds" because debris from the fire or hot liquid can contaminate the wound if the wound is open (full-thickness burns or partial-thickness burns with disrupted blisters). A clean wound results from contact burns that are no more than partial thickness in depth with intact blisters. If the skin barrier is broken, the body is susceptible to infection, and those wounds must be thoroughly cleaned as a first step in treatment. The mechanism of injury and whether the wound is clean or not can greatly influence treatment options. For instance, it typically is not acceptable to put an occlusive dressing on a wound that is not clean and free of debris and bacteria.

Electrical Burns

Electrical burns require special consideration because the electrical current enters the body at one site (the entrance wound) and then exits the body at another site (exit wound), creating two visible wounds. As the electrical current travels through the body, viable tissue and organs between the entrance and exit wounds are damaged, making it difficult to discern the extent of the burn injury. Patients with electrical injuries should receive cardiac monitoring until the physician determines that the cardiac tissue has not been damaged (Hettiarachy & Dziewulski, 2004). The etiology of an electrical injury can be high voltage, low voltage, or lightning.

According to Kidd et al. (2007), patients with electrical burns require early surgical releases and debridement to prevent further tissue damage. Surgical procedures include fasciotomies, nerve decompression, escharotomies, abdominal exploration, amputation, excision, and grafting. Early reconstruction has also been deemed beneficial to long-term outcome (Kidd et al., 2007).

Chemical Burns

Chemical burns occur most frequently in industrial settings, but they can occur from the misuse of typical household cleaners. Burns that occur from a chemical agent tend to be very deep because the burn continues to progress until all of the corrosive material is removed. It is important to keep in mind that some chemical agents need to be neutralized once in contact with the skin. A burn unit will have the appropriate first aid materials to properly treat a chemical injury and provide the best outcome for the patient (Hettiarachy & Dziewulski, 2004).

Frostbite

Although not a burn, severe *frostbite* injuries are best treated in burn centers and wound care centers. Frostbite is similar to burns in that they both involve the skin and underlying structures. Frostbite generally affects the extremities, and the severity of the frostbite depends on the temperature and the length of exposure to the cold.

Murphy, Banwell, Roberts, and McGrouther (2000) described three phases of a frostbite injury: prethaw field care, immediate hospital rewarming phase, and postthaw care phase. The only objective in the *prethaw phase* is to protect the affected area. The injured tissue should be padded and splinted in transport to a hospital. The area of frostbite should not be intentionally rewarmed until definitive rewarming can occur. The *rewarming phase* should be completed in a hospital setting and is carried out in a warm water bath of 40° C –42° C (104° F to 107.6° F) for 15–30 minutes or until thawing is completed (Arford, 2008; Murphy et al., 2000). The *postthaw phase* is devoted to minimizing the inflammatory process and preventing further tissue damage.

Most physicians wait until after the rewarming phase to assess the depth of the frostbite and the extent of injury. Historically, frostbite has been classified into four degrees.

- *First-degree frostbite* is classified as decreased sensation, edema, and redness surrounding the tissue. First-degree frostbite does not involve blistering.

- *Second-degree frostbite* is differentiated from first-degree frostbite by the presence of clear blisters. Skin remains reddened and edematous.

- *Third-degree frostbite* is characterized by the presence of hemorrhagic blisters indicating damage to the dermal layer of skin or deeper.

- *Fourth-degree frostbite* is a full-thickness wound that can involve bone, muscle, and tendon (Arford, 2008).

More recently, frostbite has been classified into superficial and deep categories. *Superficial frostbite* is tissue damage limited to the skin and underlying subcutaneous tissue. *Deep frostbite* is tissue damage extending beyond the skin and subcutaneous tissue and involving the muscle, tendon, and bone (Arford, 2008).

Injured tissues may not die immediately; therefore, it may take several days to months to determine the extent of injury. Many surgeons will allow frostbite to declare itself (the wound or injury is not progressing and all of the damaged tissue has been "declared") before taking the patient to the operating room for excision of the damaged tissue, which can take up to 3 months. Treatment in the meantime consists of daily dressing changes, hydrotherapy, and therapy to maintain range of motion (ROM). In severe cases, fingers and toes are allowed to self-demarcate or self-amputate, allowing for the retention of the greatest amount of viable tissue.

Medical Management of Acute Burns

The burn patient's medical condition will greatly direct the involvement of occupational therapy and the timing of treatment. Three distinct phases guide the treatment and care of burns: the emergent phase, the acute phase, and rehabilitation phase. The first 72 hours after a burn injury are referred to as the *emergent phase*. The *acute phase* begins after the first 72 hours and is the phase in which wound healing and closure occur. After wounds are healed, the *rehabilitation stage* begins (Serghiou, Holmes, & McCauley, 2004).

When a patient arrives at a burn center, one of the first things done is the calculation of the total body surface area (TBSA) burned using the rule of nines. The body is divided into regions, and each region is then described as a multiple of nine, which is then referred to as a percentage. The regions include the head, arms, legs, and torso. The head is 9%; each arm is 9%; each leg is 18%; and the torso is 36%. Superficial burns are not calculated as part of the TBSA burned (Kao & Garner, 1999).

The calculation of the TBSA burned percentage allows physicians to calculate the patient's fluid resuscitation and nutritional needs. Fluid resuscitation is calculated using the Parkland formula and serves as a guide for the physician to maintain hemodynamic stability in the first 24 hours after injury. The percentage of TBSA burned also allows for estimations of timing for hydrotherapy, dressing changes, and surgical treatments.

In very large burns, or burns with *circumferential eschar* (thick, inflexible burned tissue seen in full-thickness burns), of the extremities or trunk, patients are at risk of developing compartment syndromes because of generalized systemic edema. The eschar is unable to accommodate large amounts of swelling or edema, which results in decreased perfusion to underlying tissues. To prevent further tissue death, burn surgeons will typically perform echarotomies and, in extreme cases, fasciotomies to relieve the pressure of the increased edema on the underlying tissues.

Depending on the mechanism of injury, percentage TBSA burned, and affected anatomical areas burned, a patient may or may not be intubated in the field. As described by Kao and Garner (1999), a systemic inflammatory response that results from burn injuries greater than 30% TBSA can lead to intubation for airway protection. This inflammatory response can lead to decreased profusion and oxygenation to tissues and is one reason for intubation even in the absence of an inhalation injury.

If an inhalation injury is suspected, the patient will be intubated for mechanical ventilation. An inhalation injury has three components: carbon monoxide intoxication, upper-airway swelling, and acute respiratory failure (Kao & Garner, 1999). Patients with an inhalation injury will remain intubated until the swelling in the airway has subsided and the patient is able to maintain oxygenation without the assistance of a ventilator. It is important to note that although patients with an inhalation injury are typically very sick, therapy may still be indicated for splinting, positioning, and even passive ROM (PROM).

Nutrition plays a vital role in the healing process of any illness or injury. The caloric requirement for a burn patient can be estimated using the Curreri formula, but many practitioners find this estimate to be inaccurate and prefer to provide the patient with 20% more calories than the resting energy expenditure measurement indicates (Graves, Saffle, & Cochran, 2009; Kao & Garner, 1999). Indirect calorimetry has

been used in recent years to more accurately determine the number of calories burn patients need.

Many burn centers use more than one formula to estimate caloric needs. Of burn centers, 75% have reported having specific criteria for the use of nutritional protocols (Graves et al., 2009). Fluid resuscitation is initiated within the first 24 hours after injury, and nutritional needs are calculated. Patients are often given prophylactic antibiotics to prevent or minimize the risk of infection. Many burn centers have designated pharmacists who are responsible for managing and recommending medications and antibiotics appropriate for individual patients. Specifically, a pharmacist can be helpful in determining antibiotic and antimicrobial regimens based on wound culture sensitivities and alerting physicians to different drug interactions and dosages.

One very important aspect of acute burn care is effective pain management. A recent study suggested that pain is greatest during dressing changes and therapeutic procedures and is not adequately controlled with pharmacological agents (Byers, Bridges, Kijek, & LaBorde, 2001). Pain management and medications are important for occupational therapists to understand because in many cases the patient is unable to verbally acknowledge pain, and the therapist is responsible for looking for other subjective and objective signs of pain. Grimacing, changes in heart rate, respirations, blood pressure, and patient resistance should be noted throughout treatment sessions because they can be indicators of increased pain (Connor-Ballard, 2009). For patients who are intubated and sedated, therapists should always be aware of the physiological responses to the treatment and use their professional judgment when asking for patients to receive more pain medication.

An understanding of frequently used medications will help therapists determine the timing of therapeutic procedures. Morphine and fentanyl have both been studied in burn patients. The data have suggested that during wound care oral fentanyl controls pain better than oral morphine. However, no difference in pain was reported with fentanyl or morphine during therapeutic procedures (Robert et al., 2003). Intravenous fentanyl has not been well studied in acute burn patients, but it is used successfully in many burn centers. A study completed by MacPherson, Woods, and Penfold (2008) suggested that the use of ketamine and midazolam delivered through a patient-controlled analgesia machine can be an effective method of pain control during dressing changes and may be effective during other procedures as well. It may be helpful to coordinate therapeutic procedures with pain medication administration, dressing changes, or both in an attempt to make the patient the most comfortable.

The perception of pain has also been reported to be interrelated with the patient's level of anxiety (Conner-Ballard, 2009; Patterson, 1995). A study by Ferguson and Voll (2004) used music relaxation during burn rehabilitation and showed a decrease in anxiety in the group of burn patients who had music compared with the group without music. However, they were not able to show a decrease in pain perception in this study. This area may be interesting and much needed for future research. It may be helpful to try and coordinate therapeutic procedures with pain medication administration, dressing changes, or both in an attempt to make the patient more comfortable.

Management of Burn Wounds

Many times, burns can be treated by a variety of interventions. Numerous different types of dressings and wound coverings are available. Treatment interventions will often be determined by the mechanism of burn, depth, and/or the presence of infection. Typically the appropriate intervention is decided by the treating physician.

Dressings

After the TBSA burned is calculated, the burn is cleansed with tap water and gentle soap, and a dressing is applied. The type of dressing used depends on the depth of the burn and the mechanism of injury. In most cases, an antibiotic or antimicrobial cream is applied to help prevent infections, which is then followed by the application of dry gauze.

Silver-impregnated dressings are frequently used for burn wounds and have a known antimicrobial effect. Dressings containing silver have many manufacturers, and the burn surgeon will decide which particular dressing is appropriate to use. Antibiotic or antimicrobial dressings are commonly used in burn care. Most commonly, bacitracin ointment is used with superficial and partial-thickness burns, and silver sulfadiazine cream is frequently used with full-thickness burns. A large assortment of impregnated gauze dressings are used to promote healing and prevent infections, and dressings used vary from center to center. Some burns can be treated with an enzymatic debridement ointment, such as collagenase. With this method, the ointment is applied to the wound, and the enzymes remove the necrotic tissue from the skin (Salcido, 2000; see Table 15.2).

Hydrotherapy

Hydrotherapy, or whirlpool, is an effective treatment for burn wounds. The jets help to remove necrotic tissue, and the warm water is soothing to the wounds. The warm water and the jets also help to increase circulation, which is known to promote wound healing. Burns are cleansed with a mild soap while the patient is in hydrotherapy. Loosened necrotic tissue that does not completely come free can either be gently scrubbed away with a wash cloth or a sponge or it can be cut away with scissors. After whirlpool, the wounds are gently dried and dressed with the appropriate dressing.

Temporary and Permanent Wound Coverings

Homograft and xenograft are both temporary wound coverings. *Homograft* uses human cadaver skin, and *xenograft* most commonly uses skin taken from a pig. The application of a temporary graft such as homograft or xenograft allows the wound bed to prepare for permanent surgical closure or a permanent

Table 15.2. Types of Dressings and Their Indications

Wound Covering	Description	Indications	Comments
Autograft	Skin taken from one part of the body and transplanted onto another part of the same person's body.	Full-thickness burns	Most acceptable form of wound closure in burn care
Apligraf	Bilayered, constructed from human neonatal foreskin.	Unclear in burn care but has been successfully used to treat skin ulcers	
Cultured epithelial autograft	Keratinocytes and fibroblasts are extracted from a full-thickness skin biopsy and are grown for 15–21 days. The cells are then "reintegrated" on a sheet of collagen.	Extremely large burns in which not enough donor sites are available to provide skin to cover wounds	Low take rate, cells are very fragile; requires increased nursing care and prolonged immobilization; can be used in conjunction with Integra and vacuum-assisted closure
Integra	Bilayer, permanent, dermal replacement layer.	Reconstruction of complex soft tissue wounds after trauma, partial-, and full-thickness burns and vascular or pressure ulcers	Two-step process, can be used with cultured epithelial autograft and vacuum-assisted closure
Alloderm	Acellular dermal matrix made from human cadaver skin.	Used for full-thickness burns as a dermal substitute	

Source. Lineen and Namais (2008).

wound covering. These grafts "take" like an *autograft* (skin taken from one part of a person's body and transplanted to another part of the same person's body) but are rejected by the body in 7–10 days (Kao & Gardner, 1999). However, homograft and xenograft help decrease fluid loss from the wound and help prevent infection. These grafts allow the wound bed the opportunity to repair itself and granulate in preparation for autografting. Xenograft is used in clean superfi-cial and partial-thickness burns, whereas homograft is most commonly used to cover very large burns after excision (Lineen & Namias, 2008).

Biobrane and Transcyte are temporary synthetic dressings that are readily available and used in burn care. *Biobrane* is a bilayer dressing that allows cell growth and migration of epithelial cells across the wound bed. As the wound heals underneath, the Biobrane is sloughed off and should be cut away and discarded. Biobrane is permeable, which allows for burn wound exudates to be released and for the application of topical agents such as antimicrobials. Biobrane is indicated for superficial and partial-thickness burns, but it has also been used as a donor-site dressing (Lineen & Namias, 2008).

Transcyte is a bilayer, synthetic biodressing that is primarily used in deep partial-thickness and excised full-thickness burns for temporary coverage (Lineen & Namias, 2008). Transcyte has also been used in the treatment of partial-thickness burns to allow for healing without autografting, but at this time no solid research has supported this use. Like Biobrane, Transcyte will "take" to the wound bed initially and then begin to peel away as the wound heals underneath.

Permanent wound coverings include autografting, Apligraf, cultured epithelial autografts, Integra, and Alloderm. *Autografting* is the most prevalent technique used in burn wound closure; it is a procedure in which skin is taken from one part of the body (most commonly the thigh) and then surgically secured to cover the open wound. The body recognizes the skin, and the autograft adheres to the underlying wound bed, providing wound closure. The success of an autograft is determined by the amount of graft "take" (healed portions in which the graft has adhered) versus the amount of graft "loss" (portions of the wound in which graft did not adhere). Table 15.2 includes a list of the different types of dressings, their definition, and indications.

Graft loss and healing rates are not well reported in the literature. Issues such as poor nutrition, hematoma, seroma, shear, infection, burn size, and other comorbid conditions may contribute to poor healing rates and graft loss (Jewell, Guerrero, Quesada, Chan, & Garner, 2007).

Vacuum-Assisted Closure Therapy

The use of *vacuum-assisted closure (VAC) therapy* has become increasingly more popular in the treatment of partial- and full-thickness burns (Koehler et al., 2008). VAC therapy is used for a variety of reasons in burn treatment:

- Graft fixation,
- Optimization of wound bed by increasing circulation,
- Decreasing edema, and
- Residual wound closure.

Additional benefits of VAC therapy are

- Reduction of bacterial colonization (Gabriel et al., 2006),
- Early mobilization of the patient (Horch, 2004),
- Reduction of necrosis (Horch, 2004), and
- Accelerated wound healing.

Application of VAC dressings should be done by a skilled therapist and in the appropriate settings determined by the ordering physician. Frequency of dressing changes is determined by the physician and can be influenced by wound infection, amount of exudates, and the stage of healing the patient is currently in. It is also important to note that several different dressings can be used under the VAC sponge dressing, each of which has a distinct advantage and will be determined by the physician. The literature has suggested that the use of VAC therapy in burn patients may reduce wound healing time and therefore reduce costs (Koehler et al., 2008; Gabriel et al., 2006; Horch, 2004).

Surgical Treatment and Techniques

Surgery is indicated for full-thickness burn injuries or for those burns not expected to heal within a 3-week period. The first step in surgical treatment of a burn wound is excision of damaged tissue or eschar (Choi & Panthaki, 2008). A common method of removing necrotic tissue from a burn wound is a technique called *tangential excision*. In this technique, metered layers of dead tissue are removed, allowing for the retention of as much viable tissue as possible (Kao & Garner, 1999). Historically, burn wounds were not excised until the natural separation of burn eschar and viable tissue occurred (at about 3 weeks), but with the introduction of tangential excision, wounds can be excised earlier because the technique allows for the identification of viable tissue as thin layers of eschar are removed (Choi & Panthaki, 2008). With large burns, excision may require several trips to the operating room to remove all of the necrotic tissue. After successful debridement and cleaning of the burn wound (surgically or nonsurgically), the wound is ready to be covered with a skin graft, temporary graft (xenograft or homograft), or a dressing. The physician determines which covering is used, based on the status and size of the wounds and the patient's medical status.

In some cases, an autograft can be placed after the *primary excision* (usually in small burns), but in most cases homograft is surgically placed using staples, which allows the wound bed to granulate and prepare for autografting (Lineen & Namias, 2008). It also protects the wound against infection. If it is unclear whether all of the necrotic tissue was removed, or if tissue profusion is poor, nutritional status is compromised or infection is present, surgeons will not cover the wound with a permanent wound covering, fearing a poor outcome. Applying temporary dressings or coverings is ideal when the circumstances are variable; they allow the formation of a healthy wound bed.

Depending on the TBSA burned, a patient may go through *serial excision* and *serial grafting* (Choi & Panthaki, 2008). In very large burns, the surgeon not uncommonly excises and grafts the neck, hands, and antecubital regions fairly early after the burn injury, which allows for the placement of a tracheotomy tube and line placement as these areas heal. As with serial excision, a patient may return to the operating room many times for autografting before complete wound closure is obtained.

Psychosocial and Mental Health Issues

Various psychosocial issues can arise after a burn injury occurs. Early identification of these issues and treatment while the patient is in the acute care setting can be beneficial to the overall outcome (Ptacek, Patterson, & Heimback, 2002). Commonly reported psychological issues reported are depression, posttraumatic stress disorder, acute stress disorder, decreased acceptance of body image, and sleep disorders (Esselman, Thombs, Magyar-Russell, & Faurbach, 2006). Ptacek et al. (2002) found evidence of mild to moderate depression ratings in burn patients who had no previous history of depression, but these ratings tended to decrease within 10 days after injury. Esselman et al. (2006) suggested that predictors of depression in burn patients include "pre-burn affective disorders, burn characteristics, dispositional variables, and coping styles" (p. 398).

Posttraumatic stress disorder and acute stress disorder have a varying prevalence depending on the assessment tool used, sample size reported, and the timing of the assessment. They are difficult and complex disorders to diagnose and are not well studied in burn patients. As with depression, premorbid psychological disorders appear to influence the development of posttraumatic and acute stress disorders in burn patients (Esselman et al., 2006).

Body image and perceived appearance in burn patients has not been well studied. Only recently has a validated tool to measure body image among burn patients become available—the Satisfaction With Appearance Scale (Lawrence et al., 1998).

According to a study published by Boeve et al. (2002), 73% of burn patients reported a problem with their sleep after injury. Moreover, the sleep problems reported involved the quality of sleep, not the quantity of sleep. Factors influencing the quality of sleep in burn patients include frequent night waking, pain, emotional distress, and sleep hygiene practices (Boeve et al., 2002). The quality of postburn sleep should be addressed and treated to minimize potential physiological and psychological deficits.

Initial Assessments and Evaluations

Typically, an occupational therapist or burn therapist evaluates burn patients within the first 24 hours after injury. Depending on the patient's medical status, a full evaluation may not be appropriate, but the patient should be assessed for splinting needs and positioned for edema control of the hands and upper extremities. Before beginning the initial evaluation, therapists should complete a full chart review. Often, therapists see the patient before a physician has completed a history and physical, so a call to the physician or other burn team members can be helpful in completing the history. Many burn centers have standing therapy orders for every patient admitted, but therapists must often rely on their professional judgment to determine the appropriateness of therapy.

Many therapists also find it beneficial to complete the initial evaluation during a dressing change. Doing this allows therapists to observe the depth of the burns and to see the exact distribution of the burn injury. When therapists are able to see the wounds, they are better able to more accurately determine whether any precautions should be adopted to protect the injured joints. It also allows therapists to gain insight for splinting and positioning. The subjective and objective portion of the burn evaluation should include but not be limited to

- Age of burn victim;
- Burn mechanism;
- Areas burned;
- Percentage burned;
- Depth of burn;
- Joints involved;
- Social history;
- Occupation;
- Past and current medical history;
- Procedures performed on admission (e.g., escharotomies); and
- Patient and family goals if applicable.

Detailed information pertaining to the joints, ROM, and mobility or functional limitations is also included in this section. Many burn patients will not be able to participate in a functional evaluation on admission secondary to severity of the burn. This part of the evaluation should be deferred until the patient is able to actively participate in treatment. When a patient is able to participate, full assessment of activities of daily living (ADLs) should be completed and goals updated accordingly. ROM measurements should be precisely taken using a goniometer for any joint that has been affected by the burn injury. Obtaining accurate measurements on the initial evaluation are imperative, because these measurements will guide the occupational therapist's goal writing and treatment planning.

ROM Measurements and Assessment

Some burn centers have a combined occupational therapy and physical therapy evaluation form on which each discipline fills out its respective sections. Traditionally, occupational therapists are responsible for completing the hand and upper-extremity PROM and (when applicable) active ROM (AROM) measurements. Because burn dressings can be restricting, a more accurate measurement will be obtained if ROM measurement is completed in the absence of dressings. ROM measurement of a burned extremity may become more difficult because wound exudate causes a slippery surface. If the patient is sedated and unable to participate in the evaluation process, PROM measurements should be taken and recorded on the evaluation form.

It is important when obtaining hand measurement to measure joints individually and compositely. Normal total motion of the digits is 270°, and functional ROM is considered to be more than 220° (Esselman et al., 2006). In the event that damage to the extensor tendons of the hand is suspected, individual joint ROM measurements are adequate, and composite measurement should not be taken because of the risk of further injury. Some ROM limiting factors present in the initial evaluation are bulky dressings, edema, and thick, inflexible burn eschar.

In patients who are alert and able to participate in the evaluation, pain is the biggest limiting factor (Edgar & Brereton, 2004). For this reason, it is extremely important to coordinate therapy evaluations and treatment with the administration of pain medication. It is also important to fully explain to patients the rationale behind early movement and treatment, namely better outcomes with a decreased risk of contracture. The remainder of the occupational therapy evaluation should coincide with a typical occupational therapy evaluation addressing deficits as they relate to performance components and performance areas.

Occupational Therapy Treatment Planning

Special factors are considered regarding occupational therapy treatment and treatment planning depending on the patient's stage of healing. Restriction, limitations, and contraindications change as patients undergo excision and grafting and the placement of temporary biologic dressings such as Transcyte and Biobrane.

Immediately after burn injury, occupational therapy treatment focuses on splinting, positioning, AROM and PROM, and patient education. Patients are encouraged to participate in ADLs as they are able. If the patient can participate, he or she is typically taken to hydrotherapy for wound care and dressing changes, which is an ideal time to complete treatment. The warm water of the whirlpool is soothing and helps reduce pain. Dressings are removed, allowing for easier movement, and it is a perfect time to address ADLs. Patients should be encouraged to complete AROM as often as tolerated with as much pain as can be tolerated.

Immobilization of joints after autografting is essential to the healing of the graft, but the time frame is based on the burn surgeon's preferences (Edgar & Brereton, 2004). Immobilization of joints after the application of Biobrane, Transcyte, Integra, and cultured epithelial autograft is also necessary to allow for the product to adhere to the burn wound. The various manufacturers have suggested guidelines for the timeframe of immobilization after the application of these products.

Precautions and Contraindications

As with any critically ill patient, precautions and contraindications limit treatment in an acute burn injury. The most common precaution for ROM in burn patients are extensor tendon precautions for the hands.

Extensor Tendon Injuries

Because the extensor tendons of the hands lie so closely to the skin, they are at greater risk of injury when hands are burned. Unlike on other areas of the body, skin is thin on the dorsum of the hand, and it does not have a substantial amount of fat to protect underlying structures. Extensor tendon precautions should be adhered to with patients with full-thickness hand burns that cover more than half of the dorsal side of the hand and fingers, any time the occupational therapist feels that the extensor tendons or extensor hood of the fingers have been damaged, or when the patient has exposed tendon (Edgar & Brereton, 2004). It is not uncommon for tendons in the hands to be exposed after debridement of a full-thickness hand burn. In these cases, extreme caution should be used when completing ROM exercises, especially if the patient is intubated and sedated and unable to express pain to the therapist.

Extensor tendon precautions apply to the method in which PROM exercises are completed. The rationale behind the precaution is to provide each individual joint of the hand and fingers with maximal ROM without placing the extensor tendons on maximal stretch, which is done by placing the wrist in 45°–90° of extension (which provides extra slack to extensor tendons of the hand) and completing isolated joint PROM exercises. Fingers should not be bent into a composite fist because it places too much stress on the compromised tendons. The therapist should also be mindful of his or her hand placement when completing PROM exercises. The therapist grasps the lateral aspects of each phalanx distal to the joint being exercised with one hand and supports the proximal phalanx with the opposite hand. The joint is then passively moved through the full ROM.

Other Contraindications

Occupational therapists should always use their professional judgment when deciding on the appropriateness of occupational therapy. If a patient is medically unstable, then therapeutic procedures should be postponed until the patient is able to tolerate treatment. Standard precautions regarding IV lines, ventilators, and other invasive lines also apply to burn patients. Another obstacle that can limit treatment in burn patients is the presence of a tracheostomy in patients with neck and face burns, which can make ROM, splinting, and positioning challenging for therapists (Sharp, Dougherty, & Kagan, 2007). Caution must be taken when splinting over burns that are in the zone of stasis. Splinting can cause areas of increased pressure that would further decrease blood perfusion to tissue that is already vulnerable (Richard & Ward, 2005).

The formation of bone in the joints after burn and trauma injuries is called *heterotopic ossification*, and it most commonly develops in the elbow (Summerfield, DiGiovani, & Rochert, 1997). When heterotopic ossification develops, limitations in ROM lead to further functional deficits and soft tissue contractures. Treatments vary from center to center, but one study (Tsionos, Leclercq, & Rochert, 2004) has suggested that early excision of the unwanted bone growth followed by a strict splinting and continuous passive motion regime enabled increased ROM and participation in functional activities. Nonetheless, caution should be taken when working with patients who develop heterotopic ossification to ensure maximum functioning, ROM, and decreased pain.

Splinting and Positioning

It is imperative that occupational therapists assess splinting and positioning during the initial evaluation. Naturally, burned extremities are going to gravitate toward the position of comfort, and the therapist's role is to determine which extremities are in need of splinting and assess the need for different positioning techniques. Patients should be positioned in the position of function rather than the position of comfort to prevent contracture. According to Richard and Ward (2005), burn centers have no consensus in regard to splinting; many focus on activity and mobility, whereas others focus on splinting, but no data support either method.

Table 15.3 includes a list of different burn splints and positioning recommendations.

Special attention has been given to splinting and positioning techniques of the neck, hands, and shoulder secondary to the potentially devastating loss of function at these joints if not treated aggressively. Sharp et al. (2007) reported that early splinting or positioning of a neck burn before and after grafting should be a priority of burn therapists to maximize functional outcomes and prevent contracture. Splinting allows for proper positioning and consistent pressure to the healing wound, which is thought to help prevent contracture. The ideal position for splinting the hand has yet to be determined (Richard, Staley, Daugherty, Miller, & Warden, 1994), but preserving the greatest amount of function should be the goal.

Axillary burns are difficult to treat and are prone to contracture secondary to the resting position of the upper extremity, yet functional ROM of the shoulder is essential to participation in ADLs. Vehmeyer-Heeman, Lommers, Van den Kerckhove, and Boeckx (2005) described a surgical technique combined with immediate splinting the axilla in 90° of abduction after autografting, with encouraging results. The burn therapist's professional and clinical judgment is essential in determining the splinting and positioning options in burn patients, and unfortunately, very little supporting documentation is available on this topic.

Edema Management

As stated previously, systemic edema is likely in burn injuries. The effects of edema can be managed surgically by escharotomies and fasciotomies, but these procedures are invasive and not appropriate in many cases. Burn therapists are responsible for implementing edema management techniques and positioning to reduce and control edema.

Burn therapists are responsible for positioning the extremities to control and prevent edema. Pillows under the arms and legs can be an effective strategy, but more aggressive measures are often needed. An effective technique

(Text continues on p. 550)

Table 15.3. **Burn Splints and Positioning**

Joint Affected	Position of Contracture or Deformity	Position of Splinting	Splinting Materials and Positioning Devices to Consider	Considerations for Stage of Healing	Limitations to Splinting and Positioning
Mouth	Decreased vertical and horizontal opening	Maximum vertical and horizontal opening (may alternate).	Several prefabricated microstomia devices are on the market that can be adjusted vertically, horizontally, and circumferentially.	Splinting should occur beginning in the acute stage of healing through the rehabilitation phase. If autografting is not indicated, splinting should be at the discretion of the treating therapist.	Intubation
Neck	Flexion, limitations in lateral flexion and rotation	Neutral or slight extension. Pillows should be removed from under the head.	Soft collar vs. ~~hard collar for~~ prefabricated general splints. Customized thermoplastic splints. Towel roll behind neck, between scapula, or both.	Splinting is initiated in ~~the acute phase of healing~~ through the rehabilitation phase. Complete immobilization for 3–5 days after autografting.	Tracheostomy
Axilla	Adduction	90° of flexion and abduction, commonly referred to as *scaption* (upper extremity is positioned in the plane of the scapula).	Custom airplane splint made from thermoplastic material. DonJoy SCOI brace (includes shoulder; elbow, wrist, and hand); allows 30°–150° of abduction at shoulder.	Splint after autografting (3–5 days), application of CEA (≤21 days depending on burn center protocol), and Integra (follow manufacturer's guidelines) through the rehabilitation phase of healing.	Central lines and IV access lines Swan Ganz catheter

(continued)

Table 15.3.   (continued)

Joint Affected	Position of Contracture or Deformity	Position of Splinting	Splinting Materials and Positioning Devices to Consider	Considerations for Stage of Healing	Limitations to Splinting and Positioning
Elbow	Flexion	Extension.	Custom anterior-fitting elbow extension splint. Knee immobilizer cut to size.	Splint after autografting (3–5 days), application of CEA (≤21 days depending on burn center's protocol), and Integra (follow manufacturer's guidelines) through the rehabilitation phase of healing. At the first sign of contracture or loss of passive range of motion.	IV sites/lines
Wrist	Flexion	Neutral, up to 45° of extension.	Prefabricated wrist cock-up vs. custom wrist cock-up.	Generally, splinting occurs in the acute phase of healing or after autografting or wound covering through the rehabilitation phase. Splinting of the wrist is frequently combined with splinting the hand.	Circumferential burns—May need to alternate flexion and extension splints Arterial lines

Hand	Flexion, loss of web spaces	Intrinsic plus or safe position.	Custom safe-position splint. Finger extension splint or baseball glove splint (for deep palmar burns).	Deep hand burns are splinted within 24 hr of admission. Splint after autografting (3–5 days), application of CEA (≤21 days depending on burn center's protocol), and Integra (follow manufacturer's guidelines) through the rehabilitation phase of healing.	Consider tendon injuries with aggressive splinting techniques
Knee	Flexion	Extension.	Knee immobilizer. Custom posterior-fitting knee splint.	Splint after autografting (3–5 days), application of CEA (≤21 days depending on burn center's protocol), and Integra (follow manufacturer's guidelines) through the rehabilitation phase of healing.	
Ankle	Plantar flexion	Neutral.	Burn meryloperoxidase. Custom posterior foot splint.	Splinting usually begins in the acute phase of wound healing through the rehabilitation phase.	Arterial lines Risk for pressure ulcers on heal

Note. CEA = cultured epithelial autograft.

for managing upper-extremity edema is using stockinette over the burn dressings and then "hanging" it from an IV pole. To do this, the therapist will need to cut a large piece of stockinette twice the length of the patient's arm. The stockinette is then placed over the burn dressings (up to the axilla) with the extra length extending from the hand. The extra stockinette can then be tied to the hangers at the top of an IV pole next to the patient's bed. When using this technique, it is important to ensure that the extremity is well supported with pillows so that no one area is under excessive pressure.

A case study by Lowell et al. (2003) suggested that using coban wrapping is effective in controlling hand edema after skin grafting and may lead to increased hand function. This technique is widely used by burn therapists and is an effective edema management tool. One tip for su ccess with this technique is to use a small amount of lotion on the outside of the coban after wrapping to prevent the fingers from sticking together. Coban can be applied over the burn dressings and should be changed daily along with the burn dressing.

Effect of Burns on Occupational Performance

A burn injury can have a devastating effect on a person's ability to function independently and engage in his or her daily occupations. Several factors that may influence or limit a burn victim's ability to participate in ADLs and work, play, and leisure activities include

- Burn size;
- Location of burn and major joints involved;
- Depth of burn injury;
- Healing times and mechanism of wound closure;
- Presence of hypertrophic scarring and contractures;
- Edema;
- Degree of patient participation;
- Splinting regime; and
- Medical complications.

These factors are just a few of the limitations that are burn specific and should be considered when determining the extent to which a patient will be able to participate in ADLs and other functional activities. Once the patient is discharged from the hospital, frequent follow-up is necessary until the patient is able to fully participate independently in his or her daily occupations.

Patient and Family Education

As with any injury or illness, patient and family education is an important role of burn therapists. Burn therapists are responsible for training the patient in therapeutic exercises to maintain joint integrity and prevent contractures so that the patient can independently complete ADLs. In addition, therapists should teach caregivers and patients scar management techniques and functional mobility training and provide adaptive equipment and instruction when appropriate. In some burn centers, therapists are also responsible for family training in dressing changes. Burn therapists are also responsible for addressing any issues that may arise with home management skills once the patient is discharged home.

Patient and family education is essential to the successful recovery of a burn patient and should be a part of therapist's treatment from Day 1. Because of the continued pain and emotional distress that can result from a burn injury, patient rapport and trust should be the building blocks of the patient–family–therapist relationship. This trust and rapport can be established by providing the family and patient with up-to-date and accurate information regarding therapeutic procedures and practices, as well as information regarding the patient's functional status and goals.

Discharge Planning

Discharge planning for burn patients can be a difficult time for the burn team, patients, and families. The patient has often endured a prolonged hospital stay, and it can be difficult for him or her to transition to home and assume all of the care needed after a burn injury. Patients are often sent home or to rehab before complete wound closure is achieved, which results in the patient or family completing dressing changes on a daily basis (if disposition is home). If this is not possible, the patient may require frequent visits to the burn center for continued wound care on an outpatient basis. Wound care and outpatient therapy can be coordinated so that the patient does not have to make additional trips.

The following should be included in the discharge plan:

- ROM measurements at discharge (active and passive);
- ADL assessment at discharge;
- Splint schedule, if applicable;
- Home exercise program;
- Information regarding scar management and pressure garments (to be fit as an outpatient in most instances); and
- Outpatient therapy schedule.

Including these things as a part of the occupational therapy discharge plan will help ease the transition from inpatient care to outpatient care. To be successful, the discharge plan should include and consider all aspects of the patient's care and injury and include input from all members of the burn team.

References

Arford, S. (2008). Treatment of frostbite: A cold-induced injury. Journal of *Wound, Ostomy, Continence, and Nursing, 35,* 625–630.

Boeve, S. A., Aaron, L. A., Martin-Herz, S. P., Peterson, A., Cain, V., Heimback, D. M., et al. (2002). Sleep disturbance after burn injury. *Journal of Burn Care and Rehabilitation, 23,* 32–38.

Byers, J. F., Bridges, S., Kijek, J., & LaBorde, P. (2001). Burn patients' pain and anxiety experiences. *Journal of Burn Care and Rehabilitation, 22,* 144–149.

Choi, M., & Panthaki J. (2008). Tangential excision of burn wounds. *Journal of Craniofacial Surgery, 19,* 1056–1060.

Connor-Ballard, P. A. (2009). Understanding and managing burn pain: Part 1. *American Journal of Nursing, 109,* 48–56.

Edgar, D., & Brereton, M. (2004). ABC of burns: Rehabilitation after burn injury. *British Medical Journal, 329,* 343–345.

Esselman, P. C., Thombs, B. D., Magyar-Russell, G., & Faurbach, J. A. (2006). Burn rehabilitation: State of the science. *American Journal of Physical Medicine and Rehabilitation, 85,* 383–413.

Ferguson, S. L., & Voll, K.V. (2004). Burn pain and anxiety: The use of music relaxation during rehabilitation. *Journal of Burn Care and Rehabilitation, 25,* 8–14.

Gabriel, A., Heinrich, C., Shores, J., Baqai, W., Rogers, F., & Gupta, S. (2006). Reducing bacterial bioburden in infected wounds with vacuum assisted closure and a new silver dressing—A pilot study. *Wounds, 18,* 245–255.

Graves, C., Saffle, J., & Cochran, A. (2009). Actual burn nutrition care practices: An update. *Journal of Burn Care and Research, 30,* 77–82.

Hettiarachy, S., & Dziewulski, P. (2004). ABC of burns, pathophysiology, and types of burns. *British Medical Journal, 328,* 1427–1429.

Holmes, J. H. (2008). Critical issues in burn care. *Journal of Burn Care and Research, 29*(6, Suppl. 2), S180–S187.

Horch, R. (2004). Basics foundation and results of vacuum therapy in reconstructive surgery. *Zentralbl Chir, 129,* 2–5.

Jewell, L., Guerrero, R., Quesada, A. R., Chan, L. S., & Garner, W. L. (2007. Rate of healing in skin-grafted burn wounds. *Plastic and Reconstructive Surgery, 120,* 451–456.

Kao, C. C., & Garner, W. L. (1999). Acute burns. *Plastic and Reconstructive Surgery, 101,* 2482–2492.

Kidd, M., Hultman, C. S., Aalst, J. V., Calvert, C., Peck, M. D., & Cairns, B. A. (2007). The contemporary management of electrical injuries, resuscitation, reconstruction, rehabilitation. *Annals of Plastic Surgery, 58,* 273–278.

Kita, N. (2009). *Hypodermis.* Retrieved from http://plasticsurgery.about.com/od/glossary/g/hypodermis.htm

Koehler, C., Niederbichler, A. D., Jung, F. J., Scholz, T., Labler, L., Perez, D., et al. (2008). Wound therapy using the vacuum-assisted closure device: Clinical experience with novel indications. *Journal of Trauma, Injury, Infection, and Critical Care, 65,* 722–731.

Lawrence, J. W., Heinberg, L. J., Roca, R., Munster, A., Spence, R., & Fauerbach, J. A. (1998). Development and Validation of the Satisfaction With Appearance Scale: Assessing body image among burn-injured patients. *Psychological Assessment, 10,* 64–70.

Lineen, E., & Namias, N. (2008). Biologic dressing in burns. *Journal of Craniofacial Surgery, 19,* 923–928.

Lowell, M., Pirc, P., Ward, S., Lundy, C., Wilhelm, D., Reddy, R., et al. (2003). Effect of 3M Coban self-adherent wraps on edema and function of the burned hand: A case study. *Journal of Burn Care and Rehabilitation, 24,* 253–258.

MacPherson, R. D., Woods, D., & Penfold, J. (2008). Ketamine and midazolam delivered by patient-controlled analgesia in relieving pain associated with burn dressings. *Clinical Journal of Pain, 24,* 568–571.

Miller, S. F., Bessey, P., Lentz, C. W., Jeng, J. C., Schurr, M., & Browning, S. (2008). National Burn Repository 2007 Report: A synopsis of the 2007 call for data. *Journal of Burn Care and Research, 26,* 539–542.

Murphy, J. V., Banwell, P. E., Roberts, A. H. N., & McGrouther, D. A. (2000). Frostbite: Pathogenesis and treatment. *Journal of Trauma: Injury, Infection, and Critical Care, 48,* 171–178.

Patterson, D. R. (1995). Non-opioid approaches to burn pain. *Journal of Burn Care and Rehabilitation, 16*(3, Pt. 2), 372–376.

Ptacek, J. T., Patterson, D. R., & Heimback, D. M. (2002). Inpatient depression in persons with burns. *Journal of Burn Care and Rehabilitation, 23,* 1–9.

Reddy, M. (2008). Skin and wound care: Important considerations in the older adult. *Advances in Skin and Wound Care, 21,* 424–436.

Richard, R., Staley, M., Daugherty, M. B., Miller, S. F., & Warden, G. D. (1994). The wide variety of designs for dorsal hand burn splints. *Journal of Burn Care and Rehabilitation 15,* 275–280.

Richard, R., & Ward, R. S. (2005). Splinting strategies and controversies. *Journal of Burn Care and Rehabilitation, 26,* 392–396.

Robert, R., Brack, A., Blakeney, P., Villareal, C., Rosenberg, L., Thomas, C., et al. (2003). A double-blind study of the analgesic efficacy of oral transmucosal fentanyl citrate and oral morphine in pediatric patients undergoing burn dressing change and tubbing. *Journal of Burn Care and Rehabilitation, 24,* 351–355.

Salcido, R. (2000). *Enzymatic debridement: A tried and tested method.* Retrieved May 9, 2009, from http://findarticles.com/p/articles/mi_qa3977/is_200005/ai_n8891061

Serghiou, M. A., Holmes, C. L., & McCauley, R. L. (2004). A survey of current rehabilitation trends for burn injuries to the head and neck. *Journal of Burn Care and Rehabilitation, 25,* 514–518.

Sharp, P. A., Dougherty, M. E., & Kagan, R. J. (2007). The effects of positioning devices and pressure therapy on outcome after full thickness burns of the neck. *Journal of Burn Care and Research, 28,* 451–459.

Summerfield, S. L., DiGiovani, C., & Weiss, A. C. (1997). Heterotopic ossification of the elbow. *Journal of Shoulder and Elbow Surgery, 6,* 312–332.

Tsionos, I., Leclercq, C., & Rochert, J.-M. (2004). Heterotopic ossification of the elbow in patients with burns. *Journal of Bone and Joint Surgery, 86B(3),* 396–403.

Vehmeyer-Heeman, M., Lommers, B., Van den Kerckhove, E., & Boeckx, W. (2005). Axillary burns: Extended grafting and early splinting prevents contractures. *Journal of Burn Care and Rehabilitation, 26,* 539–542.

Appendix A

Common Diagnostic Tests

Helene Smith-Gabai, OTD, OTR/L, BCPR

Diagnostic tests are routinely done in hospitals to detect the presence of disease, confirm a diagnosis, or monitor response to medical treatments or are used as a screening tool. This appendix describes common diagnostic tests performed in acute care.

Biopsy

A *biopsy* is a sample of cells or tissue removed to determine whether they are normal, benign, or malignant. Biopsies are often done diagnostically to examine for the presence of disease. They are also routinely done for patients after organ transplantation to monitor for signs of rejection. A biopsy can be aspirated with a needle or performed more invasively through a surgical procedure. Biopsy carries a risk of bleeding and infection.

Blood Tests

Blood tests are used to examine specific elements dissolved in the blood. These tests may include blood counts; levels of electrolytes, oxygen, or carbon dioxide; and the presence of markers for certain conditions and diseases. Blood samples may be drawn from the venous or arterial systems. Refer to Appendix P for detail.

Computerized Axial Tomography

A *computerized axial tomography (CT)* scan involves a noninvasive imaging system in which multiple X-ray beams and computer calculations provide a cross-sectional view of the body. Images are viewed as slices; however, a spiral CT produces a three-dimensional image. A CT scan may be used with contrast to enhance differences in tissue density; however, dye may cause kidney dysfunction (Malone & Packel, 2006).

CT scans help physicians diagnose and study cancers, cardiovascular disease, musculoskeletal disorders, liver diseases, trauma, infections, or inflammatory conditions. A CT scan can also detect the presence of and differentiate between hemorrhagic versus ischemic stroke but may miss the early signs of ischemic stroke, especially in the brainstem (DeLaPaz, 2005). The information a CT scan provides may further assist with other medical procedures, such as biopsies or draining of deep abscesses or in measuring bone density. CT scan is the preferred imaging system for bone fractures and lesions (Fischbach & Dunning, 2009).

With a CT scan, the patient enters a large tube that rotates around him or her, taking radiographic images. The scan lasts approximately 30 minutes. Therapy is not limited before or after the scan because the patient is not sedated for it. However, if a CT scan is ordered to rule out a problem such as a pulmonary embolism or an extension of a cerebrovascular accident, then therapy should be deferred until the results are known. This type of scan carries a risk of radiation exposure.

Echocardiogram

An *echocardiograph* is an ultrasound device that uses high-frequency sound waves to create an image that assesses the size, structure, and movement of the heart. An *echocardiogram* also provides information on pericardial effusions, possible blood clots, tumors, arrhythmias, cardiomyopathy, aortic aneurysms, endocarditis, and heart valve functioning, as well as direction and velocity of blood flow. It may also be used to monitor response to treatment. An echocardiogram takes approximately 20 minutes. Echocardiograms have no associated risks, and activity restrictions are not necessary after an echocardiogram.

Electroencephalogram

An *electroencephalogram (EEG)* is a test that records the brain's electrical activity, commonly ordered for patients with epilepsy or seizures. Electrodes are attached to the patient's head, and the brain's electrical impulses are recorded, graphed, and measured. An EEG is also indicated for brain tumors, brain abscess, subdural hematomas, intracranial hemorrhage, encephalitis, and cerebral infarct; in the diagnosis of Parkinson's disease and Alzheimer's disease; and in confirming brain death (Fischbach & Dunning, 2009; Pagana & Pagana, 2006). An EEG can cause a seizure in someone with a seizure disorder; however, seizure is very rare.

A simple EEG can take 30 minutes; a video EEG can take 4–6 hours. Therapy is not limited before or after an EEG. Results may indicate

- *Diffuse slowing:* Nonspecific; occurs in patients with diffuse encephalopathies (e.g., dementia, metabolic encephalopathy, or anoxia);
- *Focal slowing:* Suggests localized dysfunction (e.g., focal seizure or lesion);
- *Triphasic wave:* In 50% of patients, indicates hepatic encephalopathy; in the other 50%, indicates toxic metabolic encephalopathy;
- *Epileptiform discharges:* A hallmark of epilepsy;
- *Periodic lateralized epileptiform discharges:* Associated with cerebral abscesses, anoxia, acute cerebral infarction, or mass lesions (Emerson, Walczak, & Pedley, 2005); and
- *Generalized periodic sharp waves:* May be present with cerebral anoxia or Creutzfeldt–Jakob disease.

Electromyography

Electromyography (EMG) assists with determining the source of neuromuscular weakness, identifying muscle diseases, and differentiating between myopathies and neuropathies (Pagana & Pagana, 2006). During EMG, an electrode records electrical activity of skeletal muscles at rest and during voluntary contraction. EMG may be ordered for patients with suspected polymyositis, muscular dystrophy, myopathy, hypothyroidism, sarcoidosis, Guillain–Barré syndrome, myasthenia gravis, peripheral nerve injury, multiple sclerosis, spinal cord injury, amyotrophic lateral sclerosis, or diabetic neuropathy (Pagana & Pagana, 2006). EMG is contraindicated for anticoagulated patients because of the risk of bleeding. EMG is usually done in conjunction with a nerve conduction test.

Electroneurography (Nerve Conduction Tests)

During a *nerve conduction test,* electrodes stimulate selected nerves, and the action potentials are recorded. Electroneurography measures the conduction velocity of an impulse traveling between two points. This test is used to assess peripheral nerve injuries and discriminate between nerve disease and muscle injury. A nerve conduction study is indicated for carpal tunnel syndrome, poliomyelitis, diabetic neuropathy, myasthenia gravis, Guillain–Barré syndrome, and herniated disk disease (Pagana & Pagana, 2006).

Endoscopy

Endoscopy allows direct visualization of body organs and cavities through the use of a fiberoptic lens attached to a rigid or flexible tube (Malone & Packel, 2006). Endoscopes assist with screening, diagnosis, and intervention. Images transmitted to a closed-circuit TV monitor allow visualization of areas not easily accessed (Fischbach & Dunning, 2009). A camera is inserted in one port, and additional ports may be made for insertion of instruments (i.e., for obtaining a biopsy). Common endoscopic procedures include *bronchoscopy* (respiratory system), *cystoscopy* (urinary tract), and *laparoscopy* (abdomen and pelvic area). Risks include perforation, bleeding, infection, or aspiration (Fischbach & Dunning, 2009; see Table A.1).

Table A.1. Endoscopic Surgical Procedures

Type of Endoscopy	Indication
Arthroscopy	• Tendon repair or release • Ligament repair • Meniscus removal or repair
Broncoscopy	• Visual examination of respiratory tract • Tissue biopsy • Removal of secretions and foreign objects obstructing airway • Stent placement to ensure patent airway
Cystoscopy	• Transurethral resection of prostate • Transurethral resection of superficial bladder tumors • Urethral stent placement • Removal of ureteral and bladder calculi
Endoscopic retrograde cholangiopancreatography	• Placement of stent in pancreatobiliary tree
Esophagogastroduodenoscopy	• Dilation of strictures • Placement of esophageal stents
Laparoscopy	• Cholecystectomy • Hiatal hernia repair • Inguinal hernia repair • Video-assisted colectomy
Thoracoscopy	• Wedge lung resection • Video–assisted lung resection

Source. From Pagana, K. D., & Pagana, T. J. (2006). *Mosby's Manual of Diagnostic and Laboratory Tests* (3rd ed., p. 597). St. Louis, MO: Mosby. Copyright © 2006 Mosby. Adapted with permission.

Evoked Potentials

Evoked potentials are most often performed on an outpatient basis but also may be performed on an inpatient basis. Sensory organs or peripheral nerves are electrically stimulated, providing information on specific nerve dysfunction. Electrodes are placed on the earlobes and scalp much as in an EEG. No limitations for therapy are present before or after.

Fluid Analysis

Fluid may be aspirated to determine the cause of excess fluid; to monitor for signs of infection, inflammation, or abnormal cells; or for symptom relief. For example, cerebrospinal fluid from the brain or spinal cord may be examined for the presence of meningitis, intracranial or subarachnoid hemorrhage, normal pressure hydrocephalus, systemic lupus erythematosus, or encephalitis. Synovial fluid may be aspirated from the knee, hip, shoulder, elbow, wrist, or ankle joints to determine the cause of accumulation and for pressure relief and comfort.

With *pericardiocentesis,* an accumulation of fluid (pericardial effusion) is removed from the *pericardium* (the covering around the heart). Pericardiocentesis may be indicated for infection, cardiac tamponade, systematic inflammatory diseases, or cancer. *Thoracentesis* or *pleurocentesis* is the removal of fluid from the pleural space to determine the cause of the pleural effusion or for symptom relief. Pleural effusion may be the result of heart failure, infection, inflammation, or cancer. In *paracentesis,* an excess of peritoneal fluid is removed from the abdomen. This buildup of abdominal fluid or ascites may be the result of liver dysfunction. Fluid aspiration carries the risk of bleeding, infection, or puncture.

Intravenous Urographies

An *intravenous pyelogram* is used to evaluate the kidneys, ureters, and bladder. This study may be used to assess renal size and shape, assess for kidney stones, and assess kidney function. However, it is being replaced by CT scans because CT scans are less invasive to the system.

Lumbar Puncture

A *lumbar puncture* (e.g., spinal tap) is performed by inserting a needle into the subarachnoid space (L3–L4) and collecting a sample of cerebrospinal fluid. A lumbar puncture is used to diagnose diseases of the brain or spinal cord and infectious or inflammatory conditions, such as

- Normal pressure hydrocephalus
- Subdural hematoma
- Multiple sclerosis
- Guillain–Barré syndrome
- Meningitis.

A lumbar puncture takes approximately 30 minutes, and the patient is on bedrest for 2–4 hours after the procedure.

Magnetic Resonance Imaging

Magnetic resonance imaging (MRI) is a noninvasive test that uses superconductive magnets, radio waves, and computers to provide a detailed sectional image of the body and a study of the molecular nature of tissue (Fischbach & Dunning, 2009). This scan is based on the actions of hydrogen ions within a magnetic field (Pagana & Pagana, 2006). Views can be reconstructed in any plane with a three-dimensional view (Fischbach & Dunning, 2009). MRI is used to view the brain, subarachnoid spaces, blood vessels, fat, tendons, ligaments, joints, structures of the heart, solid organs of the gastrointestinal (GI) system, kidneys, and reproductive organs.

This type of scan involves no exposure to radiation. During an MRI, the patient lies on a platform that is moved into the donut-shaped hole of the scanner. Machines that are more open for claustrophobic patients are available because patients must remain still during the scan to prevent distortion of the images. An MRI takes approximately 45 minutes. Therapy should be deferred until the results are known (e.g., if an MRI is ordered to rule out an extension of a cerebrovascular accident).

Common metal objects (scissors, electronic devices, oxygen tanks) can become lethal projectiles because of the strong magnets of an MRI scanner, and patients should be screened for these objects before entering the scan room (Fischbach & Dunning, 2009). MRIs are contraindicated for patients with pacemakers, metal implants, inner ear implants, infusion pumps, metal fragments, and cerebral aneurysm clips; patients who require continued cardiac monitoring with electrocardiograph leads; or patients who are pregnant (Pagana & Pagana, 2006).

A *magnetic resonance angiography* may be performed at the same time as an MRI. This test evaluates intracranial and extracranial vasculature and is useful in localizing ischemic lesions.

Nuclear Medicine Scans

In *nuclear medicine scans,* the patient receives a small dose of radioactive chemical tracer. A camera takes images of body structures and functions through energy coming from the tracer.

Nuclear scans are used diagnostically for cancers and injury. A *hepatobiliary iminodiacetic acid (HIDA)* scan is a nuclear scan used for looking at bile flow and areas of bile leakage. It also produces images of the liver, small intestine, bile ducts, and gallbladder. A *dual-energy X-ray absorptiometry (DEXA)* scan is used for studying bone mineral density and bone thinning.

Positron Emission Tomography

Positron emission tomography (PET) is another type of nuclear medicine imaging technique. A PET scan may be ordered for oncology, neurology, or cardiology patients. Positrons emitted from radioactive chemicals are sensed by detectors, which combine with CT to form a high-resolution image (Fischbach & Dunning, 2009; Pagana & Pagana, 2006). A radioisotope for specific organs or tissue is inhaled, injected, or ingested (Malone & Packel, 2006). Increased color denotes areas of increased uptake. These radioisotopes have a relatively short half-life to minimize radiation exposure (Malone & Packel, 2006). PET may also be combined with a CT scan.

PET scans provide information on anatomy, physiology, and metabolism, and CT and MRI scans do not. PET scans provide information on blood flow, tissue perfusion, and tissue metabolism "based on oxygen, glucose, and fatty acid utilization and protein synthesis" (Fischbach & Dunning, 2009, p. 741). PET scans are also helpful in studying cancers, coronary heart disease, myocardial infarction, stroke, epilepsy, Parkinson's disease, Huntington's disease, Alzheimer's disease, and dementia (Pagana & Pagana, 2006).

After a PET scan, patients are encouraged to drink plenty of water to flush out the radioactive material, flush twice after urinating, and wash hands thoroughly. A PET scan can take 2–4 hours to complete depending on the system being studied. *Single photon emission computed tomography (SPECT)* is a related nuclear imaging technique.

Pulmonary Function Testing

A *pulmonary function test (PFT)* is used in the diagnosis and screening of pulmonary restrictive and obstructive diseases. It measures the volume and flow of air during breathing, the strength of respiratory muscles, and how well lungs function in delivering oxygen to the blood system (lung diffusion capacity). PFTs are indicated for patients with chronic obstructive pulmonary disease, asthma, sarcoidosis, and fibrosis. Rates vary by age, gender, and body size.

A *flow volume loop* is a graphic depiction of inspiration and expiration volumes and flow rates. A spirometer is one tool used during PFTs that measures how much air is breathed in and out and how fast air is exhaled. In addition, *pulse oximetry* and *arterial blood* gas are further tests of pulmonary function. Refer to Chapter 5 for more detail.

Radioactive Isotope Scanning

Radioactive isotopes are swallowed or injected into the bloodstream. Their uptake into tissue is captured with a specialized camera. Areas of uptake are called *hot spots* or *cold spots*. Hot spots indicate areas of increased uptake, and cold spots indicate areas of decreased uptake. Radioisotope scanning may be used to examine the thyroid, liver, spleen, brain, and bone. It is also used diagnostically to detect the presence of cancerous tumors (cold spots).

Radiography

X-rays examine soft tissue and bony structures of the body. X-rays are short-wave electromagnetic vibrations that produces images in shades of white, black, and gray. Light absorption depends on the density of the structure that it passes through. Dense structures appear white, and more hollow areas appear black.

X-rays are used to detect abnormalities of the heart, lungs, gastrointestinal tract, and thyroid gland. For example, in studying cardiopulmonary structures, an X-ray may be used to determine heart enlargement or presence of fluid in the lungs. X-rays are also used to check for positioning of chest tubes and nasogastric tubes (e.g., kidney, ureter, and bladder imaging). Contrast may also be used to increase visualization of certain structures that are not evident with traditional X-ray.

Stool Cultures

Stool cultures are tested when patients have enteric disorders, severe diarrhea, abdominal bloating, and fever. The most common bowel pathogens are salmonella, shigella, Campylobacter, Yersinia, *Escherichia coli,* Staphylococcus, *Helibacter pylori,* and colostidium. Normal bacteria can also become pathologic secondary to a prolonged course of antibiotics or immunosuppression (Pagana & Pagana, 2006). Viruses, bacteria, and parasites can cause infections that can progress to toxic megacolon (Pagana & Pagana, 2006).

Cultures may also be taken to test for occult blood. Blood in stool may be because of peptic ulcer diseases (e.g., esophagitis, gastritis, ulceration), varices, inflammatory bowel diseases, gastrointestinal tumors, arteriovenous malformations, diverticulosis, hemorrhoids, or gastrointestinal surgery (Pagana & Pagana, 2006).

Therapists working with patients requiring a stool sample should observe standard precautions. If a patient is positive for *Clostridum difficile (C-diff),* wash hands with soap and water, not alcohol-based gels or foam. Refer to Chapter 12 for more information.

Transesophageal Echocardiogram

A *transesophageal echocardiogram (TEE)* is an invasive endoscopic test in which a probe is inserted through the mouth and into the esophagus and sits behind the heart. The TEE provides a clearer picture of the heart and major blood vessels than a traditional echocardiogram and is useful in determining the presence of clots, masses in the heart, valvular dysfunction, pericardial effusion, endocarditis, pericarditis, tamponade, aortic dissections, congenital heart diseases, and cardiac arrhythmias. This test takes approximately 1 hour, and therapy is usually deferred before and after the TEE because the patient is sedated. A TEE carries a risk of throat discomfort and a smaller risk of bleeding and perforation.

Ultrasound Studies

An *ultrasound* is a noninvasive procedure for studying soft tissue structures. High-frequency sound waves directed at an organ or structure are reflected back to a transducer, which produces a structural image (Malone & Packel, 2006). An ultrasound provides information on size, shape, and position of organs.

A *Doppler ultrasound* is used to study blood flow. It provides information on direction, speed, and magnitude of circulation. "For example, narrowed blood vessels produce high velocities, indicating possible stenosis or vasospasm or potential arteriovenous malformations" (Malone & Packel, p. 60). A Doppler ultrasound is also used to rule out deep vein thrombosis and provide information on veins for grafts and dialysis access grafts (Fischbach & Dunning, 2009). Therapy is usually deferred pending results of a Doppler ultrasound to rule out deep vein thrombosis.

Duplex ultrasound is a combination of real-time and Doppler ultrasonography used to study anatomical structures (e.g., blood vessels) and the blood flow through them.

Urinalysis

Urine is the by-product of metabolism and is predominantly (95%) composed of water. Blood includes most of the same substances as urine but in different concentrations (Irion & Goodman, 2009). Urine is examined for color; pH; and presence of ketones, glucose, blood, and protein. Normal urine is pale yellow; however, the color may change as the result of certain medications, foods, supplements, or conditions. Dark brown–colored urine is symptomatic of liver disease or disseminated intravascular coagulation, whereas bleeding from the kidneys or bladder turns urine red (Irion & Goodman, 2009).

A high urine pH may be caused by kidney failure, kidney tubular acidosis, urinary tract infections, hyperventilation, potassium deficiency, or vomiting. Low pH may be the result of metabolic acidosis, diabetic ketoacidosis, starvation, uremia, diarrhea, respiratory acidosis, chronic obstructive pulmonary disease, or renal tuberculosis. Ketones indicate triglyceride metabolism. Fat rather than carbohydrates is fuel for the body when glucose is not metabolized. Glucose in the urine is indicative of diabetes mellitus. *Hematuria* (blood in the urine) may be because of acute tubular necrosis, cancer, bladder or kidney stones, or urinary tract infections. Leukocyte esterase and nitrate tests are used to test for urinary tract infections (Pagana & Pagana, 2006). Urine cultures are also used to test for illegal drugs.

Therapists should follow input and output guidelines when indicated and not discard urine before measuring. Although measuring urine output is typically performed by nursing services, therapists may need to address this issue if they are working on toileting with patients. Therefore, therapists need to know that urine should not be discarded if the patient's output is being monitored. Urine output should be measured and listed on the patient's Input and Output Chart, or urine should be left on the side for nursing staff to measure later. Therapists should also be aware of urinary catheters when moving patients (refer to Chapter 10 for more information).

References

DeLaPaz, R. (2005). Computed tomography and magnetic resonance imaging. In L. P. Rowland (Ed.), *Merritt's neurology* (11th ed., pp. 67–79). Philadelphia: Lippincott Williams & Wilkins.

Emerson, R. G., Walczak, T. S., & Pedley, T. A. (2005). Electroencephalography. In L. P. Rowland (Ed.), *Merritt's neurology* (11th ed., pp. 79–88). Philadelphia: Lippincott Williams & Wilkins.

Fischbach, F., & Dunning, M. B., III (2009). *A manual of laboratory and diagnostic tests* (8th ed.). Philadelphia: Wolters Kluwer Health.

Irion, G. L., & Goodman, C. C. (2009). Laboratory tests and values. In C. C. Goodman & K. S. Fuller (Eds.), *Pathology: Implications for the physical therapist* (3rd ed., pp. 1637–1667). Philadelphia: W. B. Saunders.

Malone, D. J., & Packel, L. (2006). Clinical laboratory values and diagnostic testing. In D. J. Malone & K. L. B. Lindsay (Eds.), *Physical therapy in acute care* (pp. 31–65). Thorofare, NJ: Slack.

Pagana, K. D., & Pagana, T. J. (2006). *Mosby's manual of diagnostic and laboratory tests* (3rd ed.). St. Louis, MO: Mosby.

Appendix B
Medications

Helene Smith-Gabai, OTD, OTR/L, BCPR

Generic and Brand Names	Indication	Side Effects
Cardiovascular		
amiodarone (Cordarone, Pacerone)	Antiarrhythmic medication	Halo vision (deposits formed on the corneas of the eyes), blue-gray discoloration of the skin, sunburn, thyroid disorders, hepatoxicity, lung disease
acetylsalicylic acid (i.e., ASA or aspirin) (Aspirin, Bayer Aspirin, Ecotrin, and more)	Anti-inflammatory agent that prevents platelet adhesion and acts as a prophylaxis for thromboemboli	GI discomfort
procainamide (Pronestyl, Procan-SR, Procanbid), propafenone (Rythmol), quinidine (Cardioquin)	Antiarrhythmic medications	GI symptoms (i.e., nausea, vomiting), palpitations, rash, insomnia, dizziness
doxazosin mesylate (Cardura), terazosin HCL (Hytrin), prazosin HCL (Minipress)	Alpha-adrenergic blockers; lower blood pressure	Headache, palpitations, fatigue, nausea, weakness, drowsiness, dizziness
digoxin (Lanoxin), digitoxin (Crystodigin)	Medication for CHF and atrial arrhythmias; increases force of heart muscle contractions	Nausea, vomiting, fatigue, lethargy, weakness, headache, visual disturbances, hypotension, depression, confusion, restlessness, seizures, bradycardia, irregular heart rhythms
furosemide (Lasix), mannitol (Osmitrol), bumetanide (Bumex), torsemide (Demadex)	Diuretics; eliminate excess body fluid (decreasing blood pressure) of patients with heart failure, peripheral edema, or volume overload	Hypotension, frequent urination, weakness, fatigue, possibly decreased potassium levels
metoprolol (Lopressor, Troprol-XL), propranolol HCL (Inderal), atenolol (Tenormin), betaxolol (Kerlone), carteolol (Cartrol), carvedilol (Coreg), penbutolol (Levatol)	Beta blockers; slow heart rate and reduce blood pressure. Used as a medication for angina, HTN, and arrhythmias	Dizziness, fatigue, nausea, insomnia, weakness, slow pulse, nightmares, depression, increased glucose levels, cholesterol, sexual dysfunction, asthma attacks

(continued)

Generic and Brand Names	Indication	Side Effects
milrinone (Primacor), dobutamine (Dobutrex)	Inotrope medications; short-term use for decompensated heart failure and cardiogenic shock	Headache, nausea, palpitations, shortness of breath, allergic reaction, ventricular arrhythmia, sudden death
nifedipine (Adalat, Procardia), diltiazem (Cardizem, Dilacor), verapamil (Calan, Verelan), amlodipine (Norvasc), nicardipine (Cardene)	Calcium channel blockers; vasodilator that lowers blood pressure. Used in treatment of angina, HTN, arrhythmias	Dizziness, fainting, headache, fluid retention, palpitations, rash
nitroglycerin, isosorbide dinitrate (Isordil, Iso-Bid), minoxidil (Loniten)	Peripheral and coronary vasodilator; reduces cardiac workload. Used in treatment of angina attack	Dizziness, headache, GI symptoms (i.e., nausea, vomiting, diarrhea), increased heart rate, difficulty breathing, drowsiness, swollen ankles
clopidogrel (Plavix)	Platelet-inhibiting agent. Used for patients with ACS, PAD, recent MI, or CVA	Chest pain, abdominal pain, fatigue, diarrhea, hemorrhage, skin bruising, headache, edema, dizziness, arthralgia, upper respiratory infection
streptokinase (Streptase), urokinase (Abbokinase), alteplase (Activase, tPA; tissue plasminogen activactor), tenecteplase (TNKase), reteplase	Thrombolytics used to break down and dissolve blood clots	GI, GU, or intracranial bleeding; headache; fever; nausea; low back pain
enalapril (Vasotec), captopril (Capoten), benazepril (Lotensin), lisinopril (Prinivil, Zestral), ramipril (Altace), quinapril (Accupril)	ACE inhibitors used in treatment for HTN, heart failure Improves sympathetic heart rate and response to exercise	Headache; dizziness; hypotension; palpitations; numbness or tingling of hands, feet, or lips; persistent dry cough; skin rash; loss of taste; renal failure; edema
warfarin (Coumadin), enoxaparin (Lovenox), dalteparin (Fragmin), danaparoid sodium (Organan), ardeparin (Normiflo), hirudin (Refludan)	Anticoagulant medications used for prevention and treatment of clots	Easy bruising, excessive bleeding, joint pain, paralysis, difficulty breathing and swallowing
simvastatin (Zocor), rosuvastatin (Crestor),	Hypolipidemic agents that decrease cholesterol and LDL	GI discomfort; nausea, vomiting, and diarrhea;

Generic and Brand Names	Indication	Side Effects
lovastatin (Mevacor), fluvastatin (Lescol), atorvastatin (Lipitor), cholestyramine (Questran)	levels; used for treatment of hypercholesteremia	constipation; flatulence; myalgia; increased liver enzymes; peripheral neuropathy; insomnia; rash
Pulmonary		
albuterol (Proventil, Ventolin), terbutaline (Brethine, Brethair), pirbuterol (Maxair), levalbuterol (Xopenex)	Beta 2 agonists; short-acting bronchodilators used for COPD	Rapid heartbeat or palpitations, headache, dizziness, nausea, vomiting, diarrhea, anxiety, hives, skin rash, nervousness, tremor
aminophylline, theophylline (Theo-dur, Slo-Bid), oxtriphylline (Choledyl)	Methylxanthines used in treatment of severe COPD	GI discomfort, heartburn, insomnia, headache, tachycardia, tachypnea, irritability
beclomethasone (Vanceril), budesonide (Pulmicort), fluticasone (Flovent), triamcinolone (Azmacort), flunisolide (AeroBid)	Inhaled corticosteroids used in treatment of COPD	Nose or throat irritation, congestion, nosebleed, hoarseness, increased coughing, asthma, headache, nausea, oral thrush, back pain
formoterol (Foradil), salmeterol (Serevent)	Beta 2 agonist; long-acting bronchodilators used for COPD	Throat irritation, hoarseness, asthma, rapid heart rate, palpitations, headache, dizziness, nausea, vomiting, diarrhea, anxiety, tremors
ipratropium bronmide (Atrovent), tiotropium (Spiriva)	Anticholinergics; assist with bronchodilation in treatment of COPD	Dry mouth, blurred vision, cough, tachycardia, constipation, urinary retention, headache, dizziness, confusion, impaired memory, glaucoma
oxygen	Improves oxygenation of tissue and used in prevention and treatment of hypoxia and hypoxemia	Oxygen toxicity; may depress respiratory drive in hypercapnic patients
Neurological		
benzatropine (Cogentin), amantadine (Symmetrel)	Used in treatment of Parkinson's disease	Blurred vision; dizziness; GI symptoms; anorexia; dry mouth, nose, or throat; orthostatic hypotension; anxiety; hallucinations; tachycardia; palpitations; difficult or painful urination (especially in older men)

(*continued*)

Generic and Brand Names	Indication	Side Effects
clonazepam (Klonopin), ethosuximide (Zarontin), trimethadione (Tridione)	Antiseizure medication	Drowsiness, dizziness, weakness, unsteadiness, headache, sleep disturbances, feelings of depression, hypotension, GI symptoms, bronchospasm, respiratory depression, arthralgia, myalgia, allergic reaction
phenytoin (Dilantin)	Anti-epileptic agent used in control of generalized tonic-clonic, psychomotor, and temporal lobe seizures. Also used in prevention and treatment of seizures occurring during or after neurosurgery	Dizziness, headache, mild nervousness, confusion, GI symptoms, sleep disturbances, ataxia, decreased coordination, nystagmus, diplopia, arthralgia, skin rash, liver damage
amitriptyline (Elavil)	Antidepressant	MI, CVA, arrhythmia, orthostatic hypotension, syncope, fatigue, tachycardia, palpitations, seizure, sleep disturbances, headache, peripheral neuropathy, ataxia, tardive dyskinesia, paresthesias, hallucinations, delusions, confusion, coma
haloperidol (Haldol)	Antipsychotic agent	Blurred vision, dry mouth, weight gain, drowsiness, GI symptoms, skin rash, involuntary muscle spasms, headache, dehydration
levodopa (i.e., L-dopa), carbidopa and levodopa (Sinemet)	Used in treatment of Parkinson's disease	Dry mouth, dyskinesia, orthostatic hypotension, HTN, cardiac irregularities, syncope, dyspnea, psychotic episodes, depression, sleep disturbances, GI symptoms, GI bleeding, anorexia, UTI, dry mouth, phlebitis, back and shoulder pain
lithium, hioridatine (Mellaril), chlorpromazine (Thorazine), clozapine (Clozaril)	Antipsychotic agent	Seizure, dizziness, HTN, involuntary muscle spasms, dyspnea, fever, GI symptoms, puckering of the mouth, jitteriness, sensitivity to light

Generic and Brand Names	Indication	Side Effects
phenobarbital, carbamazepine (Tegretol)	Anticonvulsant agent	Fatigue, depression, difficulty concentrating, memory problems, dizziness, bone loss, dry mouth, GI symptoms, rash, fever
fluoxetine (Prozac), imiprimine (Tofranil), bupropion (Wellbutrin), sertraline (Zoloft)	Antidepressants	Drowsiness, blurred vision, GI symptoms, weight gain, increased appetite, orthostatic hypotension, arrhythmia, tremor
t-PA (i.e., tissue plasminogen activator)	Thrombolytic or "super-anticoagulant" that dissolves blood clots. Used only during the 3-hr window after acute CVA	GI, GU, or intracranial bleeding; headache; light-headedness; fever; nausea; chest pain; low back pain; allergic reaction
Musculoskeletal and orthopedic		
Colchicine	Used in the treatment of gout	Drowsiness, GI symptoms, hematuria, bone marrow depression, aplastic anemia, renal insufficiency
Corticosteroids such as cortisone, hydrocortisone, prednisone	Anti-inflammatory medication, also used in treatment of autoimmune and endocrine disorders	Osteoporosis, weight gain, hyperglycemia, depression, headache, restlessness, HTN, peptic ulcers, fragile skin
alendronate (Fosamax)	Used in the treatment of osteoporosis and Paget's disease	Hypokalemia, weakness, musculoskeletal pain, headache, GI symptoms, arrhythmias, HTN, and headache
azathioprine (Imuran), methotrexate (Rheumatrex, Trexall)	Disease modifying antirheumatic drugs used in treatment of arthritic disorders	Arthralgia, myalgia, alopecia, fatigue, hypotension, HTN, tachycardia, chest pain, GI symptoms, upper respiratory tract infections
salicylates/aspirin (Anacin, Bufferin), ibuprofen (Advil, Motrin), indomethacin (Indocin), naproxen (Aleve, Naprosyn), celecoxib (Celebrex)	NSAIDs	Headache, dizziness, drowsiness, hypokalemia, tinnitus, edema, gastritis, peptic ulcer disease, heartburn, nausea, vomiting

(continued)

Generic and Brand Names	Indication	Side Effects
diazepam (Valium), baclofen (Lioresal), cyclobenzaprine (Flexeril)	Antispasticity agents and muscle relaxants. Also used frequently in patients with neurological disorders such as TBI and SCI	Dry mouth, constipation, nausea, hypotension, edema, dizziness, fatigue, headache, arrhythmia
Endocrine		
insulin lispro (Humalog), insulin aspart (Novolog), insulin glulisine (Apidra)	Ultra rapid-acting insulin	Hypoglycemia, headache, nausea, confusion, trouble concentrating, drowsiness, weakness, dizziness, blurred vision, fast heartbeat, sweating, hypokalemia, rash, allergic reaction, tremor, seizure
Regular human insulin (Humulin R, Novolin R)	Short-acting insulin	Hypoglycemia, blurred vision, weight gain, allergic reaction
isophane insulin (Neutral Protamine Hagedorn or NPH)	Intermediate-acting insulin	Hypoglycemia, dizziness, sweating, irritability, headache, hunger, weight gain, hypersensitivity
isophane insulin (Novolin N, Humulin N), insulin detemir (Levemir), insulin glargine (Lantus)	Long-acting insulin	Hypoglycemia, weight gain, rash
biguanides, such as metformin (Glucophage, Riomet Fortamet, Glumetza)	Oral hypoglycemic used in treatment of Type 2 diabetes	GI symptoms, metallic taste
sulfonylureas, such as glyburide (Micronase, DiaBeta), glipizide (Glucotrol), glimepiride (Amaryl)	Oral hypoglycemic used in the treatment of Type 2 diabetes	Hypoglycemia, GI symptoms
thiazolidinediones such as rosiglitazone (Avandia), pioglitazone (Actos)	Oral hypoglycemic used in the treatment of Type 2 diabetes	Associated with liver problems
alpha glucosidase inhibitors such as acarbose (Precose), miglitol (Glyset)	Oral hypoglycemic used in the treatment of Type 2 diabetes	Flatulence, diarrhea, abdominal bloating
levothyroxine (Levothroid, Synthroid, Levoxyl, Levoxine)	Used in treatment of hypothyroidism	Insomnia, headache, irritability, HTN, tachycardia, arrhythmia, GI symptoms, weight loss

Generic and Brand Names	Indication	Side Effects
propylthiouracil (i.e., PTU), methimazole, beta-adrenergic blockers such as propranolol, potassium iodides (Pima), lidocaine hydrochloride (LidoPen), radioactive iodine (also know as sodium iodide 131)	Antithyroid medications used in treatment of hyperthyroidism	GI symptoms, arrhythmia, myalgia, arthralgia, rash, hypothyroidism, hyperkalemia
Calcium supplements such as calcium carbonate, calcium citrate (Citracal), calcium gluconate, calcitriol	Used in the treatment of hypoparathyroidism	GI symptoms
Biophosphates such as alendronate (Fosamax), etidronate (Didronel), pamidronate (Aredia)	Used in prevention of osteoporosis or bone fracture in patients with Paget's disease or bone metastases; can be used to treat hyperparathyroidism	HTN, headache, tachycardia, GI symptoms, weakness, musculoskeletal pain, hypokalemia
vasopressin (Pitressin, Pressyn)	ADH, vasopressin; regulates water retention	MI, angina, GI symptoms, fever, dizziness, headache
Gastrointestinal and genitourinary		
azathioprine (Imuran)	Immune-modulating drug used in the treatment of Crohn's disease	Increased risk of infection, fatigue, nausea, vomiting, loss of appetite, hepatoxicity
Dulcolax, FiberCon, Metamucil, Colace, Correctol	Laxatives used in treatment of constipation	Rectal bleeding, nausea, vomiting, abdominal pain or cramps, weakness, dizziness
Kaopectate, Lomotil, Immodium, Maalox, Pepto-Bismol	Used in treatment of diarrhea	Constipation, urinary retention, tachycardia, dizziness, drowsiness, headache, confusion
furosemide (Lasix)	Loop diuretic, used in treating fluid retention	Dry mouth, thirst, nausea, vomiting, drowsiness, light-headedness, weakness, easy bruising, hearing loss, skin rash, loss of appetite, jaundice, low fever

(continued)

Generic and Brand Names	Indication	Side Effects
mercaptopurine (Purinethol)	Immune-modulating drug used in the treatment of Crohn's disease	Arthralgia, bone marrow suppression, hair loss, rash, hepatic dysfunction, susceptibility to infection, nausea, vomiting, diarrhea, neoplasms, pancreatitis
esomeprazole (Nexium), omeprazole (Prilosec), lansoprazole (Prevacid), pantoprazole (Protonix), Rabeprazole (Aciphex)	Proton pump inhibitors used in treatment of ulcers and GERD	Nausea, vomiting, diarrhea, flatulence, abdominal pain, headache, weakness, fatigue, drowsiness, chest pain, dry mouth, rash
famotidine (Pepcid)	Used in prevention and treatment of ulcers (decreases acid secretions)	Headache, dizziness
promethazine (Phenergan, Anergan), prochlorperazine (Compazine), dimenhydrinate (Dramamine), Zofran	Anti-emetics used in the treatment of nausea and vomiting	Blurred vision, dizziness, drowsiness, fatigue, dry mouth, constipation, HTN, hypotension, bradycardia, tachycardia, rash, photosensitivity
metoclopramide (Reglan)	Used in the treatment of GERD and diabetic gastroparesis	Restlessness, drowsiness, fatigue, insomnia, headache, confusion, depression, Parkinsonian-like symptoms (i.e., tremor, rigidity, bradykinesia), fluid retention, impotence, hypotension, HTN, arrhythmia, heart failure, GI discomfort, incontinence, urinary frequency
ranitidine (Zantac), cimetidine (Tagamet)	Histamine-receptor (H_2) blockers inhibit acid secretion; used in the treatment of GERD	Diarrhea, dizziness, somnolence, headache, peripheral neuropathy, ataxia, diplopia, confusion, hallucinations, cardiac arrhythmias, rash, vasculitis
Oncology		
Cisplatin	Used in treatment of lung, head and neck, uterine, ovarian, testicular, and prostate cancers	Otoxicity, hypokalemia, hypomagnesemia, peripheral neuropathy
Cytarabine	Used in treatment of leukemia and lymphoma	Cerebellar toxicity

Generic and Brand Names	Indication	Side Effects
dexamethasone (Decadron)	Glucosteroid used as an anti-inflammatory agent in the treatment of lymphoma, leukemia, and multiple myeloma	Irritability, insomnia, increased appetite, heartburn, fluid retention, weakness, increased blood sugar levels, impaired wound healing
doxorubicin (Adriamycin)	Used in treatment of breast, stomach, liver, bladder, and prostate cancers; sarcoma; lymphoma; multiple myeloma; and leukemia	Myelosuppression, cardiomyopathy
ifosfamide (Ifex)	Used in treatment of ovarian, breast, testicular, and lung cancers and lymphoma	Myelosuppression, lethargy, cerebellar toxicity, urinary problems
methotrexate (Rheumatrex, Trexall)	Used in treatment of breast, uterine, head and neck, uterine, and cervical cancers and leukemia	Myelosuppression, pulmonary fibrosis, transverse myelitis, osteoporosis, cerebellar dysfunction
methylprednisolone (Solu-Medrol, Medrol)	Systemic glucocorticosteroid used in the treatment of leukemia, lymphoma, and multiple myeloma Anti-inflammatory drug also used to prevent and treat GVHD for stem cell transplantation	Cellulitis, fungal infections, easy bruising (purpura), acne, weight gain, sleep disturbances, insomnia, depression, osteoporosis, weakness, diabetes, headache, glaucoma, cataracts, salt retention, edema
tamoxifen (Nolvadex)	Used in treatment of breast cancer	Hot flashes, uterine bleeding, fluid retention
taxol (Paclitaxel)	Used in treatment of breast, lung, and ovarian cancer and AIDS-related Kaposi sarcoma	Peripheral neuropathy, parethesias, seizure, bradycardia, flulike symptoms, HTN
vincristine	Used in treatment of lymphoma, leukemia, lung, and breast cancers	Paresthesia, ataxia, foot drop, cranial nerve palsies, loss of deep tendon reflexes
Anti-infection, antifungal, and antiviral agents		
amprenavir (Agenerase), indinavir (Crixivan), abacavir (Ziagen), aztreonam (i.e., AZT), zidovudine (Retrovir), didanosine (Videx)	Antiretroviral, nucleoside reverse transcriptase inhibitors, and protease inhibitors used in the treatment of HIV	Orthostatic hypotension, GI symptoms, fatigue, drowsiness, headache, weakness, peripheral neuropathy, musculoskeletal pain

(continued)

Generic and Brand Names	Indication	Side Effects
acyclovir (Avirax), ganciclovir (Cytovene), oseltamivir (Tamiflu)	Used in treatment of common viral infections	Arthralgia, ataxia, peripheral neuropathy, GI symptoms, hypotension, HTN, arrhythmia, seizure, dizziness, headache, drowsiness
sulfamethoxazole, and trimethoprim (Bactrim, Septra)	Antibiotics used to treat various infections and in prevention of *pneumocystic carinii* pneumonia	Skin rash, GI symptoms, fatigue, headache, fever, thrombocytopenia
cilastatin and impenem (Primaxin)	Antibiotics for bacterial infections (i.e., streptococcus pneumonia, enteroccoccus, Klebsiella, and *Escherichia coli (E. coli)*	Seizures, dizziness, hypotension, GI symptoms
clotrimazole topical (Mycelex, Lotrimin)	Used in prevention and treatment of fungal infections of the mouth and gut	Bad taste in mouth
ciprofloxacin (Cipro), levofloxacin (Levaquin)	Used in the treatment of respiratory, GI, and GU infections. Also used in treating septicemia, MRSA, *E. coli,* and meningitis	GI symptoms, hepatoxicity, seizures, drowsiness, fatigue, headache, dizziness, blood glucose disorders, arrhythmia
nystatin (Mycostatin), amphotericin (Fungizone), fluconazole (Diflucan)	Used in the prevention and treatment of fungal infections	Headache, dizziness, hypotension, abdominal discomfort, arthralgia, myalgia, peripheral neuropathy
penicillin	Antibiotics used in treatment of respiratory and GU infections, sepsis, endocarditis, peptic ulcer disease, and sexually transmitted diseases	GI symptoms, seizures
streptomycin, gentamicin, neomycin	Used in the prevention and treatment of gram negative bacterial infections	Nephrotoxicity, ototoxicity
tetracycline (Sumycin)	Used in treatment of acne, chronic bronchitis, and atypical pneumonia	Dizziness, rash, fatigue, GI symptoms, ataxia

Generic and Brand Names	Indication	Side Effects
valganciclovir (Valcyte)	Antiviral medication used in prevention and treatment of cytomegalovirus	Thrombocytopenia, anemia, dizziness, fatigue, edema, convulsions, parethesias, GI symptoms, upper respiratory infection, UTI, back pain, arthralgia, depression, psychosis
vancomycin (Vancocin)	Antibiotic used in treatment of severe infections (i.e., methicillin-resistant staphylococci), which are unresponsive to conventional antibiotics	Nephrotoxicity, neutropenia, hearing loss, flu symptoms, rash, redness of skin, bruising, weakness, abdominal discomfort
Transplantation		
amlodipine (Norvasc)	Antihypertensive	Hypotension, dizziness, fatigue, fluid retention, weakness
azathioprine (Imuran)	Immunosuppressant used in transplantation; also an immune-modulating drug used in the treatment of irritable bowel disease	Bone marrow suppression, leukopenia, pancreatitis, cholestasis, anorexia, hepatotoxicity, arthralgia, hair loss, rash, susceptibility to infection, GI symptoms, neoplasms; may cause nightmares
cyclosporine (Neoral, Sandimmune, Gengraf)	Immunosuppressant used in transplantation to prevent acute rejection	Increased risk of infection, HTN, renal dysfunction, hemolytic uremic syndrome, lymphocytic proliferative syndrome, tremors, paresthesias, sodium retention, hyperkalemia, hyperglycemia, hepatic dysfunction, seizures, hirsutism, thickening of gums, elevated cholesterol, anemia, headaches; may cause gallstones. Prolonged use may lead to diabetic neurotoxicity and decreased bone density.

(continued)

Generic and Brand Names	Indication	Side Effects
muromonab-DC3 (Orthoclone OKT3)	Immunosuppressant used in organ transplantation. Used for acute rejection when nonresponsive to other immunosuppressants	Chest pain, fever, chills, GI symptoms, pulmonary edema, bronchospasm, dyspnea, pruritus, malignant lymphoma, rigor, malaise, meningitis, mental status changes, hypokalemia, anaphylaxis
mycophenolate mofetil (CellCept)	Antirejection immunosuppressant	GI symptoms, leukopenia, neutropenia, sepsis, abdominal pain, leg cramps, headache
sirolimus (Rapamune)	Antirejection immunosuppressant	Hyperlipidemia, bone marrow suppression, and thrombocytopenia in liver transplant patients with preexisting thrombocytopenia
tacrolimus (FK506, Prograf)	Antirejection immunosuppressant	Increased risk of infection, tremors, headaches, thinning hair, hepatotoxicity, neurotoxicity, HTN, hyperglycemia, hyperkalemia, GI symptoms, renal dysfunction, mental status changes, depression, headache, insomnia, photophobia, diabetes; may cause gallstones
Pain		
aspirin	Oral analgesic; used in treating headache, muscle aches, or fever	Stomach irritation; can prolong bleeding. Not for use in children or teenagers, pregnancy, or those with kidney or liver disease, asthma, high blood pressure, and bleeding disorders
acetaminophen	Oral analgesic used to relieve generalized aches and pains and reduce fevers	Associated with liver toxicity
celecoxib (Celebrex)	Cox-2 inhibitor class of NSAID used to treat pain or inflammation caused by a variety of conditions including arthritis and ankylosing spondylitis	GI and cardiovascular

Generic and Brand Names	Indication	Side Effects
fentanyl (Duragesic)	Opioid; continuous dose is delivered via a patch worn for 3 days. Used to treat chronic pain	Confusion, headache, dizziness, weakness, shallow breathing, GI symptoms, dry mouth
ibuprofen (Advil, Motrin, Nuprin)	NSAID used to treat pain and reduce fever	GI discomfort
methadone	Narcotic pain reliever used to treat pain and to reduce symptoms during drug detoxification	Hallucinations, confusions, shallow breathing, chest pain, dizziness, syncope, restlessness, sleep disturbances, dry mouth, GI symptoms
morphine (MS Contin)	Narcotic pain reliever used to treat moderate to severe pain	Seizure, confusion, memory problems, light-headedness, syncope, cold or clammy skin, shallow breathing, slow heartbeat, anxiety, GI symptoms, sleep disturbances
naproxen sodium (Aleve)	NSAID used to relieve mild to moderate pain and to reduce inflammation	GI discomfort, ulcers, internal bleeding
oxycodone (OxyContin, Roxicodon)	Narcotic pain reliever used to treat moderate to severe pain	Respiratory depression, bronchospasm, GI symptoms, hypotension, bradycardia, central nervous system depression, confusion, dizziness, seizure
Percocet	Combination of oxycodone and acetaminophen used to relieve moderate to severe pain	Shallow breathing, slow heartbeat, syncope, confusion, seizure, blurred vision, GI symptoms, dry mouth, jaundice
Vicodin	Combination of acetaminophen and hydrocodone used to treat moderate to severe pain	Shallow breathing, slow heartbeat, syncope, confusion, seizure, blurred vision, GI symptoms, dry mouth, problems with urination, tinnitus, jaundice
hydromorphone (Dilaudid)	Narcotic pain reliever used for the relief of moderate to severe pain	Nausea, vomiting, shallow breathing, slow heartbeat, seizure, convulsions, cold or clammy skin, confusion, severe weakness, dizziness, fainting

(continued)

Generic and Brand Names	Indication	Side Effects
tramadol (Ultram)	Narcotic-like pain reliever, used to treat moderate to severe pain	Seizure, skin rash, shallow breathing, weak pulse, dizziness, drowsiness, weakness, GI symptoms, blurred vision, insomnia
ketorolac (Toradol)	NSAID used short-term (≤5 days) to treat moderate to severe pain, usually after surgery	Dizziness, headache, chest pain, weakness, GI symptoms, dry mouth, problems with urination, tinnitus, jaundice

Note. ACE = angiotensin-converting enzymes; ACS = acute coronary syndrome; ADH = antidiuretic hormone; CHF = congestive heart failure; COPD = chronic obstructive pulmonary disease; CVA = cerebrovascular accident; GERD = gastroesophageal reflux disease; GI = gastrointestinal; GU = genitourinary; GVHD = graft versus host disease; HTN = hypertension; LDL = low-density lipoprotein; MI = myocardial infarction; MRSA = methicillin-resistant *Staphylococcus aureus*; PAD = peripheral artery disease; NSAID = nonsteroidal anti-inflammatory drug; SCI = spinal cord injury; TBI = traumatic brain injury; UTI = urinary tract infection.

Note. There are no generic listings for brand medications if there is no equivalent or if there are multiple listings for the same medication.

Appendix C

Bedrest Deconditioning and Prolonged Immobility

Suzanne E. Holm, MA, OTR, BCPR

Bedrest may be prescribed for people to promote medical stability, especially in cases of multiple trauma, burns, deep vein thrombosis, pulmonary embolism, and myocardial infarction. Although a prescribed length of time for bedrest varies, research has continued to advocate for early mobility, especially in the case of low back pain, myocardial infarction, and pneumonia (Moret, Aujesky, & Lamy, 2007). Early ambulation was not associated with a higher incidence of a new pulmonary embolism or deep vein thrombosis when compared with bedrest in a study with more than 3,000 patients (Aissaoui, Martins, Mouly, Weber, & Meune, 2008). Indeed, overall physical and psychological quality of life is linked to upright posture and engagement in physical activity (Acree et al., 2006; Motl & Snook, 2008).

Bedrest, which can be defined as being restricted to bed for medical purposes, and *immobility,* or limiting movement, can have deleterious effects on all body systems, including musculoskeletal, respiratory, and cardiovascular. Bedrest and immobilization can also result in secondary complications, including a decline in functional capacity. *Deconditioning,* or the reduction of functional capacity of musculoskeletal and cardiovascular systems, is well recognized as being closely linked to bedrest (Halar & Bell, 2004). Studies have indicated that musculoskeletal decline can begin in as early as 6–48 hours with up to a 40% loss of muscle strength in 1 week that is further exacerbated by elevated cortisol levels that promote additional muscle protein catabolism (Paddon-Jones et al., 2006; Storch & Kruszynski, 2008). Additionally, a study by Needham (2008) indicated that more than 45% of clients in the intensive care unit (ICU) had associated neuromuscular dysfunction as a result of prolonged inactivity and immobility, regardless of the admitting diagnosis. Early mobilization is strongly supported, especially for clients in the ICU (Bernhardt, 2008; Needham, 2008; Perme, Southard, Joyce, Noon, & Loebe, 2006). Table C.1 lists the effects of immobility on the major organ systems.

Effects of Bedrest and Immobility on Body Systems

All body systems are negatively affected by prolonged bedrest and immobility. Changes to the musculoskeletal, cardiovascular, and respiratory systems include weakness, contractures, deconditioning, hypotension, hypoventilation, and an increased risk for deep vein thrombosis formation and pneumonia. A person's metabolic homeostasis declines resulting in impaired protein and fat metabolism and bone loss. The skin is at greater risk for pressure ulcers and systemic infection. There is reduced peristalsis and increased constipation and urinary retention within the gastrointestinal and urologic systems. Psychologically, the person may experience confusion and depression with sustained immobility. The major body systems and the effects of bedrest are explored in the following sections.

Musculoskeletal System

Deconditioning caused by bedrest can be independent of the primary disease and physically debilitating in clients who attempt to resume normal active living and working (Bernhardt, Dewey,

Table C.1.   Effects of Immobility on Organ Systems

Organ System	Effects of Immobility
Musculoskeletal	Weakness, muscle and joint contracture, osteoporosis, exercise intolerance
Cardiovascular	Deconditioning, orthostatic hypotension, increased risk for thrombus formation
Respiratory	Hypoventilation, atelectasis, increased risk for pneumonia
Metabolic–endocrine	Decreased metabolic rate, impaired protein and fat metabolism, bone loss
Integumentary	Pressure ulcers, systemic infection
Neurological–psychological	Confusion, sensory deprivation, depression, impaired coping
Gastrointestinal–urologic	Constipation, reflux, urinary retention, reduced peristalsis

Thrift, & Donnan, 2004; Halar & Bell, 2004). Additional musculoskeletal system dysfunction caused by bedrest deconditioning and prolonged immobility can result in

- Reduced muscle contraction of postural muscle and shortening of collagen-containing tissues;
- Increased risk for injury to bones and joints from loss of muscle mass and diminished bone density;
- Increased risk of osteoporosis because of calcium loss (Bell, 2006);
- Deficiency in motor neuron activation;
- Reduction of blood flow to muscles, red blood cell volume, capillary network, and development of oxidative enzymes, resulting in increased muscle fatigue (Fielding & Bean, 2006); and
- Joint contractures from a decrease in the length and diameter of the muscle fibers and extensibility, an increase in intramuscular connective tissues, and a decrease in capillary density in the muscle (Bell, 2006).

Neural organization required to provide maximal voluntary muscle contraction diminishes after 6 weeks (Bell, 2006). Therefore, reduced balance and incoordination are frequently seen after prolonged bedrest, increasing the client's risk for falls and ability to compensate during functional activity.

Cardiovascular System

Cardiovascular system dysfunction from immobility can result in orthostatic hypotension, increased workload of the heart, and increased risk for thrombus formation. Additional cardiovascular dysfunction caused by deconditioning and immobility can result in

- Decreased ability of the autonomic nervous system to regulate blood volume and pressure, impaired sympathetic activation, and orthostatic intolerance;
- Recumbent posture increases central blood volume and stimulates diuresis, resulting in loss of plasma volume *(hypovolemia)*;
- Hypovolemia complications include venous stasis and blood hypercoagulability, increasing the risk for thrombogenesis (Dean, 2007);
- A recumbent position causes the blood vessels of both cardiac and smooth muscles to dilate, resulting in a decreased ability for effective contraction when upright, increasing the risk for dizziness and fainting;

- Maximal aerobic capacity diminishes 9%–12% after 7–10 days of bedrest (Convertino, Bloomfield, & Greenleaf, 1997; Kortebein et al., 2008);

- After 7 days of bedrest, stroke volume decreases 15% (Halar & Bell, 2004); and

- With immobilization, the heart rate increases 0.5 beats per minutes per day; a greater risk for tachycardia occurs with prolonged bedrest (Strax, Gonzalez, & Cuccurullo, 2004).

Pulmonary System and Respiratory Function

The respiratory and cardiovascular systems are closely linked, and prolonged immobility and bedrest will further compromise pulmonary effectiveness. Inactivity increases the risk for deep vein thrombosis formation, which can contribute to development of a pulmonary embolus. The recumbent position places extra pressure against the chest wall, reducing effective inspiration and expiration while further disrupting the oxygen and carbon dioxide balance and contributing to oxygen desaturation or hypoxemia. Additional pulmonary complications and respiratory dysfunction resulting from prolonged immobility and bedrest in the supine position include

- Limited lung expansion that reduces effective gas exchange and increases the risk for pooled or stagnant secretions (Bergquist & Neuberger, 2006);

- Reduction in the cough reflex and effectiveness, increasing the risk for pneumonia; and

- Diminished pulmonary lung flow, which increases the risk for *atelectasis* (i.e., collapse of part of the lung) and pulmonary infection (Bell, 2006).

Endocrine and Metabolic Systems

Bedrest deconditioning and immobility result in systemic metabolic and endocrine system changes, especially when complicated by traumatic injury or chronic illness. The excretion and subsequent loss of essential electrolytes may include nitrogen, sodium, potassium, phosphorus, and calcium. Electrolytes control fluid levels, acid–base balance, nerve conduction, blood clotting, and muscle contraction. Immobility and bedrest deconditioning can result in additional endocrine and metabolic system dysfunction:

- Immobility facilitates production of thyroid hormone, resulting in bone loss; decreases androgen hormone production, which also decreases bone mass; and reduces glucose tolerance, which impairs protein and fat metabolism (Marini & Wheeler, 2005);

- Physical inactivity is associated with the development of insulin resistance, dyslipidemia, increased blood pressure, and impaired microvascular function in healthy people (Hamburg et al., 2007);

- The stress response to critical illness, such as activation of the hypothalamic–pituitary–adrenal axis, can lead to increased production of glucocorticoids that contribute to increased blood glucose levels, decreased insulin action, inhibition of connective tissue and bone formation, decreased gastrointestinal absorption of calcium, and increased calciuria (Tobin & Uchakin, 2005);

- High levels of glucocorticoids are associated with immunosuppression; and

- Immobility causes cortisol levels to rise; hypercortisolemia results in proteolysis (breakdown of proteins) primarily in fast-twitch Type II white muscle fibers (Tobin & Uchakin, 2005), resulting in skeletal muscle atrophy and dysfunction.

Integumentary System

Muscle action promotes healthy and effective circulation. Immobility and bedrest deconditioning reduce circulation in soft tissues and limit tissue perfusion over bony prominences, increasing the risk for skin breakdown. Decubitus ulcers result where the tissue becomes necrotic and ulcerates. Sustained pressure over an area also reduces nerve sensitivity, which diminishes blood supply, ultimately restricting nutrients to that area. Areas susceptible to ischemia include the occipital region, scapula, elbows, sacrum, coccyx, ischial tuberosities, trochanters, and heels. The supine position also dilates blood vessels and increases perspiration. In turn, macerated or wet skin is more vulnerable to skin breakdown.

Malnourishment, which often occurs simultaneously with critical illness and bedrest, contributes to muscle protein loss and creates a negative nitrogen balance, restricting tissue health and growth. The risk for systemic infection is greater if wounds become ulcerated and infected. In severe cases, osteomyelitis or life-threatening sepsis can result.

Neurological and Psychological Systems

Immobility is linked with reduced quality of life, especially with prolonged illness or ICU hospitalization (Dowdy et al., 2005). Studies have linked bedrest deconditioning and sustained immobility with a reduction in independence for self-care skills, increased sensory deprivation, and the development of cognitive impairments that can include disorientation, depression, anxiety, confusion, or even delirium. People may also experience disturbances in a healthy sleep-and-wake cycle. The supine position alters a person's metabolic rate, temperature, and hormone function; therefore, a prolonged immobile posture will affect homeostatic mechanisms.

Gastrointestinal and Urologic Systems

Increased urinary excretion occurs when the client is placed on bedrest, especially during the first few days of immobilization, because of increased kidney circulation in the recumbent position. Many clients experience a loss of appetite, decreased gastrointestinal peristalsis, and a diminished ability to functionally eat or self-feed in the supine position. A reduction in oral intake can result in dehydration and loss of nutrition. Additionally, constipation from a reduction in peristalsis is further complicated by a decline in intestinal and calcium absorption.

Chronic Critical Illness and Long-Term Critical Care

Prolonged bedrest resulting from chronic critical illness and long-term critical care further affects the metabolic and endocrine systems, complicating changes to the musculoskeletal system. Additional chronic critical illness dysfunction caused by bedrest deconditioning and immobility can result in

- Atrophy of skeletal muscles from deconditioning and hypokinesia;
- Accelerated bone loss and systemic protein loss;
- Neuroendocrine decline in hepatic insulin-like growth factor 1 production, thyroid, and gonad function (Mesotten & Van den Berghe, 2006; Van den Berghe, 2002; Vanhorebeek & Van den Berghe, 2006), which are required for normal growth and metabolism;
- Increased susceptibility to contraction-induced tearing because of muscle fiber atrophy (Tobin & Uchakin, 2005) from muscle inactivity and hypercortisolemia; and
- Myopathy as a result of biochemical changes (e.g., protein kinase C), which can contribute to further immobility (Vattemi et al., 2004).

Implications for Occupational Therapy

Prolonged immobility significantly impairs all of the body systems and a client's ability to engage in daily activities. Clients frequently experience impaired muscle weakness, activity intolerance, hypotension, hypoventilation, and sensory deprivation. Bedrest and immobility can result in a decline in a client's functional capacity, including the ability to complete activities of daily living (ADLs). Research on specific protocols and therapeutic interventions for clients who have extended hospitalizations remain limited; researchers have indicated the need for further investigation, including development of safety parameters and therapy guidelines (Morris & Herridge, 2007). Although most research has focused on the client's physical status, the occupational therapist should seek to incorporate the client's emotional and cognitive status into the overall plan of care to optimize participation in basic ADLs (Coster, Haley, Jette, Tao, & Siebens, 2007).

Clients who require the ICU or mechanical ventilation face additional challenges regarding deconditioning and immobility. A review of studies between 1990 and 2007 by Choi, Frederick, and Hoffman (2008) examined the use of various mobility interventions (i.e., electrical stimulation, arm exercise, inspiratory muscle training) with clients on prolonged mechanical ventilation; however, the evidence on how to specifically improve mobility outcomes is limited. Stiller, Phillips, and Lampert (2004) examined the effectiveness of early mobility, including ambulation, in a study of 31 ICU patients. The results of early mobility were significant increases in both heart rate and blood pressure with mild desaturation levels. In spite of the cardiovascular changes, Stiller et al. supported the use of early mobilization. Stiller's (2007) later study provided more comprehensive guidelines when therapy is initiated for clients who have been critically ill or have had prolonged immobility to decrease the risk of pulmonary complications, decrease the duration of mechanical ventilation, decrease the length of hospitalization, and increase recovery rates.

The elderly population, especially those people with chronic conditions, is at a greater risk for loss of physical and mental well-being when hospitalized because of associated baseline inactivity, nutritional compromise, decline in cognitive functioning, possible depression, and reduced energy reserves. To facilitate function during hospitalization, research by Gillis and MacDonald (2005) recommended a hospital environment that is "elder friendly" and included frequent walking and exercise programs. A review of more than 3,000 studies by de Morton, Keating, and Jeffs (2007)

suggested that multidisciplinary intervention, which included exercise for acutely ill elderly people, may result in reduced hospitalization length of stay and cost. Gill, Allore, Holford, and Guo (2004) endorsed the use of interventions that increase clients' reserve capacity and promote compensatory strategies to minimize the progression of disability.

To minimize the deleterious effects of deconditioning and immobility, studies on elderly people in nursing facilities indicated that exposing clients to outdoor light, keeping clients out of bed, and providing structured physical activity were proactive means to promote increased functional activity (Martin, Marler, Harker, Joesphson, & Alessi, 2007). Adler and Roberts (2006) recommended the use of Tai Chi for elderly patients, especially for those with chronic illnesses, to address flexibility and activity tolerance needs. This study's recommendations could have positive implications for hospitalized clients in the acute care setting to promote functional gains.

Intervention

Occupational therapists can incorporate occupational performance skills to increase the client's tolerance for activity, in preparation for further self-care activities after bedrest deconditioning and prolonged immobility, through

- Education of client and relevant others about the positive effects of movement and activity and the consequences associated with bedrest and immobility;
- Bed positioning to increase tolerance for upright posture; promote deep breathing; and encourage functional positioning for self-feeding, eating, and safe swallowing;
- Bed positioning for engagement in basic self-care, including oral hygiene, to minimize the risk for microaspiration;
- Bed mobility to promote positioning for function, optimize sensory input, and minimize risk for skin breakdown;
- Exercise programs at bed level to include movement against gravity, isometrics when appropriate, weight-bearing activities, and integration of core muscles;

- Upper-extremity stretching and neuromuscular reeducation;
- Upper-extremity exercises to facilitate movement against gravity, functional upper-extremity use, adaptive equipment training, and coordination skills;
- Splinting to address upper-extremity range-of-motion deficits and positioning needs;
- Progressing activity from bed level or long sitting in bed, to edge of bed, then to out of bed or chair level;
- Enhancing skills for orientation, attention and concentration tasks, memory activities, and visual–perceptual abilities; and
- Incorporating the use of leisure activities, meaningful occupations, and social interaction.

Studies specifically focusing on occupational therapy intervention for clients at risk for deconditioning from prolonged immobility or hospitalization, although limited in sample size, have promoted engagement in purposeful activity and meaningful occupation. Bynon, Wilding, and Eyres (2007) developed an acute care occupational therapy pilot program that improved overall occupational performance and reduced length of stays by increasing the use of activity. Specifically, educating families on how to minimize sensory deprivation (e.g., providing glasses, hearing aids), promoting engagement in functional activities (e.g., reading the newspaper, crafts), and using public spaces (e.g., cafeteria, chapel, park) had positive outcomes (Bynon, Wilding, & Eyres, 2007). Another acute care pilot program by Eyres and Unsworth (2005) studied elderly clients and concluded that clients receiving occupational therapy services reported feeling more confident in self-care skills and experienced a greater sense of well-being with improved client family satisfaction. Further research and additional studies are needed in support of occupational therapy intervention with clients who are at risk for bedrest deconditioning and immobility.

References

Acree, L. S., Longfors, J., Fjeldstad, A. S., Fjeldstad, C., Schank, B., Nickel, K. J., et al. (2006). Physical activity is related to quality of life in older adults. *Health and Quality Life Outcomes, 30*(4), 37.

Adler, P. A., & Roberts, B. L. (2006). The use of Tai Chi to improve health in older adults. *Orthopedic Nursing, 25*, 122–126.

Aissaoui, N., Martins, E., Mouly, S., Weber, S., & Meune, C. (2008). A meta-analysis of bedrest versus early ambulation in the management of pulmonary embolism, deep vein thrombosis, or both. *International Journal of Cardiology, 137*, 37–41.

Bell, K. (2006). Complications associated with immobility after TBI. In N. D. Zasler, D. I. Katz, & R.D. Zafonte (Eds.), *Brain injury medicine: Principles and practice* (pp. 605–614). New York: Demos Medical.

Bergquist, S., & Neuberger, G. B. (2006). Altered mobility and fatigue. In I. M. Lubkin & P. D. Larsen (Eds.), *Chronic illness* (5th ed., pp. 147–178). Boston: Jones & Bartlett.

Bernhardt J. (2008). Very early mobilization following acute stroke: Controversies, the unknowns, and a way forward. *Annals of Indian Academy of Neurology, 11*, 88–98.

Bernhardt, J., Dewey, H., Thrift, A., & Donnan, G. (2004). Inactive and alone: Physical activity within the first 14 days of acute stroke unit care. *Stroke, 35*, 1005–1009.

Bynon, S., Wilding, C., & Eyres, L. (2007). An innovative occupation-focused service to minimise deconditioning in the hospital: Challenges and solutions. *Australian Occupational Therapy Journal, 54*, 225–227.

Choi, J., Frederick, J. T., & Hoffman, L. A. (2008). Mobility interventions to improve outcomes in patients undergoing prolonged mechanical ventilation: A review of the literature. *Biological Research for Nursing, 10*(1), 21–33.

Convertino, V. A., Bloomfield, S. A., & Greenleaf, J. E. (1997). An overview of the issues: Physiological effects of bedrest and restricted physical activity. *Medicine and Science in Sports and Exercise, 29*, 187–190.

Coster, W., Haley, S. M., Jette, A., Tao, W., & Siebens, H. (2007). Predictors of basic and instrumental activities of daily living performance in persons receiving rehabilitation services. *Archives of Physical Medicine and Rehabilitation, 88*, 928–935.

Dean, E. (2007). Impaired aerobic capacity/endurance associated with deconditioning (Pattern B).

In M. Moffat (Chief Ed.) & D. Frownfelter (Assoc. Ed.), *Cardiovascular/pulmonary essentials: Applying the preferred physical therapist practice patterns* (pp. 37–82). Thorofare, NJ: Slack.

de Morton, N.A., Keating, J. L., & Jeffs, K. (2007). Exercise for acutely hospitalised older medical patients. *Cochrane Database of Systematic Reviews, 1*, CD005955. Retrieved December 1, 2008, from http://mrw.interscience.wiley.com/cochrane/clsys rev/articles/CD005955/frame.html

Dowdy, D. W., Eid, M. P., Sedrakyan, A., Mendex-Tellez, P. A., Pronovost, P. J., Herridge, M. S., et al. (2005). Quality of life in adult survivors of critical illness: A systematic review of the literature. *Intensive Care Medicine, 31*, 611–620.

Eyres, L., & Unsworth, C. A. (2005). Occupational therapy in acute hospitals: The effectiveness of a pilot program to maintain occupational performance in older clients. *Australian Occupational Therapy Journal, 5*, 218–224.

Fielding, R. A., & Bean, J. (2006). Acute physiological responses to dynamic exercise. In W. R. Frontera (Chief Ed.), D. M. Slovik, & D. M. Dawson (Assoc. Eds.), *Exercise in rehabilitation medicine* (2nd ed., pp. 3–12). Champaign, IL: Human Kinetics.

Gill, T. M., Allore, H. G., Holford, T. R., & Guo, Z. (2004). Hospitalization, restricted activity, and the development of disability among older persons. *JAMA, 292*, 2115–2124.

Gillis, A., & MacDonald, B. (2005). Deconditioning in the hospitalized elderly. *Canadian Nursing, 101*, 16–20.

Halar, E. M., & Bell, K. R. (2004). Immobility and inactivity: Physiological and functional changes, prevention, and treatment. In J. A. DeLisa, B. M. Gans, N. E. Walsh, W. L. Bockenek, & W. R. Frontera (Eds.), *Physical medicine rehabilitation: Principles and practice* (4th ed., pp. 1447–1468). Philadelphia: Lippincott Williams & Wilkins.

Hamburg, N. M, McMackin, C. J., Huang, A. L, Shenouda, S. M., Widlansky, M. E., Schultz, E., et al. (2007). Physical inactivity rapidly induces insulin resistance and microvascular dysfunction in healthy volunteers. *Arteriosclerosis, Thrombosis, and Vascular Biology, 27*, 2650–2651.

Kortebein, P., Symons, T. B., Ferrando, A., Paddon-Jones, D., Ronsen, O., Protas, E., et al. (2008). Functional impact of 10 days of bedrest in healthy older adults. *Journals of Gerontology, Series A: Biological Sciences and Medical Sciences, 63*(A), 1076–1081.

Marini, J. J., & Wheeler, A. P. (2005). General supportive care. In J. J. Marini & A. P. Wheeler (Eds.), *Critical care medicine: The essentials* (3rd ed., pp. 291–310). Philadelphia: Lippincott Williams & Wilkins.

Martin, J. L., Marler, M. R., Harker, J. O., Josephson, K. R., & Alessi, C. A. (2007). A multicomponent nonpharmacological intervention improves activity rhythms among nursing home residents with disrupted sleep/wake patterns. *Journals of Gerontology Series A: Biological Sciences and Medical Sciences, 62*(A), 67–72.

Mesotten, D., & Van den Berghe, G. (2006). Changes within the GH/IGF-I/IGFBP axis in critical illness. *Critical Care Clinics, 22*(1), 17–28.

Moret, C., Aujesky, D., & Lamy, O. (2007). Complete bedrest prescription in an internal medicine ward: A dangerous treatment? *Revue Medicale Suisse, 3*(131), 2479–2482.

Morris, P. E. & Herridge, M. S. (2007). Early intensive care unit mobility: Further directions. *Critical Care Clients, 23*, 97–110.

Motl, R. W., & Snook, E. M. (2008). Physical activity, self-efficacy, and quality of life in multiple sclerosis. *Annals of Behavioral Medicine, 35*, 111–115.

Needham, D. M. (2008). Mobilizing patients in the intensive care unit: Improving neuromuscular weakness and physical function. *JAMA, 300*, 1685–1690.

Paddon-Jones, D., Sheffield-Moore, M., Cree, M. G., Hewlings, S. J., Aarsland, A., Wolfe, R. R., et al. (2006). Atrophy and impaired muscle protein synthesis during prolonged inactivity and stress. *Journal of Clinical Endocrinology and Metabolism, 91*, 4836–4841.

Perme, C. S., Southard, R. E., Joyce, D. L, Noon, G. P., & Loebe, M. (2006). Early mobilization of LVAD recipients who require prolonged mechanical ventilation. Texas Heart Institute Journal, 33, 130–133.

Stiller, K. (2007). Safety issues that should be considered when mobilizing critically ill patients. *Critical Care Clinics, 23*, 35–53.

Stiller, K., Phillips, A. C., & Lambert, P. (2004). The safety of mobilization and its effect on hemodynamic and respiratory status of intensive care patients. *Physiotherapy Theory and Practice, 20,* 175–185.

Storch, E. K., & Kruszynski, D. M. (2008). From rehabilitation to optimal function: Role of clinical exercise therapy. *Current Opinion in Critical Care, 14,* 451–455.

Strax, T. E., Gonzalez, P., & Cuccurullo, S. (2004). Physical modalities, therapeutic exercise, extended bedrest, and aging effects. In S. Cuccurullo (Ed.), *Physical medicine and rehabilitation board review* (pp. 533–584). New York: Demos Medical.

Tobin, B. W., & Uchakin, P. N. (2005). Nutritional consequences of critical illness myopathies. *Journal of Nutrition, 135,* 1803S–1805S.

Van den Berghe, G. (2002). Neuroendocrine pathobiology of chronic critical illness. *Critical Care Clinics, 18,* 509–528.

Vanhorebeek, I., & Van den Berghe, G. (2006). The neuroendocrine response to critical illness is a dynamic process. *Critical Care Clinics, 22*(1), 1–15.

Vattemi, G., Tonin, P., Mora, M., Filosto, L., Morandi, C., Savio, I., et al. (2004). Expression of protein kinase C isoforms and interleukin-1ß in myofibrillar myopathy. *Neurology, 62,* 1778–1782.

Appendix D

Energy Conservation and Work Simplification Strategies

Natan Berry, MS, OTR/L

Energy conservation improves total endurance and reserves more energy for activities that are most important or most valued. Simplifying a task and reducing the amount of effort required to complete it reduces the amount of stress produced and causes less pain. These principles allow a person to have optimal performance with minimal physical output. Many activities can be graded to decrease the amount of energy or effort needed to accomplish a task. Each day, a person begins with a certain amount of energy. Spend it too soon, and none will be left for the rest of the day. Balancing work and rest helps to ensure a person has enough energy to make it through the whole day. Please see Box D.1 for basic principles in energy conservation.

Energy Conservation Tips

- Sit for as many activities as possible.
- Allow yourself more time for each activity.
- Consider the best time of day for each activity.
- Eliminate unnecessary tasks (e.g., air drying the dishes instead of hand drying).
- Take frequent rests. Rest before getting too tired or overfatigued.
- Balance rest and activity.
- Preplan activities: Try daily schedules, weekly schedules, or both so activities can be evenly spread out.
- Store things that are used often at a level comfortable to reach to avoid excessive reaching, bending, or stretching.

- Avoid lifting and carrying heavy objects.
- When engaging in activities, use both arms (hands) in smooth, flowing motions. Avoid jerky movements.
- Remember to use pursed-lip breathing during activities that may increase your shortness of breath. *Pursed-lip breathing* is breathing in through the nose and out through gently pursed lips (i.e., smell the roses and blow out the birthday candles).

Avoid Unnecessary Motions

- Minimize steps in a task. Consider what you are going to do next.
- Use labor-saving equipment that is easy to handle and operate.
- Avoid overreaching and bending by arranging equipment and materials in your work area within easy reach.
- Slide objects; do not lift and carry.
- Use carts with wheels to substitute for carrying or lifting.
- Use good posture and body mechanics.
- Use proper breathing techniques when performing any task.
- Perform a task in the proper sequence. Repeating the same methods will increase skill and make movements more efficient and economical. For example, if you normally put on a shirt before your pants, keep that sequence consistent. Do not don pants before your shirt, deviating from your normal routine.
- Combine steps when possible (e.g., don underwear and slacks over feet at the same time before pulling both up over hips).

Box D.1.   Principles of Energy Conservation

Planning	Pacing
• Think ahead. — Think about what you are going to do and how you are going to do it. • Simplify. — Minimize steps in a task. — Combine tasks to eliminate extra work. • Organize. — Prevent extra movements and reduce clutter by organizing the work space. • Prepare. — Make sure you have needed supplies and equipment ready before starting the activity.	• Allow enough time to complete the activity without rushing. • Modify or eliminate activities that involve prolonged strain. • Body signals — Learn to recognize fatigue and stop before getting overtired. — Get adequate sleep. • During the day — Balance work and rest periods. — Take frequent breaks. — If needed, do part of a task and finish it later. — Work at a moderate pace. • During the week — Distribute heavy tasks over the course of the week. Do frequent preventive maintenance to avoid large jobs.
Prioritizing	**Positioning**
• Choose. — Do the most important tasks, and eliminate unnecessary ones. • Get help. — Hire help or assign duties to other family members (delegate). • Invest. — Use adaptive equipment, electronic appliances, computers, and other technology to help minimize exertion. — Invest in lightweight tools and equipment. — Install swing-out shelving, revolving shelves, or stackable bins. — Invest in an apron with pockets for carrying cooking items or cleaning utensils.	• Self — Sit to work as much as possible. — Avoid bending over or reaching overhead. — Use good posture and body mechanics in all activities. — Use slow, smooth movements, not fast, jerky movements, when completing tasks. • Objects — Slide rather than lift objects. — Use wheels (e.g., wheeled cart) to transport objects rather than carrying them. — Let gravity assist whenever possible. — Use long-handled tools to minimize excessive reaching and bending. • Environment — Organize storage areas. — Arrange work items within easy reach. — Have correct counter or work heights, noise level, and lighting. — Convert a first-floor room into a bedroom to avoid climbing stairs.

- Minimize trips between points. Gather all necessary items before moving between different rooms or locations.
- If available, use store scooters or wheelchairs for shopping instead of walking the aisles.
- Consider hiring someone to assist with certain activities, such as lawn care, maintenance, cooking, or cleaning.

Avoid Rushing

- Plan your schedule to allow time to engage in the task and also take rest periods.
- Work at a slowed, rhythmic, relaxed speed; work to music if necessary.
- Pace yourself.
- Spread heavy and light tasks throughout the day or week, doing heavy tasks when you have the most energy.
- Set priorities.
- Eliminate unnecessary tasks.
- Delegate jobs when appropriate.
- Plan frequent periods for rest and relaxation (both mentally and physically).

Set Up Proper Working Conditions

- Sit when able and at a proper work height. A good work height is when you do not have to reach or bend excessively.
- Avoid clutter in work areas.
- Optimally position needed materials and equipment close together.
- Organize all work areas by keeping all supplies for an activity or task stored together. Use organizing equipment (e.g., lazy susan, stacking shelves, bins).
- Ensure work areas have good lighting and ventilation.

Grooming and Hygiene

- Sit when possible.
- Have one designated area where all supplies are organized (e.g., razor, toothbrush, makeup, other toiletries).

- Consider a short, easier-to-care-for haircut.
- Wash hair while in the shower.
- Have hair done by a professional, or ask family members to help out.
- Support elbows on a counter or table top when tasks take 5 minutes or longer.
- Never force, bear down, or hold your breath when having a bowel movement. Take deep breaths in through your nose and push gently as you blow out through pursed lips.

Bathing and Showering

- Sit on a shower or tub chair or stool when showering or bathing.
- Sit to dress, undress, bathe, and dry.
- Use a long-handled bath sponge or hand towel to wash back and feet.
- Use lukewarm water to reduce steam if you have difficulty with shortness of breath, or decrease the amount of steam by turning on the cold water first and then adding hot water slowly.
- Use a shower hose extension (i.e., hand-held shower) to increase control over direction of spray.
- Install grab bars and nonslip strips to prevent falls.
- Organize shampoo, conditioner, and soap in an easy-to-reach place in the shower or bathtub.
- Have a towel and robe easily accessible. Use a towel or terry-cloth robe to pat yourself dry (or wear a terry-cloth robe until dry) instead of vigorously drying yourself off with a towel.
- If oxygen is prescribed, it should be worn while in the shower or bath.
- Avoid overexertion by taking rest breaks.

Dressing

- Designate a dressing area where all clothes can be reached easily.
- Before starting, gather all clothes and shoes together.

- Remember breathing techniques—Exhale while bending over or raising arms up.
- Wear loose-fitting, lightweight, comfortable clothing. Use suspenders if belts are too restricting.
- Sit to dress.
- Complete lower-body dressing before upper-body dressing.
  - Eliminate bending as much as possible to minimize shortness of breath. Consider using adaptive equipment to minimize bending.
  - Bring feet up toward body (e.g., can prop on stool) rather than bending down.
  - Minimize bending by crossing one leg over the other while sitting to put on socks, underwear, pants, or shoes.
  - Pull underwear and pants to knees while sitting, then stand one time to pull both items of clothing up over the hips.
  - Put on slip-on shoes using a long-handled shoehorn.
- Try to use clothing that opens in the front, preferably with zippers, hook-and-loop fasteners, or buttons. Shirts that open from the front do not require neck flexion, which can constrict the lungs, making breathing slightly more labored. Similarly, use a front-closing bra.

Kitchen Organization and Meal Planning

- Use a cart with wheels to move items from the refrigerator to the sink or counter.
- Use the counter space for sliding heavy objects rather than carrying them.
- Keep frequently used items and ingredients within easy reach; store items where they will be used. For example, keep canned goods near the electric can opener, and keep pots and pans near the stove.
- Keep heavier items where they can be slid back and forth rather than lifting and carrying. Store lighter items higher up.

- Use electric appliances to make the work easier and quicker. For example, use a blender, electric can opener, electric knife, or microwave oven.
- Stabilize or set objects down on the counter or table rather than holding them.
- Use lightweight utensils and cookware.
- Distribute the weight of heavy pots or trays over two hands rather than using one. Use oven mitts for handling hot items.
- Angle a mirror over the stove to see into the pots from a seated position.
- Use dishes that can go from preparation to oven to dinner table.
- Eat on paper plates or reuse dishes directly from the dishwasher.
- Inquire whether the grocery store delivers or whether Meals on Wheels is available in your area.

Cooking

- Cook large quantities, and freeze individual portions for later.
- Prepare part of the meal ahead of time.
- Use recipes that require short preparation time and little effort.
- Gather all necessary items before beginning meal preparation.
- Sit to prepare items and mix ingredients.
- Make one-pot meals.
- Use ready-made foods to eliminate preparation time.
- Avoid peeling and other preparations. Use packaged fresh vegetables or frozen products.
- Serve food directly from baking dish.

After-Meal Cleanup

- Rest after meals before starting to clean up.
- Have everyone clear their own place setting.
- Use a utility cart to transport items.

- Let dishes soak to eliminate scrubbing.
- Sit to wash dishes or use a dishwasher.
- Let dishes air dry.
- Use lightweight cloths or sponges rather than heavy terry cloth rags.

Housecleaning

- Clean a different room each day.
- Use a lightweight vacuum or power broom.
- Use long-handled dusters and cleaning attachments.
- Sit to dust.
- Use a mop or a dustpan with an extended handle to clean up spills on the floor.
- Use a dust mitt rather than gripping a dust rag.
- Break up chores over the whole week, doing a little each day.
- Keep cleaning supplies in the room in which you use them.
- Allow cleaning agents (foamy spray) time to do their work so that less scrubbing is required.

Bed Making

- Store bed linens near the bedroom.
- Use fitted sheets.
- Make as much of the bed as possible while still lying in it, or sit on the edge of the bed and scoot up as the covers are straightened.
- Use the clock method. Start at one end of the bed, and slowly make the bed as you move around it to the other side.

- Use a lightweight spread or comforter.
- Consider changing the sheets less often to conserve energy.
- Share the task with another person to reduce reaching.

Laundry

- If laundry area is downstairs or at the opposite end of the home, put soiled clothes in a large laundry bag and throw it downstairs or drag it to the washer.
- Use a scoop for a dry detergent rather than lifting the whole box. Put liquid in a pump container.
- Use a wheeled cart to move clothes.
- Make more frequent trips with lighter baskets of laundry rather than carrying heavy but less frequent loads.
- Sit to iron, sort clothes, pretreat stains, or fold laundry.
- Transfer wet clothes into the dryer a few items at a time.
- Use a long-handled reacher to remove clothes from the back of the washing machine.
- Remove clothes from the dryer immediately after cycle to avoid wrinkles.
- Get help to fold large items such as sheets.
- Buy clothes that are easy to wash and require little to no ironing.
- If you need to iron, try a travel iron, which weighs less than 2 pounds.
- When ironing, slide the iron rather than lifting it.
- Do not do all the laundry chores in 1 day. Spread the tasks out over several days.

Appendix E

Altered Mental Status

Judy R. Hamby, MHS, OTR/L, BCPR

An admitting diagnosis of altered mental status (AMS) is vague and provides minimal direction toward knowing the etiology or actual diagnosis. Loosely defined, *AMS* is an alteration in cognitive skills and functioning. It is generally the symptom, not the final diagnosis. Four of the main causes of AMS are progressive degrees of dementia, delirium (resulting from medical issues), metabolic encephalopathy, and depression (Flaherty & Rost, 2007; Gerstein, 2008; Leong, Jian, Vasu, & Seow, 2008). Some causes of AMS are reversible, and others indicate a progression of symptoms of a disease process, such as in Alzheimer's disease. For the patient with AMS, addressing and modifying environmental issues that mitigate performance and safety, focusing on caregiver education and prevention of secondary disabilities, should be therapeutically addressed in the acute care setting.

Clinical Features

Many clinical features of the causes of AMS are similar and can frequently be superimposed on preexisting diagnoses. Consider this scenario: A patient has a premorbid diagnosis of dementia, develops a urinary tract infection, and is then hospitalized with delirium. Overlapping cognitive issues such as hallucinations may be caused by the delirium and preexisting memory impairments resulting from dementia. Knowing the patient's premorbid functional status can enhance the therapeutic intervention that focuses on the newest symptoms that the family may not be able to manage. It also assists in understanding the impact the new deficits are having on the old and how they are affecting performance skills. Symptoms common to all four diagnoses are fluctuations in occupational performance skills as a result of decreased cognitive functioning, alertness and level of consciousness, and sleep disturbances. The differing symptoms of each diagnosis are delineated in Table E.1, and the mental dysfunction associated with the abnormal laboratory values frequently associated with AMS are delineated in Table E.2.

Dementia

The primary clinical feature of dementia is a progressive decline in mental functioning that impedes task performance. It is characterized by changes in performance skills that can affect behavior or appearance (e.g., poor hygiene, disheveled appearance) and memory impairment with at least one other deficit: aphasia, apraxia, agnosia, or executive function deficits (American Psychiatric Association, 2000a; Burns & Levy, 2006; Levy, 1998). Most types of dementia are irreversible; however, some causes of dementia are reversible, and often the progression can be slowed. See Table E.3 for the nonreversible and reversible etiologies of dementia.

Delirium

Delirium is a sudden and acute change in mental status, frequently presenting with psychomotor activity impairment and difficulty maintaining a stream of thought along with poor reasoning skills. Common perceptual disturbances include hallucinations, illusions, and misinterpretations. Motor signs such as tremor, myoclonus, and *asterixis* (irregular flapping movements of the outstretched hands) may also be present. Delirium can be superimposed on an existing dementia and is usually the result

Table E.1. **Differentiating the Diagnoses**

Symptom Presentation	Dementia	Delirium or Acute Confusional State	Metabolic Encephalopathy	Depression
Onset	Slow and insidious or stepwise in vascular dementia	Sudden and acute with precise time of onset (even with an existing dementia)	Usually during an acute illness	Can be chronic, recurrent, or an acute adjustment to a life change (adjustment disorder)
Duration	Years	Short time (usually <1 mo), but symptoms can present for months in very elderly people or if super-imposed on dementia	Variable, depending on severity of associated systemic illness	Treated, can be of short duration; if untreated, may last indefinitely
Following directions	Impaired	Impaired	Impaired	Not impaired, although may respond slowly or with "I don't know"
Orientation	Usually disoriented to time and place, not person until later stages	Variable; confusion and disorganized thinking present	Confusion and disorientation	Not disoriented
Attention	Impaired	Impaired or fluctuating attentiveness; easily distracted	Impaired	Decreased concentration
Agitation	Possible	Frequently	Frequently	Possible; may have psychomotor agitation or retardation or could be normal
Level of consciousness	Normal	Abnormal and fluctuates, ranging from motor hyper-activity to obtundation	Abnormal	Normal
Sundowning	Yes	Yes	No	No
Apraxia	Possible	No	No	No
Language	Aphasia, especially word-finding deficits	Slow, incoherent, and inappropriate, rambling, pressured speech	Usually slow	Intact, but slowed poverty of speech, pausing before answering, soft or monotone speech

Sources. American Psychiatric Association (2000b), Barrie (2002), Beers and Berkow (2000a, 2000b, 2000c), Flaherty and Rost (2007), McPherson (2007), Petersen et al. (2001), Tamura (n.d.).

Table E.2.   Laboratory Findings Associated With Mental Dysfunction

Laboratory Findings	Associated Mental Dysfunction
Low thyroxine (T4) suggestive of hypothyroidism	<ul><li>Slowness to respond</li><li>Fatigue</li><li>Depression</li><li>Apathy, can have psychosis and dementia</li><li>Confusion</li></ul>
Low thyroid-stimulating hormone (TSH) suggestive of hyperthyroidism	Symptoms may be similar to those of hypothyroidism and can additionally include<ul><li>Anxiety</li><li>Agitation</li><li>Sleeplessness</li><li>Irritability</li><li>Lability</li><li>Psychosis, mania, and paranoia (in severe hyperthyroidism or during thyroid storms)</li></ul>
Low folic acid (folate)	Depression
Low hematocrit or hemoglobin	<ul><li>Decreased attention</li><li>Irritability</li><li>Feeling depressed</li><li>Fatigue</li></ul>
Sodium	Hyponatremia<ul><li>Agitation</li><li>Confusion</li><li>Delirium</li></ul>Hypernatremia<ul><li>Lethargy</li><li>Obtundation</li></ul>
Hypokalemia (low potassium)	<ul><li>Confusion</li><li>Fatigue</li></ul>
Blood glucose (hyperglycemia and hypoglycemia)	<ul><li>Confusion</li><li>Impaired memory</li><li>Lethargy, coma, stupor</li><li>Irritability</li><li>Nervousness</li><li>Inappropriate behavior</li></ul>

(continued)

Table E.2. (continued)

Laboratory Findings	Associated Mental Dysfunction
Chloride	Lethargy
CO$_2$	Confusion
Calcium	Hypocalcemia • Drowsiness • Lethargy • Confusion • Anxiety • Mimic depression, dementia, or psychosis Hypercalcemia • Irritability
Hypoxia (low O$_2$)	• Confusion • Lethargy
High blood urea nitrogen and creatinine	Confusion
Metabolic alkalosis (increased pH, CO$_2$, and bicarbonate)	Lethargy and stupor
Respiratory acidosis	Drowsiness or, if severe, progression to stupor and coma
Vitamin B12 deficiency	Confusion

Sources. Beers and Berkow (2000a), Bertelson and Price (2004), Flaherty and Rost (2007), Miller (2008), Pereira, do Couto, and de Mendonça (2006), Petersen et al. (2001), Tamura (n.d.).

of neurological, illness, trauma, or metabolic etiologies (Leong et al., 2008), including

- Electrolyte imbalance;
- Infection (especially urinary tract infection);
- Medications (medication errors, new medication, polymedication interaction);
- Cardiac dysfunction, including myocardial infarction;
- Pulmonary dysfunction (especially hypoxia and hypercarbia);
- Endocrine crisis;
- Renal or liver failure;
- Drug or alcohol intoxication or withdrawal;

- Unfamiliar place;
- Anesthesia use; delirium is present in 1%–20% of patients older than age 70 after an elective procedure and in 35%–65% after an emergency procedure (Beers & Berkow, 2000b);
- Neurological changes such as cerebrovascular accident or traumatic brain injury (once diagnosed, will no longer be considered delirium); and
- Fracture (pain).

Metabolic Encephalopathy

Diffuse brain dysfunction is the cardinal sign of metabolic encephalopathy. Usually, diffuse

Table E.3. Etiology of Dementia

Nonreversible	Reversible
• Alzheimer's disease—Plaques • Vascular dementia—Either multi-infarct dementia or the accumulation of small-vessel ischemic changes that, over time, produce dementia. Multi-infarct dementia is irreversible dementia of stepwise character attributed to recurrent ischemic infarction • Frontotemporal dementia • Parkinson's disease • Multiple sclerosis • Long-term alcohol or drug use • HIV	• Normal pressure hydrocephalus (possibly reversible if addressed early enough) • Subdural hematoma • Folic acid, thiamine, or vitamin B12 deficiency • Thyroid dysfunction • Anemia • Depression (dementia syndrome of depression or "pseudodementia"—Dementia improves with treatment of depression; Gerstein, 2008)

motor abnormalities are present, and all four limbs are weak. Flexor or extensor rigidity might be noted as well as flaccidity in the limbs but not usually in a focal neurological distribution. Tremors, asterixis, multifocal myoclonus, seizure, and tremors may be present (Posner, Saper, Plum, & Schiff, 2007). These symptoms generally stem from a systemic process. Several etiological sources of encephalopathy are

- Anoxic or ischemic encephalopathy;
- Abnormal oxygenation;
- Sepsis;
- Electrolyte imbalance;
- Medication effects;
- Hypercapnic encephalopathy; seen in chronic emphysema with chronic respiratory acidosis, which is increased partial pressure of carbon dioxide and decreased partial pressure of oxygen causing CO_2 narcosis;
- Hepatic encephalopathy (refer to Chapter 9 for further details) resulting from chronic liver failure, portal-systemic venous shunting, or both; and
- Uremic encephalopathy, usually associated with acute renal failure.

Depression

Depression is a mood disturbance characterized by sadness, anhedonia, anxiety, irritability, and excessive concerns. Impaired cognitive skills such as decreased executive function skills, including memory, problem solving (including difficulty making decisions), and attention, can also be present (Levin, Heller, Mohanty, Herrington, & Miller, 2007). The patient may also have changes in appetite and suicidal ideation. The causes of depression are usually psychological or social factors such as a change in marital status (recently widowed or divorced), financial issues, or a reaction to an event or acute illness (e.g., an amputation or new diagnosis of Alzheimer's disease). Chronic substance abuse or physical illness may also cause depression. Depression and cognitive deficits can occur simultaneously, and the clinical implications are a higher risk for adverse physical outcomes, functional performance, and mortality (Mehta et al., 2003).

Assessment

When the occupational therapist is assessing the impact of AMS on functional performance, data should include objective outcomes that are correlated with functional skills. To maximize very limited visits, the evaluation must be focused while maintaining holistic aspects of the patient's needs. Effective occupational therapy intervention programs emerge and evolve from a continual assessment process. Clients' functional success is the desired outcome of occupational therapy and is dependent on the evaluation being accurate.

Activities of daily living (ADLs) are the crux of occupational therapy intervention in acute care and should form the basis of the evaluation. In addition to standardized tests, client factors (e.g., neuromuscular and movement-related functions and mental and sensory functions) that affect ADLs must be assessed in the context of task performance. Identifying preserved capabilities and previous habits and roles is necessary to establish a holistic picture of the patient's potential. The medical team should be notified if any symptoms of depression are noted.

Standardized assessments or screenings can be used to augment the ADL evaluation, thus objectifying findings. Commonly used assessments include the Mini-Mental Status Examination (MMSE), St. Louis University Mental Status Exam (SLUMS), Montreal Cognitive Assessment (MoCA), Allen Cognitive Levels (ACL), Geriatric Depression Scale (GDS), and Confusion Assessment Method (CAM) tests.

Mini-Mental Status Examination

The MMSE (McPherson, 2007; Tombaugh & McIntyre, 1992) is the assessment tool most commonly used by medical personnel. It evaluates short-term memory, language, attention, praxis, and orientation. However, it is not reliable for identifying mild cognitive impairment. The score usually used to indicate cognitive impairment is 23/30 (Barrie, 2002; McPherson, 2007). This test takes less than 15 minutes to administer.

St. Louis University Mental Status Exam

The SLUMS correlates highly with the MMSE and takes approximately 7 minutes to adminis-

ter. The SLUMS is more effective than the MMSE in identifying mild neurocognitive disorders (Tariq, Tumosa, Chibnall, Perry, & Morley, 2006), and it can be obtained at http://medschool.slu.edu/agingsuccessfully/pdfsurveys/slumsexam_05.pdf.

Montreal Cognitive Assessment

The MoCA is a brief screening tool that takes approximately 10 minutes to administer and is useful for detecting mild cognitive impairment (McPherson, 2007; Smith, Gildeh, & Holmes, 2007). A score of 26/30 indicates normal cognitive functioning. This test can be obtained at www.mocatest.org.

Allen Cognitive Levels

The ACL measure has long been used in the field of occupational therapy and has been validated for use with patients who are experiencing dementia (Levy, 1998). The ACL is a standardized leather-lacing task that identifies the patient's current performance level.

Geriatric Depression Scale

The GDS (Brink et al., 1982) is a brief assessment used to detect signs and symptoms of depression, and it can be obtained at www.stanford.edu/~yesavage/GDS.html. Multiple language translations are also available at this site.

Confusion Assessment Method

The CAM (Beers & Berkow, 2000b; Inouye et al., 1990) differentiates delirium from dementia. The first two symptoms and one of the last two must be present to make a positive diagnosis of delirium:

- An acute change in mental status and fluctuating symptoms
- Inattention
- Altered level of consciousness
- Disorganized thinking.

A training manual (Inouye, 2003) with testing forms can be obtained at http://elderlife.

med.yale.edu/pdf/The_Confusion_Assessment_Method.pdf.

Therapeutic Intervention

Occupational therapy intervention addressing functional performance should be tailored to the constellation of deficits the patient presents. Incorporating interventional strategies for the physical, psychological, and cognitive components into the task will improve performance. The occupational therapist can assist the patient and family with adapting to changing needs to maximize ADL performance and promote independence and safety. Dementia, however, is a chronic condition. Unless a significant change occurs in function or in the caregiver's ability to provide adequate care, the role of the acute care occupational therapist is generally to provide input into safety and performance skills strategies for the discharge disposition. The overall goals of occupational therapy in the acute care setting should be to maximize or maintain the functional capacity for task performance.

Cognitive and Behavioral Issues

Both cognitive changes, including disorientation, confusion, and attentional and memory deficits, and behavioral changes such as agitation and irritability are present in AMS, resulting in a decline in occupational performance skills. These issues must be addressed to facilitate optimal task performance. Refer to Chapter 6 for further discussion of cognitive deficits.

Agitation

Frequently, patients who are exhibiting AMS demonstrate increased agitation in an unfamiliar environment with an unfamiliar routine, which can further confuse and disorient them (Levy, 1998). Agitation can be nonaggressive or aggressive. *Nonaggressive behaviors* include attention seeking with constant requests for assistance, verbal aggression (e.g., cursing, yelling, temper tantrums), and wandering. *Aggressive behaviors* include pinching, hitting, kicking, and scratching. In the hospital setting, aggressive behaviors, wandering, or getting out of bed when the patient is unable to safely perform this task results in the patient either receiving sedating medications or being restrained. Agitated behaviors can often be traced back to the patient's inability to communicate basic needs such as needing to go to the bathroom, being in pain, or being lonely or afraid. Caregivers, including family and staff, while attempting to provide compassionate care, often lack the understanding that the patient is not capable of communicating effectively.

Assisting caregivers with determining the antecedent event of increased agitation (or any other behavior) may decrease the severity or number of episodes. Later, after the event is over, the confused patient often does not recall the content of the issue but may retain the emotions associated with an event. Emotional memories can often be the antecedent of the behavior; therefore, maintaining calm during exchanges can improve future interactions. The occupational therapist can assist in reducing the necessity of restraints by assisting the staff in using interactional and environmental strategies.

Normalcy in the daily routine can lessen agitation and other behavioral issues. Several methods to increase orientation include using clocks and calendars, opening curtains during the day, performing self-care routines at normal times, and sleeping at night with few naps during the day. In a hospital setting, normal daily activity routines such as getting dressed are generally not encouraged. The occupational therapy intervention plan of care can include incorporating a routine schedule, thus increasing feelings of competence, reducing confusion, or both.

Sensory overload in busy or loud environments may also trigger agitation behaviors. Whenever possible, the environment should be modified to be peaceful, with decreased attentional demands such as an excessive numbers of visitors or the TV being on all day.

Apraxia

Praxis and attentional deficits are frequently noted in patients with dementia. *Apraxia* is the loss or impairment of the ability to perform purposeful skilled movements; it is considered a cognitive motor disorder (Heilman & Gonzalez Rothi, 2003). The several types of praxis include *conceptual* (previously called *ideational*), *ideomotor* (inability to perform after verbal commands), and *motor* (Heilman & Gonzalez Rothi, 2003).

Setting up the task by having commonly used items in sight can alleviate symptoms of apraxia or decreased attentional skills, thus eliciting a correct response to natural environmental cues (Burns & Levy, 2006). For example,

- Gentle hand-over-hand tactile cuing may also improve initiation of tasks;
- Removing superfluous environmental objects can reduce attempts to use unnecessary tools for an ADL task;
- Directions should be concrete and contextual to improve performance;
- Using pantomime may facilitate performance if ideomotor apraxia is noted; and
- Motor learning is possible with repetition, and repetition should be used even in the hospital setting.

Therapy can structure tasks to use the intact brain pathways to access motor planning within the context of function (Heilman & Gonzalez Rothi, 2003; Jacobs et al., 1999).

Safety Judgment

The skills to make safe decisions such as procedural memory, attention, and problem solving are often impaired. Further decreasing safety judgment may be new physical limitations of which the patient is unaware and decreased knowledge of the new environment and the rules, such as calling the nurse before getting out of bed. The patient is often fearful of falling when engaged in a functional mobility task with unfamiliar people assisting in a novel manner. Assure the patient of his or her safety during activities, avoid sudden movements, and remember that the patient needs to move slowly. Modifying the environment or the daily routine so that the environment is intrinsically safer can improve patient safety. Removing bed cords that may trip the patient, turning on a

nightlight, or instituting a toileting schedule can alleviate some of the stress involved with needing to go to the bathroom.

Sundowning

Sundowning, usually associated with dementia or Alzheimer's, is a common phenomenon in patients with AMS. With sundowning, the patient experiences a decline in cognitive functioning as fatigue begins, usually in the late afternoon or early evening (hence the name). Behaviors associated with sundowning include increased agitation, psychosis, confusion, or mood swings. Families are frequently able to identify this symptom as occurring premorbidly, if provided with examples of functional performance deficits. Encourage families to address most tasks during the early part of the day to alleviate some of the functional performance issues associated with sundowning. The acute care therapy session should occur earlier in the day to maximize performance; however, an assessment of functioning late in the afternoon may yield performance skill deficits that were not noted when the patient was rested.

New Learning Deficits

According to Baxter and Baxter (2002), memory and learning are inextricably linked. Therefore, for learning to even occur, a memory must first be laid down in the brain. Humans learn by touching, doing, engaging, and experiencing cause and effect. *Explicit memory* is the recall of facts, concepts, and events, and *implicit memory* has more emphasis on motor engrams, learned and emotional responses, and procedural recall. Implicit memory provides the best opportunity for generalization into function. However, initially the patient must often use explicit memory pathways to lay down patterns that will eventually become the implicit or more reflexive strategies. An example is the patient who just had back surgery and must learn how to sit up for the first time using back precautions. The therapist first explicitly delineates the steps in succession. Eventually, with repetition, the memories of the steps blur together to form a motor memory, thus transforming it from an explicit memory into an implicit memory and then to a learned skill.

Delirium and encephalopathy commonly occur after surgical procedures such as back and hip surgeries. The role of the occupational therapist in this context is to teach adaptive techniques for functional mobility and ADL performance. Often, therapists verbalize every step of simple tasks, such as sitting up on the edge of the bed. For the patient with new learning deficits, this presents too much information, and it should be broken down into smaller chunks of information. For instance, saying "sit up" may improve performance and would be an example of using implicit memory. Reflexively, motor patterns are more beneficial, requiring less attention and, therefore, less memory. Humans develop kinesthetic memories for tasks so as not to constantly require conscious intellectual overrides. The therapist's role is to facilitate the development of appropriate kinesthetic memories using healthy movement patterns. The patient who is expected to recover is treated with the hope of developing useful strategies or redeveloping his or her capabilities (Davies, 1994). Therapists thus influence the "functional plasticity" of the brain for learning.

Caregiver education regarding methods to foster new learning must especially occur for a patient who has just had a total hip replacement or back surgery that involves multiple adaptive strategies with rigid precautions. If cognitive deficits are suspected, request that the caregiver be present for treatment sessions so that carryover can occur at home. Instruct caregivers to provide succinct verbal directions and in how to embed adaptations into normal activities and environments. Caregivers will be the most valuable resource for reinforcing instruction in the natural environment and need instruction to properly facilitate habitual carryover.

Depression

The use of occupation as a means to mental health (Legault & Rebeiro, 2001) is the very core of the occupational therapy profession. The role of the acute care occupational therapist in enabling occupation is important to optimizing functional recovery. Depression can affect cognitive functioning in the older adult, which may impede participation in rehabilitation interventions (Levin et al., 2007; Miller, 2004). If possible, treat outside the hospital room to increase socialization. Provide achievable goals to increase feelings of competence and reduce hopelessness. Feelings of hopelessness versus helplessness herald an intensification of symptoms and are frequently verbalized during a therapeutic session, when the therapist and patient have a lot of one-to-one time. If a patient expresses feelings of hopelessness, the nurse and physician should be alerted because it can be a sign of suicidal ideation.

An expectation that the patient will be capable of effectual task performance can improve the patient's perceived self-efficacy. Assure the patient that rehabilitation is a team effort or collaboration between the therapist and patient. Improving daily structure can also ameliorate feelings of helplessness.

Activities of Daily Living

In the acute care setting, the focus of intervention is typically on basic ADLs, including feeding, dressing, toileting, bathing, grooming and hygiene, and functional mobility. To optimize ADL performance, provide graded assistance, opportunities for practice, and positive reinforcement with structured ADL tasks. Visual, tactile, and verbal cues can aid in providing clues to the sequencing of steps (Nygård, 2004), reducing apraxia, and facilitating working and procedural memory. Working memory involves the patient's ability to use motor, verbal, and visual information and procedural memories to coordinate responses, acting as the overall executive of the brain to plan actions as they occur. It provides a temporary storage site for information to guide future actions.

Procedural memory is the recall of how to perform a task. Fluctuations in performance skills can be unpredictable but are often associated with fatigue resulting from overactivity the day before or earlier in the day.

Illness, cognitive fatigue, and the unfamiliar environment, tools, and routines further weaken performance, resulting in increased confusion, attention deficits, and reduced activity tolerance. Reducing the cognitive requirements by giving verbal and tactile cues can reduce fatigue, sundowning, and new learning deficits, thus increasing functional cognitive endurance. If the patient is visually impaired, using low vision strategies may improve task performance. Refer to Appendix F for low vision strategies and recommendations. Tasks of particular importance include those that contribute to health, healing, and safety such as hygiene, feeding, functional mobility, and toileting.

Feeding

Self-feeding is frequently impaired for a variety of reasons, including lack of attentional skills, praxis, or endurance (cognitive and physical) to self-feed. The patient may need to be fed to reduce malnutrition. Although self-feeding should be encouraged, nutritional intake is more important than insisting on independence. Taking food out of the hospital containers, opening utensil packages, and using normal beverage containers will increase familiarity, thus tapping into long-term procedural memory and reducing cognitive demands. If praxis skills with utensils are impaired, assist the patient with tactile cues to initiate proper usage. Reduce environmental distractors by limiting the number of visitors during meals and turning off the television, radio, or computer. Ensure that the patient has his or her dentures in, and if the patient does not use dentures, provide soft, chopped, or precut food to facilitate feeding with a safe swallow. Provide smaller, more frequent meals and ask the family to bring in favorite foods. Encourage the patient to get out of bed for all meals to improve activity tolerance and provide a sense of normalcy.

Dressing

Dressing may be impaired because of cognitive, physical, and psychological deficits and medical status. Determining the reason will assist in formulating an intervention plan. Decreased functional mobility can hinder dressing (e.g., pulling up pants, retrieving clothes) if the patient is experiencing difficulty with sitting balance or standing components. Laying out clothing and dressing from a seated, supported position may improve task performance.

Dressing requires a significant amount of activity tolerance, which may be impaired in the patient who is medically compromised. Reducing activity demands by intrinsically incorporating energy conservation and work simplification strategies may improve performance. Encourage as normal a routine as possible to decrease confusion, increase participation, or both. Routine can be especially important for the patient who is depressed, because it encourages a sense of normalcy and reduces the perception of the sick role. However, this routine may not be realistic if the patient has a scheduled medical procedure or frequent incontinence.

Toileting

Toileting and its component skills of functional mobility—cleansing, continence, and clothing management—can present hazards for the patient with AMS. Injuries occur because confused patients may also have balance deficits that increase the risk for falls when attempting to use the toilet. Episodes of bowel and bladder incontinence may also occur in the patient with AMS because of medical issues, confusion, an inability to communicate the need to go to the bathroom, or an inability to get to the bathroom in time. The patient may also forget to call for assistance because the hospital is not his or her normal environment or part of his or her routine. The therapist should assess if the patient who is unable to sequence the steps of toileting or does not recognize the tools involved in performance of the task (e.g., the patient mistakes the trashcan for the toilet).

Recognizing the cause of impaired toileting or incontinence aids the therapist in determining the most appropriate intervention. Recommendations may include structuring a toileting schedule so that the patient is taken to the bathroom every 2 hours (not just asked if he or she wants to go). Reduced liquid intake after 6:00 p.m. will reduce the number of unplanned bathroom trips, thus increasing safety. Keep a nightlight on to decrease confusion in finding the bathroom, and clearly mark the bathroom with a sign. Therapeutically addressing fall prevention by improving balance and activity tolerance can lessen the risk associated with bathroom mobility. Recommend an elevated toilet seat or bedside commode be placed over the toilet if the patient is demonstrating difficulty in sitting on or getting off the toilet.

Bathing

Performance issues during bathing can be because of pain, physical limitations, or the loss of privacy with emotional discomfort (e.g., anxiety, fear, embarrassment). These issues can increase the risk of patient and staff injury, decrease personal hygiene, and result in behavioral issues. Encourage active participation in bathing, allowing the patient to perform as much of the task as possible, reducing the invasion of personal space and privacy. Keep the room, water, and washcloths warm to reduce the discomfort of being cold that can increase resistance to bathing. Provide visual cues to aid in task performance, placing washcloths, towels, soap, and shampoo in sight. These steps can reduce deficits with memory, attention, sequencing, and praxis. If the patient is resisting bathing, put the task in context, for example, bathing is appropriate if the patient is soiled. If the patient's normal routine is to bathe in the evening, scheduling a bath at this time would be in context for the patient. Provide a shower seat to reduce activity demands and increase safety.

Grooming and Hygiene

Grooming and hygiene require a significant amount of sequencing skills. For the patient with memory and attention deficits, performance of the many steps can hinder thorough and efficient completion. Provide visual, verbal, and tactile cues to improve performance and maintain attention to each step. Grooming and hygiene tasks should be contextual; for instance, the task should occur during the normal morning routine, after breakfast, or both. Being appropriately groomed improves self-esteem; however, being disheveled and ungroomed may indicate a tendency toward self-neglect. Praxis deficits can significantly affect performance and safety of grooming and hygiene activities.

Hair care can be hindered by physical dysfunction as well as cognitive and perceptual disorders. Providing the appropriate tools (e.g., hairbrush, comb) in context (e.g., when standing in front of a mirror or before visitors arrive) can improve performance. Assist with praxis, sequencing, procedural memory, and initiation deficits by using hand-over-hand assist or demonstration to initiate the task of combing or brushing hair.

Brushing teeth presents many opportunities for apraxia, procedural memory, and sequencing deficits to become evident. Provide visual environmental cues for task performance. Placing only the necessary tools (e.g., toothpaste, toothbrush, cup) will improve sequencing and reduce environmental stimuli that can be confusing. If the patient has oral discomfort, he or she may avoid brushing teeth because of pain. Dentures are frequently misplaced, so the hospital caregiver may need to ensure they are in a safe place at night.

Pointing out that a male patient has stubble may be the catalyst for shaving, and the patient may not initiate the task without this contextual verbal cue. Recommend use of a waterproof electric shaver because it involves fewer steps to sequence and less risk of cutting oneself. Because the male patient may be used to using water as he shaves, a waterproof shaver may alleviate some of the danger in having electronics near water. However, safety razors may be contraindicated for patients on blood thinners. In addition, ensure the shaver is being properly used (i.e., used to shave facial hair only).

Functional Mobility

Functional mobility can be compromised as a result of both physical and cognitive limitations. Therefore, ensuring a safe environment in which to ambulate is vital. Conversely, many patients with cognitive impairments need a physical outlet, and walking can be a good way to distract the patient, fatigue the patient for rest, or provide an outlet for psychomotor agitation. The patient may attempt to wander or unsafely attempt to get out of bed, requiring supervision. Discerning the cause may increase safety. Reasons include looking for a bathroom, pain, escaping an environment that is distressing, or boredom. Labeling the bathroom, reducing distractors, providing pain medication, or offering beverages or something to do may result in decreased wandering behavior.

The medical illness for which the patient is hospitalized can further decrease functional mobility. Bed alarms should be turned on at all times. Structured times for walking also provide opportunities for the patient to walk with supervision. Encourage families to enroll in the Alzheimer's Association Medic Alert + Safe Return program (see www.alz.org/safetycenter), especially if the patient has a tendency to wander, possibly getting lost.

Environmental Considerations

Modify the environment to encourage active participation within the patient's capabilities. An environment with fewer distractors can enhance attention and the patient's ability to participate when not overwhelmed with environmental stimuli. Turning off the TV or radio can reduce the stimuli in the room. Occasionally, agitated patients may have a sitter in the room. The sitter should be encouraged to pursue quiet endeavors such as reading versus watching TV to reduce stimuli. Too many visitors can also contribute to increased confusion because "entertaining the guests" increases the environmental stimuli that easily fatigue the patient. Encourage few and brief visits of less than 10 minutes.

Physical Issues

Functional performance can deteriorate if the patient is physically impaired. Encourage the patient to get out of bed as much as possible because patients with AMS who are bed bound are at high risk for pressure sores, atelectasis, and deconditioning (Beers & Berkow, 2000c). See Appendix C for further information regarding bedrest deconditioning and prolonged immobility. Increase activity tolerance with light activity such as walking, keeping in mind

that cognitive deficits may be superimposed on underlying medical issues. Incorporating physical activities into normal routines at the normal time of day also facilitates occupational performance. Encourage normal sleep patterns that provide an adequate amount of sleep (Miller, 2008). Ensure that the patient's physical and sensory needs are met, such as hearing aids in and functional, glasses on and clean, hunger satisfied, and toileting needs addressed.

Family Education

Developing a partnership with family members will further enhance the care of patients with AMS. Family education regarding the nature of the diagnosis, safety needs, necessity of routines, and interactional strategies (see Box E.1) are important for all diagnoses. Families should also be educated on the transitory nature of symptoms for delirium and metabolic encephalopathy, and possibly depression, because symptoms are expected to resolve with medical treatment.

Families should encourage participation in ADLs because successful completion provides an intrinsic link to normalcy and feelings of competence (Hasselkus & Murray, 2007). Therapists can address safety concerns for medication, financial management, and driving and encourage the family to designate responsibility for these tasks before the patient is discharged. For many adults, driving represents their link to autonomy and as such is usually relinquished with hesitation. Recommend that the patient not drive until the physician clears him or her or until a formal outpatient driving evaluation has been completed. Behavioral management strategies for behaviors such as sundowning, yelling, uncooperativeness, and wandering are a primary concern and should be addressed.

Educational materials that may be helpful to caregivers include an informational brochure compiled by the Family Caregiver Alliance (2008) titled *Practical Tools and Resources for Caregivers*. The National Institute on Aging has several useful publications regarding Alzheimer's disease that can also be generalized to other dementia diagnoses.

Box E.1.   Suggestions for Encouraging Task Performance for Patients With Altered Mental Status

1. Do not argue with the patient; distract him or her from the point of contention or concern.
2. The patient will remember the emotional content of an interaction but not necessarily the actual event.
3. Use a soothing voice; do not increase voice volume. Use low tones (not necessarily volume but pitch).
4. Suggest; do not command or talk in a condescending manner.
5. When the patient is upset or agitated, change the topic or the task, and return to it later.
6. If a particular task is being resisted, try to put it into context. For instance, with bathing, go out to the garden and get dirty. The patient may then want to take a bath.
7. The fear of falling is great. Pulling may actually increase resistance. Put movement into context, and allow the patient to go at his or her own pace. Do not rush.
8. If the patient is agitated, come down to his or her eye level.
9. Introduce yourself every time you enter the patient's room.
10. Be reassuring and positive in all interactions.
11. Reduce environmental distractions whenever possible to decrease sensory overload.

Conclusion

Occupational therapists facilitate ADL performance competence through careful application of therapeutic strategies in patients with AMS. Accurate assessment should address cognitive, behavioral, and physical deficits, followed by the use of therapeutic interventions such as prudent cuing, environmental modifications, and task restructuring because these can alleviate performance deficits. The functional sequelae of delirium, dementia, metabolic encephalopathy, and depression can confound acute medical issues and should be addressed by the therapist. Fostering a partnership with the patient and caregiver facilitates improved patient functioning and ultimately a safer discharge from the hospital.

References

American Psychiatric Association. (2000a). *Delirium, dementia, and amnestic and other cognitive disorders.* In *Diagnostic and statistical manual of mental disorders* (4th ed., text rev., Code 300.11). Washington, DC: Author. Retrieved November 29, 2008, from STAT!Ref: http://online.statref.com/document.aspx?fxid=37&docid=239

American Psychiatric Association. (2000b). *Mood disorders: Depressive disorders: Major depressive disorders.* In *Diagnostic and statistical manual of mental disorders* (4th ed., text rev., Code 300.11). Washington, DC: Author. Retrieved November 29, 2008, from STAT!Ref: http://online.statref.com/document.aspx?fxid=37&docid=239

Barrie, M. A. (2002). Objective screening tools to assess cognitive impairment and depression. *Topics in Geriatric Rehabilitation, 18*(2), 28–46.

Baxter, M. F., & Baxter, D. A. (2002). Neural mechanisms of learning and memory. In H. S. Cohen (Ed.), *Neuroscience for rehabilitation* (2nd ed., pp. 321–348). Philadelphia: Lippincott Williams & Wilkins.

Beers, M. H., & Berkow, R. (Eds.). (2000a). Behavior disorders in dementia. In *The Merck manual of geriatrics* (3rd ed., pp. 371–377). Whitehouse Station, NJ: Merck Research Laboratories.

Beers, M. H., & Berkow, R. (Eds.). (2000b). Delirium. In The *Merck manual of geriatrics* (3rd ed., pp. 350–356). Whitehouse Station, NJ: Merck Research Laboratories.

Beers, M. H., & Berkow, R. (Eds.). (2000c). Depression. In The *Merck manual of geriatrics* (3rd ed., pp. 310–322). Whitehouse Station, NJ: Merck Research Laboratories.

Bertelson, J. A., & Price, B. H. (2004). Depression and psychosis in neurological practice. In W. G. Bradley, R. B. Daroff, G. M. Fenichel, & J. Jankovic (Eds.), *Neurology in clinical practice: Vol. 1. Principles of diagnosis and management* (4th ed., pp. 103–116). Oxford, England: Butterworth-Heinemann.

Brink, T. L., Yesavage, J. A., Lum, O., Heersema, P., Adey, M. B., & Rose, T. L. (1982). Screening tests for geriatric depression. *Clinical Gerontologist, 1,* 37–44.

Burns, T., & Levy, L. L. (2006). Neurocognitive practice essentials in dementia: Cognitive disabilities-reconsidered model. *OT Practice, 11*(3), CE1–CE8.

Davies, P. M. (1994). *Starting again.* Berlin: Springer-Verlag.

Family Caregiver Alliance. (2008). *Practical tools and resources for caregivers.* San Francisco: Author. Retrieved July 26, 2009, from http://caregiver.org/caregiver/jsp/content/pdfs/FCA-Harford-Practical%20Tools-Caregivers.pdf

Flaherty, A. W., & Rost, N. S. (2007). *The Massachusetts General Hospital handbook of neurology* (2nd ed.). Philadelphia: Lippincott Williams & Wilkins.

Gerstein, P. S. (2008). *Delirium, dementia, and amnesia.* Retrieved August 15, 2009, from http://emedicine.medscape.com/article/793247-overview

Hasselkus, B. R., & Murray, B. J. (2007). Everyday occupation, well-being, and identity: The experience of caregivers in families with dementia. *American Journal of Occupational Therapy, 61,* 9–20.

Heilman, K. M., & Gonzalez Rothi, L. J. (2003). Apraxia. In K. M. Heilman & E. Valenstein (Eds.), *Clinical neuropsychology* (4th ed., pp. 215–235). New York: Oxford University Press.

Inouye, S. K. (2003). *The confusion assessment method (CAM): Training manual and coding guide.* New Haven, CT: Yale University School of Medicine. Retrieved August 16, 2009, from http://elderlife.med.yale.edu/pdf/The_Confusion_Assessment_Method.pdf

Inouye, S., van Dyck, C., Alessi, C., Balkin, S., Siegal, A., & Horwitz, R. (1990). Clarifying confusion: The confusion assessment method. *Annals of Internal Medicine, 113,* 941–948.

Jacobs, D. H., Adair, J. C., Williamson, D. J., Na, D. L., Gold, M., Foundas, A. L., et al. (1999). Apraxia and motor-skill acquisition in Alzheimer's disease are dissociable. *Neuropsychologia, 37,* 875–880.

Legault, E., & Rebeiro, K.L. (2001). Case report—Occupation as a means to mental health: A single-case study. *American Journal of Occupational Therapy, 55,* 90–96.

Leong, L. B., Jian, K. H., Vasu, A., & Seow, E. (2008, September 24). Prospective study of patients with altered mental status: Clinical features and outcome. *International Journal of Emergency Medicine, 1,* 179–182. doi:10.1007/s12245-008-0049-8

Levin, R. L., Heller, W., Mohanty, A., Herrington, J. D., & Miller, G. A. (2007). Cognitive deficits in depression and functional specificity of regional brain activity. *Cognitive Therapy and Research, 31,* 211–233.

Levy, L. L. (1998). The cognitive disabilities model in rehabilitation of older adults with dementia. In N. Katz (Ed.), *Cognition and occupation in rehabilitation* (pp. 195–221). Bethesda, MD: American Occupational Therapy Association.

McPherson, S. (2007, March 9). *Aging and cognition: Assessment and behavioral interventions.* Lecture presented at Health Education Network, Atlanta, GA.

Mehta, K. M., Yaffe, K., Lenga, K. M., Sands, L., Whooley, M. A., & Covinsky, K. E. (2003). Additive effects of cognitive function and depressive symptoms on mortality in elderly community-living adults. *Journals of Gerontology, Series A: Biological and Medical Sciences, 58*(A), 461–467.

Miller, M. O. (2008). Evaluation and management of delirium in hospitalized older patients. *American Family Physician, 78,* 1265–1270.

Miller, P. A. (2004). A quick screen for depression. *Gerontology Special Interest Section Quarterly, 27,* 4.

Nygård, L. (2004). Responses of persons with dementia to challenges in daily activities: A synthesis of findings from empirical studies. *American Journal of Occupational Therapy, 58,* 435–445.

Pereira, A. F., do Couto, F. S., & de Mendonça, A. (2006). The use of laboratory tests in patients with mild cognitive impairment. *Journal of Alzheimer's Disease, 10,* 53–58.

Petersen, R. C., Stevens, J. C., Ganguli, M., Tangalos, E. G., Cummings, J. L., & DeKosky, S. T. (2001). Practice parameter: Early detection of dementia: Mild cognitive impairment (an evidence-based review): Report of the Quality Standards Subcommittee of the American Academy of Neurology. *Neurology, 56,* 1133–1142.

Posner, J. B., Saper, C. B., Plum, F., & Schiff, N. (2007). Multifocal, diffuse, and metabolic brain diseases causing delirium, stupor, or coma. In *Plum and Posner's diagnosis of stupor and coma* (4th ed., pp. 179–296). New York: Oxford University Press.

Smith, T., Gildeh, N., & Holmes, C. (2007). The Montreal cognitive assessment: Validity and utility in a memory clinic setting. *Canadian Journal of Psychiatry, 52,* 329–332.

Tamura, M. K. (n.d.). Recognizing delirium, dementia, and depression. In *Online geriatric nephrology curriculum* (chap. 36) Retrieved July 26, 2009, from www.asn-online.org/education_and_meetings/geriatrics/Chapter36.pdf

Tariq, S. H., Tumosa, N., Chibnall, J. T., Perry, M. H., III., & Morley, J. E. (2006). Comparison of the Saint Louis University Mental Status Examination and the Mini-Mental Status Examination for detecting dementia and mild neurocognitive disorder: A pilot study. *American Journal of Geriatric Psychiatry, 14,* 900–910.

Tombaugh, T. N., & McIntyre, N. J. (1992). The Mini-Mental State Examination: A comprehensive review. *Journal of the American Geriatrics Society, 40,* 922–935.

Appendix F

Low Vision: Strategies for Successful Intervention

Judy R. Hamby, MHS, OTR/L, BCPR

Low vision is defined as uncorrectable vision loss that interferes with performance of daily activities ("Low Vision Glossary," 2008). The American Foundation for the Blind has estimated that 21.2 million people in the United States have vision loss, with approximately 6.2 million elderly people (ages 65 or older) reporting difficulty seeing even with glasses (Kelly, 2008). As the population ages, that number is expected to drastically increase. The likelihood that an occupational therapist will treat a patient with low vision in the acute care setting is high because the predominant patient population is elderly.

Low vision is typically not the primary diagnosis, and it is frequently not even noted in a patient's medical history, but it may be a contributing reason for the admission. For example, could patient with diabetes see the wound on the bottom of his or her foot, or did the patient with macular degeneration fall and break a hip because it was too dark on the way to the bathroom? Low vision is important to address because it is frequently associated with an increased risk for falls (Black & Wood, 2005). Vision changes and their implications are listed in Table F.1. The acute care therapist must determine whether low vision is present to ensure effective intervention.

Anatomy

The eye is approximately the size of a table tennis ball but houses an enormous number of structures. The *sclera* is the white outermost layer of the eye, protecting and maintaining the eye's shape. The *iris,* covered by the *cornea,* is the colored structure that works like the lens of a camera, allowing images into the eye and controlling the amount of light permitted into it via the pupil. Behind the iris sits the *lens*, a clear structure that helps focus the image onto the retina. The innermost layer, the *retina,* contains nerve cells that receive the image and then transmit it via the optic nerve to the brain (see Figures F.1 and F.2 for lateral and anterior views of the eye).

Terminology

The terminology in Table F.2 can assist the clinician when evaluating, planning, and documenting information for a person who is visually impaired. The clinician should note that current classification of low vision is based on deficits in visual acuity and visual field. Other visual disturbances, such as perceptual or oculomotor deficits, are not included in current definitions of low vision.

Common Diagnoses

According to Kelly (2008), the four most common eye diseases among elderly people are macular degeneration, cataracts, glaucoma, and diabetic retinopathy. These diagnoses also appear to be the four most common eye diseases encountered in an acute care setting. Refer to Table F.3 for more information on these eye diseases.

Evaluation

Clinical evaluation of low vision is brief and pointed in the acute care setting. Generally, treatment of this chronic condition is addressed in the outpatient arena. However, occasionally,

Table F.1.	Normal Age-Related Vision Changes and Their Implications

Normal Age-Related Vision Changes	Implications
Loss of accommodation because lens becomes less flexible with age	• Dependent on glasses for seeing clearly at near distances
Slower visual adaptation	• Takes longer to adapt to lighting changes, e.g., when walking into a dimly lit hospital room from the bright hallways
More light scatter in the eye and increased difficulty with glare	• Needs lighting adjustment; modify illumination • May need sunglasses, tinted glasses, or a visor
Dry eyes	• Needs eye drops more frequently • Eyes can be more painful
Decreased sensitivity to contrast	• Color discrimination fades • Contrast is more important • Needs bolder colors • May need increased task lighting

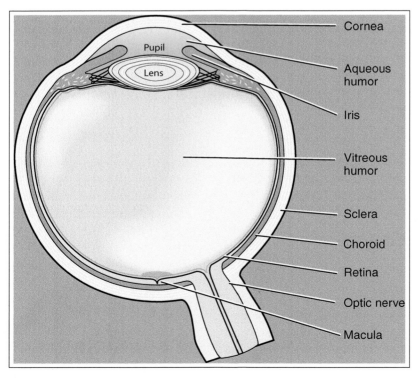

Figure F.1. Lateral view of the eye.
Source. Richard Fritzler, Medical Illustrator, Roswell, GA.

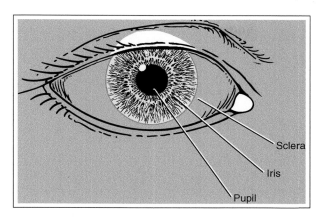

Figure F.2. Anterior view of the eye.
Source. Richard Fritzler, Medical Illustrator, Roswell, GA.

low vision interferes with basic activities of daily living (BADLs) or affects the discharge disposition sufficient to require direct intervention. If it does not affect discharge, then recommendations for outpatient referral are the most appropriate course of action. In general, an awareness of the patient's visual history and how it affects function is sufficient to adequately address acute care-related issues. Pertinent areas to evaluate are listed in Table F.4 if an evaluation and treatment are warranted (for neurological vision evaluation, refer to Chapter 6) to ensure a safe discharge, or if it would have an impact on the patient's acute care stay. Refer to Table F.5 for a list of near vision equivalencies.

Intervention

The goal of treatment is to facilitate occupational performance by maximizing usable vision through modification of objects, environments, tasks, and routines. Treatment should be initiated if it would have an immediate impact on the patient's hospitalization or discharge. A referral to low vision rehabilitation services is warranted if the patient's visual impairments continue to limit the patient's abilities after discharge. Recommended intervention strategies for the acute care setting are listed in Box F.1.

Low vision interventions generally address these five areas:

1. Maximizing usable vision
   - Using prescribed optical aids such as glasses, magnifiers (optical aids must be prescribed by an eye doctor), or both and
   - Using visual skills such as scanning or eccentric fixation.
2. Increasing "identifiability" of objects
   - Using color, contrast, auditory, or tactile methods.
3. Environmental modifications to facilitate safety and task performance
   - Adjustments to lighting and
   - Organization.
4. Adapting tasks and routines
   - Simplification;
   - Alternate methods that rely less on vision when vision is unreliable; and
   - Compensatory devices such as talking glucose meters.
5. Maximizing wellness
   - Facilitate emotional adjustment and
   - Provide resources and referral.

It would be useful to have the following items included in a low vision evaluation and treatment kit:

- Reading materials of various sizes and types (e.g., medicine bottles, book, magazine, cereal box, newspaper, hospital menu, diabetic testing supplies and syringe, name tag);
- Pocket-sized acuity chart;
- 4× magnifier;
- Gooseneck lamp for task lighting;
- Adhesive hook-and-loop fastener in various colors or electrocardiagram sticker;
- Various colors of duct tape;
- Red fingernail polish;
- Black placemat;
- Bold black markers (nonpermanent, such as those found in children's coloring kits);
- Signature guides; and
- Low vision handout, including a list of local resources.

(Text continues on p. 620)

Table F.2. Terminology	
Level and Measurement of Visual Impairment	**Functional Implications**
Normal vision 20/12–20/25	• No visual deficits • Able to read with no devices or adaptations at a normal reading speed

Near normal
    20/30–20/60
 	
    Visual field ≤50°
	• Reading speed is normal, but person must hold material closer.
	• Difficulty reading fine print; uses glasses.
	• May need to scan environment if the visual field is restricted. May be surprised by events in the periphery.

Moderate low vision
    20/70–20/160
 	
    Visual field ≤30°
	• Reading is not comfortable for an extended time.
	• Must use magnifiers.
	• If peripheral visual field is affected, then environmental scanning is required.

Severe low vision
    20/200–20/400
    Visual field ≤20°
	• Reading is slow and uncomfortable.
	• Functional mobility requires continuous environmental scanning; person will need a guide or assistive device such as a cane.
	• Often bumps into obstacles.
	• Posture is often rigid.

Profound low vision
    20/500–20/1,000
 	
    Visual field ≤10°
	• Only performs essential spot reading, but with difficulty and with electronic magnification optical devices. Requires alternative methods because vision is unreliable.
	• Assistance is required for all functional mobility.
	• Will require training with a cane or guide dog for all mobility and safety.

Near blindness
    Less than 20/1,000
    Visual field ≤5°
	• Has only light and shadow perception.
	• No reading; must rely on talking books or devices and Braille.
	• Must use cane or guide dog for all functional mobility.

Blindness Total loss (total blindness)	• No vision

Sources. Andersson and Cocciarella (2000), Medicare (2002), "New Requirements for Low Vision Rehabilitation Demonstration Billing" (2006), Warren (2008), "What Is 20/20 Vision?" (2007).

Table F3. **Eye Diseases**

Diagnosis	Primary Visual Deficit	First Symptom	Functional Implications	Acute Care Implications
Age-related macular degeneration (AMD)	Decreased central vision *Two types:* • Wet—Increasing number of blood vessels rupturing in the macula. • Dry—Macula atrophies.	Straight lines often appear wavy.	• Patient does not actually register a distinctly edged black spot (scotoma) because of perceptual completion and visual closure. Actually sees blurry, hazy, dark, or light area. • Objects appear to come in and out of view. • Difficulty seeing facial features, colors, or signs. • Central vision is impaired. • Often unable to read or see food on plate.	• Teach the patient how to use the preferred retinal locus to use eccentric vision. Training will be very brief and likely not sufficient for mastery for all tasks. Patient looks at things using the peripheral vision versus centering the object. Help the patient find the area of most acuity (e.g., 12:00, 3:00, 6:00, 9:00). • Patient will not recognize faces. • Patient may appear confused. • Frequently during the tracking evaluation, the patient will lose the visual stimuli in the center, which may be the first clue that the patient has AMD. Patients usually forget to inform doctors and therapists that they have macular degeneration when they are in the hospital for another reason. • Vision may get worse if patient has wet AMD and is on a blood thinner. • If AMD is the wet type, it may have been treated with laser coagulation therapy (older treatment) and, more recently, injection therapy with antivascular endothelial growth factor to stop the growth of the blood vessels. • There is no known cure for the dry type of AMD, but many patients take multivitamins.

(continued)

Table F.3. (continued)

Diagnosis	Primary Visual Deficit	First Symptom	Functional Implications	Acute Care Implications
Glaucoma	• Loss of peripheral vision initially, then centrally, and ultimately blindness if left uncontrolled. Glaucoma has no known cause. It is often characterized by increased fluid pressure damaging the optic nerve. It can also be caused by deterioration of retinal cells (ganglion cells). A patient may have glaucoma in the absence of increased intraocular pressure.	Patient may interpret change in vision as • Needing a change in glasses • Decreased night vision. Primary closed angle glaucoma is characterized by • Sudden onset and unilateral vision changes and pain.	May have reading vision, but with no peripheral vision, it is difficult for a person to scan the environment to see where he or she is going and avoid obstacles.	• Use low vision strategies. • Usually treated with medications to prevent pressure from building up.
Cataracts	Yellowing or a cloudiness of the lens.	Blurry vision.	• Increased sensitivity to glare. • Ghost images. • To others, the eyes appear milky or yellowish. • Decreased color vision.	*Precaution:* If head is hit, then the implant can be dislodged. Report to the doctor if patient complains of an unexplained change in vision or unilateral diplopia after a hit on the head. *Medical treatment:* Surgical intervention usually fixes the problems. Most choose to get a surgical lens implant, which eliminates the problem.

			Surgery: A small slit is made in cornea, then the lens is removed and an intraocular implant is put in its place. To have the surgery, patients must stop using blood thinners, which puts them at risk for blood clots and stroke. • Use large print and high-contrast materials.
Diabetic retinopathy	• Leaking blood vessels in the retina cause severe and progressive blurring. • Gradual central vision decrease because of macular edema or capillary dropout. • Primary complication of diabetes. Two types: • Nonproliferative (does not interfere with function) • Proliferative (interferes with functional vision).	Usually no early symptoms.	• Contrast reduced for reading; print distorted. • Decreased visual acuity; can fluctuate with changes in blood sugar levels with proliferative diabetic retinopathy. • With the nonproliferative type, fluctuations in blood sugar will not generally result in vision changes. • Decreased color vision.	• Possible retinal detachment resulting from the development of scar tissue • Use low-vision strategies. • Use large-print or talking diabetes supplies such as talking blood sugar meter and large print or clicking syringe. • Determine whether fluctuating vision shows a pattern, and plan performance of tasks and therapy accordingly. • Encourage the patient to discuss fluctuating vision patterns with the diabetes educator and the physician, because it may aid in formulating a more appropriate medication schedule.

Table F.4. **Evaluation of Performance Skills or Areas in Clients With Low Vision**

Performance Skill or Area	Evaluation	Analysis and Intervention
History	• Do you wear glasses or use magnifiers? What for? Are they necessary, and do they work? • Do you have a history of a vision loss? Why? • What is the diagnosis? • How does it affect you functionally?	• A history determines the patient's level of awareness of visual deficits. • Refer to Table F.3 for specific interventions for eye diseases. • Patient needs to wear glasses for the appropriate evaluation (e.g., patient should wear reading glasses if he or she needs them for reading task). • Wash glasses for the patient using soap and water. • If the cause of vision loss is known, then incorporate issues into intervention. • Central visual loss (e.g., because of age-related macular degeneration) will generally affect one's ability to see detail, such as when reading standard print materials or visually identifying food on a plate. It may also make the patient appear confused when he or she cannot recognize faces of staff or friends and family. • Peripheral visual field loss (e.g., from glaucoma) will generally affect balance and mobility. • Cataract surgery with lens implants may render old glasses useless for distance tasks. • Sudden vision changes after a fall may indicate a dislodged lens implant, which constitutes an ophthalmologic emergency. Call the doctor immediately.
Lighting level	• Does the light in the room bother you? • Do you prefer lights on, off, or dimmed? • Can you see better in bright or dim lights? Why?	• Patient may have more trouble with glare. • Patient may need task lighting. • Change lighting levels using the various lights in the room (e.g., direct, indirect, overhead). • Turn lights on or off according to patient's preference.

Visual field	• Can you find items in your room? • Do you tend to bump into walls or furniture? • Central visual field deficits are addressed in the visual acuity section.	• Visual field deficits may indicate an undiagnosed visual disease. • They will affect room orientation. • They will affect the patient's ability to locate call bells, bed controls, phone, food, bathroom, and so forth. • Patient will need to work on nonvisual balance strategies. • Instruct the patient in scanning strategies.
Visual acuity and contrast sensitivity	• Therapist will likely need to test grossly unless a pocket-sized acuity test is available. Near acuity is most commonly assessed through reading. • Use the following commonly available items for a functional reading evaluation (see Table F.5 for visual acuity levels correlated with font sizes and examples): — Newspaper — Magazine — Can or cereal box label — Hospital menu — Medicine bottle — Diabetes testing supplies and syringe — Name tag (front with large print and back with small print) — Asking whether patient can see the call bell and bed controls — Asking whether the patient can see and identify food on the plate — Asking whether patient can pour water into a glass or milk into a polystyrene cup.	• Therapist may need to obtain patient's glasses. • Evaluation may indicate a need for further evaluation in the hospital if the visual change is acute. • If visual changes have been gradual, refer to outpatient resources. • If patient is unable to see well, then may need to modify — The visual target (increase contrast and size, provide tactile cues) — The environment (task lighting), organization — The task (adaptive techniques) — Simplification, devices, strategies. • Provide enlarged diagrams of bed controls and other patient-operated devices or appliances. • When providing printed instructions to the patient, type them in the font size that patient is able to read (refer to Table F.5).

(continued)

Table F4. (continued)

Performance Skill or Area	Evaluation	Analysis and Intervention

	• Distance acuity
	  • Exit sign
	  • Wall clock
	  • TV
	  • Information sign-in room.	

Writing	• Write appointment. • Write phone number. • Fill out a blank check. • Write a dictated sentence.	• If the patient is unable to write, then he or she may be unable to recall items such as medication schedules, appointments, and information provided by medical professionals. Teach adaptive writing strategies such as using a bold black fine-tip pen or bold-lined paper (which can be printed off the computer for the patient). • Teach patient to enlarge writing so that he or she can read it back to himself or herself.

Basic activities of daily living	• Include skills typically evaluated in the acute care setting:
	  • Self-feeding
	  • Toileting
	  • Functional mobility (especially going to the bathroom)
	  • Signing name.
		• May need to adapt the task if vision is affecting the task.
		• Bifocals increase the risk for fall and may need to be removed before attempting steps and any distance ambulation (e.g., in the hall; Davies et al., 2001).

Navigation and way finding	• Can the patient locate the bathroom? • Can the patient navigate the room safely to avoid hazards or obstacles? • Can the patient find the bed on returning from the bathroom? • Can the patient locate and safely sit down on a chair?	• If the patient is demonstrating difficulty with this performance area, it may be indicative of a peripheral visual field deficit. • If the answer to any of the questions is no, then safety is impaired for mobility. • Instruct in room orientation. • Instruct family regarding sighted guide. • Keep things in place.

		• Instruct hospital support staff to keep things in place in the patient's room. • Instruct patient to look at baseboards for cues to where the walls end or where stairs are located. • Rope lighting along a wall can help orient patients to the bathroom.
Family support	• Is family available to assist with adaptations? • Is the family able to participate in education?	• Medicare does not pay for any adaptive equipment. If family cannot obtain the recommended devices, then the therapist must modify all tasks using readily available objects. • Signs will need to be posted to assist hospital staff with strategies if family is not available (see Figures F.3 and F.4).
Cognition	• Briefly assess memory.	• All strategies are compensatory and novel; therefore, memory must be intact to be effective. If memory is impaired, then the staff and family will need to make the environment intrinsically more accessible and safer for the patient. • Use the Mini-Mental Status Exam (Folstein, M. F, Folstein, S. E., and McHugh, 1975) or St. Louis University Mental Status Examination (Tariq, Turnosa, Chibnall, Perry and Morley, 2006).
Medical comorbidities	• Complete a thorough chart review before entering the room.	• Peripheral neuropathies will affect ability for tactile discrimination. When applying tactile identifiers, consider using rough textures (e.g., put hook-and-loop fastener on a call button). • If patient has dementia, tasks will need to be intrinsically adapted. Family must be educated. • If patient has Parkinson's disease, vision is frequently affected as part of the disease process (see Chapter 6 for further information). Tremors will affect use of hand-held optical devices. • If patient has cerebrovascular accident or traumatic brain injury, he or she may have concomitant oculomotor and perceptual deficits that will affect visual function (see Chapter 6).

(continued)

Table F.4. *(continued)*

Performance Skill or Area	Evaluation	Analysis and Intervention

Ability to adapt	• Determine insight or awareness and level of acceptance.	• Allow patient to discuss frustrations and fears regarding the loss of vision. If vision loss is acute onset (e.g., occipital stroke or sickle cell exacerbation), the fear is overwhelming and affects every interaction for the patient.
		• According to Teitelman and Copolillo (2005), the acceptance of vision impairments generally falls into the following stages:
		  — Emotional challenges: Relinquished activities, lost independence, lost spontaneity, increased effort required, and impact on social interactions.
		  — Negative emotional outcomes: Depression, stigma or embarrassment, frustration, resigned acceptance.
		  — Emotional adaptation: Cognitive restructuring, social support, adapting or retraining activities, making a contribution, faith, and genuine acceptance.

	Table F.5.		Near Vision Equivalencies

Metric Size	Snellen Equivalent (When Measured at 16 in.)	Font Size (Times New Roman)	Example
8 m	20/400	72	Legally blind
6.3 m	20/320	58	Legally blind
5 m	20/250	44	Legally blind
4 m	20/200	36	Legally blind
3.2 m	20/150	28	Low Vision
2.5 m	20/125	24	Low Vision
2.0 m	20/100	18	Low Vision
1.6 m	20/80	14	Low Vision
1.3 m	20/63	12	Near normal
1.0 m	20/50	10	Near normal
0.8 m	20/40	8	Near normal

Source. Weisser-Pike, Orli (personal communication, December 30, 2009). Reprinted with permission.

Box F.1. Low Vision Intervention Strategies

Priority issues in the hospital:

- Obtain patient's glasses, magnifiers, or both.

- Ensure call bell accessibility (place an electrocardiogram lead sticker on the call bell to allow for tactile discrimination).

- Promote self-feeding using modifications (see Figure F.3).

- Provide education to the client and relevant others about the nature of the visual impairment to increase carryover of techniques, strategies, and modifications. It is helpful to have a family member present to carry over information in the home.

- With the patient's or family member's permission, post a sign (Figure F.4) over the bed stating that the patient is visually impaired (document permission in the chart because this could be construed as a Health Insurance Portability and Accountability Act violation).

- Train the patient in self-advocacy. For example, instruct the patient to request others keep clutter to a minimum and not move things in the room, so they can be easily found where the patient left them.

- Teach navigational skills (e.g., scanning, trailing) so that the patient can find things in the hospital room and in preparation for the discharge environment.

Priority issues for discharge:

- Teach the patient to sign his or her name using a signature guide (make a temporary one of cardboard).

- Provide enlarged labels on medicine bottles if the patient is going home. If the patient has diabetes and going home, obtain a talking glucose meter and other low vision diabetes supplies. Contact the hospital diabetes educator for assistance.

- Train the patient to use a sighted guide. Train family members to be sighted guides.

- Teach room orientation skills for family, especially if discharge to an unfamiliar environment is imminent (e.g., to a subacute rehabilitation facility, another family member's home).

- Modify standard adaptive equipment (e.g., reachers, sock aids). If the patient has trouble seeing all the way to his or her feet, modify equipment using the following strategies:

— Color the edges of a sock aid, reacher, and long shoehorn or dressing stick with red fingernail polish or spray paint to increase patient's ability to see the edge of the device.

— Use a contrasting background, for example, a dark carpet or dark-colored towel on the floor, when training the patient to use a white-colored sock aid.

— Be sure to teach the patient to feel the edges of all seats (e.g., toilet, tub bench, chairs, beds) with the backs of legs before sitting.

— Mark the edges of a tub bench with a bright-colored towel. Use dark-colored duct tape or spray paint on the edges of tub benches and bedside commode armrests.

— Instruct the patient to run the reacher or dressing stick down the leg and over the foot to locate the opening of the pant leg or sock.

Box F.1.   (continued)

- Request that back braces be adapted with contrasting-color hook-and-loop fastener to assist with fastening.
- Ensure appropriate task lighting is available to maximize use of adaptive devices.
- If the patient requires magnification, all handouts should be in large print (see "Written Communication Tips" section).
- Appropriate community referral
- Ophthalmology
- Low vision resources, for example, the American Foundation for the Blind (www.afb.org/services.asp):
  - Local blind or low vision services
  - Community resources and support groups
  - Vocational rehabilitation
  - Department of Veterans Affairs services, if eligible
  - See other professional and patient-related resources in Box F.2.

Box F.2.   Low Vision Resources for Clinicians and Patients

- **Academy for Certification of Vision Rehabilitation and Education Professionals:** www.acvrep.org
- **American Academy of Ophthalmology Smart Sight Initiative:** http://one.aao.org/CE/EducationalContent/Smartsight.aspx
- **American Academy of Optometry:** www.aaopt.org
- **American Council of the Blind:** resources for persons with low vision http://www.acb.org/resources/
- **American Foundation for the Blind:** www.afb.org
- **American Occupational Therapy Association:** http://www.aota.org/Practitioners/ProfDev/CE/Aota/SPCC/LowVision.asp
- **Association for Education and Rehabilitation of the Blind and Visually Impaired:** www.aerbvi.org
- **College of Optometrists in Vision Development:** 243 N. Lindberg Boulevard, Suite 310 St. Louis, MO 63141; (888) COV-D770
- **Lighthouse International:** www.lighthouse.org and for a resource list go to https://www.lighthouse-sf.org/services/vlrc/
- **National Eye Institute, National Institutes of Health:** www.nei.nih.gov/

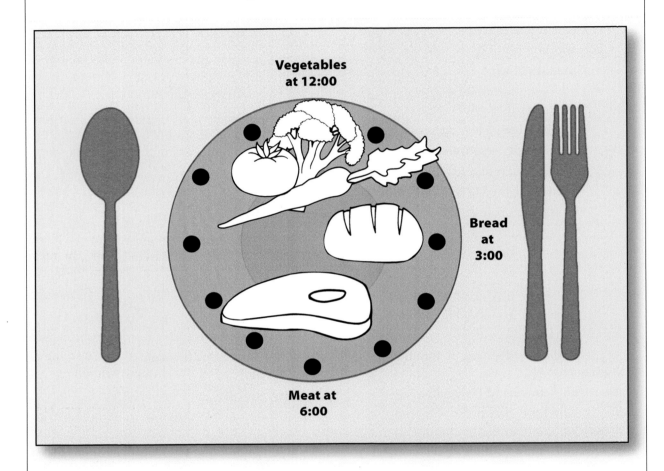

Figure F.3. Feeding poster of clock method.
Source. Richard Fritzler, Medical Illustrator, Roswell, GA.

General Communication Techniques

Occupational therapy intervention can be improved using strategies for verbal and written communication that take into consideration a patient's visual impairment. These communication strategies will improve patient understanding of education and compliance with health care recommendations.

Verbal Communication Tips

- Be clear in communicating.
  - Use specific and clear directions;
  - Use concrete terminology with specific distances and directions (e.g., "The chair is 3 feet to your left"); and
  - Do not use hand gestures (e.g., pointing to something).
- Use sound cues (e.g., tap on chair).

> ## PATIENT IS VISUALLY IMPAIRED
>
> • Introduce yourself when you enter the room.
>
> • Tell the patient everything you are doing *before* you do it.
>
> • Do not move things in the room.
>
> • Inform the patient when you are leaving.
>
> Thank you,
>
> Occupational Therapy

Figure F.4. Visually impaired patient sign.

- Do not worry about saying *look* or *see*.
- Always introduce yourself when entering, and inform the patient when you are leaving the room.
- Do not increase the volume of your voice unless the patient also has a hearing impairment.

Written Communication Tips

- Use boldface 18-point type with an ordinary typeface with uppercase and lowercase; Arial or Times New Roman are the best (Arditi, 2008; Kitchel, 2004).
- Increase spacing between lines.
- Use matte-finish white paper or light yellow paper.
- Use a black marker or gel pen when writing for the patient.
- Do not format the page in columns because it makes text navigation more difficult.

General Environmental Adaptations for the Hospital

To improve the efficacy of occupational therapy in the acute care setting, ensure that the environment is safe and conducive for learning and task performance. Using the following low vision task adaptations and modifications, ADL and functional mobility performance can be maximized to ensure successful transition to the next level of care.

Lighting

- In the hospital setting, determine which lighting is most advantageous (e.g., reading light, overhead light).
- Be aware that fluorescent light is especially difficult for patients with glare issues.
- Glare may increase distractibility, especially for those who already have difficulty concentrating. *Indirect glare* is light reflecting off surfaces such as water, highly polished floors, stainless-steel appliances (walkers), dishes, and silverware.
- Shine a light directly onto the materials when reading, writing, or eating. Be careful of burns if the light is too close to the face.
- Keep a nightlight on at night if the patient has independent bathroom privileges.
- Keep curtains or window shades pulled down during the day if glare is a problem.
- If increased lighting is required and glare is not a problem, keep curtains or blinds open so that patients can benefit from natural lighting.

Stairs

- Ability to distinguish steps depends on lighting and contrast between steps.
- Patterned carpeting can be especially difficult because it reduces the contrast between steps, making the steps look like a ramp.
- Remove bifocal and multifocal glasses before going up and down stairs because this increases falls (Davies, Kemp, Stevens, Frostick, & Manning, 2001).
- Place a tactile cue at the border of the stair railing to indicate the last step.

Hospital Room

- Do not move objects in the room; keep environments organized.
- Tape a folded 2-inch by 2-inch gauze pad, an electrocardiogram sticker, or hook-and-loop fastener on the call bell so the patient can feel it. The patient may also want another tactile adaptation on the light, TV, or radio button. Make sure it is distinguishable from the call bell.
- Use triangular pieces of hook-and-loop fastener as arrows to assist the patient in knowing in whether the head of bed is up or down.

Mobility

- Let the patient take your arm and follow next to you.
- Describe where you are going and when you are changing direction.
- Let the patient get behind you when walking in narrow spaces by placing your arm behind your back.
- Do not push the patient ahead of you.
- Do not move things in the room (post a sign).
- Explain hazards when ambulating with the patient, in the patient's room, or in the hallways.

Basic Activities of Daily Living

Following are tips for patients.

- Feeding and eating
  - Use the clock method; have someone describe the location of the food in terms of a clock.
  - Use a white plate for contrast. Put the plate on a dark surface or place mat.
  - Use the continental eating method: Cut with the dominant hand while holding the fork in the nondominant hand and using it to feed yourself. Cut with the knife going down the back of the fork rather than through the tines. Always keep your fork in the bite that was just cut and gently try to pull the bite away to determine whether it is cut completely through. Use the knife to assess the size of the bite.
- Pouring hot or cold liquids
  - For cool drinks, place the tip of your index finger over the edge of the cup or put a table tennis ball in the cup to provide contrast as it floats on the top.
  - For hot liquid and soup, use a "say when" or a table tennis ball. It will float to the top as the cup is being filled.
  - Always place the pitcher spout on the cup before pouring.
  - Pour over a sink or tray to contain spills.
- Telling time
  - Use a large-faced watch with black numbers on a white background.
  - Use a talking watch or clock.
- Applying toothpaste
  - Squirt the toothpaste directly into the mouth.
  - Put fingers around the bristles, then spread the toothpaste from end to end.
  - Squeeze toothpaste into a jar and swipe the brush over it.

— Use a travel toothbrush, which can be purchased at a department store. Put the paste in the handle and push a button to squeeze the paste up through the bristles.

- Operating appliances
  - Do not mark every setting; just pick one or two that are the most frequently used. Also mark the spot to where it must be turned.
- Clothing identification
  - Keep socks pinned together at all times. A "sock lock" can also be used.
  - Organize closets and drawers in a systematic way.
  - Label hangers with painter's tape that will easily come off when finished.
- Toileting
  - To increase the contrast between the white floor, white toilet, and clear water, use toilet bowl water bluing agent or a colored toilet seat.
  - Use good lighting in the bathroom. Keep a nightlight on all the time.
- Writing
  - Use bold-lined paper and a fine felt-tip black marker.
  - Use a signature guide.

Summary

Low vision is not usually the reason for a hospital admission; however, it can impact the disposition of the patient to the next level of care and the safety of the patient while in the hospital. Therapy focusing exclusively on low vision strategies should not be the primary issue addressed by occupational therapy in the acute care setting, but it can be the starting point for continued follow-up after the primary medical issues are resolved. The occupational therapist can evaluate and provide intervention using low vision communication strategies and environmental and task adaptations. Appropriate utilization of these techniques will facilitate ADL performance, improve patient safety and, ultimately, facilitate discharge to the next level of care.

References

Andersson, G. B., & Cocciarella, L. (Eds.). (2000). The visual system. In *Guides to the evaluation of permanent impairment* (5th ed., pp. 277–304). Chicago: American Medical Association.

Arditi, A. (2008). *Making text legible: Designing for people with partial sight.* Retrieved January 1, 2009, from www.lighthouse.org/accessibility/legible/

Black, A., & Wood, J. (2005). Vision and falls. *Clinical and Experimental Optometry, 88,* 212–222.

Davies, J. C., Kemp, G. J., Stevens, G., Frostick, S. P., & Manning, D. P. (2001). Bifocal/varifocal spectacles, lighting and missed-step accidents. *Safety Science, 38,* 211–226.

Folstein, M. F., Folstein, S. E., & McHugh, P. R. (1975). Mini-Mental State. A practical method for grading the cognitive scale of patients for the clinician. *Journal of psychiatric research, 12,* 189–198. doi:10.1016/0022-3956(75)90026-6.

Kelly, S. (2008). *Facts and figures on Americans with vision loss.* Retrieved October 12, 2008, from http://www.afb.org/Section.asp?SectionID=15

Kitchel, J. E. (2004). *Large print: Guidelines for optimal readability and APHont a font for low vision.* Retrieved January 1, 2009, from www.aph.org/edresearch/lpguide.htm

Low vision glossary. (2008). Retrieved January 11, 2009, from www.nei.nih.gov/lowvision/content/glossary.asp

Medicare. (2002). *Medicare coverage of rehabilitation services for beneficiaries with vision impairment* (Monograph No. AB-02-078, CMS Pub. 60AB). Retrieved December 28, 2008, from www.cms.hhs.gov/transmittals/Downloads/AB02078.pdf

New requirements for low vision rehabilitation demonstration billing [Monograph]. (2006). MLN Matters (Serial No. MM3816). Retrieved December 28, 2008, from www.cms.hhs.gov/MLNMattersArticles/downloads/mm3816.pdf

Tariq, S. H., Tumosa, N., Chibnall, J. T., Perry, M. H., III., & Morley, J. E. (2006). Comparison of the Louis University Mental Status Examination and the Mini-Mental Status Examination for detecting dementia and mild neurocognitive disorder: A pilot study. *American Journal of Geriatric Psychiatry, 14,* 900–910.

Teitelman, J., & Copolillo, A. (2005). Psychosocial issues in older adults' adjustment to vision loss: Findings from qualitative interviews and focus groups. *American Journal of Occupational Therapy, 59,* 409–417.

Warren, M. (Ed.). (2008). *Low vision: Occupational therapy and intervention with older adults* (rev. ed.). Bethesda, MD: American Occupational Therapy Association.

What is 20/20 vision? (2007). *Eye Digest.* Retrieved October 12, 2008, from www.agingeye.net/visionbasics/healthyvision.php

Appendix G

Bariatrics: Implications for Acute Care Practice

Judy R. Hamby, MHS, OTR/L, BCPR

introduction

The occupational therapist in the acute care setting is often faced with the challenging task of instructing patients who are morbidly obese. Given the increasing bariatric population, training in activities of daily living (ADLs) is necessary to address prevention of weight-related medical issues that arise, partially because of an inability to provide adequate self-care. Proactive ADL training will mitigate or even circumvent medical issues related to self-care deficits. Effective intervention includes instruction in conceptual strategies such as energy conservation, work simplification, and injury prevention, as well as basic and instrumental ADLs (BADLs and IADLs).

According to the Centers for Disease Control and Prevention, approximately one-third of adult Americans older than age 20 are obese (Buchwald, 2005; Foti & Littrell, 2004). The economic impact is estimated to be *almost* $100 billion, or approximately 9% of U.S. health expenditures (Bungum, Satterwhite, Jackson, & Morrow, 2003; Finkelstein, Fiebelkorn, & Wang, 2003). Provision of interdisciplinary services is critical to the efficacious provision of care to patients who are morbidly obese. If care is effectively managed, patients who are receiving bariatric surgery and patients with a comorbidity of obesity will ultimately demonstrate improved performance in BADLs and IADLs as well as take preventative measures for improved hygiene. Patient instruction in independent self-care along with encouragement to actively engage in occupation could also reduce the use of staff resources and proactively avoid complications.

Occupational therapy services dedicated to furthering quality of life in patients who are morbidly obese are vital (Clark, Reingold, & Salles-Jordan, 2007; Foti & Littrel, 2004). In 2006, the American Occupational Therapy Association [AOTA] issued a position statement regarding obesity, stating, "Occupational therapy's holistic and unique focus on occupation and daily life activities offers structured intervention and support for the management of obesity across the lifespan regardless of ability" (AOTA, 2006, p. 847). The provision of occupational therapy services to the bariatric population would serve not only patients (and their families) but also payers. By addressing the issue of occupational performance mastery to circumvent admission to higher levels of care such as assisted living facilities or nursing homes or readmission to acute care, health care costs are reduced. Attending to the patient's physical, emotional, and financial needs by proactively addressing the ADL needs of the bariatric population will ultimately improve occupational competency and quality of life (AOTA, 2007).

Morbid Obesity

According to the consensus statement put forth by the American Society for Bariatric Surgery and the American Society for Bariatric Surgery Foundation, *morbid obesity* is defined as "clinically severe obesity or extreme obesity" (Buchwald, 2005, p. 372) and a body mass index (BMI) of 35 or more if a high-risk comorbidity is present or 40 or more if no high-risk comorbidity is present (Buchwald, 2005). *BMI* is the comparison of fat matter to lean matter using a comparison of body weight to height (Foti & Littrell, 2004). A BMI of 40 or more indicates that the person is about 100 pounds overweight.

Morbid obesity often heralds the advent of many other diseases (Buchwald, 2005; Foti & Littrell, 2004) such as diabetes; renal failure; cardiovascular disease (e.g., hypertension, peripheral vascular disease, heart attack); arthritis, especially in weight-bearing joints;

and pulmonary disease (e.g., asthma, sleep apnea). It can also portend neurological diseases (e.g., stroke, carpal tunnel syndrome), vascular disorders (e.g., peripheral vascular disease, venous insufficiency), psychological disorders (e.g., history of abuse, substance abuse, anxiety, eating disorders, body schema disturbances, depression), and endocrine disorders (e.g., cancer, fetal abnormalities, male hypogonadism). The research is unclear regarding the reason for the rise in morbid obesity, but several reasons have been proposed, including childhood-related issues, poor understanding of proper diet, lack of exercise, and technology-related inactivity.

Because of the high-risk complications of morbid obesity and for cosmetic reasons, bariatric surgery has become increasingly popular. However, acute care therapists are frequently called on to work with patients for whom morbid obesity is a comorbidity, not the reason for admission (e.g., stroke, orthopedic surgery). In general, the intervention in the acute care setting is similar for both these populations, with a few

differences. The bariatric surgery patient is generally in better health and is mobile but may have incision precautions. The morbidly obese patient who is hospitalized is generally in poorer health and less active. In the acute care setting, occupational therapists rarely provide postoperative intervention to the bariatric surgery patient unless complications have occurred, because patients generally stay for only a few days. In this case, the intervention does not change from that for the patient who is morbidly obese.

Intervention

The specific issues that should be addressed by occupational therapy are listed in Tables G.1 and G.2, including patient-centered strategies and caregiver-centered interventions. Caregiver interaction can mitigate many problems if addressed proactively. Injury to both the caregiver and patient is preventable and is paramount to intervention. See Box G.1 for additional information.

Table G.1. **Patient-Centered Intervention in Bariatrics**

Performance Area	Clinical Intervention	Adaptive Devices or Strategies
Discharge planning	• Assess need for further therapy in later levels of the continuum of care (see Appendix M for further information). • Address needs for specialized bariatric equipment and specialized services. • Assess safety concerns. • Provide therapy sufficient for the patient to make functional gains, which will facilitate admission acceptance to rehabilitation facilities. • Ensure weight restrictions are maintained. Durable medical equipment is available that can accommodate >900 lb.	• Bariatric beds • Bariatric bathroom equipment • Bariatric mobility devices • Lift equipment
Basic activities of daily living		
Dressing	• Upper- and lower-body dressing. • Clothing resources to improve self-image and hygiene.	• Reacher • Sock aid • Shoehorn • Cuff and collar extenders

Table G.1.   (continued)

Performance Area	Clinical Intervention	Adaptive Devices or Strategies
Toileting	• Cleansing. • Clothing management. • Bedpans.	• Bidet • Toilet aid • Reacher • Bariatric bedpans can be obtained at www.comfortpan.com
Hygiene	• Bathing strategies. • Maintenance of healthy skin. • Regular skin inspections (with mirrors as needed) • Strategies to reduce moisture • Clothing choice.	• Long sponge brush • Hand-held shower • Long mirrors • Hair dryer (use on a cool setting to dry between skin folds) • Non-cornstarch-based powders
Functional mobility	• Bed mobility. • Getting out of chairs. • Widening doorways.	• Leg lifter • Bed risers (can also be used on easy chairs with 4 legs) • Offset door hinges • Remove door jams
Performance skills	Morbidly obese patients frequently demonstrate generalized debility; increasing activity tolerance and general strengthening will intrinsically improve the patient's ability to perform activities of daily living (ADLs): • General strengthening • Maximization of activity tolerance • Therapeutic exercise and reconditioning program • Injury prevention.	• Active range of motion (with and without weights) • Aerobic exercises • Energy conservation and work simplification strategies • Body mechanics
Psychosocial and lifestyle restructuring	Encourage engagement in • Exercise and conditioning programs • Leisure activities • Coordinating diet, exercise, and personal goals.	Include the family in these discussions
Home management	• Cooking. • Cleaning.	
Community access	• Automobile. • Community mobility.	• Seat belt extenders • Small steering wheels • Scooters

Table G.2. Caregiver-Centered Issues in Bariatrics

Clinical Issues	Strategies

Transfer techniques	• Must establish trust with the patient. Time spent in preparatory strategies and rapport building will be invaluable.
	• Bed mobility
	  — Use trapeze bars on beds to assist with bed mobility.
	• Bed controls
	  — Most Hill–Rom beds can be positioned into a full bed-chair position. Before the bed is placed in the chair position, remove the footboard. Then the bed can be lowered all the way to the floor, allowing the patient to stand up from a chair position.
	  — Keep the head of the bed up.
	  — When scooting a patient up in the bed, put the bed in Trendelenburg position to go downhill.
	• Out-of-bed functional mobility
	  — Use extra-long gait belts when transferring patients who are obese.
	  — Instruct the patient to perform multiple repetitions of knee extension when seated on the edge of the bed to ensure at least basic strength. Perform a manual muscle test. Be aware that the patient's functional strength relative to weight may still be inadequate to sustain a functional stand (Dionne, n.d.). Once standing, encourage the patient to weight-shift back and forth before moving away from the bed. Only once sufficient strength to ambulate has been established should mobility or transfers occur.
	  — If unsure about sustainable strength, have someone following with a chair or remove the footboard from the bed and ambulate around the bed. The first suggestion is the safest; however, it is not always feasible.
	  — Sliding boards are often unsafe for the bariatric patient (Dionne, n.d.).
	  — Common mechanical lift systems
	    ▪ *Sling lifts (Hoyer)*—Most commonly used device. The sling must be rated for the patient's weight.
	    ▪ *Stand-and-rise systems (Sara lift)*—Difficult to use if the patient's legs are excessively large; however, it allows the patient to bear weight on his or her own legs for standing tasks.
	    ▪ *Ceiling-mounted lifts (Arjo)*—Permanently mounted in one room and therefore not available to the general hospital population.
	  — *Stretcher chair or lateral transfer devices (Barton)*—Usually reclines flat, allowing for level lateral transfers. Once the patient is on the chair, it is then moved into the chair position. Caution with any gaps between the surfaces.
	  — Air mattress sliders, slide glide transfer devices, or sliding sheets (Airpal)—Reduces friction during lateral supine transfer between level surfaces.
	  — Caution with any gaps between the surfaces.

Table G.2. **(continued)**

Clinical Issues	Strategies

Bariatric equipment in the hospital	All equipment should be wide enough to accommodate girth and rated for appropriate weight.
	
	• Beds
	  — Frequently too high to safely get up or sit back down, so a platform may be needed (appropriately weight-rated)
	  — Beds are difficult for the bariatric patient to roll over in because of the patient's girth to bed-width ratio. If the bed is not wide enough, the patient may need to scoot over to the edge rather than use a standard log roll. However, strongly encourage the appropriate bed size to maximize patient mobility and prevent skin breakdown.
	• Ambulation devices (walkers, canes)
	• Wheelchairs
	• Chairs in the room
	• Floor-mounted toilets are the safest. If the room has only a wall-mounted toilet and the patient weighs more than 400 lb, a bariatric bedside commode over the toilet is recommended.

Precautions specific to bariatric patients	• Weight limits on durable medical equipment—Use equipment that is rated for higher weights.
	• Toilets—Discuss with your facilities management department the weight limits of floor versus wall-mounted toilets. Most wall-mounted toilets have a weight limit of approximately 400 lb. These toilets can fall off the wall.
	• Do not be cajoled into getting the patient to the bedside commode quickly if the patient has not been out of bed. Establishing mobility status when the patient is in a rush to go to the bathroom is hazardous.
	• Incision precautions
	  — Consider using an abdominal binder. Two or three can be combined to fit the girth appropriately. It is also possible to cut off a section of the binder so that it fits the trunk appropriately.
	  — Reaching down to address instrumental or basic activities of daily living may increase stress on incisions and cause dehiscence. Consider using long-handled adaptive devices.
	• Generalized weakness can increase potential for falls. Strength relative to size may not be sufficient for safe mobility.

Advocacy for the morbidly obese patient to maximize quality of life	• Resources should be provided and are abundant, especially for the patient who is Internet active, using keyword searches such as *obesity, bariatric,* or *plus size.* • Encourage compassionate attitude. • Encourage well-balanced nutritious meals.

Box G.1.   Activities of Daily Living for the Bariatric Patient

Dressing Techniques

Pants and Undergarments

Use a reacher to put on pants and underwear. Grab the waistband and thread the pants over your foot. Once you can reach the waistband, repeat the process to put pants over the other foot. Put both undergarments and pants on over your feet, then stand and pull them up at the same time. Sit down to dress.

Socks

Use a sock aid to put on socks. If your foot is frequently damp, wide, or swollen, use a soft or wide sock aid. If feet are damp, sprinkle powder in the sock aid to make the foot slide easier.

- Slide the sock on with the bottom of the sock on the rounded part;
- Pull the sock tight against the end, and stop at the rope knots;
- Put your toe into the opened sock and point down;
- Pull on both ropes with equal strength until the sock is all the way on; and
- The sock aid will come out of the sock once it is over the heel.

Cuffs and Collars

If cuffs and collars are too small, use extenders.

Shoes

If you have trouble reaching your shoes to put them on or tie them, several options include wearing slip-ons, shoes with Velcro® fasteners, or shoes with elastic shoelaces. The elastic shoelaces can be tied before putting them on, making the shoes into slip-ons. Use a long-handled shoehorn to get your shoes on.

Clothing

Many resources are available to purchase clothing in larger sizes.

Hygiene

Good hygiene is important to avoid body odors, and maintaining healthy skin is also critical for hygiene and health.

Some hints for a good cleaning regimen follow:

- Bacteria produce odor and irritation and grow in warm, dark, moist places, such as skin folds. Of these three conditions, the only one that can be controlled is the amount of moisture in skin folds.
- Odors can develop anywhere skin touches skin, not just in the groin and underarm areas, especially under the stomach, behind the knees, in the navel, and under breasts.
- Use a germicidal soap to assist in eliminating the bacteria, then rinse thoroughly so that soap residue will not lead to irritation.

Box G.1. (continued)

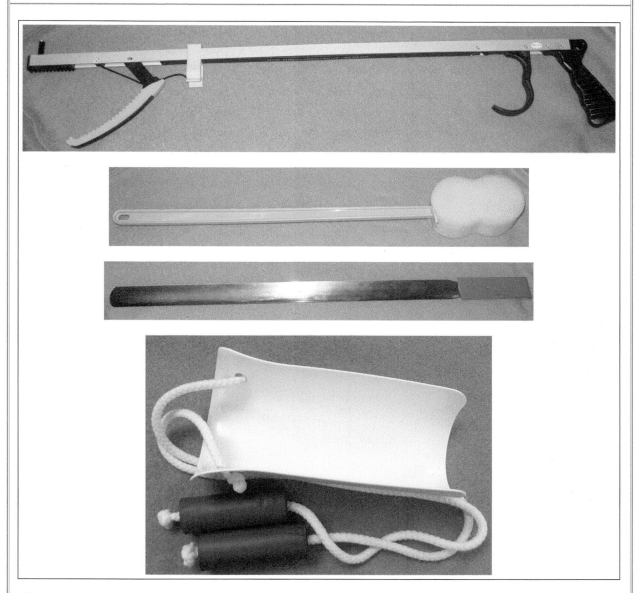

Figure G.1. Adaptive equipment used in bariatrics.

- Dry thoroughly, especially between all skin folds. You may want to consider using a hair dryer on a low, cool setting to assist in the drying process. Do not use a hot dryer, which can burn skin.
- To best clean the navel, use a cotton swab and hydrogen peroxide. Again, dry thoroughly.
- Avoid cornstarch-based powders; use Sween® cream. If this cream is not available, an acceptable option would be a noncaking cornstarch powder.
- Check your skin on a weekly basis, especially skin folds. If needed, ask a family member or friend to check areas you cannot see, or use a mirror.

(continued)

Box G.1.   *(continued)*

- Clothing choices can also contribute to moisture control.
  - Cotton absorbs moisture, and polyester locks it in.
  - Wearing properly fitting cotton underwear is important. Consider wearing a panty liner or pad to absorb excess moisture
  - Tight clothes can cause skin irritation and should be avoided.
- Freshen up during the day, using baby wipes to control odor if needed.
- Mitchum antiperspirant is especially made for people who sweat a lot.

Bathing

Hard-to-reach areas can make washing more difficult. Here are a few suggestions.

- Use a long-handled sponge for areas that are hard to reach, such as your back and legs.
- Sit to make reaching these areas easier and to save energy.
- If stepping into the tub is getting difficult, use a transfer tub bench (see Figure G.2). The bench has two legs outside the tub, and two inside. Sit on the end, slide back, and swing your legs over the edge. If you are having trouble getting your legs over the edge, use a sheet to help by putting it around the foot and pulling your leg over the edge of the tub. A shower seat is another option for those who are able to step into the tub or who have a shower stall but want to sit down.

Check the weight limit on the bath seat before buying. Most benches available in stores have a limit of 250–300 pounds. Benches rated for higher weights can be bought from medical supply stores. The manufacturer provides this information.

- Use hand-held shower sprayer to help rinse all areas.
- Place items on a shelf so they can be easily reached in the shower.
- Clean the shower sponge by either putting it in the dishwasher or boiling it for about 5 minutes at least once a week.

Toileting

Reaching to cleanse after going to the bathroom can be very difficult. Several ideas for maintaining good hygiene follow.

- Use a toilet aid to hold toilet paper or flushable wet wipes to extend your reach.
- A *toilet aid* is a set of tongs (see Figure G.3). Put the end of the toilet paper between the tongs to hold the paper, then wrap the toilet paper around the tongs. Once you are done wiping, pull the tongs apart so that the toilet paper can fall in the toilet. Carry a small, wide-mouthed bottle filled with bleach water in which the toilet aid will fit. The toilet aid can then be cleaned after every use.
- Wet wipes might allow for quicker cleaning.
- A portable bidet fixture can be installed on your toilet to further cleanse this hard-to-reach area. Most portable bidets fasten to the sink faucet, with a hose extending to the toilet. When the water is turned on, it squirts up, providing a refreshing cleaning. A squeeze bottle can also be used.

Box G.1.   (continued)

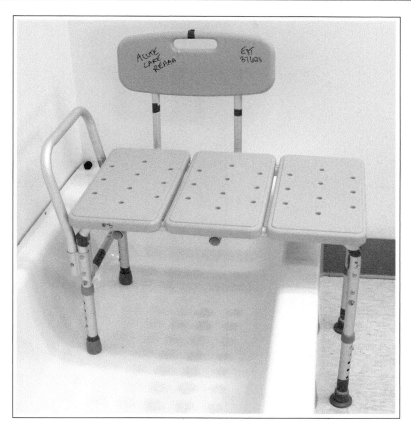

Figure G.2. Transfer tub bench.

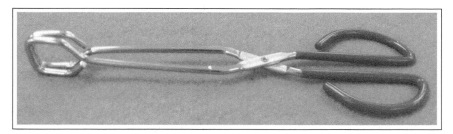

Figure G.3. Toilet aid.

- If the patient is having trouble getting up from the toilet, place a bedside commode over the toilet (without the pail), providing a higher seat and armrests, or use an elevated toilet seat with an oblong opening (see Figure G.4).

(continued)

Box G.1.   (continued)

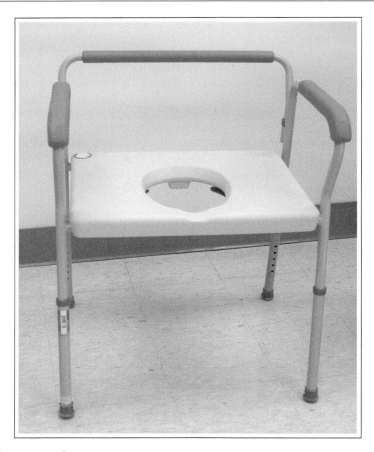

Figure G.4. Bedside commode.

Home Management

Cooking can be tiring and provides opportunities for injury. Here are some suggestions:

- Sit while preparing food.
- To improve reach, install pullout shelving, use a reacher, and adjust work heights to avoid fatiguing or painful positions. One way to do this is to place a cutting board on top of a pulled-out drawer near the sink so that you can easily cut food while seated.
- To sit in front of a cabinet that does not have room for your feet, open the cabinet doors and move things around to give your feet room.
- To reduce the weight of items that you need to carry, use lighter items such as aluminum pans rather than cast iron or use a rolling cart to transport items.
- Gather all work supplies and ingredients before starting your food preparation.
- For easy meal preparation, make a double batch of food and freeze the extra portions.

Box G.1. (continued)

Cleaning can be one of the most tiring and painful activities people do. The following are several ways to make cleaning easier.

- For low areas, use long-handled tools, such as a mop, to clean tubs and long-handled dusters, and long-handled dustpans so that you do not have to stoop.
- Use a reacher to pick up items on the floor.
- Use a heavy-duty footstool to reach high items. Check for weight limits.
- Sit to iron, wash dishes, and fold clothes.
- Use a utility or gourmet cart to carry things.
- Time-saving strategies can also decrease fatigue.
  — Keep cleaning supplies on each floor of your home.
  — Spread out the cleaning by doing one room each day instead of a marathon cleaning session on Saturday morning. This method will also make weekends more enjoyable, leaving more time for active leisure pursuits.
  — Keep the house clutter-free, reducing the time needed to clean the house because you will not have to straighten before cleaning.
  — To reduce the time spent making beds, straighten the sheets and blankets by pulling them tight before you get out of the bed. Once you get out of the bed, make each side completely before switching sides.
- Make a list of 10-minute chores that you have been putting off. Post it on the refrigerator or by the phone. When you have 10 free minutes, go to the list. This makes the to-do list less overwhelming.

Preventing injury is key to maintaining an active lifestyle. Apply the following strategies when lifting or moving things.

- When trying to pick up an item, whether small or large or heavy or light,
  — Keep your back straight, and squat instead of bending over;
  — Bring the item close to your body, and test the weight before picking it up;
  — Lock your arms around the item before picking it up;
  — Use the strength in your legs instead of your arms;
  — Rather than twist, turn your body all the way around;
  — If at all possible, push, do not pull, items; and
  — Ask for help if something is too heavy.

Mobility in the Community

Community access is very important for maintaining an active lifestyle.

- If getting your leg into the car is difficult, use a leg lifter (see Figure G.5).
- Scooters can be purchased for personal use.

(continued)

Box G.1.   (continued)

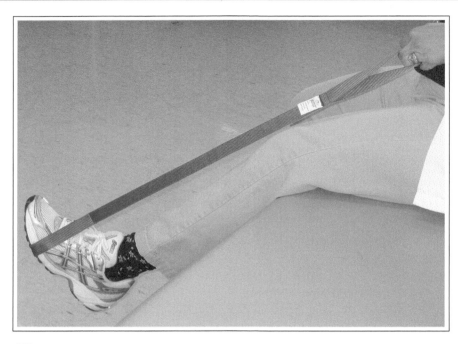

Figure G.5. Leg lifter.

- Standard seat belts are often too small. Obtain seat belt extenders.

Mobility in Your Home
Bed Mobility
Getting out of bed can be hard if your stomach muscles are weak or you have had surgery.

- Use the log roll method.
  — *Step 1:* Turn on your side.
  — *Step 2:* Swing your legs over the edge of the bed.
  — *Step 3:* Push up on your arms.

Widening Doors
If doors need to be widened, either have the door jams removed, or install offset or swing-away door hinges, widening the opening by about 2 inches.

Getting Out of a Chair
Getting out of a chair that is too narrow or low can be hard. Use the following steps to get out of a chair:

- *Step 1:* Scoot forward to the edge of the chair.
- *Step 2:* Bring your feet as close to the chair as possible and lean forward.
- *Step 3:* Push off with your arms to stand up.

Box G.1.   (continued)

If you cannot get up from your favorite chair, put it on risers. The higher the chair, the easier it is to get out of. If you have a choice of chairs, sit in the highest. The next best option is a wide chair with armrests. Check the weight rating of all chairs with the manufacturer before buying.

Resources

- *Occupational and physical therapy:* Call your local hospital to contact an occupational therapist regarding difficulty with self-care or home management tasks or a physical therapist for difficulty with mobility-related issues such as walking or getting up from a chair.
- *Adaptive equipment:*
  — http://www.pattersonmedical.com/ or 1-800-323-5547 for adaptive equipment and offset door hinges
  — www.amplestuff.com or 866-486-1655 for self-care adaptive equipment and smaller steering wheels
  — www.adaptiveaccess.com/offset_hinges.php or 281-856-9332 for offset door hinges.
- *Tips:* www.plussizeyellowpages.com or call 1-877-KellyBliss for tools, tips, and techniques for healthy living, including links for clothing.

Clothing

Women

- **Absolute Women (sizes 14–30):** www.absolute-woman.com/awcloth.htm
- **Making It Big on Line (sizes 22–44):** www.makingitbigonline.com or 877-644-1995
- **Silhouettes, Hanover Direct, Inc.:** www.silhouettes.com or 888-651-8337
- **Coldwater Creek (sizes 1X–3X):** www.coldwatercreek.com or 800-510-2808
- **Just My Size (sizes 1X–4X):** www.justmysize.com or 800-261-5902
- **B&Lu (trendy clothing sizes 14–30):** www.bandlu.com or 888-992-9899
- **Catherine's (sizes 16W–34W):** www.catherines.com
- **The Avenue:** www.avenue.com or 800-441-1362
- **Junonia:** www.junonia.com or 800-JUNONIA.

Men

- **Think Big:** www.thinkbig.com or 800-767-0319
- **Big and Tall by Kramers (sizes 1X–8X):** 800-527-5677
- **Sizewise:** www.sizewise.com/links/mens.html
- **Big & Tall direct:** http://www.bigtalldirect.com/index_768.htm or 800-214-9686
- **Big Guys (sizes 2X–7X):** www.bigguys.com.

Source. Handout used with permission from WellStar Health System Rehabilitation Department. Written by Judy R. Hamby, MHS, OTR/L, BCPR.

References

American Occupational Therapy Association. (2006). AOTA's societal statement on obesity. *American Journal of Occupational Therapy, 63*, 847–848.

American Occupational Therapy Association. (2007). Obesity and occupational therapy [Position Paper]. *American Journal of Occupational Therapy, 61,* 701–703.

Buchwald, H. (2005). Consensus conference statement: Bariatric surgery for morbid obesity: Health implications for patients, health professionals, and third-party payers. *Journal of the American College of Surgeons, 200,* 593–604.

Bungum, T., Satterwhite, M., Jackson, A. W., & Morrow, J. R. (2003). The relationship of body mass index, medical costs, and job absenteeism. *American Journal of Health Behavior, 27,* 456–462.

Dionne, M. (n.d.). *Transfer key: Bariatric ergonomics mechanical transfer section.* Retrieved January 3, 2009, from www.bariatricrehab.com/transferkey. html

Finkelstein, E. A., Fiebelkorn, I. C., & Wang, G. (2003). National medical spending attributable to overweight and obesity: How much, and who's paying? *Health Affairs Web Exclusive.* Retrieved December 15, 2008, from http://content.healthaffairs.org/cgi/content/full/hlthaff.w3.219v1/DC1

Foti, D., & Littrell, E. (2004). Bariatric care: Practical problem solving and interventions. *Physical Disabilities Special Interest Section Quarterly, 27,* 1–3, 6.

Appendix H

The Dizzy Patient

Judy R. Hamby, MHS, OTR/L, BCPR

The order for occupational therapy states, "Dizzy patient—evaluate and treat." Where do you start? More than 3% of emergency room (ER) visits are by patients with a primary complaint of dizziness or vertigo (Kerber, Meurer, West, & Fendrick, 2008; Newman-Toker et al., 2008), accounting for 8 million visits per year. In patients older than age 70, dizziness is the most frequent reason provided for a physician visit (Clendaniel, 2001). According to Clendaniel (2001), ER visits in patients with a primary complaint of dizziness include diagnoses as listed in Table H.1.

A medical and neurological workup to rule out a stroke or brain tumor is typically the reason for admission. However, if the computerized tomography scan is negative, the admitting doctor may or may not know exactly where to start with intervention. Physical and occupational therapists are often consulted to provide input regarding the patient's functional level in determining rehabilitation options, safety for discharge, or a definitive diagnosis. The admitting physician may seek input from other specialist consultants such as a neurologist or ear, nose, and throat doctor (*otolaryngologist*).

Central vs. Peripheral Causes of Dizziness

Although most causes of dizziness are peripheral, it is important when determining the primary cause to differentiate between a central or medical etiology. The differences between central and peripheral etiologies of dizziness, as well as treatment suggestions, are listed in Table H.2. However, other causes of dizziness can include

- *Vascular insufficiencies,* such as stenosis or occlusion of carotid arteries or vertebrobasilar insufficiency, which is characterized by poor blood flow to the posterior portion of the brain. It can manifest as drop attacks, especially when the patient extends his or her neck backward (e.g., when washing hair or reaching for items on an overhead shelf). Symptoms may last a few minutes or hours and are usually considered a warning sign of stroke. Symptoms vary but usually include the same signs as a transient ischemic attack with the exception of drop attacks characterized by sudden generalized weakness.

  A Vertebral Artery Compression Test is usually performed; however, it is recommended that only an experienced therapist perform this test. The patient should be in supine position with the neck held in extension and rotation for 30 seconds. Nystagmus, nausea, or vertigo is a positive sign. However, the final position of this test is also the final position for the Dix–Hallpike test, which evaluates for benign paroxysmal positioning vertigo (BPPV). Therefore, an alternative that will differentiate between the two would be to perform the test in sitting position. Instruct the patient to sit and flex forward at the hips, then extend and rotate the neck, which allows the patient to keep the head vertical, thus eliminating the etiology of BPPV (change in head position against gravity; Cohen & Gavia, 1998).

- *Cardiac insufficiencies (low ejection fraction):* Recommend a cardiology consult if dizziness symptoms are noted with
  — Arrhythmias or palpitations;
  — Orthostatic hypotension;
  — Perspiration;
  — Pallor; or
  — Syncope.

Table H.1.   **Emergency Room Diagnoses of Dizziness**

Reason	%	Diagnoses (%)
Otological	24	• Benign paroxysmal positional vertigo (48) • Miscellaneous diagnoses (33) • Ménière's disease (19)
Medical etiology	32	• Cardiac (56) • Medications (19) • Abnormal lab values (17) • Infections (8)
Unlocalized	42.3	• Unknown (64) • Psychogenic (13) • Aging (13) • Posttraumatic (10)
Central etiologies	1.7	• Cerebrovascular accident (35) • Migraines (16) • Miscellaneous (49)

- *Autonomic neuropathy,* especially if patient has diabetes. Request that endocrinology or internal medicine consult.

- *Lab abnormalities:*
    - Blood sugar levels (hypoglycemia or hyperglycemia)
    - Potassium (can cause arrhythmias)
    - Sodium (can be related to dehydration or kidney disease)
    - White blood cells (can indicate infection)
    - Increased cerebral–spinal fluid pH (can cause calcium changes and resultant nystagmus)
    - Calcium level (changes muscle activity of eyes).

- *Medications that can cause dizziness:*
    - Chemotherapy drugs
    - Antibiotics (e.g., gentamycin, streptomycin)
    - Diuretics given to kidney patients
    - Tranquilizers
    - Antihypertensives (can cause presyncopal light-headedness)
    - Anticonvulsants.

Evaluation

Use the evaluation format provided in Box H.1 to determine the necessity and type of intervention warranted. The Vestibular Disorders Activities of Daily Living Scale (Cohen & Kimball, 2000) is also a valuable tool; it consists of 28 questions regarding personal care, mobility, and instrumental activities of daily living. It is rated on a 10-level ordinal self-report scale.

Patient Resources

- Vestibular Disorders Association (www.vestibular.org)
- Self-care handout (see Box H.2).

Table H.2. **Differentiating Central and Peripheral Dizziness**

Clinical Presentation	Central Dizziness	Peripheral Dizziness
Onset	• Sudden onset, or slow onset if etiology is tumor growth • Usually accompanied by headache • Moderate symptoms overall	• Sudden or gradual onset • Severe symptoms • No headache
Functional abilities	• No standing or walking • May have other neurological symptoms	• Bedridden initially but can walk and stand a little • Disequilibrium in busy or dark environments • Motion sensitivity
Nausea	Moderate nausea	Severe nausea and vomiting
Description of dizziness	Vertigo • "I'm spinning" • "Head is spinning" • "Light-headed" • Perceived tilt	• Oscillopsia—"Room is spinning (moving)" or objects seem to move back and forth
Consistency of symptoms and duration	• Symptoms are continuous and not dependent on position • Does not subside	• Seconds, minutes, or days (with BPPV, usually <1 min) • Symptoms are positional and usually worse with affected ear down • Symptoms fluctuate and usually decrease as etiology clears • Recurrent, intermittent, or both if Ménière's or BPPV • Relieved by staying still
Hearing	Usually no hearing loss	Can have any or all of these symptoms: • Tinnitus (ringing in the ears) • Decreased hearing

(continued)

Table H.2. (*continued*)

Clinical Presentation	Central Dizziness	Peripheral Dizziness
		• Ear pain • Ear fullness
Vision	• Sometimes associated with diplopia • Walks like a robot to minimize visual disturbances • Symptoms persist even with eyes closed unless they are the result of cranial nerve involvement that causes diplopia • Can have blurry vision if the cerebellum is infarcted because of poor vestibular ocular reflex, which controls retinal slip (the movement of a visual image across the retina)	• Generally no diplopia, but patient reports blurry vision with position changes • Head turns with eyes open toward affected side increase blurriness and feelings of oscillopsia • Symptoms reduce with eyes closed

Nystagmus	• Usually in the same direction, but can be any direction—horizontal, vertical, or rotary
	• Starts immediately with testing
		• Horizontal, vertical, or rotary (torsional) and can change directions with changes in body or head position
		• Starts after delay once causative positioning is achieved
		• Describes nystagmus in terms of the direction of the fast beat of the nystagmus and which eye or eyes are moving (the eyes may be going in different directions):
		  — Downbeat
		  — Upbeat
		  — Torsional
		  — *Geotrophic* (if patient is lying on his or her side, and the fast beat is going down toward the floor)
		  — *Ageotrophic* (if patient is lying on his or her side, and the fast beat is going up toward the ceiling)
		• Increases with gaze toward involved side and decreases with visual fixation

Falls	Falls and nystagmus to same side as affected ear	Falls to same side as nystagmus (same side as lesion)
Weakness or quality of movement	Not associated with weakness	• Generalized weakness in all extremities • Ataxia
Causes	• BPPV resulting from loose otoliths ("stones" in the ear canal) • 8th cranial nerve lesion • Aging (because of loss of sensation, especially decreased proprioception in lower extremities resulting from peripheral neuropathies, and low vision causing increased reliance on diminished vestibular system) • Vestibular neuronitis • Otitis • Ménière's, which is sometimes associated with dehydration and is recurrent and hereditary • Drug induced — Alcohol — Antibiotics — Furosemide — Quinidine — Quinine — Aspirin	• Brainstem lesion • Cerebellar lesion • Acoustic schwannoma • Drugs (barbiturates or diphenylhydantoin, an antiepileptic medicine) • Vertebral dissection • Stroke, transient ischemic attack • Traumatic brain injury • Trauma—Whiplash • Migraines • Multiple sclerosis (rare)
Recommendations and treatment	• Provide ADLs handout to minimize potential for injury (see Box H.2) • Request ENT consult • Recommend immediate vestibular rehabilitation (e.g., physical therapist or occupational therapist with vestibular rehabilitation training) with expected positive outcomes	• Provide with ADLs handout to minimize potential for injury (see Box H.2) • Request neurology consult • Request vestibular rehabilitation; however, central etiology is not as amenable to therapy; habituation exercises can make symptoms tolerable

(continued)

Table H.2. **(continued)**

Clinical Presentation	Central Dizziness	Peripheral Dizziness
	• If patient has persistent diplopia, consider patching one eye. If patching alleviates all symptoms, recommend immediate referral to a neuro-ophthalmologist	• If the patient is not safe for discharge home, recommend either inpatient rehabilitation or subacute rehabilitation
	• If patient is not safe for discharge home, recommend either inpatient rehabilitation unit or subacute rehabilitation	• Durable medical equipment or adaptive devices:
	• DME or adaptive devices:	— Reacher
	— Reacher	— Transfer tub bench or shower seat
	— Transfer tub bench or shower seat	— 3-in-1 commode
	— 3-in-1 commode	— Sock aid
	— Sock aid	— Long shoehorn
	— Long shoehorn	— Long sponge brush
	— Long sponge brush	It is recommended that only a clinician with experience and further education in the treatment of vestibular disorders provide the following treatment interventions (if indicated):
	• Medication—Antivert, Valium, or both are generally prescribed but they markedly diminish the effectiveness of rehabilitation efforts	• BPPV—Epley maneuver (only trained therapist)
		• Brandt–Daroff desensitization exercises (only trained therapist)
		• Medication—Antivert, Valium, or both are generally prescribed, but they diminish the effectiveness of rehabilitation efforts. These medications are not recommended unless the patient is unable to function without medication.

Note. ADLs = activities of daily living; BPPV = benign paroxysmal positional vertigo; DME = durable medical equipment; ENT = ear, nose, and throat.
Sources. Clendaniel (2001), Flaherty and Rost (2007), Honrubia (2000), Keshner (2007).

Box H.1.   **Vestibular Evaluation**

Chart review:

- History and physical
- Pending consults (e.g., ear, nose, and throat doctor vs. neurologist vs. neurosurgeon)
- Lab values
- Radiological reports
- Medications list (especially if any new medications).

Patient evaluation (complete the following interview before initiating the performance portion of the evaluation, which requires getting out of bed):

- Symptoms and history of onset (including whether the patient recently had a virus, exertion induced).
- Ocular range of motion: Test in all directions.
- Nystagmus
  - Nystagmus beats away from side of dysfunction (documented in terms of direction of fast phase of beat).
  - Rolling tests—Do rolls elicit nystagmus or dizziness?
  - Rapid head movement from side to side—Does this elicit nystagmus or dizziness?
  - Saccades.
- Falls
  - Direction of fall
  - Precipitating event (e.g., head position, particular task)
  - Number of falls
  - Injuries associated with falls.
- Functional mobility
  - Head turns during ambulation
  - Turning around
  - Fluidity of mobility.
- Recent changes in hearing, vision (low vision), or both: near and distance acuity.
- History of anxiety, panic attacks, or agoraphobia associated with hyperventilation. Fear and distress about the symptoms, however, are normal.
- Past medical history (especially Parkinson's disease, cerebrovascular accident, or cardiac dysfunction, such an arrhythmia).
- Oscillopsia versus vertigo
  - Oscillopsia (visual world is spinning)
    - Can you read road signs while driving and see faces when walking?
    - Is the room spinning?
  - Vertigo (sense of movement when not actually moving)
    - Are you spinning?
    - Which direction—around or linear?

Activities of daily living (ADLs), including tasks that require head movement, functional mobility, and bending down (e.g., brushing teeth, walking to bathroom, donning socks).

Box H.2. Precautions for Self-Care With Vestibular Issues

Dressing

- Do not lean over.
- Bring your feet up to you to put on shoes, pants, and underwear.
- Use long-handled equipment for dressing, including a reacher for pants and underwear, a long-handled shoehorn, and a sock aid.
- Squat to pull up pants rather than leaning over to grasp the waistband.

Grooming and Hygiene

- Sit for all grooming and hygiene tasks.
- Use a manual toothbrush rather than an electric toothbrush.
- Do not lean head back to shave; consider using an electric shaver.
- Do not lean down to shave legs.
- Be extra careful with mascara application.
- Do not lean your head over to blow-dry your hair.

Bathing

- Sit for bathing.
  - *Tub:* Use a bath seat with a back.
  - *Shower stall:* Use a bath seat with a back or a bedside commode without the pail.
- Bring feet up to wash them vs. leaning down, or use a long-handled sponge.
- Do not bend your head backward or forward to wash hair.
- Do not stand to wash your groin area. Prop your foot on the edge of the tub to wash.
- Use a long shower hose.
- Have someone with you when getting in and out of the shower.

Toileting
- Do not stand to cleanse.
- Sit for urinating.
- Pull pants up to the thighs before standing to pull all the way up.
- Put a bedside commode without the pail over the toilet to raise the seat height.

Home Management

- Sit whenever possible.
- Take extra care with loading the dishwasher and washer or dryer, especially when turning or leaning over.
- Ask for help.
- Keep pathways clear of obstacles.
- Remove area rugs because they are a tripping hazard.

Box H.2. (continued)

- Keep stairs clear and use the handrail.
- Do not remove items from or place items in a hot oven.
- Use plastic or paper products rather than glassware if you must carry items.
- Take extra care when carrying hot food items. Slide them on a countertop, or Use a rolling cart.

Driving

- Do not drive until dizziness is gone.
- Avoid parking decks because the turns can increase dizziness.
- When riding in a car as a passenger, keep eyes focused on the dashboard to avoid increased dizziness with moving objects.

Miscellaneous

- Hold onto a stable surface to stabilize yourself when leaning over.
- Feel surfaces you are about to sit on using the backs of your legs, and reach for the surface with your arms to ensure safe sitting.
- Get your balance before changing positions (e.g., lying down to sitting to standing).
- Use a reacher–grabber to pick things off the floor or high shelves.

References

Clendaniel, R. A. (2001, September). *Evaluation and management of individuals with dizziness and balance disorders.* Lecture presented at Advanced Rehabilitation Services, Marietta, GA.

Cohen, H. S., & Gavia, J. A. (1998). A task for assessing vertigo elicited by repetitive head movements. *American Journal of Occupational Therapy, 52,* 644–649.

Cohen, H. S., & Kimball, K. T. (2000). Development of the Vestibular Disorders Activities of Daily Living Scale. *Archives of Otolaryngology—Head and Neck Surgery, 126,* 881–887.

Flaherty, A. W., & Rost, N. S. (2007). *The Massachusetts General Hospital handbook of neurology* (2nd ed.). Philadelphia: Lippincott Williams & Wilkins.

Honrubia, V. (2000). Quantitative vestibular function tests and the clinical examination. In S. J. Herdman (Ed.), *Vestibular rehabilitation* (2nd ed., pp. 105–171). Philadelphia: F. A. Davis.

Kerber, K. A., Meurer, W. J., West, B. T., & Fendrick, M. A. (2008). Dizziness presentations in U.S. emergency departments, 1995–2004 [Abstract]. *Academy of Emergency Medicine, 15,* 744–750.

Keshner, E. A. (2007). Postural abnormalities in vestibular disorders. In S. J. Herdman (Ed.), *Vestibular rehabilitation* (3rd ed., pp. 54–75). Philadelphia: F. A. Davis.

Newman-Toker, D. E., Hseih, Y.-H., Camargo, C. A., Pelletier, A. J., Butchy, G. T., & Edlow, J. A. (2008). Spectrum of dizziness visits to US emergency departments: Cross-sectional analysis from a nationally representative sample. *Mayo Clinic Proceedings, 83,* 765–775.

Appendix I

Safe Patient-Handling Techniques

Sharon K. Hennigan, MA, OTR/L, CHT

Occupational therapists working in the acute hospital setting may perform evaluation and treatment tasks that require the use of manual transfer techniques with their patients. These manual transfers and maneuvers place occupational therapists at risk for musculoskeletal injuries. The research on musculoskeletal injuries sustained by occupational therapists during the delivery of patient care services is limited. Incidences of injuries, practice areas in which injuries may occur, how occupational therapists manage these injuries, and changes in practice areas are not well defined in the occupational therapy literature (Darragh, Huddleston, & King, 2009).

The nursing profession has proactively gathered these data and used them to develop safe patient-handling protocols and techniques, which have led to the development of mechanical lifting devices. In addition, federal agencies continuously assess injury rates among health care providers and provide workable guidelines to reduce the incidence of injuries among these workers. This appendix, reviews current literature and guidelines and provide occupational therapists with resources to assist in reducing their exposure to injuries that may occur during patient transfers and therapy sessions.

Incidence of Injuries Among Health Care Providers

Nurses and personal care employees have the highest prevalence of work injuries (Collins, Wolf, Bell, & Evanoff, 2004). The U.S. Bureau of Labor Statistics (BLS; 2007) reported that nursing aids, orderlies, and attendants sustained 49,480 injuries in 2006, involving an average of 94 days off from work. Lifting and moving patients were the primary source of these injuries. The BLS reported that hospitals accounted for more than 4 in 10 injuries, with general medical and surgical hospitals accounting for most of these injuries.

According to the BLS (2007) report, the highest rate of injury was to the trunk, with 43 of 100,000 full-time employees reporting injuries to this body area. The back or spine was the most common part of the trunk for which workers reported injuries. Upper-extremity injuries were the second most common, with 30 of 100 full-time employees sustaining injuries to this body region.

Hospital patients are often dependent on others for their physical needs and rely on health care providers to assist them in performing their self-care activities. Health care providers have reported musculoskeletal injuries when transferring patients and assisting them with their self-care tasks. Multiple factors (Collins et al., 2004; Darragh et al., 2009; Lipscomb, Trinkoff, Brady, & Geiger-Brown 2004) contribute to these injuries, including

- Transferring patients on and off of stretchers, repositioning patients in bed, and transporting patients in a bed or stretcher;
- Patients' age and weight—a documented problem since the 1970s when the National Institute for Occupational Safety and Health (NIOSH) began reporting health care provider injuries—particularly because patients' physical size is increasing and people are living longer, requiring more physical assistance;
- Patients' limited ability to follow instructions during transfers or assist with their own self-care activities because they are combative or have reduced cognitive skills;
- Patients' balance, coordination, and vision deficits, which affect their ability to assist with transfers;

- Health care providers' insufficient physical size and strength to manage dependent patients by themselves or with teams of health care providers and possible overestimation of their ability to safely perform patient transfers;

- Inadequate staffing of nursing personnel and health care providers to participate in team transfers;

- The number of hours health care providers spend in direct patient care, which can lead to fatigue and use of awkward postures and movement patterns, including working consecutive work shifts, working 8 or more hours per work shift, and performing repeated manual lift tasks and awkward postures and movements during these extended work hours;

- Length of time during the work shift spent providing direct patient care tasks compared with nonpatient care tasks, such as paperwork, committee assignments, or supervisory duties;

- Surgeries or medical conditions that may require early patient mobility, because these patients demonstrate limited strength and endurance and require the physical assistance of health care providers to begin moving from bed to toilet, bed to chair, and bed to walking with assistive devices; and

- Patients' fear, anxiety, or distrust of health care providers during the transfer maneuver.

Injuries Among Nursing Personnel

High-risk patient handling is defined as using awkward and static postures and forceful movements during manual lifts with patients that create significant biomechanical and postural stress on the spine and upper extremities. An example of this type of maneuver is assisting a patient with moving from a supine position to a seated position while in the bed. The nursing staff may attempt this maneuver by himself or herself, and the patient may have limited strength to assist during the maneuver. The nurse or nursing aide bends at the spine and reaches with the arms around the patient's upper body or uses the pull sheets under the patient, then twists at the spine and pulls the patient up in the bed. The nurse or nursing aide may repeat these postures and movements from one side to the other side of the bed as the patient is assisted in moving up in the bed. The nurse or nursing aide raises the head of the bed and may repeat these postures and movements again to situate the patient in a comfortable, seated position.

These postures and movements create physical stressors to the muscles, tendons, ligaments, and joints of the spine, upper body, and arms, where the weight and force of the patient's body are distributed through the employee's body. These stressors can lead to the onset of musculoskeletal injuries and cumulative conditions.

Nursing is ranked as one of the top 10 occupations that experience work-related musculoskeletal injuries. A belief exists in the nursing profession that practicing good body mechanics will protect nurses from musculoskeletal injuries (Powell-Cope, Hughes, Sedlak, & Nelson, 2008); however, strong evidence has shown that body mechanics alone is not a safe practice, despite continued manual patient handling techniques being taught in nursing schools (Linton & van Tulder, 2001; Nelson & Baptiste, 2004). Nelson and Baptiste (2004) described the consequences of using high-risk patient handling techniques:

- Nursing staff working with musculoskeletal injuries who have reduced physical capacities that can affect patient safety and comfort during manual lifting techniques;

- Reduced available staff to respond and assist with patient care tasks;

- Using high-risk handling techniques that may lead to patient injuries, such as falls from dropping patients;

- Bruising of the patient's body areas when gripped to manually move the patient; and

- Disruption of skin integrity when using patient handling techniques, including ulcers and skin tears.

Staffing shortages in nursing are complicated by nursing personnel transferring to jobs in which the risk of injuries is less and nurses leaving the profession because of chronic musculoskeletal conditions. The staff shortages are addressed by using temporary nursing staff and providing overtime for current staff. Using temporary nursing staff may not be effective because these employees should be trained in all aspects of their job requirements, including safe handling techniques and resources. The training may be hurried because of the need to respond to patient care demands. As a result, these employees may not know or understand how to obtain assistance from colleagues to perform patient-handling techniques, and this scenario may lead to an injury to the temporary employee or patient. Providing overtime for current nursing staff increases the physical demands on their bodies with limited rest breaks for recovery. This solution may also lead to safety issues for the health care provider and patient.

Injuries Among Physical and Occupational Therapists

Cromie, Robertson, and Best (2000) performed a survey of physical therapy colleagues to gather insight into the prevalence of work injuries in the physical therapy profession and its impact on practice. They found that the most serious work-related injuries were associated with the low back, followed by the neck and upper-back region. The third most commonly reported area of complaint was the thumb.

The clinical practice areas most frequently left by respondents were neurology and rehabilitation. More than 17.7% of the therapists who reported musculoskeletal disorders changed areas of practice or left the profession because of symptoms (Cromie et al., 2000), which may suggest that therapists remove themselves from a particular work environment after experiencing musculoskeletal symptoms or leave the profession because of the severity of their symptoms. This study revealed that 60% of respondents had moderately severe symptoms and, of those, 40% reported difficulty performing daily tasks and leisure activities (Cromie et al., 2000).

Most respondents used some type of aid to reduce stress on their bodies (Cromie et al.,

2000). A common solution to reduce postural strain on the spine was using an adjustable-height bed or treatment table. The therapists also selected treatments or modalities for their patients' treatments that reduced stress to their bodies. For example, a therapist may choose electrotherapy over a manual technique for a patient's treatment so as to manage his or her own symptoms. Therapists need to assess their workloads, personal factors, and specific work tasks to determine ways to reduce stress on their bodies.

Little research is available specific to work-related injuries incurred by occupational therapists during the course of patient care tasks and the steps taken to reduce or eliminate future injuries. According to Darragh et al. (2009), occupational and physical therapists are at similar risk for work-related injuries and developing work-related musculoskeletal disorders. Both professions reported working more than 35 hours per week, with more patient care responsibilities, which led to increased musculoskeletal injuries and symptoms. The body areas reported by therapists to be injured or experience musculoskeletal symptoms included the low back, hand, shoulder, and neck.

Therapists continue working in direct patient care, even though their work tasks aggravate their symptoms (Darragh et al., 2009). Therapists treat their own injuries or symptoms, alter their own work practices, or access colleagues for treatment. Because therapists are capable of managing their own injuries and symptoms, they may be reluctant to report these injuries to their managers. However, more than 50% of both professional groups reported changing or were considering a change in practice areas because of injuries or musculoskeletal symptoms (Cromie et al., 2000; Darragh et al., 2009).

Health Care Facility Safety Guidelines

Ergonomics is the science of designing equipment and creating workflow patterns that keep workers safe from injuries. Workers may try to fit into their work environment by using awkward postures and inefficient workflow movements and patterns to complete their job tasks. In addition, workers may not use available equipment or have access to equipment that can reduce these static postures and repeated body movements. Any one of these factors or combinations of all three can lead to musculoskeletal symptoms and injuries. Federal agencies such as NIOSH and the Occupational Safety and Health Administration (OSHA) have provided guidelines to improve patient-handling techniques for the safety of health care workers. Health care companies and institutions are using these guidelines to assess their patients' needs and implement solutions to reduce and eliminate health care provider injuries and ensure patient safety.

National Institute for Occupational Safety and Health

NIOSH began assessing and reporting work-related injuries of health care workers in the early 1970s and published guidelines in 1977 for evaluating occupational safety and health programs in hospitals. As a result, hospitals formed safety and health committees that addressed the following items (NIOSH, 1988):

- Inspecting workplaces for health and safety hazards;
- Regularly reviewing accident rates, results of prevention activities, and other relevant data;
- Preparing information for workers on identified hazards;
- Organizing educational classes;
- Reviewing safety and health aspects for new construction and renovated facilities; and
- Investigating accidents.

Hospitals and health care facilities have many types of workers. Along with NIOSH, various agencies have addressed the different environmental factors that health care workers may come into contact with while working in this setting. OSHA has created a set of guidelines that can assist hospital administration and employees with creating a safe work environment.

Occupational Safety and Health Administration

OSHA has produced guidelines and a learning module to guide employers and employees within the various health care settings on steps to create a safe work environment leading to increased patient safety. In its *HealthCare Wide Hazards Module—Ergonomics* (OSHA, 2009), OSHA identified areas needing to be addressed in a facility's safety and health program:

- *Management leadership and employee participation:*
  - Initial and ongoing training of employees related to injury prevention;
  - Methods of transfer and lifting to be used by all staff and compliance with these techniques; and
  - Written procedures for employees to report early signs and symptoms of any musculoskeletal disorder or injury.
- *Workplace analysis:*
  - To identify existing and potential hazards within the workplace and determine methods to correct the hazards. Work tasks are assessed for duration, frequency, and magnitude of exposure to ergonomic stressors that include force, repetition, awkward postures, vibration, and contact stress.
- *Accident and record analysis:*
  - Analysis of injury and illness logs or records to identify patterns of injury that occur over time. This step includes reviewing OSHA 300 logs, OSHA 301 forms, and Workers' Compensation documents.
- *Hazard prevention and control:*
  - Providing adequate staffing, ongoing assessment of patient needs, and no-lift policies and
  - Proper selection of, training in, and use of assistive equipment or devices used to care for patients and within the work environment.

The OSHA (2009) module discusses engineering controls and solutions as modifications to the physical environment and provides employees with proper assistive devices and equipment to reduce excessive lifting hazards. Selecting proper equipment depends on the specific needs of the physical facility, patients, staff, and management. Devices and equipment may include

- Rolling shower chairs that allow a patient to be transported in the chair to be toileted and showered, thereby reducing the number of lifts by the employee;

- Shower stalls that allow shower chairs to be pushed in and out on a level floor surface;

- Toilet seat risers that equalize the height of the wheelchair and toilet, permitting a lateral transfer and eliminating vertical lifting of the patient from the wheelchair to the toilet;

- Mechanical lift equipment that lifts patients who cannot support their own weight and requires no manual pumping by the employee;

- Overhead track-mounted patient lift equipment that provides patient mobility without manual lifting;

- Lateral transfer devices to move a patient from bed to gurney and eliminate the use of multiple staff members and draw sheets; and

- Walking belts or gait belts with handles that provide stability for an ambulatory patient, allowing health care workers to hold the belt and support the patient. These belts should not be used to vertically or horizontally lift the patient.

The OSHA (2009) module also discusses administrative controls and solutions that address management and employees' responsibilities for implementing ergonomic and safety programs. Examples of these controls and solutions include

- Accurately recording employee and patient injuries and illnesses;

- Identifying and treating injured employees early;

- Providing light-duty or no-lifting work restrictions during the recovery periods for injured employees;

- Systematically monitoring injured employees to identify when they are ready to return to full duty; and

- Continual education and training programs for management and employees on the facility's ergonomic stressors, controls, and solutions. Training should be provided at the time employees are hired and repeated at regular intervals. OSHA has recommended the training include but not be limited to these ergonomic controls and solutions:

   — Employees should never lift alone.

   — Employees should use mechanical assistance or perform team lifts.

   — Employees should receive training in how and when to use mechanical devices.

   — The number of lifts per health care employee per day should be limited.

   — Employees should keep the patient as close to his or her body with all lifts and movements.

   — Employees should avoid lifting with their spine in a rotated or twisted position.

Evidence-Based Practice Interventions and Challenges

Nelson and Baptiste (2004) summarized current evidence for ergonomic interventions that may reduce nursing personnel injuries. Their article reflected greater descriptions of engineering controls, administrative controls, and behavioral or work practice controls. These controls, although beneficial for occupational therapists, may not easily fit into treatment plans for patients.

Engineering Controls

Engineering controls are preferred because permanent changes are made to eliminate risks at the identified source. They may consist of changes in the physical environment, layout of the space, and tools and equipment used to perform the job tasks. These controls focus on physical modifications to patient rooms, bathrooms, beds, and patient handling equipment and devices. The physical environment should be free of barriers that restrict the health care provider's ability to easily move the patient and related medical and mobility equipment within the confines of the patient's room. An example of this solution is a rolling shower chair that allows the health care provider to transport the patient into the bathroom. The shower area would permit entrance of the patient and shower chair. This solution can reduce the number of manual lifts required of the health care provider to perform a bathing task with the patient.

Another solution is a mechanical device that lifts a patient from bed to chair. These devices are becoming more available in hospital settings. Gait belts remain a commonly used solution to guide a patient through a functional activity. Gait belts are not used to manually lift and move a dependent patient.

Despite the advantages of such equipment, barriers to its use exist (Nelson & Baptiste, 2004) that may include

- Patient aversion to the equipment;
- Unstable or operationally difficult-to-use equipment;
- Storage issues or location of equipment in an inconvenient place;
- Poor maintenance and cleaning of equipment;
- Health care staff's time constraints to perform patient care tasks;
- Inadequate numbers of available mechanical equipment;
- No staff training on how and when to use the mechanical equipment;
- Space restrictions within patient care areas to maneuver mechanical equipment; and
- Weight limitations of the mechanical equipment.

These barriers do not excuse occupational therapists from using mechanical devices and gait belts. It is important that the therapist assess each patient's needs and reassess the patient as he or she makes progress in the treatment plan, accessing the necessary equipment and support staff for patient and therapist safety. The therapist may plan to use patient-handling equipment during the initial session and, as the patient progresses in strength and confidence, reduce the use of the equipment. The therapist may need to plan for help from a colleague or assistant, depending on the patient's physical abilities. The therapist should always have a gait belt on the patient because the patient's status can change, requiring fluctuating levels of assistance during transfers and mobility tasks.

Administrative Controls

These types of controls include developing and implementing no-lift policies, performing ergonomic assessments of patient care needs, and using patient lift teams. *No-lift, zero-lift, minimal-lift,* or *lift-free policies* or *safe patient handling and movement* are terms that apply to facility policies that strongly encourage health care providers to avoid manual handling of patients. These policies require administration and management to ensure proper equipment is available, maintained, and in sufficient quantities to meet the needs of the patient population. No-lift policies require health care workers to assess the patient's physical and cognitive status and medical conditions to determine the safest method to move him or her. These policies are effective if the following items are in place (Nelson & Baptiste, 2004):

- Management support;
- Availability of mechanical equipment;
- Equipment maintenance;
- Employee training and retraining; and
- Culture of safety.

A culture of safety requires a collective attitude and agreement by management and employees to share in the responsibility of creating and implementing safe handling policies. This culture requires that management and employees actively participate in using the available ergonomic controls and solutions, providing a safe environment for themselves and for the patients (Nelson & Baptiste, 2004).

Another administrative control is ergonomic assessment patient protocols. Methods used to handle and transfer patients vary among the various health care facilities. A fall risk protocol is an example of an ergonomic assessment patient protocol. It defines the patient's physical and cognitive status and medical conditions that place him or her at risk for a fall. Each facility defines the steps health care providers use to keep these patients safe and how and when to use available safety equipment.

The third administrative control is using patient lift teams. A *lift team* is defined as two physically fit people, competent in lifting techniques, who work together to perform high-risk patient transfers (Nelson & Baptiste, 2004). Team members are selected on the basis of having no prior history of musculoskeletal injuries and are considered physically fit. After selecting team members, these individuals are trained to work together and to use mechanical lift devices. The lift teams are believed to be effective in reducing nursing back injuries (Nelson & Baptist) because they

- Eliminate lifts that are uncoordinated;
- Are matched for body size and shape similarities;
- Reduce fatigue of the floor nursing staff;
- Use mechanical devices; and
- Are trained to lift and work together.

The challenge in creating nursing lift teams is the limited pool of nurses who are able to pass a physical exam and have no history of musculoskeletal injuries. Nursing shortages may place more work on the available lift teams. In addition, the lift team cannot address all patient-handling activities, such as repositioning a patient in bed, assisting with toileting tasks, or dressing a patient, duties typically performed by floor nursing staff.

Occupational therapists in the acute hospital setting should be knowledgeable in both facility and departmental no-lift policies and procedures. They should seek training in the safe use of mechanical lift devices and discuss with department leaders how and when to use this equipment during patients' treatment sessions. Departmental algorithms may exist that determine when and how a therapist should obtain assistance with physical or manual treatment techniques. Rehabilitation departments may use a modified version of lift teams. Multidisciplinary teams can coordinate treatment together in one session with the patient. It is important that these team members routinely work together and effectively communicate with each other during manual patient handling interventions.

Behavioral Controls

These controls may also be known as *work practice controls*. They include training in

- Body mechanics to be used throughout all job activities;
- Joint protection principles for employees;
- Manual patient lifting techniques;
- Proper use of lifting equipment and devices; and
- Use of unit-based peer leaders (Nelson & Baptiste, 2004).

Student nurses and therapists attend classes on proper body mechanics and manual lifting techniques. This training has been shown to sometimes be ineffective in changing work practices and eliminating injuries (Linton & van Tulder, 2001; Nelson & Baptiste, 2004). It is more effective to train staff in the use of mechanical handling equipment and emphasize proper body mechanics when using this equipment. Changing habits is the primary focus of behavioral controls. Nurses and therapists have relied on manual handling techniques while being fully aware of the injuries and symptoms they or peers sustain in using these techniques. As mechanical handling equipment becomes available, it becomes the responsibility of management and unit leaders to facilitate a behavior or cultural change among staff to choose to use this equipment over manual lifting techniques.

General Body Mechanic Principles

Occupational therapists newly employed in the acute hospital setting will typically participate in the new employee training related to proper body mechanics and lifting techniques. This training should include learning to assess a patient's needs and accessing resources and equipment before initiating a transfer with the patient.

An example of how to use this training could be at the close of a treatment session, when the therapist is assisting the patient back to the bed. The patient is fatigued after the therapy session and lacks enough strength to make this maneuver by himself or herself. The patient has moved toward the edge of the wheelchair but is having difficulty rising out of the chair. The therapist is using a wide stance and is bending at his or her knees but needs to bend further down to reach the gait belt around the patient's waist. As the patient rises, he or she hesitates and is slightly off balance. The therapist may need to assist the patient into a standing position, performing a vertical lift. In completing the patient's transfer back into bed, the patient may stumble, and the therapist may twist his or her back to prevent the patient from falling, while also directing the patient into a seated position onto the bed. The therapist in this situation can reduce the risk of injury and stress for the patient and himself or herself by assessing the patient's physical abilities before beginning this transfer. The therapist would identify the patient's need for additional assistance at the close of the session, leading to the use of a mechanical device, assistance from colleagues, or both to transfer the patient back to bed.

When a therapist performs a patient-handling technique, the following body position is used to maintain the body in a position of stability and strength:

- Feet planted flat on the ground;

- Wearing supportive shoes that offer shock absorption abilities;

- Knees slightly flexed;

- Feet, knees, and hips in alignment with each other;

- Spine maintained in its natural S posture, obtained by
  — Slightly tightening abdominal muscles;
  — Slightly tightening buttock muscles;
  — Keeping the shoulders over or aligned with the hips; and
  — Pulling the neck back, slightly flexed (imagine the ears in alignment with the shoulders);

- Elbows flexed to approximately 90°; and

- Palms of the hands facing each other.

When performing dynamic movements and static postures, the closer the body stays to this position, the stronger it is during the maneuver or position. Along with body posture, general body mechanic principles that can reduce the force of patient's weight to the therapist's body are to

- Plan ahead and obtain help from colleagues, equipment, or both on the basis of the patient's needs;

- Maintain a base of support with the feet and legs throughout the maneuver;

- Keep the knees bent during the maneuver;

- Pivot with the feet and avoid twisting the spine; and

- Keep the patient's weight close to the therapist's body during the maneuver.

Occupational therapists should assess and reassess their own physical abilities as they engage in patient care activities and be proactive with their own health and safety. The following list may help therapists understand their physical abilities, when to seek assistance from colleagues, and the type of assistance that may be needed to safely perform patient care activities:

- Therapist's body size and weight;

- Patient's body size and weight;

- Therapist's general health and physical abilities;

- Therapist's current musculoskeletal injuries and symptoms; and

- Therapist's current fatigue level.

References

Collins, J. W., Wolf, J., Bell, J., & Evanoff, B. (2004). An evaluation of a "best practices" musculoskeletal injury prevention program in nursing homes. *Injury Prevention, 10,* 206–211.

Cromie, J. E., Robertson, V. J., & Best, M. O. (2000). Work-related musculoskeletal disorders in physical therapists: Prevalence, severity, risks and responses. *Physical Therapy, 80,* 336–351.

Darragh, A. R., Huddleston, W., & King, P. (2009). Work-related musculoskeletal injuries and disorders among occupational and physical therapists. *American Journal of Occupational Therapy, 63,* 351–362.

Linton, S., & van Tulder, J. W. (2001). Preventive interventions for back and neck pain problems: What is the evidence? *Spine, 26,* 778–787.

Lipscomb, J., Trinkoff, A., Brady, B., & Geiger-Brown, J. (2004). Healthcare system changes and reported musculoskeletal disorders among registered nurses. *American Journal of Public Health, 94,* 1431–1435.

National Institute for Occupational Safety and Health. (1988). *Guidelines for protecting the safety and health of health care workers* (Pub. No. 88–119). Washington, DC: Author. Retrieved July 5, 2009, from http://www.cdc.gov/niosh/docs/88-119/

Nelson, A., & Baptiste, A. S. (2004). Evidence-based practices for safe patient handling and movement. *Online Journal of Issues in Nursing, 9.*

Occupational Safety and Health Administration. (2009). *HealthCare wide hazards module—Ergonomics.* Retrieved July 4, 2009, from www.osha.gov/SLTC/etools/hospital/hazards/ergo/ergo.html

Powell-Cope, G., Hughes, N. L., Sedlak, C., & Nelson, A. (2008). Faculty perceptions of implementing an evidence-based safe patient handling nursing curriculum module. *Online Journal of Issues in Nursing, 13,* 1–14.

U.S. Bureau of Labor Statistics. (2007). *Charts 10, 22, 31 and 37.* Retrieved July 10, 2009, from http://www.bls.gov/iif/oshbulletin2006.htm

Appendix J

Pain Management Through Traditional and Complementary Approaches

Suzanne E. Holm, MA, OTR, BCPR

Pain control assessment and intervention is a top priority in the acute care hospital setting. Therapists frequently work with patients who have postoperative and acute pain issues and who may also have underlying chronic pain. Not only is pain a top concern for many patients in the hospital setting, but also approximately 80% of patients report acute pain after surgery (Apfelbaum, Chen, Mehta, & Gan, 2003). Pain experiences outside of the hospital setting are also of concern. The Centers for Disease Control and Prevention's (CDC's) National Center for Health Statistics indicated that 1 in 4 adults reported a day-long period of pain in the past 30 days, and almost 60% of adults older than age 65 stated that the pain lasted 1 year or longer (CDC, 2006). Therefore, more often than not, the occupational therapist will evaluate and treat patients with pain management issues.

Both acute and chronic pain can adversely affect appetite, sleep, energy levels, and mood. In postoperative and acute pain situations, pain is frequently managed through a pharmacological approach. Therefore, adequate analgesic management is essential, and good pain control is associated with improved recovery times, reduced hospital stays, and increased individual and nurse satisfaction (Polomano, Dunwoody, Krenzischek, & Rathmell, 2008). Although acute pain can be a protective mechanism, uncontrolled or chronic pain can be debilitating and impede full participation in the healing and rehabilitative process. Long-term chronic pain issues may benefit from the incorporation of nonpharmacologic strategies (e.g., body-based pain management approaches, physical agent modalities) in addition to pharmacological intervention.

Finding the balance between the patient's report of satisfactory pain management and the patient's ability to actively participate in mobility and self-care, learn new compensatory strategies, and recall precautions is a frequent challenge experienced by practitioners in the acute care setting. Overmedication with pain medications, muscle relaxants, or anti-anxiety medications can have adverse consequences; resulting in patient lethargy or diminished alertness; confusion; and, often, slower recovery times. However, untreated or undertreated pain can diminish effective vascular circulation, place increased demands on oxygen needs, compromise the immune system, and increase the risk for venous thrombosis (Koo, 2003; McMain, 2008); therefore, effective and individualized pain management is essential.

Pain Categories and Interventions

Occupational therapists will benefit from understanding the pain mechanism of injury and both pharmacological and nonpharmacological pain management techniques to facilitate functional engagement in activities and mobility for patients who experience acute pain, chronic pain, or both. Assessment of a person's baseline level of pain or the report of any breakthrough pain experienced with activity is usually completed through a client self-reporting tool. *Pharmacological* pain management ranges

659

from traditional oral analgesics to more invasive techniques, like continuous peripheral nerve blocks. *Nonpharmacological* interventions include body-based pain management, physical agent modalities, cognitive–behavioral modifications, and visualization and muscle relaxation techniques.

Mechanism of Injury

Pain is usually categorized according to the mechanism of injury, which includes nociceptive and neuropathic pain. An additional category, known as *psychogenic pain*, or pain stemming from behavioral or emotional reasons, is beyond the scope of this section. *Nociceptive pain* indicates that an injury has occurred to superficial or deep structures. The body's nervous system is responding to nerve injury and tissue damage through stimulation of nociceptors (i.e., pain receptors). Examples of nociceptive pain include pain from surgery or trauma, pain from burns, and arthritic pain.

Neuropathic pain typically involves damage to the peripheral or central nervous system; usually, no localized area of damage or injury is present. Neuropathic pain is often described as radiating, burning, or aching, with clients frequently reporting dysesthesias (e.g., burning or tingling sensations). Pain may also follow a nerve distribution. Examples of neuropathic pain conditions include postherpetic neuralgia, diabetic neuropathy, complex regional pain syndromes, and central nervous system damage.

Duration of Pain

Both acute and chronic pain can be classified according to duration. *Acute pain* typically signifies a quick onset related to nociceptive pain from injury, trauma, or surgery. As the body heals, the pain usually dissipates over time. *Chronic pain* is a more complex syndrome and can be associated with pain lasting more than 3 months, a longer-than-expected healing time, or an unknown source of pain.

Assessment of Pain

Pain assessment requires the client's pain to be systematically assessed and the intervention documented, noting the level of effectiveness. Use of a client self-reporting tool is the most widely accepted method. However, an effective assessment can be affected by a client's cognitive or communication impairments, cultural differences, and the assessor's subjectivity (McMain, 2008). Therefore, skilled observation of a client's behavioral or physiological status is essential when a nonverbal assessment is required.

Pharmacology

Acute nociceptive pain is usually treated through the use of oral analgesics; however, the use of anti-anxiety or antiseizure medications may also be incorporated. This section provides an overview of frequently used medications. Oral pain medications, common uses, and side effects are listed in Table J.1.

Oral Analgesics

Oral analgesics are usually a first-line defense for pain management after surgery or trauma for nociceptive pain. Oral pain medications can include

- *Nonaspirin pain relievers:* Address minor pain, but without anti-inflammatory properties. An example is acetaminophen. In 2009, the U.S. Food and Drug Administration (FDA, 2009) issued a final rule for new labeling to notify consumers about the safety risks with use of acetaminophen and nonsteroidal anti-inflammatory drugs, including stomach bleeding and liver damage.

- *Anti-inflammatory drugs:* Reduce inflammation and swelling and relieve pain. Examples include aspirin (e.g., acetylsalicylic acid) and aspirin with acetaminophen. Aspirin thins the blood, and precautions should be used with people who are pregnant; have bleeding disorders, peptic ulcer disease, or kidney disease; or have uncontrolled blood pressure (FDA, 2009).

- *Nonsteroidal anti-inflammatory drugs (NSAIDs):* Used to address pain, reduce inflammation, and decrease fever. Examples include ibuprofen, ketoprofen (e.g., Orudis), and naproxen (e.g., Naprosyn, Aleve).

Table J.1. Oral Pain Medications, Common Uses, and Side Effects

Oral Analgesics	Uses	Side Effects
Aspirin	Anti-inflammatory for headache, muscle aches, fever	Stomach irritation; can prolong bleeding; not for use in children or teenagers; women who are pregnant; or those with kidney and liver disease, asthma, high blood pressure, or bleeding disorders
Acetaminophen	For generalized aches and pains; not anti-inflammatory	Associated with liver toxicity; caution for those with kidney or liver disease or with alcoholism
Ibuprofen	Lasts longer than aspirin; anti-inflammatory	Caution for those with kidney or liver disease or with alcoholism; may irritate the stomach
Naproxen sodium	Lasts longer than aspirin; anti-inflammatory	Possible stomach irritation; typically higher in cost
COX–2 inhibitors	Reduces inflammation	Possible gastrointestinal and cardiovascular side effects

NSAIDs work by stopping prostaglandins by blocking two enzymes, cyclooxygenase–1 and cyclooxygenase–2 (i.e., COX–2). *Prostaglandins* are hormone-like substances that control physiological functions (e.g., inducing fever, raising or lowering blood pressure). The enzymes, especially COX–2, promote the production of prostaglandins, which can activate the body's inflammatory response.

- *Opioids and morphine derivatives:* Frequently used to treat short-term severe acute pain, cancer pain, and chronic nonmalignant pain (Chou et al., 2009). Examples include morphine and morphinelike drugs like codeine. Additional examples include oxycodone (e.g., OxyContin, Percocet, Tylox, Roxicodone, Roxicet), hydrocodone and acetaminophen (e.g., Lortab, Vicodin), meperidine (e.g., Demerol), Fentanyl, or Percocet (oxycodone and acetaminophen). Opioids have sedative effects that may impair alertness. People who use opioids may develop a physical dependence on the medication. Common acute side effects include nausea, vomiting, itching, and constipation. With chronic use, people may experience hormonal and immune system changes and *hyperalgesia*, or increased sensitivity to pain, that may ultimately contribute to further disability and increased medical costs (Manchikanti & Singh, 2008).

Additional Pharmacology Used in Pain Management

Additional medications have been found to be effective in pain management, although pain management may not be their primary use. Off-label use pharmacology for pain control includes

- *Antidepressants and anti-anxiety medication:* Can be used to relieve pain and improve sleep by influencing the amount of serotonin or norepinephrine released; for example, diazepam (e.g., Valium) is sometimes used in relieving low back pain.

- *Antiseizure medications (anticonvulsants):* May be used in the treatment of neuropathic pain to influence the amount of neurotransmitters, especially gamma-aminobutyric acid and glycine. Gabapentin (e.g., Neurontin) has been found to be effective in reducing neuropathic pain associated with multiple sclerosis, postherpectic neuralgia, and diabetic neuropathy (Mao & Chen, 2000; Rose & Kam, 2002).

- *COX-2 inhibitors:* Have been used in the treatment of arthritis but remain under investigation for cardiovascular complications and risks, including myocardial infarction (Howes, 2007). Specifically, COX-2 inhibitors block cyclooxygenase-2 with fewer gastrointestinal side effects compared with traditional nonsteroidal anti-inflammatory drugs (NSAIDs). Examples include celecoxib (e.g., Celebrex) and rofecoxib (e.g., Vioxx) for chronic pain. Vioxx was withdrawn from the market in 2004 because of the associated high risk of heart attack and stroke.

Nonoral and Invasive Pharmacological Pain Management

In the treatment of chronic pain, interventions typically include more invasive approaches and the use of nonoral pharmacology. Possible interventions for nonoral pain management include patient-controlled analgesics, implanted drug delivery systems, epidurals, nerve blocks, and transdermal patches.

In acute pain management, patient-controlled analgesia (PCA) is a method by which the client can self-administer a premeasured dose of a narcotic solution that is delivered intravenously or subcutaneously. The medication is preprogrammed for amount and timing of delivery (e.g., 1 mg of morphine no more than once every 8 minutes). The PCA is typically used in postoperative situations and may facilitate effective pain management while limiting possible overuse. However, patients who are unable to use the pain button mechanism because of confusion, paralysis, or reduced alertness or patients who are unwilling to manage their own pain control would not be candidates for PCA.

Epidural injections are anti-inflammatory steroids that are injected into the epidural space to reduce the amount of inflammation of nerve roots exiting the spine. The epidural space is located between the dura sac and the vertebral wall. The *dura sac* surrounds the nerve roots and contains cerebrospinal fluid. The *vertebral wall* contains fat and small blood vessels. Epidural injections are frequently used in the management of chronic back pain. An extensive literature search by Parr, Diwan, and Abdi (2009) reviewed the use of lumbar interlaminar epidural injections for management of low back pain or leg pain related to disc herniation and concluded that the outcome evidence for short-term pain relief was positive.

Peripheral nerve blocks are also known as *intercostal nerve blocks, stellate ganglion blocks,* or *trigger point injections.* Blocks are used for pre- or postoperative analgesia to avoid opioid systemic effects, address acute pain control, and provide treatment of neuralgic pain. An injection, usually an anesthetic and a steroid, is given to block pain or sensation from a specific region. For example, a femoral nerve block can be used for pain control with femoral neck or shaft fractures, total hip arthroplasties, or total knee arthroplasties. An interscalene brachial plexus block can be used for pain management in shoulder surgery.

Continuous peripheral nerve blocks (CPNBs) are also known as *perineural local anesthetic infusions.* This technique is used for ongoing analgesic needs (3–5 days), especially for postoperative pain associated with orthopedic surgery. Anesthesia is delivered to the peripheral nerves that supply the affected surgical site through a portable infusion pump and catheter. Typically, people receiving CPNB report fewer episodes of insomnia and less breakthrough pain at night and express greater satisfaction with postoperative recovery (Ilfeld & Enneking, 2005). Nerve blocks require the therapist to be aware that changes in muscle sensation and strength frequently occur and that extremities may initially require extra support or protection to minimize client fall risk.

An implanted intrathecal drug delivery system is also known as a *pain pump* or *spinal pump* or as *intrathecal drug delivery (IDD).* A surgically implanted pump delivers pain medication (usually morphine or hydromorphone) to the intrathecal space around the spinal cord through a catheter. The pain medication goes directly to the opioid receptors in the spinal cord, minimizing systemic side effects. Intrathecal Baclofen therapy uses a similar procedure but is for clients with severe spasticity to reduce spasms and rigidity.

Spinal cord stimulation is a minimally invasive procedure that blocks nociceptive pain, typically chronic back or leg pain, using epidural electrodes at the spinal cord. Van Buyten's (2006) summary of research studies concluded that more than 60% of people with failed back surgery syndrome who had a spinal cord stimulation intervention experienced more than 50% pain relief, especially with early placement of dual-lead, dual-channel systems. Kuchta, Koulousakis, and Sturn (2007) found similar results for pain relief (52% reported pain relief for more than 3 years) with spinal cord stimulation placement in more than 1,300 patients.

A fentanyl transdermal system, also known as a *pain patch* or a *transdermal pain patch,* is a delivery system for opioid analgesics (typically fentanyl) that is applied directly to the skin where it is slowly absorbed into the bloodstream. It is used with people who have chronic moderate to severe pain; people with cancer pain are the primary users. The matrix fentanyl membrane patch has a silicone matrix with a rate-controlling membrane that maintains a more constant medication concentration over a 72-hour period.

Nonpharmacological Pain Management

Clients and families benefit from education regarding pain pathways, pain cycles, and pain management techniques that can provide a sense of control over pain sensations and pain perceptions. Nonpharmacological treatment approaches can be used to address both acute and chronic pain issues. In occupational therapy, nonpharmacological approaches can be integrated into treatment to further facilitate engagement in occupational performance areas, skills, and patterns. In addition to a decline in participation in self-care and instrumental activities of daily living (IADLs), the therapist should be mindful of additional deficits that

accompany ongoing, chronic pain issues, including decreased flexibility, impairments in posture and balance, and diminished activity tolerance (Stanos, McLean, & Rader, 2007).

Müllersdorf and Söderback's (2002) review of the literature regarding occupational therapy interventions used in long-term pain management cited the use of many nonpharmacological treatments, including adaptation of the environment, arts and crafts, assistive devices, biofeedback, body mechanics training, ergonomics, joint protection, relaxation techniques, and stress management. Body-based pain management approaches are listed in Table J.2.

Additionally, Müllersdorf and Söderback's (2002) research specifically supported the use of occupational therapy with clients who experience chronic pain to address education, limitations in activity performance, patient discouragement, issues related to dependency, and needs related to occupation. Rochman and Kennedy-Spaien (2007) promoted additional intervention areas for occupational therapists working in pain management, including the use of portable pain control modalities (e.g., cold packs, self-massage), retraining in proper body mechanics, education on both the pacing of activities and incorporating breaks into daily routines, assertive training, and muscle reeducation that includes relaxation. Physical agent modalities used in pain management are listed in Table J.3.

In framing both alternative and complementary approaches to pain management, the biopsychosocial model, developed by Engel (1977), is commonly used to address the integral psychological and social aspects related to chronic pain. This model encourages independence through activity and function, rather than focusing on pain and dysfunction, and incorporates a multidisciplinary team approach (Simmonds & Peat, 2002). Approaches used in the biopsychosocial model can include cognitive–behavioral psychotherapy, mind–body treatments, and the integration of physical modalities. Specifically, cognitive–behavioral therapy increases the individual's perception of pain by increasing awareness of what contexts and behaviors influence pain so that chronic pain can be more adequately controlled. Cognitive–behavioral therapy approaches also include distraction strategies

Table J.2. Body-Based Approaches Used in Pain Management

Approach	Description
Exercise	Includes ROM, stretching, strengthening, and cardiovascular activity to build the immune system, improve cardiovascular health, and increase self-esteem.
ROM	Used to lengthen skin, fascia, ligaments, and muscles as a precursor to further muscle strengthening and retraining; increases blood flow and minimizes contractures (Stanos, McLean, & Rader, 2007).
Muscle conditioning	Improves overall function and stability while decreasing pain through strengthening, endurance, and muscle re-education.
Acupuncture or acupressure	Works through stimulation of specific points on the body through the use of fine needles or pressure. Treatment focuses on restoration of health.
Hydrotherapy	Water therapy can decrease stress on joints during exercise, improve circulation, and relax muscles. Hydrostatic forces can reduce edema and improve cardiopulmonary status (Stanos et al., 2007).
Massage	Used to enhance circulation, relaxation, and endogenous (e.g., from within the body) opioid release and improve venous return and lymphatic drainage.
Mobilization and manipulation	Mobilization includes the use of soft-tissue techniques to enhance joint ROM; manipulation also includes the use of forces to increase joint movement beyond a restriction (Stanos et al., 2007).
Tai Chi, Qigong, and yoga	Mind–body approaches that can enhance coordination and overall well-being through specific postures or movement patterns that incorporate breathing and relaxation techniques.

Note. ROM = range of motion.

such as listening to music; reading a book; praying; or playing video, number, or word games (e.g., counting backward by 3s, word anagrams). Cognitive–behavioral modifications used in pain management are listed in Table J.4.

In using a visualization technique, the client incorporates both deep breathing and the general or specific release of tension while imagining being engaged in a favorite activity or at a preferred location, like relaxing at the beach. Progressive muscle relaxation incorporates deep breathing and the purposeful tensing and release of tension in the major muscle groups, usually performed in a systematic order. With regard to meditation practices, mindfulness-based stress reduction incorporates meditation techniques with martial arts training to promote healing. Dr. Jon Kabat-Zinn at the University of Massachusetts Medical Center (Center for Mindfulness, n.d.) developed this form of meditation, and it is frequently used with clients who experience chronic pain. Suggestions for visualization and muscle relaxation techniques are given in Table J.5.

Additionally, the National Center for Complementary and Alternative Medicine (2007), which is part of the National Institutes of

Table J.3.   **Physical Agent Modalities Used in Pain Management**

Modality	Description
Transcutaneous electrical nerve stimulation (TENS)	The use of mild electronic impulses to block pain messages (inhibits nociceptive C-fibers by stimulating A-fibers) and to release endorphins. Typically used with chronic pain.
Electrical stimulation	Use of high-voltage pulsed galvanic stimulation to block pain messages, reduce muscle spasm, and minimize edema
Ultrasound	Use of deep heat primarily over joint tissues to facilitate stretching
Superficial heat and cold	Used to desensitize an area and minimize muscle spasms. Ideally should not be used >15–20 min at a time. Heat should not be used in the acute phase of an injury.

Table J.4.   **Cognitive–Behavioral Modifications Used in Pain Management**

Cognitive–Behavioral Approach	Description
Biofeedback	Use of an external device (like electromyography) to alter a physiological response through graded feedback.
Hypnosis	Being guided into an altered or focused state of consciousness through use of a specialized trained clinician (often a psychologist) to permit the mind to open to beneficial suggestions. Self-hypnosis can also be used.
Imagery and visualization	Also known as *guided imagery,* this method incorporates relaxation through the use of a picture or image or one's imagination while focusing on additional senses such as auditory or sensory, to shift attention away from the pain.
Distraction	Management of pain by directing attention elsewhere, including the use of television, radio, or music.
Progressive muscle relaxation	The use of controlled breathing and stretching to reduce pain and promote overall relaxation. Can also include relaxation breathing or deep-breathing exercises.
Meditation	A type of intervention that promotes deeper relaxation or a greater awareness; can have an effect on pain by decreasing anxiety and stress.

Table J.5. Suggestions for Visualization and Muscle Relaxation Techniques

Suggestion	Description
Visualization	Start with a short (5-min) time frame, and gradually increase the time to 15–20 min. Arrange for the client to be undisturbed and positioned comfortably laying in bed or sitting in a chair. Have the client close his or her eyes and cue him or her to breathe slowly and deeply. Have the client think of a place that is calm and peaceful.
	Suggested scenario: "You are lying on a warm, sandy beach. Feel the gentle breezes touching your skin, hear the ocean as it meets the shore, smell the saltwater in the air. Feel the sand running through your fingers. Listen to the waves coming in and out, in and out. . . . Feel your body sinking into the warm sand . . . . Feel the warmth of the sun and see the beautiful colors of the sunset. . . . Imagine the ocean washing away your worries, leaving you feeling cleansed and relaxed. Spend a few minutes savoring the peacefulness of this place . . . all its sound, smells, textures, and sights. Slow your breathing with the movement of the waves, and let your muscles relax and feel heavy. Let the waves carry away any tension. When you are ready, take a deep breath and, as you exhale, slowly open your eyes."
Muscle relaxation	Start with a short (5-min) timeframe, and gradually increase the time to 15–20 min. Arrange for the client to be undisturbed and positioned comfortably. Instruct the client to close his or her eyes and take 3 deep breaths, breathing in through the nose and out through the mouth. Focus on breathing out more than on breathing in. Cue the client to return to breathing if the mind is wandering or he or she has difficulty focusing.
	Suggested scenario: "Close your eyes. Tighten the muscles in your face, scrunch them up, and then let your face and mouth smooth out and relax.
	Relax your brow. Let your head and neck relax deeper into the pillow, sinking into it.
	Now tighten the muscles in your shoulders and arms. Hold it . . . and then let your shoulders and arms relax.
	Make a tight fist with your hands, hold it . . . and then open your hands letting them relax by your sides.
	Sink deeper into the pillow. Your body is feeling heavy.
	Take a deep breath and let it out. Breathe out the tension.
	Now tighten the muscles in your stomach and back, hold it . . . and then let your stomach and back relax. Let your body sink into the bed [or chair].
	Now tighten your buttocks, hold it . . . and then let the tension go out of your pelvis and buttocks. Take a deep breath and let it out.
	Tighten the muscles in your thighs and legs, hold it . . . and then let your thighs and knees relax.
	Now tighten the muscles in your ankles, feet, and toes, hold it . . . and then let them relax.
	Your body is getting heavy and warm.
	Stay in this position for a few minutes feeling comfortable and relaxed. When you are ready, slowly open your eyes and stretch."

Table J.5.   (continued)

Suggestion	Description
Simple deep breathing	Have the client sit quietly with his or her shoulders relaxed. Cue the client to breathe out slowly through gently pursed lips for a count of 3–5. Then cue the client to pause for 1–2 counts, neither inhaling nor exhaling. Cue to inhale slowly, through the nose, if possible, while expanding the belly for a count of 2. Then exhale slowly again. Ideally, the client should work up to exhaling the breath twice as long as inhaling the breath.

Health, has classified nontraditional pain management into five approaches: (1) alternative medical systems (e.g., acupuncture), (2) mind–body therapies (e.g., biofeedback, hypnosis), (3) biologically based therapies (e.g., herbal medicine), (4) energy therapies (e.g., Reiki, healing touch), and (5) manipulative or body-based methods (e.g., massage therapy, chiropractic).

Occupational therapists working with clients who have pain management issues should seek to incorporate meaningful occupations and activities whenever possible, guide clients in setting short- and long-term goals, help to establish a daily routine that will integrate coping strategies and pacing activities, and include some aspect of play, music, laughter, or art.

Additional nontraditional pain management approaches that are beyond the scope of this book include animal-assisted therapy; aromatherapy; art therapy; the use of herbs, vitamins, and diet; hyperbaric oxygen treatments; magnets; music; prayer; and psychotherapy.

References

Apfelbaum, J. L., Chen, C., Mehta, S. S., & Gan, T. J. (2003). Postoperative pain experience: Results from a national survey suggests postoperative pain continues to be undermanaged. *Anesthesia and Analgesia, 97,* 534–540.

Center for Mindfulness in Medication, Health Care and Society. (n.d.). *30 years of international distinction.* Retrieved September 23, 2010 from http://www.lib.wsc.ma.edu/webapa.htm.

Centers for Disease Control and Prevention. (2006). *New report finds pain affects millions of Americans.* Retrieved July 2, 2009, from www.cdc.gov/nchs/pressroom/06facts/hus06.htm

Chou, R., Fanciullo, G. J., Fine, P. G., Adler, J. A., Ballantyne, J. C., Davies, P., et al. (2009). Clinical guidelines for the use of chronic opioid therapy in chronic noncancer pain. *Journal of Pain, 10,* 113–130.

Engel, G. (1977). The need for a new medical model: A challenge for biomedicine. *Science, 196,* 129–136.

Howes, L. G. (2007). Selective COX–2 inhibitors, NSAIDs, and cardiovascular events—Is celecoxib the safest choice? *Therapeutics and Clinical Risk Management, 3,* 831–845.

Ilfeld, B. M., & Enneking, F. K. (2005). Continuous peripheral nerve blocks at home: A review. *Anesthesia and Analgesia, 100,* 1822–1833.

Koo, P. J. S. (2003). Acute pain management. *Journal of Pharmacy Practice, 16,* 231–248.

Kuchta, J., Koulousakis, S., & Sturn, V. (2007). Neurosurgical pain therapy with epidural spinal cord stimulation (SCS). *Acta Neurochirugica Supplement, 97,* 65–70.

Manchikanti, L., & Singh, A. (2008). Therapeutic opioids: A ten-year perspective on the complexities and complications of the escalating use, abuse, and nonmedical use of opioids. *Pain Physician, 11*(2, Suppl.), S63–S88.

Mao, J., & Chen, L. L. (2000). Gabapentin in pain management. *Anesthesia and Analgesia, 91,* 680–687.

McMain, L. (2008). Principles of acute pain management. *Journal of Perioperative Practice, 18,* 472–478.

Müllersdorf , M., & Söderback, I. (2002). Occupational therapists' assessments of adults with long-term pain: The Swedish experience. *Occupational Therapy International, 9,* 1–23.

National Center for Complementary and Alternative Medicine. (2007). *What is CAM?* Retrieved April 7, 2009, from http://nccam.nih.gov/health/whatiscam/overview.htm

Parr, A. T., Diwan, S., & Abdi, S. (2009). Lumbar interlaminar epidural injections in managing chronic low back and lower extremity pain: A systematic review. *Pain Physician, 12,* 163–188.

Polomano, R. C., Dunwoody, C. J., Krenzischek, D. A., & Rathmell, J. P. (2008). Perspectives on pain management in the 21st century. *Journal of PeriAnesthsia Nursing, 23*(1, Suppl.), S4–14.

Rochman, D., & Kennedy-Spaien, E. (2007). Chronic pain management: Approaches and tools for occupational therapy. *OT Practice, 12*(13), 9–15.

Rose, M. A., & Kam, P. C. (2002). Gabapentin: Pharmacology and its use in pain management. *Anaesthesia, 57,* 451–462.

Simmonds, M. J., & Peat, J. H. (2002). Rehabilitation therapies in pain and disability management: An activity-driven biopsychosocial model of practice. In C. D. Tollison, J. R. Satterthwaite, & J. W. Tollison (Eds.), *Practical pain management* (3rd ed., pp. 120–135). Philadelphia: Lippincott Williams & Wilkins.

Stanos, S. P., McLean, J., & Rader, L. (2007). Physical medicine rehabilitation approach to pain. *Medical Clinics of North America, 91,* 721–759.

Van Buyten, J. (2006). Neurostimulation for chronic neuropathic back pain in failed back surgery syndrome. *Journal of Pain and Symptom Management, 31,* 25–29.

U.S. Food and Drug Administration. (2009). *Aspirin for reducing your risk of heart attack and stroke: Know the facts.* Retrieved July 5, 2009, from www.fda.gov/Drugs/EmergencyPreparedness/BioterrorismandDrugPreparedness/ucm133431.htm

Appendix K

Evidence-Based Practice

Natan Berry, MS, OTR/L

Evidence-based practice (EBP) creates a framework for valid, accurate, and meaningful interventions in occupational therapy practice. Best practice can occur in implementing effective interventions when therapists work with research evidence, clinical knowledge, and clinical reasoning in collaboration with clients (Dunn & Ball, 2008). EBP seeks to incorporate evidence obtained from a scientific method into clinical practice. Clinicians can thus better engage in best practices and increase the validity of the interventions they choose. EBP is "the conscientious, explicit and judicious use of current best evidence in making decisions about the care of the individual patient. It means integrating individual clinical expertise with the best available external clinical evidence from systematic research" (Sackett, Rosenberg, Muir Gray, Haynes, & Richardson, 1996, p. 71).

Using EBP not only ensures better-quality and more effective treatment, but it can also help validate what occupational therapists do as a profession. Using evidence to support occupational therapy services makes insurance companies and other third-party payers more likely to reimburse for occupational therapy services (Wells, 2007). This appendix describes some of the steps and procedures to achieve EBP.

Evidence-Based Practice and Occupational Therapy

Since EBP was first introduced in 1996, its focus has evolved into a systematic use of best practice with an emphasis on client centered-care and coordination among all practitioners and administrators working with the client (Bondoc & Burkardt, 2004). EBP is compatible with the *Occupational Therapy Practice Framework* (2nd ed.; AOTA, 2008a), which supports a client-centered approach to planning interventions and using the best available evidence to support practice. The American Occupational Therapy Association (AOTA) in its *Centennial Vision* has challenged practitioners to produce research that demonstrates the effectiveness of occupational therapy in six areas, including rehabilitation and productive aging (Gutman, 2008), two common practice areas in acute care.

AOTA (2008b) has supported use of evidence-based literature and its application to practice. AOTA has advocated the use of studies and sources that are high in quality, rigor, and clinical relevance (AOTA, 2008a), and it has dedicated a section of its Web site to evidence-based practice and research, which includes a variety of tools, including the Evidence Brief Series. This section reviews information related to a variety of practice areas relevant to acute care practice (e.g., traumatic brain injury, geriatrics, Parkinson's disease, stroke, multiple sclerosis, substance abuse disorders). In addition, AOTA also has available a list of Critically Appraised Topics and Papers on health conditions and areas of practice, Web-based EBP resources, and an EBP *Resource Directory*. Even with these resources, individual clinicians should be proactive and well versed in doing their own search for evidence to support best practice patterns (Taylor, 2000).

Challenges

Therapists face several challenges in incorporating EBP into acute care. For example, frequent productivity expectations can limit EBP implementation because it can take valuable time that therapists simply do not have. Al-Almaie and Al-Baghli (2005) found that the biggest barriers to practicing EBP by physicians were lack of training (72.9%), facilities (34.4%), and time (29.2%). Young and Ward (2001) also found that lack of time was considered an important barrier to incorporating EBP. In addition, occupational and physical therapists have also cited time constraints as a barrier to EBP (Jette et al., 2003; Taylor, 2000).

Because EBP was only introduced in the mid-1990s, universities have only recently started incorporating EBP into curricula. Training in, familiarity with, and confidence in being able to search databases tend to be associated with younger therapists who are inexperienced. However, new therapists may not yet have a grasp of the gaps in knowledge and practice.

Another challenge with EBP is that many older therapists may not have learned how to complete research or apply research to practice. Therapists who have always done things a certain way may have trouble adjusting to newer techniques and prefer to continue with routine approaches and interventions. One form of collecting and using information without the practitioner's awareness is *tacit knowledge* (Pollock & Rochon, 2002), which is knowledge that is embedded in one's thinking process. Practicing therapists base therapeutic interventions on current knowledge and previous experience. Thus, they select interventions without consciously thinking about whether evidence exists to support their choice, a further barrier to EBP.

Searching for Evidence

For therapists to actively find evidence, they need to know what specifically they are seeking, which is done by formulating a research question and identifying the situation about which they are seeking information. In formulating a research question for EBP, three elements must be included: (1) situation, (2) intervention and comparison, and (3) outcomes. The literature is reviewed to determine which interventions are currently available, how they compare with each other, how they can be implemented, and what the expected outcomes are (Lou, 2002).

Over the past several years, EBP has become an accepted provision of therapy services. Concurrently, an ever-increasing amount of evidence has also become available. Accessibility has increased because of the advent of the Internet, which allows clinicians to access literature and full-text journals from anywhere in the world, although often at a cost if the practitioner is not associated with a hospital that has a medical library with access to these databases.

Although books, non–peer-reviewed journals, and professional magazines are acceptable sources of information, it is best to seek information from peer-reviewed journals and publications, because peer-reviewed journals have a higher level of authenticity and are better scrutinized by experts in the field (Lou, 2002). Applying peer-reviewed results to clinical practice should lead to better outcomes because the evidence supports it.

When searching for evidence on the Internet, it is important to note the differences between using general search engines, such as Google, and electronic bibliographic databases, such as CINAHL or Medline. A Google search may show results not necessarily written by experts, and the information provided may be inaccurate and not trustworthy. One frequently used example is Wikipedia, an online encyclopedia. Although the information listed in Wikipedia articles appears credible and accurate, it cannot be considered a credible or reliable source, because all articles can be edited by anyone. Although information obtained through search engines may be accessed more quickly, using scholarly databases can bring results that are more reliable because they can be filtered to show only peer-reviewed articles. Occupational therapy is a skilled profession and requires a higher standard of practice, so research should be from reliable and credible sources. Various databases that may assist the acute care therapist in searching for evidence to support best practice are listed in Table K.1.

In evaluating Web sites, several questions must be addressed in determining whether the information listed is trustworthy and helpful. Is the Web site relevant to what you are looking for? Is the information current and presented by a reliable organization? When was the information

(Text continues on p. 674)

Table K.1. Helpful Databases for Doing a Literature Search

Database	Focus	Availability	Web Site
AgeLine	Older adults and aging	Free	www.aarp.org/research/ageline/
CINAHL	Publications from nursing and the allied health professions, including occupational therapy	Subscription	www.ebscohost.com/cinahl/
Cochrane Library	Database collection that contains independent evidence to inform health care decision making; Consists of systematic reviews, technology assessments, and clinical trials	Subscription	www3.interscience.wiley.com/cgi-bin/mrwhome/106568753/HOME?CRETRY=1&SRETRY=0
ERIC	Education literature	Free	www.eric.ed.gov/
Medline	Compilation of medical- and biomedical-related publications from the National Library of Medicine	Free	www.nlm.nih.gov/medlineplus/
OTDBASE	Occupational therapy journal literature search service based in Canada	Subscription	www.otdbase.org/
OT Search	Bibliographic database covering the literature of occupational therapy and its related subject areas hosted by AOTA	Subscription	www1.aota.org/otsearch/
OT Seeker	Database of abstracts of systematic reviews and randomized controlled trials relevant to occupational therapy	Free	www.otseeker.com/
OvidSP	Collection of medical and health subjects; users can search multiple databases at once	Subscription	http://gateway.ovid.com/
PsycINFO	Abstracts of international literature in psychology and related behavioral and social sciences	Subscription	www.apa.org/psycinfo/
PubMed Central	Digital archive of biomedical and life sciences journal literature from NIH	Free	www.pubmedcentral.nih.gov/

(*continued*)

<table>
<tr><td colspan="4" align="center">*Table K.1.*   (*continued*)</td></tr>
</table>

Database	Focus	Availability	Web Site
SUM-Search 2	Selects the best resources for your question, formats your question for each resource, and makes additional searches based on results	Free	http://sumsearch.uthscsa.edu/

Note. AOTA = American Occupational Therapy Association; NIH = National Institutes of Health.
Source. From Lou, J. Q. (2002). Searching for the evidence. In M. Law (Ed.), *Evidence-based rehabilitation* (pp. 72–94). Thorofare, NJ: Slack. Copyright © 2002 by Slack, Inc. Adapted with permission.

Table K.2.   **Additional Evidence Resources**

Resource	Description	Web Site
AARP	Identifies and provides links to >300 major or unique libraries, clearinghouses, databases, directories, bibliographies, and Web metasites around the world that focus on aging or closely allied subjects	www.aarp.org/research/internet_resources/
Google Scholar	Search across many disciplines and sources—peer-reviewed papers, theses, books, abstracts, and articles—from academic publishers, professional societies, preprint repositories, universities, and other scholarly organizations	http://scholar.google.com
National Center for the Dissemination of Disability Research	Provides access to the Cochrane Library free of charge in areas associated with disseminating disability research	www.ncddr.org/cochrane/
Guidelines for using McMaster Qualitative review form	How to critically review qualitative studies	www.srs-mcmaster.ca/Portals/20/pdf/ebp/qualguidelines_version2.0.pdf
Guidelines for using McMaster Quantitative review form	How to critically review quantitative studies	www.srs-mcmaster.ca/Portals/20/pdf/ebp/quanguidelines.pdf
Psychological Database for Brain Impairment Treatment Efficacy	Database that catalogs studies of cognitive, behavioral, and other treatments for psychological problems and issues occurring as a consequence of acquired brain impairment	www.psycbite.com/

Table K.3. Levels of Evidence for Occupational Therapy Outcomes Research

Level of Evidence for Design	Definition
I	Randomized controlled trial
II	Nonrandomized controlled trial—2 group
III	Nonrandomized controlled trial—2 group (1 treatment), pretest and posttest
IV	Single-subject design
V	Narratives; case studies
Sample size	
A	$N \geq 20$ per condition
B	$N < 20$ per condition
Internal validity	
1	*High internal validity:* No alternate explanation for outcome
2	*Moderate internal validity:* Attempt to control for lack of randomization
3	*Low internal validity:* 2 or more serious alternative explanations for outcome
External validity	
a	*High external validity:* Participants represent population, and treatments represent current practice
b	*Moderate external validity:* Between high and low
c	*Low external validity:* Heterogeneous sample without being able to understand whether effects were similar for all diagnoses or treatment does not represent current practice

Note. The format of level coding is design + sample size + internal validity + external validity. For example, a study coded as IIA2a is a 2-group or 2-condition nonrandomized controlled trial design with a sample size of 20 or more participants per condition, with moderate internal validity in which an attempt was made to control for lack of randomization and with high external validity in which both participants represented the population under study (e.g., stroke) and treatments represented current practice (e.g., Bobath neurodevelopmental treatment).

Source. From Lieberman, D., & Scheer, J. (2002). AOTA's Evidence-Based Literature Review Project: An overview. *American Journal of Occupational Therapy, 56,* 346. Copyright © 2002 by the American Occupational Therapy Association. Reprinted with permission.

last updated? Is the information presented clearly in a well-organized manner? Is the author or source reputable and credible? Is the information presented based on evidence or on opinion? Government (.gov), educational institution (.edu), and organization (.org) domains are generally more reliable sources of information than commercial sites (.com). Refer to Table K.2 for a list of additional Internet resources.

One obstacle to searching for evidence using databases is that the therapist may be confronted with too many results. To help narrow search results, search terms should be as specific as possible. In addition, the therapist can use the Boolean term "AND" to connect two keywords and limit publication years, language, and publication type. Broadening search terms using "OR" between two keywords, including all publication types and searching for older articles, are helpful when initial results are too few. Once research articles are located through a literature search, they will still need to be judged for validity, reliability, and applicability (Lou, 2002).

Levels of Evidence

When reviewing literature, the different levels of evidence with regard to design, sample size, internal validity, and external validity need to be evaluated (Lieberman & Scheer, 2002). McMaster University has useful guidelines for evaluating qualitative and quantitative evidence (Law et al., 1998; Letts et al., 2007) in the literature. The best level of evidence (also known as the gold standard) is a randomized controlled trial (Level I) with a sample size of 20 or more (Level A), high internal validity (Level 1), and high external validity (Level a; Lieberman & Scheer, 2002). A study coded *IA1a* is considered the most reliable and valid research study possible.

Another research design method includes *cohort studies,* which refers to studies with a group of people who experience the same or similar situations. Although similar to randomized controlled studies, cohort studies are more limited because more variables need to be considered. *Quantitative studies* and *qualitative studies* differ in the way in which they are conducted, the way in which their evidence is presented, and the method by which reliability and validity are established. Therapists need an understanding of how to read and interpret both kinds of research. Levels of evidence useful in EBP are listed in Table K.3.

Application to Practice

Once research is accessed, reviewed, weighted, and found to be applicable to practice, it should then be implemented. Information should be shared and reviewed with fellow colleagues, including discussion of incorporating research findings into practice. Once findings are implemented, outcomes should be reevaluated to ensure efficacy and best practice.

Providing EBP in the acute care setting is a challenge. Practitioners are confronted with time constraints, limited access to databases, and inadequate training and education in obtaining evidence. AOTA is working toward increasing accessibility to relevant evidence. Occupational therapists working in acute care should check whether their hospital has a medical library that can be used. Some hospitals even allow access remotely so that research does not necessarily have to be done during work hours. These resources can help therapists confront the challenges and barriers of incorporating EBP in acute care. Having literature that illustrates the importance of EBP can also allow hospitals to be more accepting of using work time to complete research. Applying EBP in acute care is certainly feasible, and by overcoming some of the barriers listed here, occupational therapists can provide better care that meets patients' needs, supports occupational therapy's efficacy, and validates the profession.

References

Al-Almaie, S. M., & Al-Baghli, N. (2005). Barriers facing physicians practicing evidence-based medicine in Saudi Arabia. *Journal of Continuing Education in the Health Professions, 24,* 163–170.

American Occupational Therapy Association. (2008a). *AOTA's evidence-based practice resources: Using evidence to inform occupational therapy practice.* Retrieved September 28, 2010, from http:// www.

aota.org/Educate/Research/EBP-Resources-2010. aspx

American Occupational Therapy Association. (2008b). Occupational therapy practice framework: Domain and process (2nd ed.). *American Journal of Occupational Therapy, 62,* 625–683.

Bondoc, S., & Burkardt, A. (2004). Evidence-based practice and outcomes management in occupational therapy. *OT Practice, 9*(20), CE1–CE8.

Dunn. W., & Ball, J. (2008). Development of evidence-based knowledge. In M. Law & J. MacDermid (Ed.), *Evidence-based rehabilitation: A guide to practice* (pp. 15–34). Thorofare, NJ: Slack.

Gutman, S. A. (2008). From the Desk of the Editor— State of the journal. *American Journal of Occupational Therapy, 62,* 619–622.

Jette, D. U., Bacon, K., Batty, C., Carlson, M., Ferland, A., Hemingway, H. D., et al. (2003). Evidence-based practice: Beliefs, attitudes, knowledge, and behaviors of physical therapists. *Physical Therapy, 83,* 786–805.

Law, M., Stewart, D., Pollock, N., Letts, L., Bosch, J., & Westmorland, M. (1998). *Guidelines for critical review form: Quantitative studies.* Hamilton, ON: Author. Retrieved April 12, 2009, from www.srs-mcmaster.ca/Portals/20/pdf/ebp/quanguidelines. pdf

Letts, L., Wilkins, S., Law, M., Stewart, D., Bosch, J., & Westmorland, M. (2007). *Guidelines for critical review form: Qualitative studies* (Version 2.0). Hamilton, ON: Author. Retrieved April 12, 2009, from www.srs-mcmaster.ca/Portals/20/pdf/ebp/qualguidelines_version2.0.pdf

Lieberman, D., & Scheer, J. (2002). AOTA's evidence-based literature review project: An overview. *American Journal of Occupational Therapy, 56,* 344–349.

Lou, J. Q. (2002). Searching for the evidence. In M. Law (Ed.), *Evidence-based rehabilitation* (pp. 71–94). Thorofare, NJ: Slack.

Pollock, N., & Rochon, S. (2002). Becoming an evidence-based practitioner. In M. Law (Ed.), *Evidence-based rehabilitation* (pp. 31–46.). Thorofare, NJ: Slack.

Sackett, D. L., Rosenberg, W. M. C., Muir Gray, J. A., Haynes, R. B., & Richardson, W. S. (1996). Evidence-based medicine: What it is and what it isn't. *British Medical Journal, 312,* 71–72.

Taylor, M. C. (2000). *Evidence-based practice for occupational therapists.* Oxford, England: Wiley.

Wells, J. K. (2007). Application of the occupational therapy practice framework and evidence-based practice in a clinical situation. *Indian Journal of Physiotherapy and Occupational Therapy, 1*(1).

Young, J. M., & Ward, J. E. (2001). Evidence-based practice in general practice: Beliefs and barriers among Australian GPs. *Journal of Evaluation in Clinical Practice, 7,* 201–210.

Appendix L

Ethics

Helene Smith-Gabai, OTD, OTR/L, BCPR

Occupational therapists working in acute care make ethical decisions in dealing with daily challenges. In today's managed care environment of limited resources, conflicts can arise among hospital policies, rules, and culture, which can conflict with therapists' values and their focus on client-centered care (Hammell, 2007). Knowledge and understanding of ethical principles can help therapists resolve difficult ethical dilemmas and the conflicting pressures seen in practice.

Making ethical decisions is a learned process based on bioethical principles, professional codes of conduct, reflection, and clinical judgment. However, most ethical dilemmas are situation specific. No professional code of ethics can guarantee that the best decision will always be made. Ethical conflicts often arise because of differences in stakeholders' values, requiring the application of a combination of ethical theories and principles (Kassberg & Skar, 2008). The American Occupational Therapy Association (AOTA) has developed a code of ethics that promotes a high standard of professional behavior, increases ethical awareness, and upholds the core values of the profession (AOTA, 2010).

Ethical Theories and Principles

Various ethical theories are relevant to health care, because no one theory is applicable to every situation or conflict. Having an understanding of various theories and principles can assist therapists in identifying and framing the type of ethical conflict they are facing. The two most applicable ethical theories to health care are deontology and teleology. Two other additional ethical principles are religious ethics and pragmatism.

Most bioethical guidelines are based on Beauchamp and Childress's (2001) *Principles of Biomedical Ethics*, which include respect for autonomy, nonmaleficence, beneficence, and justice (Gabard & Martin, 2003; McCormick, 1998):

- *Respect for autonomy* generally refers to informed consent and awareness that patients have the capacity to make their own decisions.
- *Nonmaleficence* refers to doing no harm (e.g., the Hippocratic Oath) through omission or commission. This principle also refers to health care provider competency.
- *Beneficence* refers to promoting good. This principle goes hand in hand with *nonmaleficence*. Health care providers have an obligation to act in ways that benefit the patient or prevent the patient from being harmed. Beneficence may have implications for issues regarding patient safety that are in conflict with patient autonomy.
- *Justice* refers to equality and fairness in accessibility to treatment and allocation of resources.

Deontology

The *deontological ethical approach* is based on a combination of both rights ethics and duty ethics. The focus is on making decisions based on duty without consideration of the consequences or outcome, taking a certain action because it is your moral duty and the "right thing to do" (Barnitt, Warbey, & Rawlins, 1998). *Deontology* encompasses *rights ethics, duty ethics,* and *virtue ethics.* It respects individual patients' rights, dignity, and autonomy in making their own health care decisions. In duty and virtue ethics, the health care provider and the patient in concert consider what their moral duty is in making and implementing health care decisions. The emphasis is on intent, not just outcomes.

Today, when patients are more proactive, better informed, and more knowledgeable about their heath conditions, health care professionals take a more collaborative and client-centered approach that is less paternalistic. In deontology, clinicians' primary responsibility is to their patients. As stated earlier, Beauchamp and Childress (2001) have laid out a list of basic ethical duties for practitioners that have been adopted by most medical and health care professional codes of ethics.

Rights Ethics

In *rights ethics*, human rights are the most important issue and the basis of the U.S. political and legal system. Human rights convey dignity and authority because each person should be counted as a moral equal (Gabard & Martin, 2003). Ensuring patients' privacy, protection, and confidentiality is an important issue in health care. For example, these issues and rights ethics can be supported through patients' informed consent and adherence to the Health Insurance Portability and Accountability Act (HIPAA) standards.

Duty Ethics

Duty ethics are based on actions that are in accordance with morals and principles of duty. Action is based on the means, not the ends or outcome. Duty should always be carried out, even when it does not promote the greater good.

Virtue Ethics

Acting in accordance with *virtue ethics* means acting as the person you aspire to be. Virtue ethics is based on moral motivations, personal relationships, and moral aspirations. Most people want to lead virtuous lives, self-actualize to the best of their abilities, and achieve excellence for the higher good. In virtue ethics, health care providers should be people of practical wisdom, place their patients' needs before their own, and be not only technically competent but also of good character (Summers, 2009).

Teleology

Teleology is based on *utilitarianism (consequentialism)*, in which the outcome is the most important factor (Barnitt et al., 1998). Ethical decisions are based on what is best for most people, regardless of individual rights.

Utilitarianism is based on the principle that the ends justify the means. What is best for the greater good, the greater society, is the correct course of action even if it violates the rights of the individual. The rights of each person are equally weighted on the basis of which action produces the most good for the most people.

In *rule utilitarianism*, the right course of action is that which conforms to a set of rules adopted by society. Two sets of rules may be compared to see which one would be of greatest benefit to society. Rule utilitarianism considers interrelated rules as a contextually based code of conduct because some rules apply only to certain settings or particular professions. Consequences are measured with regard to sets of established rules.

Health care policymakers and managers' focus may be more utilitarian, with an emphasis on using and maximizing resources for the most clients. Policymakers develop rules, policies, and procedures in creating an environment that is equitable and safe for the provision of services to the most people. The utilitarian emphasis here is on outcomes.

Religious Ethics

In *religious ethics*, morals, virtues, ideals, and principles are based on religious beliefs. Patients' religious views may affect how they respond to their illness and make decisions about their health care. Therefore, therapists should respect differing religious views and should not impose their religious beliefs on their patients.

Pragmatism

Pragmatism is not based on utilitarianism or rights, duty, virtue, or religious ethics. Pragmatism is action based on responsible and good moral judgment. Moral principles are viewed as general guidelines. Decisions are based on whichever approach is the most appropriate for the situation or context, not on a rigid set of rules (Gabard & Martin, 2003).

Ethics and the Current Health Care System

Both deontology and utilitarianism ethical theories have a place in health care decision making and can be combined in health care practice. For example, the American Hospital Association first developed a patient's bill of rights in the 1970s that supported the dignity and individual rights and values of patients. This bill of rights has since been updated and is now called the *Patient Care Partnership*, which outlines the patient's expectations, rights, and responsibilities as a client (American Hospital Association, 2003).

Along with the patient's bill of rights, the *Institutional Review Board* procedures of informed consent were formulated to protect the rights of individual patients while keeping the outcome of the greater good in mind. These types of documents, policies, and procedures blend morals, values, and ethics protecting the individual within the larger framework or context of health care public policy, health care institutes, and delivery of health care services.

The current system of health care in the United States (at the time of the writing of this book) is *managed care,* a purchased system of health care delivery that controls for cost, access, quality, and quantity of care to its members. This health care system was adopted to control spiraling costs; however, it has also affected the delivery of occupational therapy services and increased pressure on productivity (Lopez, Vanner, Cowan, Samuel, & Shepherd, 2008). Institutions want quality standards to remain high while at the same time they expect their health care providers to do more with less.

Many stakeholders are involved in managed care, including patients, health care providers, hospitals, laboratories, plan administrators, stockholders (in for-profit companies), and the federal and state governments (Medicare and Medicaid). Managed care appears to have a teleological ethical approach, in which care is provided on the basis of what is best for the most people, with a focus on outcomes. However, ethical conflicts may be inherent because of the structure and practices of individual managed care programs and the relationship among all stakeholders and their differing values. Managed care practices (Dombeck & Olsan, 2002) may include

- *Gag rules:* Physicians are limited in what information they are allowed to relay to their patients about treatment options or testing.
- *Incentives:* Physicians are provided with financial incentives to limit health care expenditures for the plan. For example, physicians may receive a bonus for ordering less expensive or less frequent tests.
- *Withholds:* A *withhold* is the opposite of an *incentive.* The managed care organization withholds money, penalizing physicians who order too many tests or expensive procedures.
- *Gatekeeper:* The primary care physician who controls access to all tests and specialty referrals. Incentives and risk sharing may influence the gatekeeper.
- *Risk sharing:* Cost of health care expenditures is controlled through risk of financial loss shared between physicians and insurers. Physicians may be influenced by pressure from administrators or colleagues to cut costs.
- *Capitation and fee for service:* Physicians are paid only a prescribed fee (set price) per visit or procedure, no matter what the actual cost of care is. Physicians increase their productivity by seeing more patients in less time and ordering less expensive tests and treatments (Jecker & Braddock, 2008).

Each of these practices, although improving efficiency and cost, can undermine patient–health care provider relationships and Beauchamp and Childress's (2001) bioethical principles. Patient autonomy may be violated if patients are denied care they deem necessary or are denied access to relevant information, undermining and preventing them from making fully informed health care choices (Agich, 2009). Autonomy concerns issues of trust, veracity, and rights ethics because patients may feel they have no alternatives as a result of economic, medical, and social circumstances that limit their free choice in health care decision making (Agich, 2009).

According to Hedgecoe (2006), physicians may also feel they lack the freedom (*autonomy*) to uphold bioethical principles. They may face pressure from managed care plans, superiors, or colleagues to cut costs by limiting patient access to information or expensive tests and procedures. In addition, physicians may also feel pressure from patients or families to provide certain treatments or referrals denied by their plan coverage, which may lead them to engage in the practice of deceptive coding or fraud.

Despite these challenges, managed care seems to function within a teleological or utilitarianism system of ethics through financial responsibility. According to the Medicine as a Profession Managed Care Ethics Working Group Statement (Povar et al., 2004), it is essential that the relationship between all stakeholders be based on respect, truthfulness, fairness, and compassion. All parties must have a covenant of trust. In addition, health care decision making and resource allocation should be shared by all parties on the basis of transparency, well-informed knowledge, and public dialogue to shape policy.

Health Care–Related Ethical Issues

According to Gabard and Martin (2003), health care professionals face four types of health care–related ethical issues: (1) compliance, (2) moral disagreements, (3) moral vagueness, and (4) ethical dilemmas. *Compliance* is knowing what is right and doing what is right. *Moral disagreements* are disagreements about what is moral or what is the moral or right decision in a given situation. *Moral vagueness* includes situations that are not clear, how to frame the moral issue, or what a specific moral value implies. *Ethical dilemmas* are when two or more moral issues are in conflict without an obvious course of action.

However, Finch, Geddes, and Larin (2005) have grouped health care–related ethical issues into three broad groups:

1. *Patient themes:* Informed consent, confidentiality, treatment effectiveness, and quality of life issues;
2. *Professional themes:* Veracity, competence, professional boundaries, and collegiality; and
3. *Miscellaneous:* Fees and billing, conflict of interest, societal well-being, and allocation of scarce resources.

Occupational Therapy Code of Ethics and Ethics Standards

The *Occupational Therapy Code of Ethics and Ethics Standards* (AOTA, 2010) is a guide for high standards of professional behavior, responsibilities, and competency that supports the core values and attitudes of the profession (Lopez et al., 2008). The code of ethics is based on seven core values of occupational therapy (Slater, 2008):

1. *Altruism:* Unselfish concern for the welfare of others;
2. *Equality:* Impartiality, fairness, respect for diversity, and an awareness of the fundamental human rights and opportunities of all people;
3. *Freedom:* Self-determination to choose between autonomy and societal membership and affirming the rights of people to pursue goals that have personal and social meaning to them;
4. *Justice:* Provision of professional services to all needing occupational therapy services and abidance of laws governing professional practice;
5. *Dignity:* Respecting the uniqueness and inherent worth of all people;
6. *Truth:* Veracity, truthfulness, accountability, and authenticity in all professional dealings; and

7. *Prudence:* Actions governed by rational thought, discretion, moderation, and reflection.

Occupational therapists are also expected to uphold the following professional behaviors (Slater, 2008):

- *Honesty:* With themselves and others; being self-aware of skills and limitations;
- *Communication:* Being conscientious and truthful in all forms of communication;
- *Ensuring the common good:* Being socially responsible;
- *Competence:* Including seeking out opportunities to increase professional competence;
- *Confidential and protected information:* Sharing information only on a need-to-know basis;
- *Conflict of interest:* Upholding integrity in all interactions; maintaining impartiality, nonexploitation;
- *Impaired practitioner:* Ensuring safety of others when a therapist cannot competently perform his or her professional duties even with accommodation;
- *Sexual relationships:* Considered forms of misconduct;
- *Payment for services and other financial arrangements:* Specific outcomes are not guaranteed nor is payment received on the basis of promises of successful outcomes; and
- *Resolving ethical issues:* Using all available resources to identify and resolve ethical conflicts.

The *Occupational Therapy Code of Ethics and Ethics Standards* includes the following principles (AOTA, 2010):

- *Beneficence:* Concern for the safety and well-being of recipients of occupational therapy services, including advocating for patients to receive needed services and promotion of public health, safety, and well-being;
- *Nonmaleficence:* Avoidance of inflicting harm, client exploitation, and relationships or activities that compromise professional judgment and objectivity, ensuring patient safety, and taking action when colleagues' skills are impaired and at risk of causing harm;
- *Autonomy and confidentiality:* Respecting recipients of occupational therapy services and ensuring their rights, including the individual's right to refuse services, and protecting all forms of confidential communication (e.g., written, verbal, electronic);
- *Duty:* Maintaining high standards of competence including adherence to AOTA standards of practice, having the appropriate credentials for the services that are provided, and engaging in evidence-based practice;
- *Procedural justice:* Adhering to government laws and association policies that guide professional practice and keeping a record of information relating to professional activities;
- *Veracity:* Providing accurate information, including credentials, qualifications, education, training, and experience; disclosing any conflicts of interest; refraining from using communications that are fraudulent or deceptive; and accepting responsibility for actions that may reflect poorly on the profession; and
- *Fidelity:* Treating other professionals and colleagues with respect, fairness, discretion, and integrity.

Resolving Ethical Conflicts

Health care providers are expected to base their clinical and ethical decisions on professional values and societal norms (Finch et al., 2005). Each ethical situation needs to be considered on its own merits, including the therapist's moral obligations, responsibilities, and consideration of outcomes that will most benefit his or her patients. Addressing ethical conflicts is a process that is situation specific (AOTA, 2008). Many models of ethical decision making exist, and most models involve similar steps (Gabard & Martin, 2003; Horowitz, 2002):

1. Gather all relevant facts and information.
2. Identify the type of ethical dilemma.

3. Analyze the problem on the basis of ethical theories and principles; consult the *Occupational Therapy Code of Ethics and Ethics Standards,* (as a guideline for professional conduct).

4. Identify all applicable laws.

5. Consider all options and practical approaches.

6. Consult with colleagues or others (without violating confidentiality).

7. Implement the selected action.

8. Evaluate outcomes

Refer to Figure L.1 for an illustration of a model that can assist therapists in navigating the ethical decision-making process. In addition, Kornblau and Starling proposed the Clinical Ethics and Legal Issues Bait All Therapists Equally (CELIBATE) method, which guides therapists through a 10-step process of addressing ethical and legal issues related to practice (cited in Denend & Finlayson, 2007).

Having a clear understanding of the *Occupational Therapy Code of Ethics and Ethics Standards* can assist therapists in determining the type of ethical conflict they may be facing and in framing a resolution. Refer to AOTA's Web site (www.aota.org) for more information on the *Code of Ethics* and the process for filing an ethics complaint. All ethical decisions and choices have both good and bad consequences. Violations of ethical standards can lead to reprimand, sanctions, or legal recourse. If disciplinary action is required, it is the responsibility of AOTA, the National Board for Certification in Occupational Therapy, or state regulatory boards, depending on the type of violation (Slater, 2008).

Implications for Occupational Therapy

Occupational therapy is a moral and ethical helping profession. Occupational therapists have an obligation not just to their patients but also to the institution in which they work, their profession, and themselves. Issues can arise if hospital or third-party payer policies conflict with occupational therapy practice patterns including client-centered care (Hammell, 2007). In addition, therapists have the obligation to do good and do no harm, but these concepts are complex and challenging in a hospital setting in which the time to work with patients, and resources, may be limited.

Acute care therapists face many ethical dilemmas, which can be similar to other areas of occupational therapy practice. For example, therapists may have to prioritize which patients are seen and whether patients are treated individually or in groups. According to a study by Foye, Kirschner, Wagner, Stocking, and Siegler (2002), occupational therapists working in rehabilitation identified three areas of ethical conflicts: (1) reimbursement pressures, (2) conflicts around goal setting, (3) and patient or family refusal of team recommendations. Additional areas identified included

- *Patient confidentiality:* Disclosing information to families or other team members;
- *Personal or professional boundaries:* Accepting gifts from patients;
- *Veracity:* Disclosing patient prognosis or efficacy of treatment;
- *Informed consent:* If patient has limited capacity or limited decision-making skills;
- *Patient or family demanding therapy:* When the patient is no longer appropriate, therapy has plateaued, or the patient is demanding equipment that is not medically necessary;
- *Therapist's responsibility with knowledge of unsafe patient behavior;* and
- *Family's role in decision making* (Foye et al., 2002).

Clinical uncertainty or pressure from other professionals may also affect ethical decision-making skills (Healy, 2003). Ethical issues can also arise because of billing issues; documentation; cultural differences; equipment refusals; legal issues; or even observing a coworker engaging in unethical, immoral, or illegal activities. Differences in opinion may occur among the therapist, patient, family, and other health care providers about what is in the patient's best interest (Kassberg & Skar, 2008).

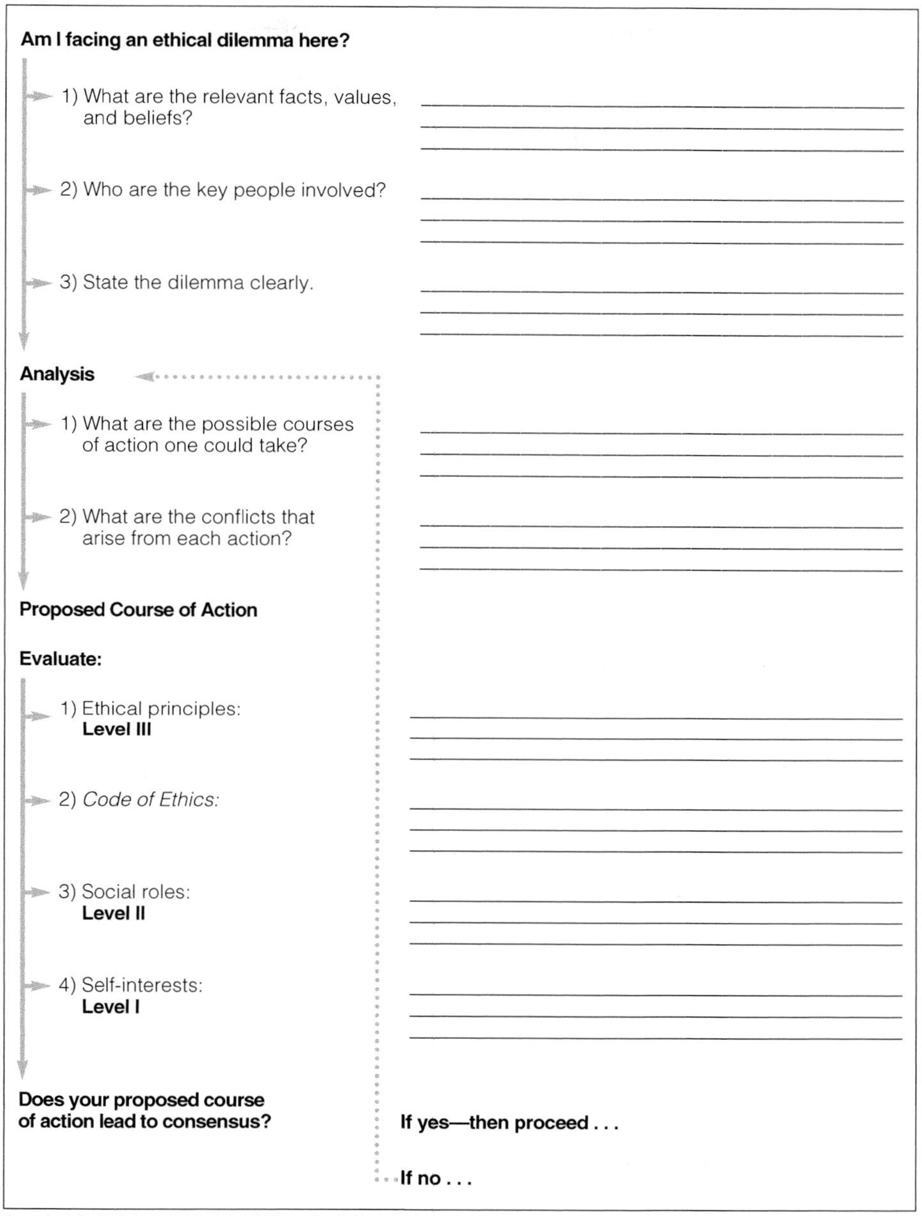

Am I facing an ethical dilemma here?

1) What are the relevant facts, values, and beliefs? _____

2) Who are the key people involved? _____

3) State the dilemma clearly. _____

Analysis

1) What are the possible courses of action one could take? _____

2) What are the conflicts that arise from each action? _____

Proposed Course of Action

Evaluate:

1) Ethical principles: **Level III** _____

2) *Code of Ethics:* _____

3) Social roles: **Level II** _____

4) Self-interests: **Level I** _____

Does your proposed course of action lead to consensus?   If yes—then proceed . . .

If no . . .

FIGURE 23.1. Model for Ethical Decision Making.

Figure L.1. AOTA Model for Ethical Decision Making.
Source. Slater, D. Y. (Ed.). (2008). *Reference guide to the occupational therapy ethics standards* (p. 135). Bethesda, MD: AOTA Press. Copyright © 2008 by the American Occupational Therapy Association, Inc. Reprinted with permission.

Health care providers have an obligation to act in ways that benefit the patient and promote good (beneficence). However, ethical issues can arise even in the routine task of making discharge recommendations. For example, a patient may expect to return home after hospitalization, but the family wants a nursing home placement because they feel unable to meet the patient's physical needs. In contrast, a family may want the patient to return home, but the health care team recognizes that the home environment is unsafe.

In addition, a recommendation in favor of nursing home placement may be devastating for the patient, and the patient may refuse this disposition, even though it is unsafe for him or her to return home (Moats, 2006). What is the obligation of the occupational therapist in this situation? Occupational therapists are members of a health care team, employees of the hospital, and advocates for patients. The recommendation for nursing home placement may be beneficent, but it can also be paternalistic, and it may violate the patient's autonomy (rights ethics). If a patient wishes to return home, the occupational therapist may be able to facilitate this process by addressing safety issues through recommendations for adaptive equipment, home modifications, community resources (e.g., Meals on Wheels), an emergency response system (e.g., LifeLine®), referral to a home health agency, or caregiver education.

Occupational therapists should be open to and aware of ethical conflicts around them, be knowledgeable of the profession's code of ethics and professional behaviors, and have an understanding of the ethical decision-making process. These recommendations will assist therapists in making decisions that uphold their integrity and competence, as well as support the rights of others, and promoting the high standards of the profession. Ethical theories and principles assist occupational therapists with stating and resolving ethical conflicts, organizing their moral reflections, and justifying principles of their professional behavior and duties (Gabard & Martin, 2003).

Ethical decision making is a complex and dynamic process that is challenging because there are no easy answers. It can be emotionally uncomfortable, with no one correct approach that all stakeholders can agree on or outcome that will make them happy. However, applying ethical theories and principles can help occupational therapists make these difficult and challenging decisions that not only benefit patients but also complement the institutional environment and culture in which they work.

References

Agich, G. J. (2009). Respecting the autonomy of old people living in nursing homes. In E. E. Morrison (Ed.), *Health care ethics: Critical issues for the 21st century* (2nd ed., pp. 184–200). Sudbury, MA: Jones & Bartlett.

American Hospital Association. (2003). *The patient care partnership*. Retrieved May 17, 2009, from www.aha.org/aha/issues/Communicating-With-Patients/pt-carepartnership.html

American Occupational Therapy Association. (2010). Occupational therapy code of ethics and ethics standards (2010). *American Journal of Occupational Therapy, 64* (Suppl.), S17–S26.

Barnitt, R., Warbey, J., & Rawlins, S. (1998). Two case discussions of ethics: Editing the truth and the right to resources. *British Journal of Occupational Therapy, 61,* 52–56.

Beauchamp, T. L., & Childress, J. F. (2001). *Principles of biomedical ethics* (5th ed.). New York: Oxford University Press.

Denend, T. V., & Finlayson, M. (2007). Ethical decision making in clinical research: Application of CELIBATE. *American Journal of Occupational Therapy, 61,* 92–95.

Dombeck, M. T., & Olsan, T. H. (2002). Ethics and managed care. *Journal of Interprofessional Care, 16,* 221–233.

Finch, E., Geddes, E. L., & Larin, H. (2005). Ethically-based clinical decision-making in physical therapy: Process and issues. *Physiotherapy Theory and Practice, 21,* 147–162.

Foye, S. J., Kirschner, K. L., Wagner, L. C. B., Stocking, C., & Siegler, M. (2002). Ethical issues in rehabilitation: A qualitative analysis of dilemmas identified by occupational therapists. *Topics in Stroke Rehabilitation, 9,* 89–101.

Gabard, D. L., & Martin, M. W. (2003). *Physical therapy ethics*. Philadelphia: F. A. Davis.

Hammell, K. W. (2007). Client-centred practice: Ethical obligation or professional obfuscation? *British Journal of Occupational Therapy, 70,* 264–266.

Healy, T. C. (2003). Ethical decision making: Pressure and uncertainty as complicating factors. *Health and Social Work, 28,* 293–301.

Hedgecoe, A. M. (2006). It's money that matters: The financial context of ethical decision-making in modern biomedicine. *Sociology of Health and Illness, 28,* 768–784.

Horowitz, B. P. (2002). Ethical decision-making challenges in clinical practice. *Occupational Therapy in Health Care, 16,* 1–14.

Jecker, N. S., & Braddock, C. H., III (2008). *Managed care*. Retrieved June 29, 2009, from http://depts.washington.edu/bioethx/topics/manag.html

Kassberg, A.-C., & Skar, L. (2008). Experiences of ethical dilemmas in rehabilitation: *Swedish occupational therapists' perspectives. Scandinavian Journal of Occupational Therapy, 15,* 204–211.

Lopez, A., Vanner, E. A., Cowan, A. M., Samuel, A. P., & Shepherd, D. L. (2008). Intervention planning facets—Four facets of occupational therapy intervention planning: Economics, ethics, professional judgment, and evidence-based practice. *American Journal of Occupational Therapy, 62,* 87–96.

McCormick, T. R. (1998). *Principles of bioethics.* Retrieved July 22, 2009, from http://depts.washington.edu/bioethx/tools/princpl.html

Moats, G. (2006). Discharge decision-making with older people: The influence of the institutional environment. *Australian Occupational Therapy Journal, 53,* 107–116.

Povar, G. J., Blumen, H., Daniel, J., Daub, S., Evans, L., Holm, R. P., et al. (2004). Ethics in practice: Managed care and the changing health care environment [Medicine as a Profession Managed Care Ethics Working Group Statement]. *Annals of Internal Medicine, 141*(2), 131–136.

Slater, D. Y. (Ed.). (2008). *Reference guide to the occupational therapy ethics standards* (2008 ed.). Bethesda, MD: AOTA Press.

Summers, J. (2009). Theory of healthcare ethics. In E. E. Morrison (Ed.), *Health care ethics: Critical issues for the 21st century* (2nd ed., pp. 3–40). Mississauga, ON: Jones & Bartlett.

Appendix M

Discharge Planning: A Consultative Partnership

Judy R. Hamby, MHS, OTR, BCPR

Discharge planning is one of the primary responsibilities of the acute care occupational therapist. It is a complex process that involves the therapist's critical reasoning skills, experience, appreciation for client and contextual factors, and knowledge of health care guidelines and disposition options. Determining the best possible disposition requires an honest discourse among therapist, medical team, case manager, family, and patient. Although the discharge planning strategies used in the acute care setting are rapid and sometimes only implicitly involve the patient, they do set the stage for the resumption of occupations after discharge (Jette, Grover, & Keck, 2003; Robertson & Finlay, 2007). Essentially, two models of discharge planning are currently used in the acute care setting: autonomy promotion and risk avoidance (Moats, 2006; Moats & Doble, 2006).

Stakeholder Viewpoints

The autonomy promotion philosophy is more in line with the fundamental tenets of occupational therapy in empowering autonomous decision making; however, it does not always completely address the patient's safety and quality of life. The second philosophy of risk avoidance is much more paternalistic in nature, and the patient's wants are often overlooked, thus undermining self-determination. However, although neither is optimal in isolation, on occasion each philosophy has its place. Discharge recommendations are important because they can have a profound effect on a patient's quality of life and sense of self-sufficiency (Moats, 2007; Moats & Doble, 2006; Robertson & Finlay, 2007).

Stakeholders' Discharge Criteria

Discharge decisions should be based on input from all team members involved in the patient's care while keeping in mind that each team member has his or her own professional criteria on which those recommendations are based. Unfortunately, conflict or uncertainty as to which disposition is most appropriate may arise. In addition, each team member responds to different kinds of pressure when making these types of decisions. For example, physicians are pressured to discharge patients quickly to free up beds and reduce costs. Case managers and social workers are more aware of the reality of the patient's financial situation and right to self-determination. Therapists make recommendations first and foremost on the basis of the patient's current functional status and rehabilitation needs. Most important, patients usually just want to return home, whether this is the safest option or not. These viewpoints do not always converge, making disposition planning difficult and, thus, necessitating negotiation among the different stakeholders (Huby, Brook, Thompson, & Tierney, 2007). In actuality, the physician makes the final determination regarding patient discharge in conjunction with the patient and family (Huby et al., 2007; Wilding & Whiteford, 2007).

Impact of the Medicare Prospective Payment System

All stakeholders consider many factors when determining discharge disposition, including the patient's medical stability, cognition, functional level, and rehabilitation potential. However, prevention of readmission is also necessary to consider (Robertson & Finlay, 2007). In 1983, the federal government mandated the Medicare Prospective Payment System as a means to control health care spending. Hospitals' reimbursement became a set fee per patient on the basis of the patient's diagnostic-related group, regardless of actual cost of services (American Hospital Directory, 2008).

This change encouraged hospitals to shorten hospital stays. Patients no longer have the luxury of staying in the hospital until they complete rehabilitation. With patients living longer and hospital stays becoming shorter, discharged patients are often sicker and frailer than years ago. The constraints of the prospective payer system greatly influence recommendations, occasionally causing a patient's needs to collide with the realities of the health care system. Poor decisions may contribute to readmission, failure to achieve full recovery, and client dissatisfaction (Robertson & Finlay, 2007). In addition, shortened hospital stays, increased acceptance of risk tolerance, and varying levels of staff experience may result in patients being discharged home with unmet needs (Bowles et al., 2008). Balancing safety and levels of risk for the patient and the hospital (in this age of litigation) and respecting the patient's autonomy in a collaborative manner can be difficult. This balancing act is where the art and science of therapy meet.

Role of the Occupational Therapist

The occupational therapist's responsibility is to provide input and make discharge recommendations. Therapists are usually expected to make their recommendations during the initial assessment (Jette et al., 2003) with limited knowledge of a patient's true level of function in his or her home environment, thus placing the onus of gathering information regarding the patient as quickly as possible on the therapist. It is incumbent on the therapist to make the appropriate recommendation in conjunction with the other members of the health care team. Presenting the stakeholders with the disposition options

and rationale for each improves educated decision making and assists in formulating safer and more autonomous decisions (Moats, 2007), thus bridging the gap between the clinician's and patient's viewpoints (Russell, Fitzgerald, Williamson, Manor, & Whybrow, 2002). Ultimately, however, unless the patient has been deemed incompetent, the decision is between the patient and the physician.

It is paramount that the therapist facilitate discharge and not impede the institution's ability to get the patient to the next level of care. Doing so will prevent the patient from becoming a permanent resident of the hospital. Stating discharge recommendations in a positive light rather than a negative light will assist with this process. For example, writing "the patient is not safe for discharge" hinders the effort, but, conversely, indicating how the patient could be safe facilitates the discharge process. An example of a constructive recommendation would be "the patient will require moderate physical assistance and supervision at home because of decreased performance of basic activities of daily living [BADLs], functional mobility, and safety." The medical team can better determine a safe disposition if specific safety concerns are identified, such as inaccurate medication management or meal preparation safety issues. Communicating these concerns or issues provides other team members with constructive information that can be woven into the disposition plan rather than restrictive information that hampers planning.

Sometimes discharge recommendations need to be modified when new facts come to light; however, safety should not be compromised. Despite contextual barriers that therapists face daily (e.g., evaluating in a contrived environment or the brevity of the evaluation), clinical reasoning is used to make quick determinations of what can be accomplished while the patient is in the hospital and what needs to be addressed in other settings. This reasoning is challenging because therapists' critical reasoning and clinical decision-making skills are exercised in an environment that can be incompatible with the core values of holism and client centeredness. The therapist must listen to the needs of the family and patient, both explicitly and implicitly—not only what is being said but also what is being demonstrated, including anxiety responses, fear, or lack of participation. The relationship between the therapist and the patient should be collaborative in nature (Ludwig, 2004). The role of the acute care occupational therapist is consultative, not authoritative.

In addition, the therapist's level of experience influences the process significantly, providing a filter through which therapists make discharge recommendations (Jette et al., 2003). Experience includes previous employment in different settings, awareness of the requirements for admission to different settings, and level of comfort with a particular diagnostic category. Experience also implies an awareness of community resources and the therapist's opinions and biases regarding those resources. Figure M.1 shows a discharge planning algorithm to assist therapists in making discharge recommendations.

Discharge Issues

Many issues can affect discharge and must be addressed to determine appropriate recommendations. Thorough assessment can yield the primary and mitigating issues that affect the disposition plan. This would prevent inappropriate recommendations and facilitate a disposition that would maximize safety and functional outcomes.

Primary Issues

In making discharge recommendations, the primary issues therapists need to address are

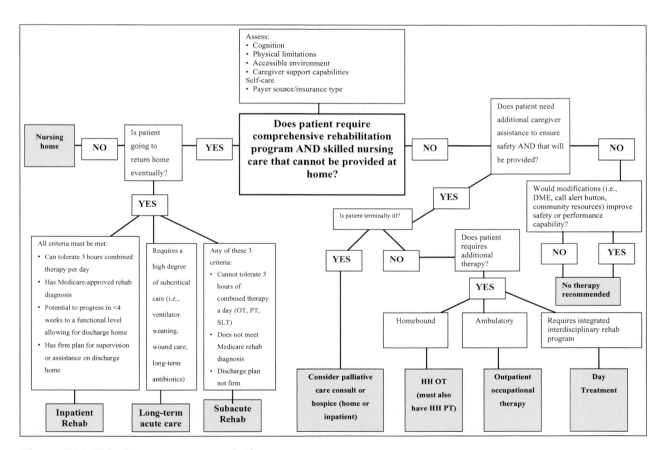

Figure M.1. Discharge recommendations.

Note. Home is loosely defined as the patient's living arrangements or situation before hospitalization. May include independent living in the patient's own home, nursing home, relative's home, or homeless shelter. DME = durable medical equipment; HH = home health; OT = occupational therapist; PT = physical therapist; SLP = speech–language pathologist.

- Patient's function and level of disability:
  — Disparity between prior and current level of functioning
  — Prognosis for recovery (rehabilitation potential)
  — Acute or chronic nature of deficits (has the patient learned to adapt over time?)
  — Level of motivation to participate;
- Patient's and family's desires and needs;
- Patient's life context, including caregiver support and the caregiver's ability to provide the necessary level of care;
- Health care regulations and institutional procedures;
- Resource availability and accessibility, including payer source (reimbursement issues); and
- Adaptive devices or durable medical equipment needs. (Jette et al., 2003)

Regulations and resources are ultimately the final determinants.

Mitigating Factors

Therapists need to determine the setting that best promotes the client's safe participation in daily occupations and take into consideration the interaction among the environmental context, the patient's abilities, and an educated prognosis. Several mitigating factors affect the discharge planning process:

- *Primary caregivers:* Caregivers' capabilities to physically, emotionally, and logistically provide care must be addressed.
- *Frail elderly patients who are cognitively intact:* Often, frail elderly patients rely on others to advocate for their needs and make arrangements on their behalf (Huby et al., 2007). However, they may have a definite opinion about their desired disposition. The very act of the patient appointing a proxy decision maker perpetuates the paternalistic model in which a negotiated decision-making process must ensue (Moats, 2007). Frail elderly patients are at risk for injury from falls or inability to take care of their basic needs such as food preparation or

bathing. If the plan is for the patient to go home alone, consider recommendations for durable medical equipment, day programs, an alert system (e.g., Life Alert), Meals on Wheels, or home health services (a home health aide is not a stand-alone service).

- *Cognitive deficits:* Consider a graded decision-making process that empowers the patient to participate (as he or she is able), thus advocating for the patient's wishes to be considered (Moats, 2007). Decisions that can be made by the patient should be honored, if possible—for instance, the general location of a facility or what personal possessions to bring from home.
- *Patients who are deemed incompetent:* To maintain a client-centered approach, the actual client may shift from the patient to the family, who will advocate for the wishes and needs of their loved one. However, it is still important to include the patient in the decision process to preserve dignity and provide purpose and meaning to life (Moats, 2007). Safety must ultimately be the deciding factor in any discharge plan for the patient who is deemed incompetent. Only a judge can declare a person incompetent, but that decision is usually based on the documentation of medical professionals. It is important to differentiate *incompetent* from *lacks capacity.* Many patients lack the capacity to make decisions, such as in dementia, but are not actually declared incompetent. The social worker and doctor will be the primary professionals to facilitate this procedure.
- *Chronic disability:* Patients with chronic diseases will frequently identify strategies to maintain basic needs and safety and often do not return to total independence. Modified independence with occasional support may be sufficient for the patient to return to a level of ability that is congruent with a safe discharge disposition (Russell et al., 2002).
- *Home safety:* Judgments made regarding patient safety while the patient is still in the hospital and not in his or her normal home environment further complicate safety

assessments. Recommendations should be provided for environmental modifications and equipment that maximize home safety. However, it is difficult to gauge a patient's true level of safety once he or she is home without direct observation or to gauge whether the patient will actually comply with recommendations.

Disposition Sites

The potential disposition sites in the full continuum of care are described in Table M.1. Also consider that decisions regarding certain disposition sites may have psychosocial and emotional ramifications, causing feelings of guilt and uncertainty in families. Family members may have made unrealistic promises that patients would not go to a nursing home (even for a short rehabilitation stay). Assisting the family to pragmatically evaluate the needs of their loved one and their own needs and capabilities, along with a clear description of the options, may facilitate the discharge process for the family (Fink, 2004) and ameliorate some of these emotions. Sharing the results of the occupational therapy evaluation and the implications for safety, independence, and quality of life can further delineate the patient's needs for the family. In the case of the frail elderly patient or the progressively declining patient, the hospitalization may even be an opportunity to make a realistic needs assessment.

Another factor to consider is that most facilities and Medicare require the patient to have been in the hospital for a 3-day qualified stay, not admitted for observation. *Observation* is defined as a 23-hour hospital admission. This observation period is used to medically monitor the patient to ascertain whether a longer inpatient admission is medically necessary ("Outpatient Observation Services," 2009).

Inpatient Rehabilitation Unit Regulations

Further complicating the disposition recommendation are governmental guidelines from the Centers for Medicare and Medicaid Services

(CMS; 2008) regarding admission to an acute inpatient rehabilitation setting. CMS requires that 60% of those patients admitted to an inpatient rehabilitation facility must fall into one of 13 diagnostic categories. This rule is informally called the "60% rule" (CMS, 2008). If the facility is not in compliance, then CMS funding would cease, essentially shutting down the rehabilitation unit. The medical conditions that qualify for admission (CMS, 2008) include

- Stroke;
- Congenital deformity;
- Major multiple trauma;
- Fracture of femur (hip);
- Spinal cord injury;
- Amputation;
- Brain injury;
- Burns;
- Neurological disorders, such as multiple sclerosis, motor neuron diseases, polyneuropathy, muscular dystrophy, and Parkinson's disease;
- Active polyarticular rheumatoid arthritis, psoriatic arthritis, and seronegative arthropathies resulting in significant functional impairment of ambulation and other activities (ADLs);
- Systemic vasculidities with joint inflammation resulting in significant functional impairment of ambulation and other ADLs;
- Severe or advanced osteoarthritis (osteoarthrosis or degenerative joint disease) involving two or more weight-bearing joints (elbows, shoulders, hips, or knees, but not counting a joint with a prosthesis) with joint deformity and substantial loss of range of motion, atrophy of muscles surrounding the joint, and significant functional impairment of ambulation and other ADLs; and
- Knee or hip replacement surgeries meeting one of the following criteria: bilateral knee or hip joint replacement surgery, body mass index higher than 50, and older than age 85.

(Text continues on p. 697)

Table M.1. Disposition Sites

Disposition Site	Requirements for Admission	Goals	Potential Discharge Sites
Acute care	Medically unstable	• Assure medical stability • Initiate rehabilitation • Determine disposition	• Inpatient rehabilitation • Long-term acute care • Subacute rehabilitation • Day treatment • Traditional outpatient care • Home with or without home health services including PT, OT, SLP, RN, and aide • Nursing home • Hospice

Hospice	• Inpatient hospice requirements:
	  • Terminally ill with <6 mos to live
	  • Acute medical intervention or nursing care for palliation of symptoms
	• In-home or nursing home hospice requirements:
	  • Terminally ill with <6 mos to live
		• Comfort measures
		• Usually minimal to no provision of rehabilitation
			• Home with or without home health services. If the hospice deems therapy appropriate, it will be provided

Nursing home	• Admission requires a 3-day hospitalization for a qualified reason (must be medically necessary to be in the hospital; provision of acute therapy services alone does not make the hospitalization medically necessary; Birmingham, 2008) • Indicates no, or very limited, goals for rehabilitation • Family is unable to care for patient at home because of the intensity of care required	• Patient safety • Assistance with ADLs	• Hospice (can also be at the nursing home) • Home with or without home health services including PT, OT, SLP, RN, and aide

Table M.1.   **(continued)**

Disposition Site	Requirements for Admission	Goals	Potential Discharge Sites
Long-term acute care	• Hospital-based inpatient care for those who require extended stays • Subcritical care provided, but the patient still requires a high level of skilled care because of medical complexity of illness, but is not critically unstable • Patient may be ventilator dependent initially but admitted for ventilator weaning • Most patients are referred from intensive care unit settings—stable but too sick for general floor care • A nurse evaluates patient referrals in conjunction with medical director of long-term acute care	• Not specifically for PT, OT, or SLP, but usually incorporates an interdisciplinary team approach and uses appropriate rehabilitation therapies to maximize patient functioning • Patient is anticipated to be in recuperative process or receiving palliative care (palliation of symptoms such as pain or constipation)	• Hospice • Nursing home • Inpatient rehabilitation • Subacute rehabilitation • Home with or without home health services including PT, OT, SLP, RN, and aide
Home health	• Requires 1–3 disciplines for therapies • Treatment is not as intensive as rehabilitation facility (patients are not seen daily) • OT, SLP, or aide not considered a stand-alone therapy. PT or nursing must also be ordered, at least in the beginning • Usually a multidisciplinary treatment model • Homebound; usually only able to leave for medical appointments • Provides for client-centered care because patients are in their own normal environment	• Maximize patient and caregiver carryover of therapeutic intervention • Support for the family • Especially beneficial for the patient with dementia because of the familiarity of the environment	• Day treatment • Traditional outpatient • Can go to subacute rehabilitation facility or nursing home directly from home, but must be admitted within 30 days of hospital discharge

(continued)

	Table M.1. (continued)		
Disposition Site	**Requirements for Admission**	**Goals**	**Potential Discharge Sites**
Subacute rehabilitation or skilled nursing facility (SNF)	• Admission requires a 3-day inpatient hospitalization for a qualified reason (must be medically necessary to be in the hospital; provision of acute therapy services alone does not make the hospitalization medically necessary; Birmingham, 2008) • Might be housed in a nursing home or occasionally on a separate wing • Therapies are provided at an intensity of <3 hr/day (usually closer to 1.5 hr/day) • An acute care occupational therapy evaluation is not required for admission; however, it may augment information the SNF needs to justify reimbursement levels. The SNF does have 5 days to justify the admission • Interdisciplinary team • Maximum length of stay is 100 days. Days 1–20 are fully paid by Medicare, and days 21–100 require a copay (approximately $135/day; Birmingham, 2008). If the patient has been in a SNF within the past 60 calendar days, the day count continues from the last day of the preceding admission • The patient must be admitted to the SNF within 30 days of hospital discharge to be eligible for benefits	• Goal-oriented, comprehensive inpatient care that does not depend heavily on high-tech monitoring, surgical intervention, or complex diagnostic procedures • Allows for slower progression	• Inpatient rehabilitation • Home with or without home health services including PT, OT, SLP, RN, and aide • Day treatment • Traditional outpatient

Table M.1.   (continued)

Disposition Site	Requirements for Admission	Goals	Potential Discharge Sites
Inpatient rehabilitation facility or unit	• A discharge plan is identified for home, family's homes, or personal care home with 24-hour care available. Nursing home not an acceptable disposition • Patient must tolerate ≥3 hr of therapy daily • Patient requires 24-hr nursing care • Patient is medically stable • Patient has been screened and approved for admission by the medical director • Must qualify via one of the 13 diagnostic categories unless admission is considered under the 40% allowable rule (rare) • Patient demonstrates willingness and motivation to participate in an intensive rehabilitation program • Usual length of stay is 7–28 days	• Patient demonstrates potential for functional improvement in a reasonable time frame	• Traditional outpatient • Day treatment • Home with or without home health services including PT, OT, SLP, RN, and aide • Assisted living facility

Day treatment program	• Provides cognitive, physical, and behavioral intervention for patients who require an integrated multimodal rehabilitation program
	• Cohesive interdisciplinary treatment team:
	  • Case manager
	  • Doctor
	  • Neuropsychologist
	  • OT
	  • PT
	  • Nurse
	  • SLP
		• Typically focuses on patient's awareness and treatment of his or her impairments and their impact on return to normal functioning
		• Addresses:
		  • Community reintegration
		  • Return to work or school
		  • Instrumental activities of daily living
			• Traditional outpatient

(continued)

Table M.1.   (continued)

Disposition Site	Requirements for Admission	Goals	Potential Discharge Sites
Traditional outpatient	• Medically stable • Living at home • Requires 1–3 disciplines in a multidisciplinary format	• Extensive family education performed to improve carryover and prepare the patient for final discharge from therapies	• Typically the last level of the continuum of care

Note. ADLs = activities of daily living; OT = occupational therapist; PT = physical therapist; RN = registered nurse; SLP = speech–language pathologist.

Table M.2.   Community Resources

Specialized Services	Sources and Web Sites
Adaptive devices or durable medical equipment (free or low cost and loaner services)	• Area churches • Each state has a service for adaptive devices. Internet search phrase: *assistive technology loan services* and name of state • Nonprofit organizations • Classified ads
Elder care referral source	• www.aplaceformom.com (free service)
Geriatric care manager	• www.caremanager.org
Hand therapist (certified)	• www.htcc.org • www.asht.org
Low vision therapists and services for people with visual impairments	• http://forms.lighthouse.org/hny/search
Neuro-ophthalmologist	• http://www.nanosweb.org/i4a/pages/index.cfm?pageid=3280
Neuro-optometrist	• www.nora.cc
Neuropsychologist	• www.nanonline.org/NAN/Membership/Directory/Search.aspx • www.theaacn.org/diplomates/database/view.php
Pulmonary rehabilitation	• www.emphysema.net/Rehab-Support/Rehab/pulrehab10.htm
Stroke rehabilitation (inpatient)	• National Stroke Association's Guide to Choosing Stroke Rehabilitation Services: www.stroke.org/site/DocServer/Choose _Rehab_Provider.doc?docID=1121 This resource is especially helpful if the patient had a stroke while traveling and must now find a rehab center in his or her own city.
Vestibular rehabilitation therapists (certified)	• www.vestibular.org
Vocational rehabilitation specialists	• Use keyword search *vocational rehabilitation* and name of state

Community Resources

In addition to having an understanding of the different discharge disposition settings and programs, an awareness of available community resources is invaluable as the patient enters the rehabilitation continuum. Assisting the patient with locating resources and the appropriate type of therapist may be the most helpful service provided. Web sites of helpful community resources are listed in Table M.2, and the questions in Figure M.2 can assist the patient or family member when trying to find a qualified therapist.

Questions				
Name				
Phone number				
Address				
Do you take my insurance?				
What is your primary specialty? (It is especially important to distinguish between therapists specializing in orthopedic and therapists specializing in neurological disorders.)				
How many years of experience do you have?				
How many patients have you treated in the past year with this diagnosis?				
Are you certified in this specialty? If not, what specialties are you certified in?				
What is a typical treatment plan?				
What is your philosophy of care?				
What are your hours?				
What is the estimated cost of the service?				
Other/comments:				

Figure M.2. Finding a qualified therapist.
Source. Judy R. Hamby

Summary

Discharge planning is an important and multifaceted decision, often made in a pressured, fast-paced environment with limited patient interaction and superficial knowledge of patients' and families' wants and needs. At times, the disparity between the patient's desires and needs is a wide chasm to bridge. Presenting needs in terms of the patient's quality of life can have a profound effect in arbitrating the conflicting viewpoints, furthering the collaborative relationship and contributing to safety. Ultimately, the safety of the disposition plan is the final determinant of discharge and should be the primary consideration because many factors contribute to discharge recommendations.

References

American Hospital Directory. (2008). *Medicare prospective payment system*. Retrieved August 12, 2008, from www.ahd.com/pps.html

Birmingham, J. (2008). Understanding the Medicare "extended care benefit" a.k.a. the 3-midnight rule. *Professional Case Management, 13*(1), 7–16.

Bowles, K. H., Ratcliffe, S. J., Holmes, J. H., Liberatore, M., Nydick, R., & Naylor, M. (2008). Post-acute referral decisions made by multidisciplinary experts compared to hospital clinicians and the patients' 12-week outcomes. *Medical Care, 46*(2), 158–166.

Centers for Medicare and Medicaid Services. (2008). *Inpatient rehabilitation facility prospective payment system*. Retrieved March 22, 2009, from www.cms.hhs.gov/MLNProducts/downloads/InpatRehabPaymtfctsht09-508.pdf

Fink, J. L. W. (2004). Long-term care: Helping families make the best decision. *Hospital Nursing, 34*(6), 18–20.

Huby, G., Brook, J. H., Thompson, A., & Tierney, A. (2007). Capturing the concealed: Interprofessional practice and older patients' participation in decision-making about discharge after acute hospitalization. *Journal of Interprofessional Care, 21,* 55–67.

Jette, D. U., Grover, L., & Keck, C. P. (2003). A qualitative study of clinical decision making in recommending discharge placement from the acute care setting. *Physical Therapy, 83,* 224–236.

Ludwig, F. M. (2004). Occupation-based and occupation-centered perspectives. In K. F. Walker & F. M. Ludwig (Eds.), *Perspectives on theory for the practice of occupational therapy* (pp. 373–442). Austin, TX: Pro-Ed.

Moats, G. (2006). Discharge decision-making with older people: The influence of the institutional environment. *Australian Occupational Therapy Journal, 53,* 107–116.

Moats, G. (2007). Discharge decision-making, enabling occupations and client-centred practice. *Canadian Journal of Occupational Therapy, 74,* 91–101.

Moats, G., & Doble, S. (2006). Discharge planning with older adults: Toward a negotiated model of decision making. *Canadian Journal of Occupational Therapy, 73,* 303–311.

Outpatient observation services. (2009). In *Medicare benefit policy manual*. Retrieved June 22, 2009, from www.cms.hhs.gov/manuals/downloads/bp102c06.pdf

Robertson, C., & Finlay, L. (2007). Making a difference, teamwork and coping: The meaning of practice in acute physical settings. *British Journal of Occupational Therapy, 70,* 73–80.

Russell, C., Fitzgerald, M. H., Williamson, P., Manor, D., & Whybrow, S. (2002). Independence as a practice issue in occupational therapy: The safety clause. *American Journal of Occupational Therapy, 56,* 369–379.

Wilding, C., & Whiteford, G. (2007). Occupation and occupational therapy: Knowledge paradigms and everyday practice. *Australian Occupational Therapy Journal, 54,* 185–193.

Appendix N

Blood Disorders

Helene Smith-Gabai, OTD, OTR/L, BCPR

The average heart pumps 1.3 gallons (5 liters) per minute, or approximately 1,900 gallons (7,192 liters) of blood each day (Eckert, 2007). Seventy-eight percent of blood is water, and 22% is solids. Blood contains red cells, white cells, platelets, and plasma and is the body's main transport vehicle for carrying nutrients, oxygen, and waste material through the body. Blood is formed through a process called *hematopoiesis*. Stem cells within bone marrow differentiate to become specific blood cells (red blood cells [RBCs], white blood cells [WBCs], or platelets). When blood cells mature and are functional, they are released into the bloodstream. The average adult body has 10 pints of blood, accounting for 7% of total body weight (Leukemia & Lymphoma Society [LLS], 2006).

RBCs account for approximately half of blood volume and have a lifespan of 80–120 days (Abrahams, 2009; LLS, 2006). The main function of RBCs is transportation of oxygen and carbon dioxide to and from the lungs. Hemoglobin, the protein within RBCs, picks up and transports oxygen throughout the body.

WBCs account for approximately 1% of blood volume (Abrahams, 2009). Unlike RBCs, WBCs leave blood vessels and enter tissue (LLS, 2006). WBCs fall into different categories and are classified as neutrophils, monocytes, eosinophils, basophils, or lymphocytes. Each plays an important role in the body's immune system response and protects against infection.

- *Neutrophils* (*granulocytes*) and *monocytes* destroy bacteria and fungi.
- *Eosinophils* fight infection caused by parasites.
- *Basophils* are associated with allergic reactions (i.e., hives, allergies, asthma, hay fever).
- *Lymphocytes* are WBCs, located primarily in the lymph nodes and the spleen, that travel throughout the lymphatic system and are composed of T cells, B cells, and natural killer cells (LLS, 2006). Refer to Chapter 12 for more information on the immune system.

An additional type of cells are *blast cells,* which are immature white blood cells normally found in marrow but not in blood. Blast cells found in the bloodstream may be indicative of acute leukemia.

Platelets are responsible for blood clotting and have a lifespan of 10 days. Platelet disorders are associated with either a low platelet count (thrombocytopenia) or a high platelet count (thrombocytosis). *Plasma* is the medium for blood cells and is predominately composed of water containing dissolved gases, minerals (e.g., iron), carbohydrates, hormones (e.g., thyroid hormone), vitamins (e.g., folic acid), enzymes, protein (e.g., albumin), fats, antibodies, and coagulation factors (e.g., gamma globulin; LLS, 2006).

Most blood disorders are the result of an impairment in blood composition. The most common symptoms of hematologic disorders include edema (i.e., lymphedema, pulmonary edema, or cerebral edema), congestion, infarction, thrombosis, embolism, splenomegaly, bleeding, bruising, or shock (Peterson & Goodman, 2009). Blood disorders often compromise the amount of oxygen that circulates throughout the body to tissues and organs (i.e., the brain) can affect cardiopulmonary function, or may increase the risk of bleeding (Abrahams, 2009; Peterson & Goodman, 2009). Refer to Appendix P for detail on blood counts, implications, and precautions.

Common blood disorders are listed in Table N.1.

Table N.1. Common Blood Disorders

Disorder	Etiology	Symptoms	Medical Management
Sickle cell disease: Blood cells are misshapen (crescent shaped) and stiff.	Genetic	• Anemia • Pallor • Weakness • Dyspnea • Jaundice • Chronic nonhealing lower-extremity ulcers • Enlarged spleen • Tachycardia • Paresthesias • Intense pain • Tissue ischemia or infarction • Retinopathy • Delayed puberty	• Medication (e.g., hydroxyurea, corticosteroids, antibiotics) • Oxygen support • Hydration • Psychosocial support • Partial RBC exchange
Hemophilia	Genetic disorder in which the clotting factors (VIII, IX, or XI) are deficient.	• Bleeding with trauma, or after surgery • Pain • Petichia, purpura, ecchymosis • Hematoma • Bleeding into joints • Hematuria • Chronically swollen joints • Joint deformity • Disorientation • Tachypnea • Hypotension • Tachycardia • Convulsions • Intracranial bleeding	• Stopping active bleeding • Factor replacement therapy • Pain management
Anemia	Shortage of RBCs because of low RBC production, high RBC destruction, or abnormal RBC maturation	Symptoms depend on the type of anemia.	Treatment based on type of anemia

Table N.1. (continued)

Iron-deficiency anemia		Fatigue, tachycardia, dyspnea on exertion, headache, dizziness, irritability, cold intolerance, dysphagia, pallor, delayed healing, inflammation of the mouth and tongue	Diet that includes iron-rich foods, iron supplements, and nutritional counseling
Vitamin B_{12} anemia		Anorexia, diarrhea, nausea, mouth ulcers, paleness, ataxia, impaired sensation, spasticity, hyperactive reflexes	Supplements and nutritional counseling
Folic acid anemia		Symptoms similar to B_{12} deficiency but without neurologic involvement	Supplements and nutritional counseling
Aplastic anemia		Fatigue, dyspnea, bleeding gums, hematuria, pallor, fever, infection, petichia, sore throat	Treatment of underlying cause, blood product transfusion, bone marrow transplant or stem cell transplant
Hemolytic anemia		Fatigue, weakness, nausea, vomiting, fever, jaundice, decreased urine output	Blood transfusion, corticosteroids, fluid replacement, splenectomy
Post-hemorrhagic anemia		• *20%–30% blood loss:* Dizziness, hypotension, tachycardia with exertion • *30%–40% blood loss:* Dyspnea, cold clammy skin, hypotension, tachycardia, decreased urine output, loss of consciousness • *40%–50% blood loss:* Shock, may be fatal	Control of bleeding source, fluids, blood and blood product transfusion, supplemental oxygen

(*continued*)

Table N.1. (continued)

Disorder	Etiology	Symptoms	Medical Management
Polycythemia	Excessive production of RBCs, platelets, myelocytes	• Increased blood viscosity • Increased risk of thrombus formation and bleeding • Headache, dizziness, blurred vision, vertigo, venous thrombosis, GI bleed, epitaxis, paresthesia in hands and feet, enlarged spleen	Phlebotomy, interferon, hydro-oxyurea, antiplatelet therapy, smoking cessation, fluid restriction
Polycythemia vera	Etiology unknown		
Secondary polycythemia	High erythropoietin levels (from altered stem cells or tumors), chronic hypoxemia (may be seen in patients with COPD, cardiopulmonary disease, high altitudes)		
Relative polycythemia (temporary rise in RBCs)	Dehydration, excessive vomiting, diarrhea, burns, excessive diuretic use		
Disseminated intravascular coagulation	Associated with severe infection, pancreatic cancer, prostate cancer, SLE, trauma, tissue acidosis, burns, shock	• Results in both hemorrhage and thrombus (SAH, CVA) • Bleeding of gums, blood in urine, hemoptysis, or GI • Cyanosis • Gangrene • Acute tubular necrosis • Dysrhythmias • MI • PE • AMS	• Requires immediate medical attention • Treatment aimed at treating underlying cause • Hemodynamic and oxygen support, blood product transfusion • Can be life threatening

Table N.1. (continued)

Disorder	Etiology	Symptoms	Medical Management
		• Renal failure • Respiratory failure • Organ failure	
Thrombotic thrombocytopenic purpura	• Etiology unknown • Associated with viral and bacterial infections, estrogen use, autoimmune disorders	• Hemolytic anemia • Thrombocytopenia • Fatigue • Weakness • Fever • Petichia • Headache • Confusion • Altered level of consciousness • Hemiparesis • Seizures • Acute renal failure	• Plasmapheresis • Plasma exchange • Antiplatelet agents • Immunosuppressants • Corticosteroids • Fall risk prevention • Splenectomy
Thalassemia	• Genetic disease • Body does not produce enough hemoglobin • Disease can be mild or severe • Short life expectancy in severe disease	• Can be asymptomatic in mild cases • Mild or severe anemia • Susceptible to infection • Growth failure • Bone deformities, brittle bones, osteoporosis • Enlarged spleen • Jaundice • Complications from heart failure and liver damage	• Blood transfusions • Folic acid supplements • Iron chelation therapy • Infection prevention • Splenectomy • Bone marrow or stem cell transplantation

Note. AMS = altered mental status; COPD = chronic obstructive pulmonary disease; CVA = cerebral vascular accident; DOE = dyspnea on exertion; GI = gastrointestinal; MI = myocardial infarction; PE = pulmonary embolism; RBC = red blood cell; SAH = subarachnoid hemorrhage; SLE = systemic lupus erythematosus.

Source. West, M. P., Paz, J. C., & Vashi, F. (2009). Vascular system and hematology. In J. C. Paz & M. P. West (Eds.), *Acute care handbook for physical therapists* (3rd ed., pp. 219–262). St. Louis, MO: W. B. Saunders. Adapted with permission.

Blood Transfusions

Blood transfusions are necessary to replace blood volume, maintain proper coagulation, and ensure good oxygen delivery to tissues when the blood system is compromised (West et al., 2009). Transfused blood may be patient donated or from a voluntary blood donor. Transfused blood products may include whole blood (blood cells and plasma), packed red blood cells, platelets, fresh frozen plasma, albumin, blood factors, or fibrinogen (West et al., 2009). RBCs are transfused to treat anemia; platelets, to treat bleeding from thrombocytopenia; and fresh frozen plasma and cryoprecipitate (cryo), to treat patients with poor clotting factors (e.g., hemophilia, liver disease; LLS, 2006). Blood transfusions generally require 3–4 hours for completion.

Certain conditions require different amounts of blood products. Table N.2 lists the average units required per condition.

Although screening has significantly improved over the past 2 decades, the risk of transmission of viruses and infections through transfusion still exists (LLS, 2006). The current U.S. blood supply undergoes 12 tests to screen for 7 infectious diseases: syphilis, HIV–1, HIV–2, human T lymphocytotropic virus (HTLV–1), HTLV–2, hepatitis B, and hepatitis C (LLS, 2006). Currently, the risk of transmission of HIV through transfusion is 1 in 2 million, and the risk of transmission of hepatitis C is 1 in 3 million (LLS, 2006).

Before a transfusion, both donor and recipient are matched for compatibility through the ABO system (inherited properties of their red blood cells). Blood is classified as Types A, B, AB, or O depending on its antigens. Blood type is also classified as either positive or negative depending on the rhesus antigen (Rh factor). However, even if matched, the risk of transfusion reaction is still present (see Table N.3). ABO compatibility and leukoreduction (removal of WBC) minimizes this risk. If a transfusion reaction occurs, the transfusion is stopped, and the blood is returned to the blood bank for inspection to determine the cause of the reaction (LLS, 2006).

Potential Transfusion Reactions

Additional complications of transfusion may include transmission of viruses such as cytomegalovirus (CMV), bacterial infections, and graft versus host disease (GVHD). Refer to Chapter 12 for information on CMV and Chapter 11 for information on GVHD. The patient's body may

Table N.2. Conditions Requiring Use of Blood Products

Condition	Red Blood Cells	Platelets	Plasma
Accident victim	4–100 units		
Kidney transplant	2 units		
Liver transplant	10 units	10 units	20 units
Heart transplant	4–6 units		
Adult open heart surgery	2–6 units	1–10 units	2–4 units
Sickle cell disease	10–15 units periodically to treat severe complications		
Cancer treatment	2–6 units	6–8 units daily for 2–4 weeks	
Leukemia	2–6 units	6–8 units daily for 2–4 weeks	
Bone marrow transplantation	1–2 units given every other day for 4 weeks	6–8 units daily for 4–6 weeks	

Source. American Red Cross. (2009). *Blood usage.* Retrieved March 22, 2009, from www.givelife2.org/aboutblood/bloodusage.asp Copyright © 2009 by American Red Cross. Adapted with permission.

also produce antibodies in response to the donor blood in a phenomenon called *alloimmunization* (LLS, 2006). With this condition, symptoms are generally not immediate; however, greater care is taken in donor selection for future transfusions (LLS, 2006).

It takes approximately 12–24 hours for hemoglobin and hematocrit levels to increase after a transfusion (West et al., 2009). Therapists are advised to defer treatment for the first 15 minutes the patient is being transfused because transfusion reactions generally occur within

Table N.3. **Transfusion Reactions**

Reaction	Cause	Symptoms	Onset
Fever (most common reaction; responsible for >90% of transfusion complications)	Patient's antibodies are sensitive to transfused blood products	• Chills, low-grade fever (>1° F), headache, nausea, vomiting, muscle pain, cough, hypotension, tachycardia, tachypnea, SOB • Treatment involves stopping the transfusions and removing donor leukocytes from blood • Symptoms usually transient	During transfusion and ≤24 hr after transfusion
Allergic (second most common reaction)	Sensitivity to transfused products (occurs in ~1%–3% of transfusions)	• Hives, rash, tachypnea, chest pain, wheezing, mucosal edema • Occurs more often with fresh frozen plasma and platelet transfusions • Can lead to cardiac arrest • Treated with antihistamines and corticosteroids • Transfusion is halted and then slowly resumes after hives resolve	Within minutes after beginning transfusion
Septic	Blood products are contaminated with bacteria (rare with current screening protocols)	• Rapid-onset high fever, hypotension, chills, headache, cramps, back pain, chest pain, SOB, renal failure, shock • Treated with antibiotics	Within first 30 min of transfusion
Anaphylactic	Patient with IgA deficiency develops IgA antibodies in response to the transfused product (very rare reaction)	• Hives, wheezing, bronchospasm, swelling of larynx, nausea, bloody diarrhea, cramps, anxiety, abrupt hypotension, shock • Can lead to cardiac or respiratory arrest • Transfusion immediately discontinued, and epinephrine and corticosteroids given	Within seconds of beginning of transfusion

(continued)

Table N.3.   (continued)

Reaction	Cause	Symptoms	Onset
Hemolytic (associated with destruction of transfused RBCs; rare complication)	Incompatibility between patient's blood and blood products (ABO incompatibility)	• Fever, chills, nausea, vomiting, headache, tachycardia, tachypnea, dyspnea, hypotension, cyanosis, bleeding, chest pain, kidney damage, or renal failure • Can lead to cardiac arrest • Mortality rate 17%–60% • Transfusion immediately terminated and measures taken to maintain blood pressure and prevent bleeding	Within minutes to hours after transfusion
Transfusion-related acute lung injury	Blood product antibodies are reactive with patient's granulocytes	• Chills, fever, hypotension, cyanosis, hypotension, pulmonary edema, severe hypoxia • Symptoms may range from mild SOB to symptoms of ARDS	Several hours after transfusion

Note. ARDs = acute respiratory distress syndrome; IgA = immunoglobulin A; RBCs = red blood cells; SOB = shortness of breath.
Sources: Leukemia & Lymphoma Society (2006); Peterson and Goodman (2009); West, Paz, and Vashi (2009).

that period (West et al., 2009). Even though nurses regularly monitor patients' vitals during transfusions, therapists should still be aware of potential transfusion reactions. Therapists may also assist by covering the patient with blankets to ease any chills. Therapy may be engaged in at bedside level, because out-of-bed activities are generally deferred while the patient is being transfused. However, if assisting the patient out of bed, consult first with medical staff. Always follow the facility's blood transfusion policies and procedures, and report any signs of complications to medical staff.

References

Abrahams, P. (2009). *Physiology*. London: Amber Books.

American Red Cross. (2009). *Blood usage.* Retrieved March 22, 2009, from www.givelife2.org/aboutblood/bloodusage.asp

Eckert, J. (2007). Cardiopulmonary disorders. In B. J. Atchison & D. K. Dirette (Eds.), *Conditions in occupational therapy: Effect on occupational performance* (3rd ed., pp. 195–218). Baltimore: Wolters Kluwer.

Leukemia & Lymphoma Society. (2006). *Blood transfusion.* Retrieved March 22, 2009, from http://promosearch.lls.org/search/?sp_a=sp10036b6c&sp_f=ISO-8859-1&sp_q=Blood+transfusion&sp-x-1=collection&sp-p-1=phrase&sp-q-1=

Peterson, C., & Goodman, C. C. (2009). The hematologic system. In C. C. Goodman & K. S. Fuller (Eds.), *Pathology: Implications for the physical therapist* (3rd ed., pp. 678–741). St. Louis, MO: W. B. Saunders.

West, M. P., Paz, J. C., & Vashi, F. (2009). Vascular system and hematology. In J. C. Paz & M. P. West (Eds.), *Acute care handbook for physical therapists* (3rd ed., pp. 219–262). St. Louis, MO: W. B. Saunders.

Appendix O

National Patient Safety Goals and Related Safety Techniques

Marcy D. Bearden, MS, OTR, and Natan Berry, MS, OTR/L

The Joint Commission Safety Standards

Marcy D. Bearden, MS, OTR

The Joint Commission is an organization committed to improving the safety and quality of care within the health care system, which it accomplishes through a health care accreditation process that focuses on performance improvement. In 1910, Ernest Codman, MD, proposed that patients should be tracked through their hospital stay, and at the end, it would be determined whether the treatment was effective. If treatments were not effective, then the health care organization was to determine why and then improve on the treatment so that similar cases in the future could be treated successfully. In the next 10 years, minimum standards would be developed for hospitals, and surveys of hospitals would begin. It was not until 1951 that The Joint Commission was actually formed by the merging of several health care–related associations. Over the next 50-plus years, the organization continued to develop its standards and continued to offer accreditation to health care organizations.

The National Patient Safety Goal program was developed in 2002 (effective January 1, 2003) to help accredited organizations focus on the most critical issues related to patient safety. National Patient Safety Goals (NPSG; see Table O.1) were developed on the basis of the specific program that is accredited (e.g., long-term care,

hospital, home care). The purpose of this section is to identify the NPSG that are specific not only to the hospital setting but to occupational therapy.

An awareness of the NPSG is essential for therapists working in the hospital setting because the hospital's accreditation depends on the implementation of and improvement in the goals listed. Although the list in Box O.1 is not a complete list of the hospital-specific goals, all the goals that occupational therapists should be aware of are listed and should be considered when treating patients. Departments should hold annual educational meetings to inform therapists of updates and changes made to the previous year's goals. These goals are reviewed annually by The Joint Commission's Patient Safety Advisory Group, and changes and revisions are made on the basis of a review of the literature to identify potential patient safety issues. The 2011 National Patient Safety Goals are now available online at www.jointcommission.org/standards_information.

Safety Information

Natan Berry, MS, OTR/L

Bathroom Safety

- To prevent burns, set your water heater so that the water is no hotter than 115° F.
- Install grab bars in your shower and tub and by the toilet. Grab bars should be attached to structural supports in the wall. If you are unable to install grab bars on your walls, grab bars with suction cups can be affixed to a wall surface that is structurally sound.

Table O.1. National Patient Safety Goals

NPSG	Implementation and Rationale	Occupational Therapists Putting It Into Action
Goal 1: Improve the accuracy of patient identification.	Use at least 2 patient identifiers when providing care, treatment, or service to • Reliably identify the person or patient. • Match the patient to the service or treatment.	Always check the patient's arm band before beginning treatment to verify name and medical record number. Other patient identifiers may be telephone number, birth date, or other patient-specific information. The room number is *not* a patient identifier.
Goal 2: Improve the effectiveness of communication among caregivers.	Orders and test results given over the phone or verbally are to be recorded and then read back to verify accuracy. • Reduces error by ensuring that the recipient of the order understood the order. • Improves patient safety. • Includes a "do not use" abbreviation list. • Ensures accuracy and consistency in documentation.	This goal applies to therapists taking phone orders and verbal orders for treatment or clarification orders for services already in progress. Always repeat the order after it is written or entered into the electronic chart to verify accuracy. Most computer-based order systems have a place to indicate that the telephone or verbal order was read back and verified. A "do not use" abbreviation list should be published at all accredited hospitals.
Goal 7: Reduce the risk of health care–associated infections.	Comply with the World Health Organization's and Centers for Disease and Control and Prevention hand hygiene guidelines. • Reduce transmission of infectious agents from staff to patients. • Implement evidence-based practices to prevent multidrug-resistant infections.	Practice appropriate hand hygiene and contact precautions, and clean all equipment between patient contacts.
Goal 9: Reduce the risk of patient harm resulting from falls.	Implement a fall reduction program. • Evaluate the patient's risk of falling and take action to reduce the risk of falling.	Therapists can gather important information during the initial evaluation that is also relevant to a fall evaluation. A fall evaluation might include • Fall history • Medication review

Table O.1. (continued)

		• Gait and balance screening • Assessment of walking aids • Environmental assessment. Many hospitals have a fall prevention form on which this information is recorded.
Goal 13: Encourage patients' involvement in their own care as a patient safety strategy.	Identify ways in which patients and their families can comfortably report concerns. • Communicate all aspects of care and treatment so that the patient and family know what to expect.	Patients should always be involved in the establishment of goals and the treatment plan.
Goal 16: Improve recognition and response to changes in a patient's condition.	A method should be in place through which staff can request assistance from trained professionals when a patient's status is deteriorating. • Early response to worsening conditions may reduce cardiopulmonary arrest and mortality.	Therapists should be aware of the patient's response to treatment and know when help is needed.

- Never use a towel rack or soap holder that is grouted into ceramic tile as a substitute for a grab bar, because both can be pulled out.
- Install a raised toilet seat or place a bedside commode (without the bucket) over the toilet to provide added height and arm rests to facilitate pushing up from a seated position.
- Install a hand-held shower to ease showering or bathing.
- If the bathroom door is too narrow for a walker or wheelchair, consider removing the door and installing a pocket door to maximize space.
- If living alone, consider bringing a cell phone or cordless phone with you into the bathroom in case of an emergency.

- Install a tub seat, tub transfer bench, or tub grab bar if you have difficulty getting into or out of the bathtub.
- Add nonslip surfaces (e.g., mat or appliqué) to the bottom of the tub or shower.
- Use only bath mats with nonskid bottoms.
- Ensure the floor and feet are dry when exiting the tub or shower.
- Place a shelf in an easy-to-reach location for easy access to soap and shampoo.
- Use lever handles instead of knobs to turn the water on and off in the tub, shower, or sink to minimize stress on hand and wrist joints.
- If you need to use the bathroom in the middle of the night, use nightlights in the hallway or bathroom for safety. Consider using a bedside commode.

General Home Safety

- Remove throw rugs from around the house or tack them down securely because they can be trip hazards.
- Increase the amount of lighting throughout the house, especially in hallways leading to the bathroom and entrances to the house.
- Have a bench near the entrance to the house for resting and setting down packages.
- Make sure seat surfaces are not too low but are easy to get up from.
- Have a LifeLine® or other medical alert system installed near your bed or worn around the neck or wrist in case of an emergency.
- Keep a telephone within easy reach in the most often occupied areas of the home (e.g., bedroom, den, kitchen).
- Place a list emergency phone numbers near every phone.
- Move frequently used items to easy-to-reach areas. If you need to retrieve something on a high shelf, use a long-handled reacher or a stool to step on instead of a chair.
- Ensure passageways have no electrical or telephone cords to trip over.
- Do not overload outlets or extension cords.
- Turn off appliances when not in use.
- Always stay in the kitchen when using the stove, oven, or any appliance that requires electricity or gas.
- Make sure pan handles are turned toward the center of the stove when cooking.
- Keep a fire extinguisher in the kitchen, and learn how and when to use it.
- Make sure to have smoke alarms on every floor and routinely check that they are in good working order.
- Store poisonous, flammable, or dangerous chemicals and cleaners in a secured cabinet and away from heating units.
- Keep cabinet doors and drawers closed when not in use.
- Install lever handles on all doors and easy-to-grasp handles on all drawers and cabinets.

- Get up slowly after sitting or lying down.
- Keep track of all medications and the labeled containers in which they came.

Fall Prevention

Having a fall can be stressful and cause increased fear of future falls. Being prepared for this possibility can greatly help how you react to and recover from a fall. According to the Centers for Disease Control and Prevention (2002), the 4 important steps for fall prevention are regular exercise, home safety, checking visual acuity and function, and having health care providers review medications.

1. Begin a regular exercise program.
   - Engage in exercises that improve strength, balance, and coordination (e.g., yoga, Tai Chi, Qigong).
2. Make your home safer.
   - Remove items (clutter) that may be tripped over from floors or entranceways.
   - Remove or tack down throw rugs.
   - Keep floor surfaces smooth but not slippery (i.e., avoid using floor polish or wax).
   - When entering a room, be aware of differences in floor levels or thresholds.
   - Keep items at a convenient height to avoid stepping on a step stool or chair to retrieve them.
   - Use grab bars in the bathroom near the toilet, tub, or shower.
   - Use nonslip mats in the tub or shower.
   - Improve lighting throughout your home, but avoid glare.
   - Have a light switch at both the top and the bottom of staircases.
   - Make sure staircases are well lit and have handrails.
   - Place fluorescent strips or a contrasting color on stair edges for easier viewing.
   - Fix loose or uneven steps.
   - Never go up and down stairs carrying items that block your vision or put you off balance.

- Arrange furniture for easy maneuverability within or between rooms.
- Make sure no electrical or telephone cords are in your way to trip over.
- Watch out for pets that may jump on you or try to walk between your legs.
- Avoid going barefoot. Wear shoes with treads.
- Wear low-heeled supportive shoes.
- Keep emergency numbers near each phone.
- Wear an alarm device.

3. Have your vision checked.
   - Vision should be checked at least once a year. Vision changes and poor vision can result in a fall.

4. Have your health care provider review your medicines.
   - If you are taking many medications, they may interact and cause an adverse reaction or drowsiness or dizziness that can lead to falls.

Suggestions for Getting Up From a Fall

- Remain calm.
- Scan your body for any injuries. If injured, immediately call for help. Having an emergency alert system or a working cell phone with you is important for this reason.
- If you are not injured, look for a sturdy piece of furniture, such as an arm chair, sofa, or staircase. Do not attempt to stand up just yet.
- Roll onto your side in the direction of the furniture that you are headed for. Start with your head, and then move your shoulders, arms, hips, and finally your legs.
- Make sure you are steady, and then crawl or drag yourself over toward the furniture.
- Place your hands on the furniture and slide one of your legs forward so that it is flat on the floor.
- Push up with your arms and legs, and then pivot your bottom over and into the seat.
- Sit and rest for several minutes before trying to get up again.
- Seek medical attention if you experience pain, lost consciousness, are bleeding, cannot remember why or how you fell, or have other medical concerns.

Reference

Centers for Disease Control and Prevention. (2002). *Preventing falls among seniors*. Retrieved July 16, 2009, from http://www.cdc.gov/ncipc/duip/spotlite/falls.htm

World Health Organization. (2009). *Guidelines on hand hygiene in health care*. Retrieved March 1, 2011, from http://www.who.int/patientsafety/information_centre/documents/en/index.html

Appendix P
Laboratory Values

Helene Smith-Gabai, OTD, OTR/L, BCPR

In acute care, occupational therapy is contraindicated or the therapeutic approach is modified for an array of medical reasons. In addition to consulting the patient's nurse before initiation of evaluation or treatment, it is imperative to verify lab values. Lab values indicate the patient's overall health and provide information about why occupational performance may be affected or reasons why therapy should be deferred. Lab values are used to screen or establish a diagnosis, rule out a condition, monitor therapies and medications, or establish a prognosis (Irion & Goodman, 2009; Pagana & Pagana, 2006).

Abnormal values will often be listed with the letters *L, H,* or *C* next to them, indicating whether the value is *low, high,* or *critical,* respectively. Therapy is not contraindicated with most abnormal lab values; however, therapy is normally deferred with critical lab values. If occupational therapy is not contraindicated, then therapy can be modified by decreasing repetitions, intensity, and amount of resistance or incorporating more rest breaks (Hergenroeder, 2006; Irion & Goodman, 2009). Therapists should always consider the total clinical picture when determining the effectiveness and appropriateness of engaging in therapy. Figure P.1. includes the traditional shorthand notation for the basic metabolic panel (BMP) and a complete blood count (CBC), often found in charts along with their normal reference ranges.

The values given in this chapter are general guidelines, and they vary between sources. If a section has no therapist considerations listed, then no specific therapy guidelines exist. Therapists should weigh the risks and benefits of patients engaging in therapy when lab values are outside the normal range. Rely on good communication with medical staff and sound clinical judgment in determining

patient appropriateness for therapy because patient safety is the ultimate consideration. Appendix P.A. can also assist readers in understanding units of measurements used in reporting laboratory values.

Complete Blood Count

A CBC is one of the most commonly ordered tests. It examines components of a blood sample, including the white blood cell (WBC) count, platelets, red blood cell (RBC) count, hemoglobin, and hematocrit. The CBC is used to screen for diseases, make a diagnosis, or monitor medical treatments and effects of drug dosages. Refer to Appendix N for information on blood and blood count disorders.

Venous puncture is the usual method for obtaining a CBC blood sample. Superficial veins such as the basilic, cephalic, or median cubital veins are the most common sites for venous puncture; however, veins in the hand or wrist or the femoral vein may also be used (Pagana & Pagana, 2006). Blood samples may also be drawn from an indwelling venous catheter.

White Blood Cells or Leukocytes

Purpose	Normal Range	Abnormal Values	Critical Values
Indicates immune system status, infection, or inflammation.	5,000–11,000/mm³	*Leukocytosis:* >11,000/mm³ *Leukopenia:* <5,000 mm³	<2,000/mm³ or >30,000/mm³

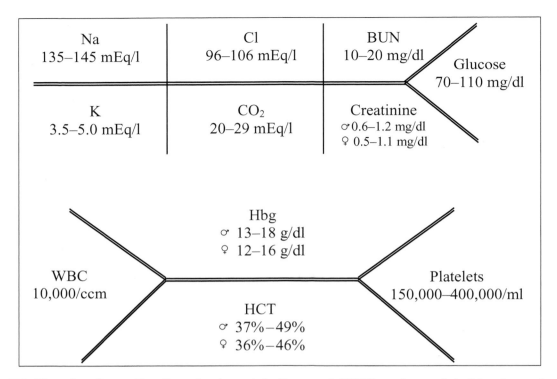

Figure P.1. Shorthand notation for a basic metabolic panel (BMP) and complete blood count (CBC), along with their reference ranges. A BMP (top) lists values for sodium, chloride, blood urea nitrogen (BUN), potassium, carbon dioxide, creatinine, and glucose. A CBC (bottom) lists values for white blood cells (WBCs), hemoglobin (Hbg), hematocrit (HCT), and platelets.

Clinical Implications

Value	Implication
<500/mm³	Extremely dangerous, may be fatal.
<1,000/mm³	Defer therapy.
<4,000/mm³	Neutropenic precautions observed. Includes strict hand washing; wearing a gown, gloves, and face mask; and disinfecting any equipment brought into the room. Reverse isolation may be observed.
<5,000/mm³ with fever	Consider deferring therapy, as patients are at increased risk of infection.
>5,000/mm³	Light or resistive exercise (as tolerated).
11,000/mm³ with fever	Use caution when exercising.

Sources. Fischback & Dunning (2009); Garritan, Jones, Kornberg, & Parkin (1995); Hergenroeder (2006); Irion & Goodman (2009).

A. *Leukocytosis* is caused by bacterial infection, inflammation, leukemia, malignancy, trauma, drugs, hemorrhage, stress, burns, dehydration, pneumonia, or tissue injury or necrosis.

B. *Leukopenia* is caused by bone marrow disorders or depression, aplastic anemia, pernicious anemia, HIV infection, autoimmune diseases, radiation or chemotherapy, drugs, alcoholism, or diabetes.

Therapist Considerations

- Observe standard precautions and good hand hygiene with leukopenia (WBC <5,000) because of the risk of infection and possible protective isolation.

- Donning a mask and gloves may be required before entering the patient's room.

- The presence of infection may increase patient's oxygen demand and utilization, thereby affecting occupational performance. Use caution with activities that further increase oxygen demand (e.g., mobilization; Stiller, 2007).

C. *Neutropenia* is a low count of neutrophils (a type of WBC that fights infection). Patients with neutropenia are at risk for nosocomial infections (Irion, 2004). Neutropenic precautions include strict hand washing; wearing a gown, gloves, and face mask; and disinfecting any equipment brought into the room.

Therapists who are sick should not treat these patients. Therapists should note that patients leaving their hospital room may have reverse isolation precautions.

Community neutropenic precautions focus on limiting exposure to infection, including avoiding crowds and people who are ill, frequently washing hands, cooking all foods thoroughly, avoiding foods that contain raw eggs or raw fish, avoiding take-out foods for which the method of preparation is unknown, using gloves for gardening, washing hands after handling pets, and avoiding pet feces.

D. *Pancytopenia* is an excessive shortage of all blood cells (WBCs, red blood cells [RBCs], platelets). Precautions include avoiding fresh fruit or vegetables, avoiding shaving with razor blades, no flossing of teeth or taking aspirin or nonsteroidal anti-inflammatory drugs (NSAIDs), and being vigilant for signs of infection (Fischback & Dunning, 2009).

Hemoglobin

Purpose	Normal Range	Abnormal Values	Critical Values
Measures blood's capacity to carry oxygen.	*Males:* 13–18 g/dl *Females:* 12–16 g/dl	<8 g/dl	*<5 g/dl:* May result in heart failure or death.
Hemoglobin gives arterial blood its bright red color.			*>20 g/dl:* Can lead to increased blood viscosity, clogging of capillaries, or tissue ischemia.

Source. Fischback & Dunning (2009).

Clinical Implications

Abnormal hemoglobin values can indicate extent of anemia or polycythemia, as well as patient response to certain treatments. Increased hemoglobin levels may be caused by chronic obstructive pulmonary disease (COPD), congestive heart failure (CHF), dehydration, polycythemia vera, or living in high altitudes. Causes of low hemoglobin include chronic renal failure, cirrhosis, burns, hyperthyroidism, and certain systemic diseases (e.g., sarcoidosis, systemic lupus erythematosus, leukemia).

Therapist Considerations

Low hemoglobin means the heart has to work harder to ensure sufficient oxygen can be transported to the rest of the body. With hemoglobin values less than 8 g/dl, a blood transfusion may be ordered; consider deferring therapy. With hemoglobin levels between 8–10 g/dl, light exercise is appropriate, but vitals should be closely monitored as patients may have poor activity tolerance. Resistive exercise can be incorporated into the plan of care with hemoglobin values more than 10 g/dl (Garritan, Jones, Kornberg, & Parkin, 1995; Irion & Goodman, 2009).

Hematocrit

Purpose	Normal Range	Abnormal Values	Critical Values
Measures the percentage of red blood cells in total blood volume.	*Males:* 37%–49% *Females:* 36%–46%	<25%	<20% or >60%

Clinical Implications

Value	Implication
<20%	Can result in cardiac failure or death
<25%	Defer therapy
25%–30%	Activities of daily living and light exercise as tolerated
30%	Add resistive exercise
>60%	Associated with spontaneous blood clotting

Sources. Fischbach & Dunning (2009); Garritan, Jones, Kornberg, & Parkin (1995).

The hematocrit value assists in diagnosing abnormal hydration levels, anemia, and polycythemia (Hergenroeder, 2006). Increased hematocrit levels may be caused by polycythemia vera, secondary polycythemia, erythrocytosis, acclimation to high altitudes, heavy cigarette smoking, chronic lung disease, or a congenital heart defect. As the viscosity of blood increases, it may hinder blood flow to the brain or increase the risk of clotting. Decreased hematocrit may be caused by anemia; hemodilution; blood loss (i.e., gastrointestinal [GI] bleed); or iron, folic acid, and B12 deficiencies.

Therapist Considerations

Symptoms of low hemoglobin and hematocrit include weakness, fatigue, tachycardia, dyspnea on exertion, and heart palpitations and decreased exercise tolerance, requiring close monitoring of vitals and rest breaks (Hergenroeder, 2006).

Red Blood Cells or Erythrocytes

Purpose	Normal Range	Abnormal Values
Reflects the number of red blood cells in blood and their capacity to transport oxygen and nutrients throughout the body.	*Males:* 4.5– 5.3 mcl *Females:* 4.1– 5.1 mcl	*Males:* >5.72 mcl *Females:* >5.03 mcl

Clinical Implications

Abnormal values may be indicative of *anemia* (decreased number of RBCs) or *polycythemia* (increased number of RBCs). Anemia may be caused by blood loss, destruction of RBCs, decreased production of RBCs (resulting from a deficiency of iron, Vitamin B12, or folic acid, which are necessary for RBC production), chemotherapy, leukemia, multiple myeloma, or systemic lupus erythematosus. Symptoms of anemia include weakness, fatigue, dizziness, dyspnea on exertion, palpitations, and rapid pulse.

Polycythemia may be caused by polycythemia vera, dehydration, severe diarrhea, chronic heart disease, poison, or pulmonary fibroses. Symptoms include headache, dizziness, blurred vision, mental status changes, and sensory disturbances in hands and feet.

Therapist Considerations

Anemic patients may have decreased endurance and aerobic capacity. Patients with polycythemia are at an increased risk for stroke and thrombosis. Check with facility policy regarding treatment while patients are being transfused; low-level or bedside activity may be permissible. Refer to Appendix N for information on transfusion reactions.

Platelets

Purpose	Normal Range	Abnormal Values	Critical Values
Responsible for clotting blood by forming platelet plugs.	150,000–400,000/µl	*Thrombocytosis:* >1 million/µl *Thrombocytopenia:* <150,000/µl	<20,000/µl

Clinical Implications

Value	Implication
<20,000/µl	Consider deferring therapy; may exhibit spontaneous bleeding, skin bruising (ecchymosis), or prolonged bleeding time; no teeth brushing.
20,000–50,000/µl	Light active range of motion (no passive range of motion), light activities of daily living (ADLs), and ambulation okay.
<50,000/µl	No resistive exercise; ambulation and ADLs okay.
50,000/µl	Resistive exercise okay.
50,000–80,000/µl	Minimal resistive exercise, low-intensity progressive resistive exercise, ambulation, and ADLs okay.
80,000–150,000/µl	Moderate resistive exercise, ambulation, and ADLs okay.
>150,000/µl	No activity restrictions.

Sources. Garritan, Jones, Kornberg, & Parkin (1995); Hergenroeder (2006); Malone & Packel (2006).

Thrombocytosis may be caused by inflammation (e.g., rheumatoid arthritis, pancreatitis), infection, iron deficiency, polycythemia vera, renal failure, cancer, splenectomy, trauma, acute blood loss, or heart disease. *Thrombocytopenia* may be caused by viral or bacterial infections, nutritional deficiency, drugs, radiation and chemotherapy, bone marrow disease (e.g., aplastic anemia, leukemia, multiple myeloma), HIV, coagulation disorders, disseminated intravascular coagulation, liver disease, or prosthetic heart valves.

Therapist Considerations

Patients with thrombocytopenia are at risk for bleeding easily from mucosal surfaces, including gums, nose, GI tract, respiratory tract, and uterus (Hergenroeder, 2006). Patients are also at higher risk for bruising and bleeding under the skin and for postsurgery bleeding, including into the central nervous system and GI tract. Massive bleeding occurs only with coagulation factor deficiency.

Activities of daily living (ADLs) modifications for patients with thrombocytopenia can include using a soft toothbrush for brushing teeth and avoiding flossing. Gently wipe but avoid blowing the nose. Avoid using tampons, shaving with a straight razor, and getting tattoos or body piercings. Also avoid taking aspirin, engaging in contact sports, or using heavy machinery. The skin and mouth should be inspected daily.

Basic Metabolic Panel

The BMP is useful in screening for diabetes and renal disease. As with a CBC, blood samples for BMP are also collected through venous puncture. A BMP measures electrolyte levels, acid–base balance, renal function, and blood sugar levels. Electrolyte balance is important for various body functions, including nerve conduction, muscle contraction, cardiac conduction, blood coagulation, and maintenance of proper fluid balance in the body (Malone & Packel, 2006). *Electrolytes* are ions of essential elements, which enter the body through diet and fluids but exit through urine, stool, or sweat. An electrolyte imbalance can have a profound effect on multiple body systems, activity tolerance, and ability to engage in occupations. Therapists should be aware of any fluid restrictions before treating patients.

Sodium

Purpose	Normal Range	Abnormal Values	Critical Values
Determinant of fluid volume in the body. Facilitates nerve conduction, neuromuscular function, and glandular secretion.	135–145 mEq/l	*Hypernatremia:* >145 mEq/l *Hyponatremia:* <135 mEq/l	≤110 mEq/l >160 mEq/l

Clinical Implications

Eighty-five percent of sodium in the body is found in blood and lymph fluid. Abnormal sodium values can cause cells to either shrink or expand. Swelling cells can lead to neurological dysfunction. *Hypernatremia* is a high sodium level caused by dehydration; limited water intake; profuse sweating or decreased antidiuretic hormone; diabetes insipidus; diarrhea; hyperventilation; or excessive intake of sodium bicarbonate, sodium chloride, or corticosteroids. Hypernatremia can also result in hypovolemia. Symptoms of hypernatremia may include mental status changes, confusion, agitation, muscle irritability, hyperreflexia, ataxia, convulsions, hypertension, tachycardia, excessive weight gain, oliguria, thirst, pulmonary edema, dry flushed skin, dyspnea, or respiratory arrest.

Hyponatremia, or a low sodium level, may be caused by excessive infusion, increased water intake, increased levels of antidiuretic hormone, renal disease, excessive sweating, hyperglycemia, or congestive heart failure. Symptoms may include oliguria, nausea, vomiting, abdominal cramps, muscle twitching, weakness, lethargy, confusion, apathy, hypotension, tachycardia, seizures, or coma.

Therapist Considerations

When working with patients, be aware of any fluid restrictions. Refer to Table P.1 for information on hypervolemia and hypovolemia.

Table P.1. Causes, Signs, and Symptoms of Hypervolemia and Hypovolemia

Fluid Status	Potential Cause	Signs and Symptoms
Hypervolemia	• Excess IV fluid • Congestive heart failure • Cirrhosis • Renal failure or nephrotic syndrome • Low-protein diet • Steroid use	• Pitting peripheral edema • Shortness of breath • Anasarca • Jugular venous distension • Hypertension • Tachycardia • Dyspnea • Acute weight gain • Edema • Rapid breathing
Hypovolemia	• Limited oral intake • Dysphasia, neglect, dementia, coma • Loss from vomiting, diarrhea	• Dry mucous membranes • Orthostatic hypotension • Tachycardia

Table P.1. (continued)

Fluid Status	Potential Cause	Signs and Symptoms
	• Diabetes • Burns • Hemorrhage • Renal failure • Abdominal surgery • Nasogastric drainage • Diuretics • Excessive sweating • Pancreatitis • Intestinal obstruction	• Tachypnea • Oliguria • Altered mental status • Rapid weight loss • Thirst • Sunken eyeballs

Sources. "Fluids and Electrolytes" (2006), Malone and Packel (2006), Polich and Paz (2009).

Potassium

Purpose	Normal Range	Abnormal Values	Critical Values
Potassium is important for neuromuscular function, action potentials, and cardiac muscle contraction and conductivity. K^+ lab values provide information on the renal and adrenal systems and acid–base imbalances. Potassium is controlled by the renal system and is excreted in urine.	3.5–5.0 mEq/l	*Hyperkalemia:* >5.0 mEq/l *Hypokalemia:* <3.5 mEq/l	<2.5 mEq/l or >6.6 mEq/l

Clinical Implications

The heart muscle is especially susceptible to potassium imbalances, which can lead to arrhythmias or cardiac arrest. *Hyperkalemia* may be caused by renal disease or failure, Addison's disease or excess Vitamin D, diabetic ketoacidosis, hypoxia, acidosis, crush injuries, burns, or medications (e.g., nonsteroidal anti-inflammatory drugs, heparin, angiotensin-converting enzyme inhibitors, beta blockers). Hyperkalemia can also be caused by excessive potassium intake secondary to oral potassium supplements or blood transfusions (Malone & Packel, 2006). Symptoms may include abdominal cramps, nausea, diarrhea, muscle weakness, flaccid paralysis, paresthesias, fatigue, irritability, anxiety, electrocardiogram changes, cardiac arrhythmias (tachycardia initially, then bradycardia), or cardiac arrest.

Hypokalemia can be caused by diarrhea, vomiting, diuretics, nasogastric suctioning, Cushing's syndrome, metabolic alkalosis, chronic renal disease, digoxin, or corticosteroid therapy. Symptoms may include paralytic ileus, decreased peristalsis, abdominal distension, constipation, muscle weakness, fatigue, leg cramps, paresthesias, disorientation, dizziness, hypotension, decreased strength of cardiac contractions and dysrhythmias (sinus bradycardia, atrial tachycardia, atrioventricular block, and ventricular tachycardia or fibrillation), and cardiac or respiratory arrest.

Therapist Considerations

It may not be appropriate or advantageous to exercise patients with hypokalemia or hyperkalemia. Exercise can worsen hyperkalemia (Irion & Goodman, 2009). If levels are less than 3.2 mEq/l or more than 5.0 mEq/l, consider deferring therapy secondary to risk of arrhythmia or tetany. Check with medical staff before treating. Potassium oral medication is fast acting, but patients may still require close monitoring (Garritan et. al., 1995). No restrictions on therapy are necessary once potassium levels are corrected (Hergenroeder, 2006).

Chloride

Purpose	Normal Range	Abnormal Values	Critical Values
Chloride level is controlled by the renal system and secreted by the stomach as hydrochloric acid. It is important for water and acid–base balance and facilitates exchange of O_2 and CO_2 in red blood cells.	96–106 mEq/l	*Hyperchloremia:* >108 mEq/l *Hypochloremia:* <96 mEq/l	<80 mEq/l or >115 mEq/l

Clinical Implications

Chloride levels provide information on acid–base balance and hydration. Levels fluctuate with fluid status (water and sodium). *Hyperchloremia* may be caused by dehydration, hypernatremia, hyperventilation, or anemia. Symptoms include weakness, lethargy, and deep and rapid breathing. *Hypochloremia* may be caused by severe vomiting or diarrhea. Symptoms include tetany, shallow depressed breathing, muscle weakness, and twitching.

Bicarbonate

Purpose	Normal Range	Critical Values
Important for acid–base balance; works as a buffer to keep pH within optimal range.	22–26 mEq/l	<10 mEq/l or >40 mEq/l

Clinical Implications

Low levels of bicarbonate are associated with disorders resulting in metabolic acidosis (i.e., diabetic ketoacidosis).

Carbon Dioxide

Purpose	Normal Range	Abnormal Values
Measure of CO_2 in blood; used to evaluate pH level and electrolyte status.	20–29 mEq/l	May result in alkalosis or acidosis.

Clinical Implications

Carbon dioxide is a waste product of metabolism that is exhaled through the lungs. High levels of carbon dioxide may be indicative of a respiratory disorder. Elevated levels may be a result of diseases that cause respiratory acidosis (e.g., COPD, pneumonia) or metabolic alkalosis (e.g., Cushing's syndrome, alcoholism). Decreased levels may be a result of diseases that cause respiratory alkalosis (e.g., hyperventilation, liver failure) or metabolic acidosis (e.g., diabetes, dehydration, heart or kidney failure).

Blood Urea and Nitrogen

Purpose	Normal Range	Critical Values
Blood urea and nitrogen are formed in the liver as a result of dietary protein breakdown and is excreted in urine. Evaluates excretory function of kidneys and metabolic function of the liver.	10–20 mg/dl	>100 mg/dl

Clinical Implications

Elevated blood urea and nitrogen (BUN) levels may indicate renal disorder requiring dialysis. Typically caused by reduction in renal blood flow, it may also be increased by intake of dietary protein or increased protein catabolism. Patients with malnutrition or liver disease may have decreased BUN levels; however, patients with hepatorenal syndrome may have normal BUN levels. Elevated BUN levels may be present in patients with CHF, diabetes mellitus, myocardial infarction (MI), burns, or cancer. Symptoms of elevated BUN levels may include confusion, disorientation, or convulsions. Low BUN levels are uncommon and are usually associated with malnutrition, low-protein diets, overhydration, or liver disease.

Creatinine

Purpose	Normal Range
Measurement of kidney function. Creatinine is a by-product of muscle metabolism.	*Males:* 0.6–1.2 mg/dl *Females:* 0.5–1.1 mg/dl

Clinical Implications

Elevated creatinine may indicate renal disorder requiring dialysis. Elevated levels may also be present in patients with urinary tract obstruction, myasthenia gravis, rhabdomyolysis, hyperthyroidism, CHF, muscular dystrophy, and chronic kidney disease resulting from high blood pressure or diabetes mellitus. Common causes of elevated creatinine include polynephritis, acute tubular necrosis, and glomerulonephritis. Symptoms of elevated creatinine include fatigue, shortness of breath, confusion, or feeling dehydrated.

Therapist Considerations

Renal failure can affect occupational performance. There are no specific activity guidelines.

Glucose

Purpose	Normal Range	Abnormal Values	Critical Values
Measure blood sugar levels.	70–110 mg/dl (fasting)	*Hypoglycemia:* <60 mg/dl *Hyperglycemia:* >250 mg/dl *Prediabetes:* 110–200 mg/dl *Diabetes:* >126 mg/dl	<60 mg/dl or >300–350 mg/dl

Clinical Implications

Hypoglycemia may be caused by an insulin overdose, insulinoma, skipped meals, or overexertion in exercise. Symptoms may include headache, weakness, shakiness, clamminess, impaired muscle control, blurred vision, or difficulty responding to commands. Patients with glucose levels lower than 70 milligrams/deciliter are usually given a quickly absorbable carbohydrate snack (e.g., orange juice). Glucose levels are then rechecked after 15 minutes.

Hyperglycemia can be caused by diabetes mellitus or stress. Glucose levels higher than 300–350 milligrams/deciliter can lead to diabetic ketoacidosis (Hergenroeder, 2006). Symptoms of hyperglycemia may include acetone breath, rapid pulse, nausea, vomiting, weakness, dehydration, or coma.

Therapist Considerations

Overexertion of a patient with low blood sugar levels (<60 milligrams/deciliter) may lead to a hypoglycemic reaction. Defer therapy if the patient is hypoglycemic and needs carbohydrates. Avoid exercising patients before mealtime and after insulin because both can result in reduced blood sugar levels (Irion & Goodman, 2009). Until blood sugar level is corrected, defer therapy for patients with blood glucose levels of 300 milligrams/deciliter or more.

Additional Electrolytes of Interest

Electrolytes included in a BMP generally include sodium, potassium, and chloride. However, testing of additional electrolytes may also be warranted and can include magnesium, calcium, and phosphate levels.

Magnesium

Purpose	Normal Range	Abnormal Values	Critical Values
Facilitates transport of proteins, sodium, potassium, and calcium. Important for neuromuscular function and use of adenosine-triphosphate (ATP) and stimulates parathyroid hormone secretion.	1.8–2.5 mEq/l	*Hypermagnesemia:* >2.5 mEq/l (rare) *Hypomagnesemia:* <1.8 mEq/l	<0.5 or >3.0 mEq/l

Clinical Implications

Hypermagnesemia may be caused by renal disease or failure, hyperparathyroidism, or hypothyroidism. Symptoms include nausea, vomiting, diarrhea, hypotension, respiratory depression, bradycardia, heart block, lethargy, drowsiness, or muscle weakness or flaccid paralysis.

Hypomagnesemia may be caused by chronic diarrhea and vomiting, use of diuretics, chronic alcoholism, or eating disorders. Symptoms can include arrhythmias, hyperactive deep tendon reflexes, hypotension, weakness, muscle spasms, numbness, tetany, lower-extremity cramps, confusion, delusions, or seizures.

Calcium

Purpose	Normal Range	Abnormal Values	Critical Values
Necessary for cell permeability, blood coagulation, muscle contractions, and bone and teeth formation; important for cardiac conductivity. Ninety-nine percent of calcium is stored in bones and teeth.	9–11 mg/dl	*Hypercalcemia:* >11 mg/dl *Hypocalcemia:* <8.5 mg/dl	<7 mg/dl (tetany) >12 mg/dl (coma)

Clinical Implications

Hypercalcemia may be caused by hyperparathyroidism, excess Vitamin D, calcium supplements, bone cancer, sarcoidosis, or respiratory acidosis. Symptoms can include nausea, vomiting, constipation, dehydration, abdominal or muscle cramps, fatigue, lethargy, drowsiness, muscle weakness, muscle flaccidity, heart block, convulsions, irritability, confusion, numbness or tingling of fingers, or pathological bone fractures.

Hypocalcemia may be caused by respiratory alkalosis, rhabdomyolysis, malignancy, chronic renal insufficiency, alcoholism, poor diet, or pancreatitis. Symptoms may include hypoten-sion, fatigue, hyperreflexia, tetany, convulsions, arrhythmias, seizures, anxiety, confusion, or irritability.

Phosphate

Purpose	Normal Range	Abnormal Values
Assists with neuromuscular regulation and cellular metabolism. Phosphate is necessary for bone formation.	2.5–4.5 mg/dl	*Hyperphosphatemia:* >4.5 mg/dl *Hypophosphatemia:* <2.5 mg/dl

Clinical Implications
Hyperphosphatemia may be caused by renal failure, uremia, hypoparathyroidism, or hypocalcemia. Symptoms may include flaccid paralysis and muscle weakness or, if patients have hypocalcemia, then seizures and tetany may also be present.

Hypophosphatemia may be related to hyperparathyroidism, hypercalcemia, or poor control of diabetes. Symptoms may include weakness, paresthesia, dysphagia, hyperventilation, weak pulse, and bone pain.

Clinical Implications
Concern for risk of bleeding with high values. Increased prothrombin time may be the result of Vitamin K deficiency; liver disease; biliary obstruction; Zollinger–Ellison syndrome; celiac disease; disseminated intravascular coagulation; or deficiency of factors II, V, VII, or X.

Therapist Considerations
If levels are elevated or critical, consult with medical staff before treating. Modify therapy to prevent patient falls and injury.

Coagulation Panel

A coagulation panel tests for clotting time of plasma. When a patient's blood is sufficiently anticoagulated for his or her condition, it is considered to be at a therapeutic level. Hypercoagulability can be caused by platelet abnormalities (e.g., arteriosclerosis, diabetes), clotting system abnormalities (e.g., CHF, immobility, prosthetic heart valves), or venous thrombosis (e.g., stasis).

Prothrombin Time

Purpose	Normal Range	Critical Value
Tests for coagulation and monitors oral anticoagulation therapy (warfarin).	12–15 s	>20 s for patients who are not anticoagulated

Partial Thromboplastin Time

Purpose	Normal Range
Tests for coagulation and monitors anticoagulation therapy (heparin).	30–40 s

Clinical Implications
A concern for risk of bleeding exists with high values. Elevated levels may be the result of malabsorption disorders, hemophilia, cirrhosis, or heparin therapy.

Therapist Considerations
If levels are elevated or critical, consult with medical staff before treating. Modify therapy to prevent patients from falling or injuring themselves and avoid interventions that include excessive resistance.

Activated Partial Thromboplastin Time

Purpose	Normal Range	Critical Value
More sensitive version of partial thromboplastin time. Test used to monitor low molecular-weight heparin (LMWH); a more expensive but quicker anticoagulation medication.	21–35 s	>70 s

Clinical Implications

Prolonged activated partial prothrombin time is associated with hemophilia, heparin or warfarin therapy, Vitamin K deficiency, liver disease, and disseminated intravascular coagulation.

International Normalized Ratio

Purpose	Normal Range	Abnormal Value	Critical Value
Developed in response to differences between labs in measuring coagulation times. Values are more uniform.	0.9–1.1	>3.5	>5

Clinical Implications

The therapeutic international normalized ratio (INR) takes several days to reach (Irion, 2004). Therapeutic INR ranges from 2–3 for patients who are anticoagulated for atrial fibrillation, coronary artery disease, cerebrovascular disease, deep vein thrombosis, or left ventricular assistive device or patients who have had a MI. The INR for mechanical heart valves ranges from 2.5–3.5. With an INR of more than 5, the risk of bleeding is increased, and patients may be on bedrest precaution (Hergenroeder, 2006).

Therapeutic Considerations

Patients with a high INR (>3.5) are at increased risk for bleeding. Consult with medical staff before treating. During therapy, use extreme caution to prevent falling or injury to patient. See Table P.2 for INR therapeutic levels.

Table P.2. International Normalized Ratio (INR) Therapeutic Levels

Oral Anticoagulation Begun 2 wk Before Surgery	INR	Target
Non–hip surgery	1.5–2.5	2.0
Hip surgery	2.0–3.0	2.5
Deep vein thrombosis prevention	2.0–3.0	2.5
Prevention of recurrent deep vein thrombosis	2.5–4.0	3.0
Prevention of systemic embolism in patients with atrial fibrillation	2.0–3.0	2.5
Cardiac stents	3.0–4.5	3.5
Prevention of arterial thrombosis, patients with mechanical heart valves	3.0–4.5	3.5

Source. Fischbach and Dunning (2009).

D-Dimer

Purpose	Normal Value
Confirms clotting and used in testing hypercoagulability. Used in diagnosis of deep vein thrombosis, disseminated intravascular coagulation, and pulmonary embolism and to screen for acute myocardial infarction. Produced by action of plasmin on cross-linked fibrin. Measures amount of fibrin degradation.	<250 pg/l

Clinical Implications

Elevated levels may indicate disseminated intravascular coagulation, deep vein thrombosis, pulmonary embolism, MI, renal failure, liver failure, malignancy, or preeclampsia in late pregnancy. D-dimer values are increased with tissue plasminogen activator (t-PA) administration.

Therapeutic Considerations

A negative test is associated with absence of deep vein thrombosis.

Arterial Blood Gas Analysis

Arterial blood gas analysis assesses cardiopulmonary function, oxygen and carbon dioxide in the blood, and acid–base regulation. It looks at values for pH, partial pressure of oxygen and carbon dioxide, and bicarbonate and oxygen saturation levels. An arterial blood gas analysis might be ordered for patients with breathing problems or lung disorders. As opposed to other blood samples drawn from the venous system (e.g., CBC, BMP), arterial blood gas is collected from the arterial system.

pH

Purpose	Normal Range	Abnormal Values	Critical Values
Measures acid–base balance of blood.	7.35–7.45	*Acidosis:* <7.35 *Alkalosis:* >7.45 *Seriously impaired cell function:* <7.2 or >7.55	≤7.20 or ≥7.60 <6.8 or >7.8 incompatible with life

Clinical Implications

Partial pressure of carbon dioxide ($PaCO_2$) and pH have an inverse relationship. When $PaCO_2$ increases, pH decreases, leading to respiratory acidosis. When pH increases and $PaCO_2$ decreases, the result is respiratory alkalosis. Refer to Table P.3 for information on acid–base disorders.

Table P.3. **Acid–Base Disorders**

Disorder	Etiology	Signs and Symptoms
Respiratory acidosis (CO_2 retention) pH <7.35 $PaCO_2$ >45 mm Hg HCO_3_ >26 mEq/L *Renal compensation:* Metabolic alkalosis	• Hypoventilation • Central nervous system depression (drugs, trauma) • Airway obstruction • Mechanical ventilation • Chronic bronchitis • Pneumonia • Sleep apnea • Cardiac arrest	• Diaphoresis • Tachycardia • Disorientation or confusion • Headache • Lethargy • Cyanosis • Ventricular fibrillation • Asterixis • Hypertension or hypotension • Coma
Respiratory alkalosis pH >7.45 $PaCO_2$ <35 mm Hg HCO_3_ <22 mEq/L *Renal compensation:* Metabolic acidosis	• Hyperventilation • Drugs • Hypoxia • Hepatic failure • Sepsis	• Light-headedness • Muscle twitching • Cardiac arrhythmia • Anxiety and agitation • Paresthesias
Metabolic acidosis (decompensated) pH <7.35 HCO_3_ <22 mEq/L $PaCO_2$ Normal *Renal compensation:* Respiratory alkalosis	• Bicarbonate depletion • Endocrine disorders (e.g., diabetic ketoacidosis) • Intestinal malabsorption • Renal disease • Hepatic disease • Chronic alcoholism • Malnutrition	• Headache • Lethargy • Nausea, vomiting, diarrhea • Muscle twitching • Cardiac arrhythmia • Convulsions • Coma
Metabolic alkalosis (decompensated) pH >7.45 HCO_3- >26 mEq/L $PaCO_2$ >45 mm Hg *Renal compensation:* Respiratory acidosis	• Loss of potassium (with diuresis) • Prolonged vomiting or gastric suctioning • Use of steroids • Massive blood transfusions • Cushing's disease • Excessive intake of antacids or bicarbonate of soda • Respiratory insufficiency • Hypocholeremia or hypophosphatemia • Excessive IV fluids	• Restlessness • Confusion • Agitation • Tetany • Nausea, vomiting, diarrhea • Convulsions • Paresthesias • Cyanosis • Apnea

Note. HCO_3^- = bicarbonate ion; $PaCO_2$ = partial pressure of carbon dioxide.

Sources. "Fluids and Electrolytes" (2006); Garritan, Jones, Kornberg, & Parkin (1995); Irion & Goodman (2009); West, Paz, & O'Leary (2009).

PaCO$_2$

Purpose	Normal Range	Critical Values
Measure of partial pressure of carbon dioxide in arterial blood (reflects how much carbon dioxide is dissolved in the blood).	35–45 mm Hg	<20 or >70 mm Hg

Clinical Implications

PaCO$_2$ is affected by pulmonary function. This test reflects how well carbon dioxide is able to move out of the body. Patients with COPD may be carbon dioxide retainers.

Therapist Considerations

Any problems with oxygenation will affect occupational performance. Therapists should not increase oxygen for patients who are carbon dioxide retainers without first consulting medical staff, because increases in oxygen may result in depression of the respiratory system. Refer to Chapter 5 for more detail. Care should be taken not to overexert patients, because overexertion will increase oxygen demand. Pursed-lip breathing and activity in an upright position assists with carbon dioxide clearance. Encourage use of the incentive spirometer.

Bicarbonate

Purpose	Normal Range	Critical Values
Measures amount of bicarbonate dissolved in arterial blood. Bicarbonate is important for acid–base balance and works as a buffer to keep pH levels within normal limits.	22–26 mEq/l	<10 mEq/l or >40 mEq/l

Clinical Implications

Abnormal bicarbonate levels indicate a metabolic problem, either metabolic acidosis or metabolic alkalosis. Low levels are associated with disorders resulting in metabolic acidosis (i.e., diabetic ketoacidosis).

Partial Pressure of Oxygen

Purpose	Normal Range	Abnormal Value	Critical Value
Partial pressure of oxygen found in arterial blood. Measures the pressure of oxygen dissolved in the blood.	80–100 mm Hg	*Hypoxemia:* <80 mm Hg	<40 mm Hg

Clinical Implications

Initial signs of hypoxemia (<80 mm Hg) include mental status changes, tachycardia, and light-headedness, which can progress to incoordination, restlessness, cardiac arrhythmias, and cardiac arrest.

Therapist Considerations

Therapists should monitor vital signs, treat to patient tolerance, and instruct patient in breathing exercises.

Oxygen Saturation

Purpose	Normal Range	Abnormal Value
Percentage of oxygen carried by hemoglobin, measured noninvasively with a pulse oximetry probe on a finger, earlobe, or forehead. Provides information on oxygenation status.	97%–99%	<90%

Clinical Implications

Oxygen saturation of less than 84% reflects an oxyhemoglobin saturation that is greatly reduced, and if untreated, can eventually lead to respiratory failure. Oxygen saturation of 90% is equal to PaO_2 of 60 mm Hg using the oxyhemoglobin dissociation curve. A finger oxygen saturation monitor may not always accurately measure blood oxygen levels because it can be affected by different external factors, including cold hands or nail polish (Schutz, 2001). Refer to Chapter 5 for more information.

Therapist Considerations

Physicians may set individual parameters below 90% for select patients. Monitor oxygen demands and modify activities when needed. Deep breathing and upright positioning assists with oxygenation and carbon dioxide removal (Garritan et. al., 1995).

Cardiac Enzymes and Markers

When the heart muscle is damaged, cardiac enzymes are released into the vascular system. Cardiac enzyme markers are therefore useful in diagnosis of MI.

Creatine Kinase

Enzyme	Purpose	Reference Range	Clinical Implication
Creatine kinase (CK)	Marker for heart attack or other muscle damage. Measures the presence of the enzyme creatine phosphokinase in blood. Also known as CPK.	*Males:* 38–174 U/L *Females:* 26–140 U/L	CK levels begin to rise within 2–4 hr of injury and peak within 14–24 hr. Levels usually return to normal within 48–72 hr. Increased CK may also be present with myocarditis, open-heart surgery, or cardioversion. A ratio of CK-MB to total CK >2.5–3.0 is suggestive of myocardial infarction (MI).
CK-MB	Enzyme found in cardiac muscle. CK-MB is a marker for acute MI or myocardium injury.	0.00–0.06	Elevated CK-MB may be seen with angina, myocarditis, MI, Duchenne's muscular dystrophy, subarachnoid hemorrhage, shock, chronic renal failure, carbon monoxide poisoning, and Reye's syndrome. After a MI, elevated levels of CK-MB appear after 6–12 hr and remain for 18–32 hr. A negative CK-MB ≥48 hr indicates the patient did not have an MI.

Therapist Considerations

If levels are elevated, vitals should be closely monitored along with frequent rest breaks. Defer therapy and consult with medical staff if patient presents with signs or symptoms of angina, hypotension, dysrhythmias, or heart attack.

Cardiac Troponin

Purpose	Normal Range	Critical Value
Proteins specific to cardiac muscle tissue. They are released with muscle injury or infarction.	Troponin I <0.35 ng/ml Troponin T <0.2 ng/ml	Troponin I >1.5 ng/ml

Clinical Implications

Troponin tests (either Troponin I or Troponin T) are usually ordered along with other cardiac biomarker tests (e.g., CK-MB). Elevations in either test may indicate acute MI, myocarditis, or unstable angina. Increased levels appear 4–6 hr after injury with Troponin I and 4–8 hr after injury with Troponin T. Levels peak at 12 hr for Troponin I and at 12–48 hr for Troponin T. Levels may not return to normal for 3–10 days with Troponin I and for 7–10 days with Troponin T.

Therapist Considerations

Consult with medical staff before treating because therapy may be inappropriate.

C-Reactive Protein

Purpose	Normal Value	Abnormal Value
C-reactive protein is produced in the liver and indicates an inflammatory condition.	<1.0 mg/dl	0.3–20 mg/dl

Clinical Implications

Risk factors for C-reactive protein (CRP) are similar to risk factors for heart disease, including obesity, sedentary lifestyle, high blood sugar, and elevated triglycerides. CRP is not usually found in normal healthy people. A more sensitive version of CRP, *high sensitivity CRP* or *hs-CRP,* is a more specific marker of risk for heart disease and MI. CRP is also useful in detecting infection and transplant rejection.

Brain Natriuretic Peptide

Purpose	Normal Value	Abnormal Values
Hormones secreted by the heart when volume overload is present; used for differential diagnosis of congestive heart failure.	*No heart failure:* <100 pg/ml	*Mild heart failure:* 100–300 pg/ml *Moderate heart failure:* 300–700 pg/ml *Severe heart failure:* >700 pg/ml

Clinical Implications

Values greater than 100 pg/ml indicate presence of CHF (Irion, 2004). Brain natriuretic peptide levels increase as heart failure worsens.

Myoglobin

Purpose	Normal Range
Released into the bloodstream during ischemia or in cases of muscle inflammation or trauma.	0–0.09 µg/ml

Clinical Implications

Myoglobin is an early diagnostic marker for acute MI. Myoglobin can be detected as soon as 2 hr after the onset of chest pain and peaks in 4 hr.

Nutritional Status

This section reviews laboratory values that reflect blood levels of glucose, vitamins, proteins and lipids; all are used as a gauge of nutritional status and health.

Hemoglobin A1C

Purpose	Normal Range	Abnormal Value	Glucose Control
Used in monitoring diabetes; provides information on longer-term blood glucose control than BMP glucose level. Hemoglobin A1C (HbA1C) is the measure of average blood glucose concentration over several weeks or months.	4%–6%	>7%	*Good:* 2.5%–5.9% *Fair:* 6%–7% *Poor:* >7 %

Clinical Implications

People with diabetes with good blood glucose control are close to a hemoglobin A1C of 6%. Patients with levels lower than 5% have the lowest rates for cardiovascular disease.

B12

Purpose	Normal Ranges	Abnormal Value
B12 is necessary for production of red blood cells and is found in animal protein.	*Adults:* 280–1,500 pg/ml *>Age 60:* 110–770 pg/ml	<100 pg/ml

Clinical Implications

B12 deficiency is associated with pernicious anemia, malabsorption disorders (e.g., inflammatory bowel diseases), hypothyroidism, and Sollinger–Ellison syndrome and after a gastrectomy or resection. Excessive B12 levels (rare) are associated with leukemia, chronic renal failure, hepatitis, cirrhosis, polycythemia vera, CHF, diabetes, COPD, and obesity.

Folic Acid

Purpose	Normal Range
Necessary for red and white blood cell function and DNA production. Folate is produced in the intestines and stored in the liver and can be found in eggs, milk, yeast, liver, leafy vegetables, and fruits.	3–13 ng/ml

Clinical Implications

Low levels of folic acid are associated with poor diet, malnutrition, alcoholism, hypothyroidism, hemolytic anemia, megaloblastic anemia, Vitamin B6 deficiency, celiac disease, inflammatory bowel diseases, intestinal resection, drugs, and liver disease.

Albumin

Purpose	Normal Range	Abnormal Values	Critical Value
Used to detect the liver's ability to synthesize proteins and is an indicator of nutritional status.	3.5–5.5 g/dl (half life = 21 days)	<3.0 g/dl is associated with nutritional compromise. <2.8 g/dl is associated with generalized edema and poor wound healing.	<1.5 g/dl

Clinical Considerations

Albumin keeps fluid from leaking into tissues. Low albumin levels (2.0–2.5 g/dl) are associated with edema and possibly hypotension. Below-normal levels of albumin may be the result of liver disease, malnutrition, Crohn's disease, infection, inflammation, nephritic syndrome, thyroid disease, digoxin toxicity, or burns. Low levels are also associated with prolonged hospital stay. Elevated albumin levels may indicate dehydration.

Therapist Considerations

Skin integrity may be compromised with decreased albumin levels (i.e., skin weeping may be noted).

Prealbumin

Purpose	Normal Range	Abnormal Values
Used to monitor nutritional status of those receiving parenteral nutrition or hemodialysis. It is a preferred marker of nutritional status.	19–38 mg/dl (half life = 3 days)	*<10 mg/dl:* Patient at significant nutritional risk, associated with poor wound healing. *0–50 mg/dl:* Associated with severe protein depletion. *50–100 mg/dl:* Associated with moderate protein depletion. *100–150 mg/dl:* Associated with mild protein depletion.

Clinical Considerations

Critically ill patients have increased nutritional needs, and the body will deplete its own tissue to survive with malnutrition. Patients with decreased nutritional status have muscle atrophy and delayed wound healing.

Lipid Profiles

Lipid profiles are a group of tests used to measure the risk for developing coronary artery disease (e.g., MI, atherosclerosis). This panel traditionally includes tests for low-density lipoprotein cholesterol (bad cholesterol), high-density lipoprotein cholesterol (good cholesterol), triglycerides, and total cholesterol.

Low-Density Lipoprotein	High-Density Lipoprotein	Triglycerides	Total Cholesterol
<70 recommended if at high risk for atherosclerotic heart disease. *<100* recommended if patient has heart disease or diabetes. *<130* recommended if patient has ≥2 risk factors for heart disease. *<160* recommended if 1 or 0 risk factors are present.	*>40:* recommended *>60:* low risk for heart disease	*<150:* recommended *<100:* desirable *150–199:* moderate risk *200–499:* high risk *>499:* very high risk *>1,000:* at risk for pancreatitis	*<200:* recommended *200–239:* borderline to moderate risk *240:* high risk

Liver Function Tests

Liver function tests are used in detecting liver disease. The liver usually filters toxins and bacteria from the bloodstream. With liver dysfunction, these substances can reach other organs, resulting in multiorgan dysfunction syndrome (Irion & Goodman, 2009).

Alanine Amino Transferase

Purpose	Normal Range	Critical Value
Alanine amino transferase (ALT) is an enzyme predominantly found in the liver with smaller concentrations found in the heart, muscle, and kidney. The ALT test is used to diagnose liver disease and to monitor treatment for hepatitis and cirrhosis.	*Males:* 10–40 U/L *Females:* 7–35 U/L	*>9,000* U/L found in alcohol-acet-aminophen syndrome

Clinical Implications
ALT is released into the bloodstream with hepatocellular damage. Elevated ALT may be a result of alcoholic cirrhosis, metastatic liver tumors, infectious or viral hepatitis, biliary obstruction, pancreatitis, MI, polymyositis, severe burns, shock, or mononucleosis. ALT may also be elevated as a result of muscle injury. People with increased ALT levels should not donate blood.

Therapist Considerations
Patients with active liver disease may present with extreme fatigue and should not be overexerted; incorporate energy conservation principles for all activities when appropriate.

Alkaline Phosphatase/Serum Glutamic-Pyruvic Transaminase

Purpose	Normal Range
Alkaline phosphatase is an enzyme made mostly in the liver and bone and to a smaller degree in the kidneys, intestines, and placenta. Alkaline phosphatase tests for gallbladder, liver, or bile duct disease. It is also associated with obstruction of the biliary tract.	30–126 U/L

Clinical Implications

Elevated levels may be the result of liver tumors, biliary obstruction, hepatocellular cirrhosis, biliary cirrhosis, cholestasis, hepatitis, mononucleosis, diabetic hepatic lipidosis, Gilbert's syndrome, chronic alcoholism, hyperparathyroidism, rheumatoid arthritis, Paget's disease, osteomalacia, Vitamin D deficiency, MI, CHF, Hodgkin lymphoma, myelogenous leukemia, cancer of the lungs or pancreas, colitis, peptic ulcer disease, sarcoidosis, amyloidosis, or chronic renal failure. Decreased alkaline phosphatase levels (*hypophosphatesemia*) may be the result of malnutrition or protein deficiency.

Aspartate Aminotransferase/Serum Glutamic-Oxaloacetic Transaminase

Purpose	Normal Range	Critical Value
Enzyme found in the liver, heart, lungs, skeletal muscle, kidney, brain, pancreas, and spleen. Traditionally used as a test for differential diagnosis of chest pain and heart and liver disease.	*Males:* 14–20 U/L *Females:* 10–36 U/L	>20,000 U/L in alcohol–acetaminophen syndrome

Clinical Implications

Aspartate aminotransferase (AST) is found in tissues of high metabolic activity. This enzyme is released into the bloodstream with damage to cells. The higher the number of damaged cells, the higher the AST level. In MI, AST levels are 4–10 times normal values. Causes of elevated AST include hepatitis, cirrhosis, mononucleosis, hepatic necrosis, Reye's syndrome, hypothyroidism, polymyositis, toxic shock syndrome, dermatomyositis, crush and traumatic injuries, pulmonary embolism, gangrene, hemolytic anemia, brain injury, and cardiac catheterization. Decreased levels are found with hemodialysis, Vitamin B6 deficiency, or azotemia.

Bilirubin

Purpose	Normal Levels	Critical Value
Measures bilirubin levels in the blood. Bilirubin is the by-product of RBC breakdown and is removed from the body by the liver.	*Direct bilirubin (circulates freely in bloodstream):* 0.1–0.3 mg/dl *Indirect bilirubin (protein bound):* 0.2–0.8 mg/dl *Total bilirubin:* 0.1–1.0 mg/dl	>12 mg/dl

Clinical Implications

Increased levels are the result of the liver's inability to remove bilirubin from the body or by increased hemolysis. Elevated total bilirubin with jaundice may be caused by liver damage, hemolysis, hepatitis, cirrhosis, mononucleosis, bile or hepatic duct obstruction, sickle cell disease, pernicious anemia, transfusion reaction, CHF, or pulmonary embolism. Direct bilirubin is associated with liver damage or obstruction and may be caused by choledocholithiasis, pancreatic head cancer, or Dubin–Johnson syndrome. Indirect bilirubin is associated with increased hemolysis and may be caused by hemolytic anemia, hemorrhagic pulmonary infarcts, trauma with large hematoma, or Gilbert's disease.

Ammonia

Purpose	Normal Range
Tests for severe liver disease, diagnoses Reye's syndrome, and monitors patients on hyperalimentation therapy.	15–60 µg/dl

Clinical Implications

Ammonia is the end-product of protein metabolism. When the liver is damaged, its ability to convert ammonia into urea is impaired and ammonia accumulates, leading to hepatic encephalopathy. Symptoms of hepatic encephalopathy include confusion, lethargy, tremors, and changes in mental status and acuity. Elevated ammonia levels may also be caused by Reye's syndrome, cirrhosis, hepatic coma, renal disease, GI infections, GI bleeds, or total parenteral nutrition.

Additional Labs

In obtaining a clearer clinical picture of their patient's health and medical status, physicians may order additional laboratory tests such as tests of thyroid function, T-cell counts, and blood alcohol levels.

Thyroid-Stimulating Hormone

Purpose	Normal Range	Abnormal Value	Critical Value
Test of primary hypothyroidism	0.4–4.2 mU/L	<0.1 mU/L (risk for atrial fibrillation, stroke)	<0.1 mU/L (indicative of primary hyperthyroidism)

Clinical Implications

Thyroid-stimulating hormone (TSH) is a hormone produced in the pituitary gland. A low level of TSH may be the result of an overactive thyroid gland (*hyperthyroidism*) or Graves disease. Symptoms of hyperthyroidism may include anxiety, irritability, tremors, weight loss, muscle weakness, atrial fibrillation, goiter, low tolerance for heat, and accelerated loss of calcium from the bones. Protrusion of the eyes is associated with Graves disease.

A high level of TSH may be the result of an underactive thyroid gland (*hypothyroidism*) or Hashimoto's thyroiditis. Symptoms of hypothyroidism may include a slower metabolism, sensitivity to cold, bradycardia, constipation, slow cognitive processing, and fatigue and is also associated with anxiety, depression, and musculoskeletal injuries (Irion & Goodman, 2009).

- T3 (triiodothyronine) is a related test for hyperthyroidism. *Normal value:* 80–200 ng/dl
- T4 (thyroxine) is a related test for hypothyroidism and hyperthyroidism. *Normal value:* 4.5–11.5 µg/dl.

Therapist Considerations

Refer to Chapter 8 for more detail on TSH and therapy guidelines.

CD4

Purpose	Normal Range	Abnormal Value
T-cell count; T cells help the body fight diseases or harmful substances.	500–1,600	<200

Clinical Implications

In HIV/AIDS testing, a CD4 count <200 indicates that the body's immune system is no longer strong enough to prevent illness and infection. Higher-than-normal T cells may be a result of leukemia, multiple myeloma, or mononucleosis.

Therapist Considerations

Observe standard precautions.

Ethanol

Purpose	Normal Value	Abnormal Value	Critical Value
Measurement of blood alcohol level.	<10 mg/dl	>80 mg/dl: Positive for most drunk driving laws	<300 mg/dl

Clinical Implications

Measures intoxication and blood alcohol levels:

- *50–100 mg/dl:* Slower reflexes and impaired visual acuity
- *100 mg/dl:* Central nervous system depression, impaired motor and sensory function, impaired cognition; cutoff level for driving under the influence
- *140 mg/dl:* Decreased blood flow to brain
- *>300 mg/dl:* Coma
- *400 mg/dl:* Death.

Therapist Considerations

Check with medical staff before evaluation or treatment because the patient may be on protocols to manage delirium tremens or have additional alcohol withdrawal symptoms.

References

Fischbach, F., & Dunning, M. B., III. (2009). *A manual of laboratory and diagnostic tests* (8th ed.). Philadelphia: Wolters Kluwer Health.

Fluids and electrolytes. (2006). In *Atlas of pathophysiology* (2nd ed., pp. 28–35). Philadelphia: Lippincott Williams & Wilkins.

Garritan, S., Jones, P., Kornberg, T., & Parkin, C. (1995, Winter). Laboratory values in the intensive care unit. *Acute Care Perspectives*, pp. 7–11.

Hergenroeder, A. L. (2006). Implementation of a competency-based assessment for interpretation of laboratory values. *Acute Care Perspectives, 15*(1), 7–15.

Irion, G. (2004). Lab values update. *Acute Care Perspectives, 13*(1), 1, 3–5.

Irion, G. L., & Goodman, C. C. (2009). Laboratory tests and values. In C. C. Goodman & K. S. Fuller (Eds.), *Pathology: Implications for the physical therapist* (3rd ed., pp. 1637–1667). Philadelphia: W. B. Saunders.

Malone, D. J., & Packel, L. (2006). Clinical laboratory values and diagnostic testing. In D. J. Malone & K. L. B. Lindsay (Eds.), *Physical therapy in acute care* (pp. 31–65). Thorofare, NJ: Slack.

Pagana, K. D., & Pagana, T. J. (2006). *Mosby's manual of diagnostic and laboratory tests* (3rd ed.). St. Louis, MO: Mosby.

Polich, S., & Paz, J. C. (2009). Fluid and electrolyte imbalances. In J. C. Paz & M. P. West (Eds.), *Acute care handbook for physical therapists* (3rd ed., pp. 437–440). St. Louis, MO: W. B. Saunders.

Schutz, S. (2001). Oxygen saturation monitoring by pulse oximetry. In D. J. Lynn-McHale & K. K. Carlson (Eds.), *AACN procedure manual for critical care* (4th ed.). Retrieved May 1, 2009, from http://classic.aacn.org/AACN/practice.nsf/Files/PO1/$file/ch%2014%20PO.pdf

Stiller, K. (2007). Safety issues that should be considered when mobilizing critically ill patients. *Critical Care Clinics, 23*, 35–53.

West, M. P., Paz, J. C., & O'Leary, K. (2009). Respiratory system. In J. C. Paz & M. P. West (Eds.), *Acute care handbook for physical therapists* (3rd ed., pp. 47–86). St. Louis, MO: W. B. Saunders.

Appendix P.A.

Units of Measurement

C	Celsius
cc	cubic centimeter
cg	centigram
cm	centimeter
cm H_2O	centimeter of water
cu	cubic
dl	deciliter
g	gram
h	hour
IU	international unit
ImU	international milliunit
IμU	international microunit
k	kilo
kg	kilogram
l	liter
mcg	microgram
mEq	milliequivalent
mEq/l	milliequivalent per liter
mg	milligram
ml	milliliter
mm^3	cubic millimeter
mM	millimore
mm Hg	millimeter of mercury
mm H_2O	millimeter of water
mmol	millimole
mol	mole
mOsm	milliosmole
mμ	millimicron

mU	milliunit
mV	millivolt
ng	nanogram
nm	nanometer
nmol	nanomole
Pa	pascal
pg	picogram (or microgram)
Pl	picoliter
Pm	picometer
Pmol	picomole
s	seconds
SI units	international system of units
μ	micron
μ^3	cubic micron
μlU	microinternational unit
μl	microliter
μm^3	cubic micrometer
μg	microgram
μmol	micromole
μU	microunit
U	unit

Source. Pagana and Pagana.

Index

Note: Page numbers in italics indicate figures, tables and boxes.